# SURGICAL PEDIATRIC OTOLARYNGOLOGY

# Surgical Pediatric Otolaryngology

EDITED BY


**William P. Potsic, M.D.**

Director, Division of Pediatric Otolaryngology
The Children's Hospital of Philadelphia

Professor of Otorhinolaryngology—Head and Neck Surgery
University of Pennsylvania School of Medicine
Philadelphia, Pennsylvania

**Robin T. Cotton, M.D.**

Director, Pediatric Otolaryngology
Children's Hospital Medical Center

Professor of Otolaryngology—Head and Neck Surgery
University of Cincinnati College of Medicine
Cincinnati, Ohio

**Steven D. Handler, M.D.**

Associate Director, Division of Pediatric Otolaryngology
The Children's Hospital of Philadelphia

Professor of Otorhinolaryngology—Head and Neck Surgery
University of Pennsylvania School of Medicine
Philadelphia, Pennsylvania


**with 137 figures in 900 parts**


1997
Thieme
New York • Stuttgart

Thieme Medical Publishers, Inc.
381 Park Avenue South
New York, NY 10016

*Surgical Pediatric Otolaryngology*
William P. Potsic, M.D.
Robin T. Cotton, M.D.
Steven D. Handler, M.D.

Library of Congress Cataloging-in-Publication Data

Surgical pediatric otolaryngology : head and neck surgery / edited by
William P. Potsic, Robin T. Cotton, Steven D. Handler.
p. cm.
Includes index.
ISBN 0-86577-153-7. — ISBN 3-13-103691-5
1. Otolaryngology, Operative. 2. Pediatric otolaryngology.
I. Potsic, William P. II. Cotton, Robin T. (Robin Thomas), 1941– .
III. Handler, Steven D. (Steven Douglas), 1946– .
[DNLM: 1. Otorhinolaryngologic Diseases—in infancy & childhood—
atlases. 2. Otorhinolaryngologic Diseases—surgery—atlases.
3. Otolaryngology—methods—atlases. WV 17 S962 1997]
RF51.S87 1997
617.5′1059′083—dc20
DNLM/DLC
for Library of Congress 96-33076
CIP



**Important note:** Medical knowledge is ever-changing. As new research and clinical experience broaden our knowledge, changes in treatment and drug therapy may be required. The authors and editors of the material herein have consulted sources believed to be reliable in their efforts to provide information that is complete and in accord with the standards accepted at the time of publication. However, in view of the possibility of human error by the authors, editors, or publisher of the work herein, or changes in medical knowledge, neither the authors, editors, publisher, nor any other party who has been involved in the preparation of this work, warrants that the information contained herein is in every respect accurate or complete, and they are not responsible for any errors or omissions or for the results obtained from use of such information. Readers are encouraged to confirm the information contained herein with other sources. For example, readers are advised to check the product information sheet included in the package of each drug they plan to administer to be certain that the information contained in this publication is accurate and that changes have not been made in the recommended dose or in the contraindications for administration. This recommendation is of particular importance in connection with new or infrequently used drugs.



Printed in the United States of America

5 4 3 2 1

TMP ISBN 0-86577-153-7
GTV ISBN 3-13-103691-5

*This atlas is dedicated to those children who have taught us and to all those children in the future who may benefit from these efforts.*

# ▸ Contents

# PART V THE NECK (LARYNX, TRACHEA, AND ESOPHAGUS)



# PART VI THE SALIVARY GLAND

## PART VIII FACIAL TRAUMA

# ▶ Preface

The idealized traditional method of teaching surgery involves a one-on-one interaction between the teacher (experienced surgeon) and the student (who may be a resident, fellow, or practitioner). Unfortunately, this scenario occurs mainly in large teaching centers and rarely in the general practice of surgery. We decided to write this atlas because many practitioners find themselves considering an operation that they have only seen or perhaps one that they performed some time ago. This atlas is intended to help those surgeons learn (or re-acquaint themselves with) the basic steps in the more common procedures performed in pediatric otolaryngology.

Most surgeons are visual and spatial in their orientation. For this reason, the atlas relies heavily on the wonderful drawings of Susan Shapiro Brenman. These illustrations are so clear that they lead the reader through the procedures even without the accompanying text. The adage that "one picture is worth a thousand words" is demonstrated in this atlas. Each step of the surgical procedure is clearly demonstrated. The text accompanying the illustrations is organized in small, concisely worded steps. Extensive references to the illustrations in the written description enable the surgeon to refer to a specific drawing for clarification of a written instruction and vice-versa.

We have assumed that the operating surgeon already has knowledge concerning the etiologies and various treatment plans of the diseases for which a specific operation is being planned. The surgeon who desires more in-depth information about a specific disease process should consult one of the many excellent comprehensive textbooks of pediatric otolaryngology and/or the current literature.

Our efforts focused on the procedures that comprise the majority of surgeries performed by pediatric otolaryngologists. We have left out uncommon procedures intended for esoteric, rare conditions. The techniques described and illustrated here are easy to follow; they are regularly performed by us in our clinical practice. While the procedures described here are certainly not original or new, our combined experience of more than 60 years of surgery has allowed us to discover and incorporate modifications of procedures that streamline, optimize, and make our surgical efforts more effective and efficient. The results from these procedures have been rewarding. We have found them easy to teach to our residents and fellows, and our trainees have found the same in helping others.

In short, we feel that this atlas can serve as a reference for the surgeon who infrequently performs pediatric otolaryngologic procedures, or as a "workhorse" for those who concentrate more of their efforts in the field. In either case, we hope that these techniques will help you to obtain the same satisfying results that we have been privileged to enjoy.

The authors gratefully acknowledge the invaluable help of Beth Ann B. McCullough in the preparation of this atlas. Susan Shapiro Brenman's illustrations bring clarity and depth to our operative descriptions. The contributions of acknowledged experts in their areas—Dr. Bruce Gantz (cochlear implantation) and Dr. Rodney Lusk (functional endoscopic sinus surgery) are greatly appreciated. Avé McCracken and Brian Hogley of Thieme have labored long and hard to bring this atlas to fruition. We are grateful for their efforts. Lastly, we would like to thank our families for their support and encouragement in this undertaking. Without it, this atlas could not have happened.

*William P. Potsic, M.D.*
*Robin T. Cotton, M.D.*
*Steven D. Handler, M.D.*

# Introduction

## ANESTHESIOLOGY AND AIRWAY MANAGEMENT

Cooperation between the otolaryngologist and the anesthesiologist is absolutely essential to a safe and successful result in pediatric otolaryngology. Anesthetic management must take into consideration the anatomic, physiologic, and pharmacologic differences between children and adults. It must be understood that the airway of a child is proportionately different from an adult's and is more prone to obstruction. The child's nose is small and the nasal airflow may be obstructed by congested mucosa or adenoid tissue. The child's tongue is relatively large and has a tendency to obstruct the pharynx along with hypertrophic tonsils that may also fold into the oropharynx. Laryngeal structures are soft and may tend to collapse on inspiration (laryngomalacia), and the floor of the mouth and tongue may obstruct a child's larynx, which is located higher in the neck than in the adult. The subglottic region in the child is narrow, and the soft areolar tissues are susceptible to edema from inflammation or from what would appear to be minor trauma. Endotracheal intubation must always be performed with minimal trauma and should be limited to a small enough tube to avoid injury from compression of the subglottic tissue.

The otolaryngologist and anesthesiologist must plan together before starting any procedure, and potential airway difficulties should be anticipated. A carefully planned operation can minimize the risk of the procedure as well as permit the timing of the administration of drugs to limit the duration of the anesthetic. The goal of anesthesia in the otolaryngic patient is to provide adequate analgesia and amnesia. Immobility is very important to enable precise microscopic surgery such as in the ear and larynx. The anesthetic technique should minimize obstruction of the operative field (e.g., nasotracheal intubation for surgery in the oral cavity), but the anesthesiologist must also protect the airway from secretions and blood, which are often present in the pharynx during head and neck surgery. Attention to the airway in otolaryngic surgery must pervade preoperative, operative, and postoperative management.

Preoperative medications are commonly used to reduce anxiety and to provide general comfort for patients who may or may not be discharged immediately after recovery from their surgery and anesthetic. Selection of drugs for premedication may vary with the preferences of the anesthesiologist, but consideration of the patient's respiratory status must be foremost. Patients with moderate-to-severe degrees of airway obstruction or neurologic dysfunction may need their premedication altered or completely withheld. For example, patients with adenotonsillar enlargement may suffer complete airway obstruction and become severely hypoxic because they fail to be aroused to breathe when the *usual* doses of sedatives are given pre- or postoperatively. Patients with laryngeal obstruction who are already hypoxic, hypercapnic, and exhausted from the strain of breathing may suddenly decompensate with the administration of sedatives.

Most surgical procedures for young children are performed using general anesthesia, but because of the extreme vascularity of head and neck structures, injection of local anesthetics containing epinephrine for vasoconstriction is often desirable. The amount of epinephrine permitted for each patient will depend on the condition of the patient, the anesthetic agents to be utilized and any other medications (e.g., cocaine) that are used.

Otologic surgery presents a challenge to the degree of cooperation between the otolaryngologist and the anesthesiologist. A myringotomy and tube placement are performed using inhalation anesthesia administered by mask. Coordination of position for exposure and sterility is essential. The airway must be maintained with the head turned and immobile while the otolaryngologist performs the procedure. The surgeon must be alert to the airway and be ready and willing to return the patient's head to the midline position, whenever needed, to reestablish airway control.

For tympanomastoid surgery, the patient is intubated with an endotracheal tube. During the last 20 to 30 minutes of tympanoplasty surgery, before the graft is placed, the anesthesiologist is frequently asked to terminate the use of nitrous oxide to facilitate positioning and maintenance of the graft. In addition, muscle relaxant medications need to be withheld if intraoperative monitoring of facial nerve function is being performed.

Surgery in the oral cavity can be made easier by use of a nasotracheal tube, but when access to the nasopharynx is needed, a curved oral RAE tube can be positioned and secured to the lower lip to provide the best exposure.

Exposure for nasal surgery is facilitated by oral tracheal intubation. Appropriate adjustment of the anesthetic agents is necessary to permit the use of intranasal cocaine for mucosal constriction, and injection of a solution of 1:400,000 to 1:100,000 epinephrine for vasoconstriction. Frequently, the nasal cavity is packed after nasal surgery, thus making immediate postoperative management dependent on the oral airway.

Upper aerodigestive tract surgery creates the demand for perhaps the greatest degree of cooperation by all professionals involved. The safest and most complete examination of the larynx, tracheobronchial tree, and esophagus is obtained with a general anesthetic. Maintenance of the proper plane of anesthesia is essential to permit observation of respiratory dynamics through the laryngoscope and bronchoscope.

Laser surgery of the aerodigestive tract requires careful attention to prevent an airway fire. Smaller than normal endotracheal tubes are required for surgical exposure, and covering the endotracheal tube with aluminum tape or using a nonflammable metal tube is necessary. The inhalation gases should be limited to mixtures that do not support combustion. Jet ventilation or insufflation without an endotracheal tube provides maximum exposure but requires extensive cooperation to ensure adequate ventilation and optimal surgical results.

Most surgery in the head and neck area involves movement of the head as well as the larynx and trachea, which can cause postintubation subglottic edema in some patients. Secure fixation of an endotracheal tube that fits loosely within the subglottic space can avoid this complication. A loose fit can be insured by having an audible leak of air around the tube at a ventilation pressure less than 20 cm of water.

On some occasions, it may be prudent to perform an elective tracheotomy to avoid emergency postoperative manipulation of the airway when respiratory difficulties are likely. This may be the case where surgery in the oral cavity is likely to produce extensive oropharyngeal edema. Patients having major craniofacial reconstruction and those with massive facial trauma may also require a tracheotomy to facilitate the surgery and to safely manage the postoperative airway.

Because children with Down syndrome often require surgery for otolaryngologic problems (e.g., tonsillectomy and adenoidectomy, myringotomy and tube placement, etc.), attention must be paid to the fact that many of these children have atlantoaxial instability. Both the anesthesiologist and otolaryngologist must be aware of this potential problem, must evaluate these patients preoperatively, and limit manipulation (especially flexion) of the neck during any surgical procedure.

## ▶ AUDIOLOGY

Pediatric audiology is an essential part of pediatric otolaryngology. Audiologic technology and knowledge have advanced to the point where no child is too young or too uncooperative to have a complete audiologic assessment. Pediatric audiology requires a full armamentarium of pure tone audiometry, tympanometry, and evoked response audiometry. Special lesion-localizing tests and central auditory batteries may be needed in specific instances.

Audiometric testing of the pediatric patient challenges the audiologist to apply all available techniques appropriate for a child's age and diagnostic requirements. Close cooperation between the audiologist and otolaryngologist is necessary to correlate the clinical findings with the interpretion and application of the test results to the clinical situation.

## ▶ RADIOLOGY

Pediatric radiology offers a full range of techniques that can be used for any selected situation: plain radiography, polytomography, arteriography, computed tomography (CT), and magnetic resonance imaging (MRI). Children often require special techniques and methods to obtain a useful study. Patient immobility is essential to CT and MRI imaging, and children may require sedation or a general anesthetic to facilitate these examinations.

Communication between the otolaryngologist and the radiologist is mandatory to obtain the maximum benefit from the requested study. The otolaryngologist must give the radiologist a good clinical summary of the patient so that the proper study is performed. This helps the radiologist to interpret the study and helps the otolaryngologist to plan his/her treatment. The findings encountered in any operative procedure should be communicated to the radiologist so that a correlation can be made between the radiographic and physical findings.

## ▶ HEAD AND NECK ONCOLOGY

Neoplasms of the head and neck in children are usually of mesenchymal origin as opposed to the epidermal-derived lesions found in adults. Consequently, the management of children's tumors and the role of the pediatric otolaryngologist are quite different from those prescribed for adults. The pediatric otolaryngologist is part of a multidisciplinary team that also includes an oncologist, radiotherapist, radiologist, and pathologist. This team approach and combined therapy have resulted in significant improvement in survival and cure rates of childhood malignancies.

While surgical excision remains the treatment of choice for benign lesions, radical surgery is rarely recommended as the primary treatment for pediatric neoplasms. However, a biopsy of the lesion is almost always required to make the diagnosis. Most often this biopsy is incisional in nature and does not involve extirpative surgery. The cure of these lesions ultimately rests upon the success of radiation therapy and chemotherapy. In rare instances, radical surgery may be indicated for "salvage" of patients after radiation therapy and chemotherapy. Occasionally, the surgeon will be asked to perform a "second-look procedure" to rebiopsy an area to measure the efficacy of treatment and to determine if there is any residual tumor after radiation and/or chemotherapy.

# PART I

# THE EAR

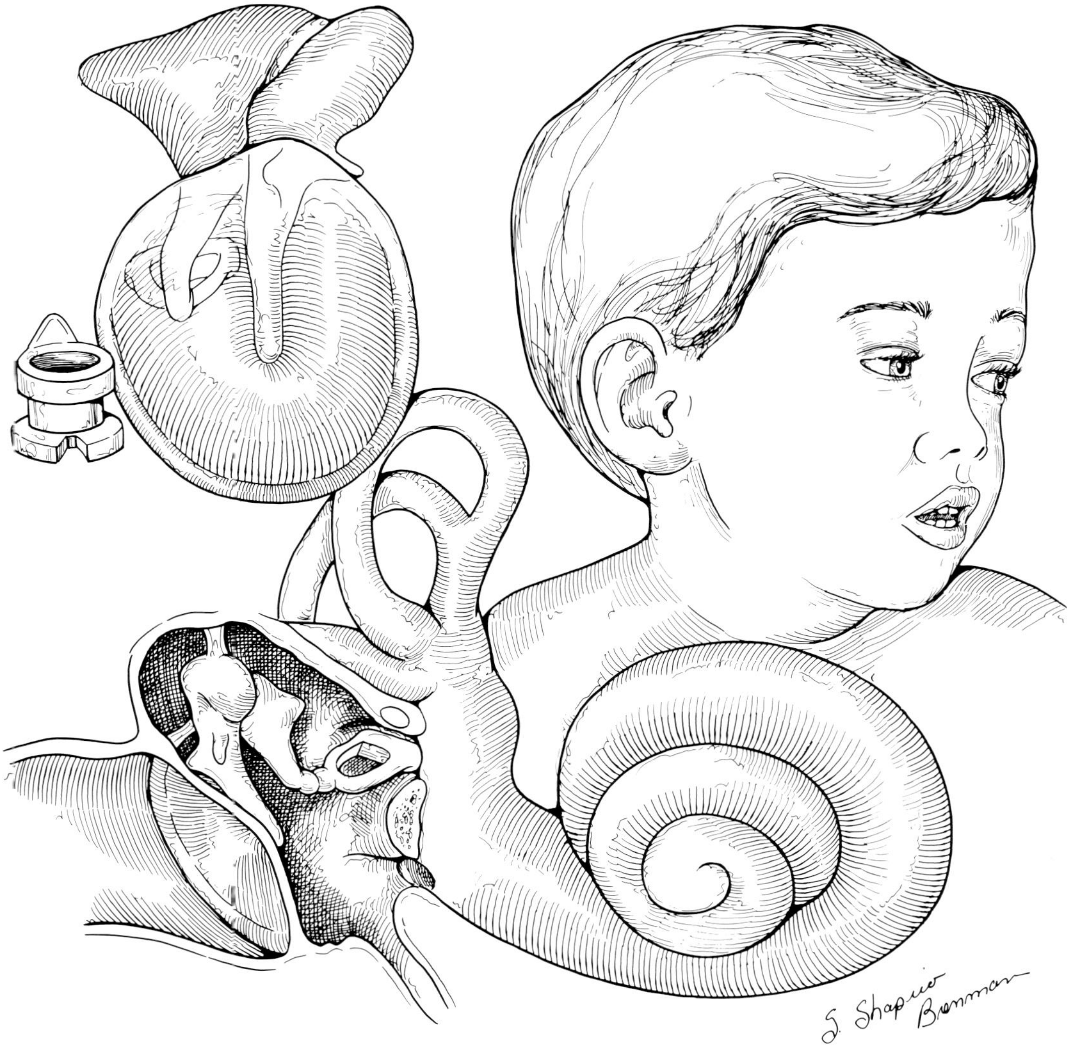

# 1 ▶ Otitis Media with Effusion

Otitis media with effusion (OME) is one of the most common chronic conditions of childhood. The primary complications of OME are (1) conductive hearing loss, (2) recurrent acute otitis media, and (3) middle ear atelectasis and cholesteatoma formation.

## ▶ 1-1 MYRINGOTOMY WITH TUBE PLACEMENT

### Indications

Myringotomy and tube placement is indicated (1) when fluid has been present for 8 to 12 weeks, despite medical therapy, causing a significant conductive hearing loss; (2) when recurrent acute otitis is debilitating by its frequency and severity; or (3) when atelectasis (tympanic membrane retraction) with fibrous adhesion, ossicular erosion, or cholesteatoma formation is imminent.

### Preoperative Evaluation

The preoperative evaluation requires a complete pneumatic otoscopic examination and audiologic evaluation. Radiography is rarely, if ever, helpful.

### Operative Technique

1. General anesthesia is administered by mask. The head is turned to the side opposite the ear being operated upon.
2. The largest speculum that will fit in the external meatus is placed in the ear. Wax is cleared from the external meatus to provide visualization of the entire tympanic membrane.
3. An incision, slightly larger than the medial flange of the tympanostomy tube to be used, is made in the anterior-superior quadrant parallel to the malleus and half the distance between the malleus and annulus (Fig. 1–1**A**).
4. Fluid is aspirated from the middle ear with a 5 French suction cannula, preferably without touching the tympanic membrane.
5. The anterior medial flange of the tube is inserted in the incision and the posterior flange is rotated into the incision with an alligator forceps or suction tip (Fig. 1–1**B–D**).
6. The lumen and area around the tube are aspirated free of blood. Antibiotic-containing ear (or eye) drops can be placed in the ear to prevent reaccumulation of blood and subsequent plugging of the tube.
7. When a prominent anterior bony canal impairs visualization of the anterior-superior quadrant, the incision and tube can be placed in the anterior-inferior or posterior-inferior quadrant of the tympanic membrane (TM) in a similar fashion. In some instances, it may be easier to perform a radial incision in the tympanic membrane.

Large flanged or "T" tubes are used in patients in whom standard tubes extrude prematurely or in those instances where it is felt that a child will need 3 to 5 years of middle ear ventilation. These tubes can be placed in a fashion similar to that used when inserting standard tubes, except that they require a larger myringotomy incision.

### Complications

1. Purulent otorrhea
2. Early extrusion
3. Permanent perforation
4. Granuloma
5. Tympanosclerosis
6. Cholesteatoma

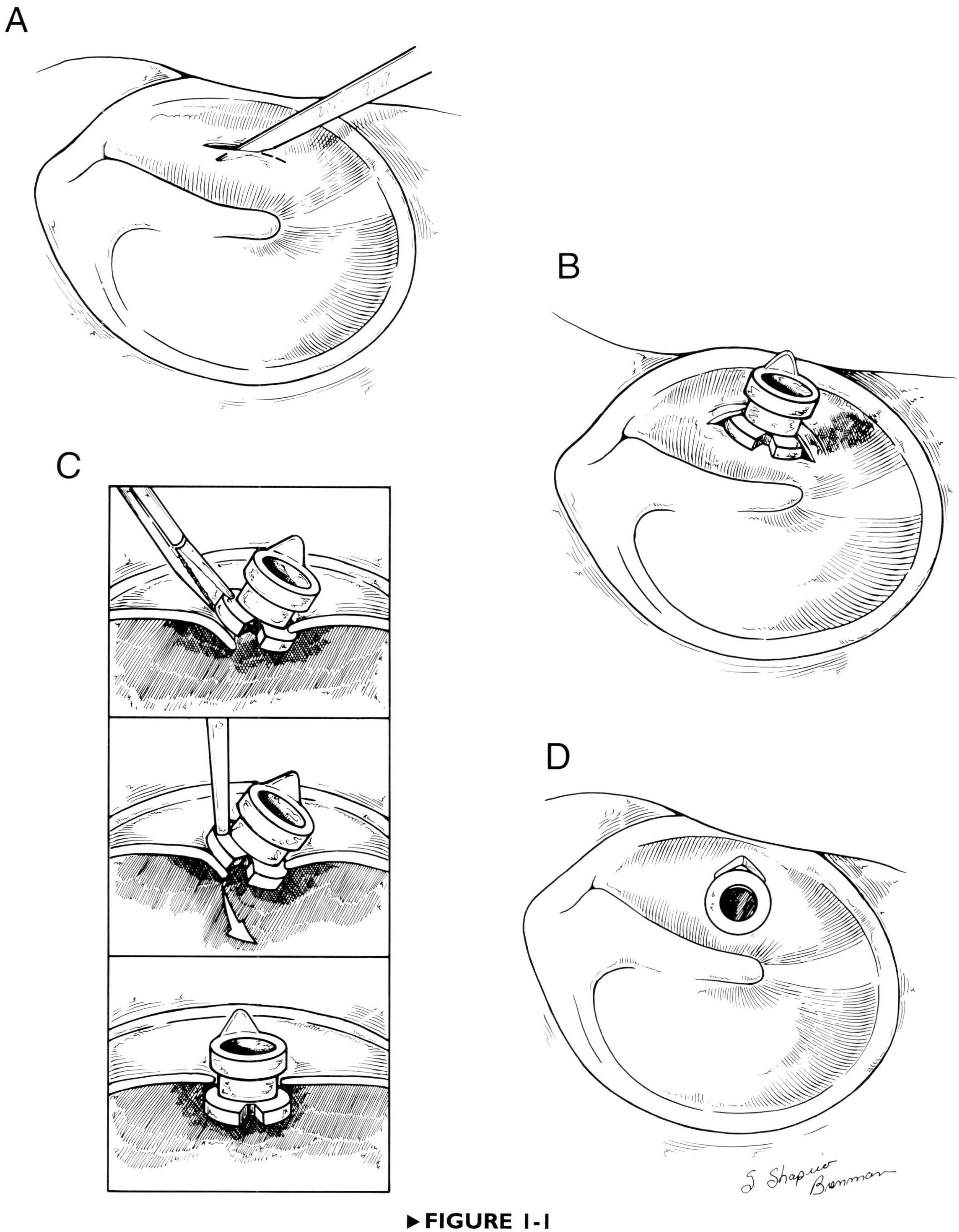


▶ **FIGURE 1-1**

# 2 ▸ Acute Otitis Media (AOM)

Acute otitis media (AOM) is one of the most common head and neck infections of childhood. Most episodes respond to antimicrobial therapy. However, in cases of suspected resistant organisms, poor response to antimicrobial therapy, or complications (such as meningitis or facial nerve paralysis), aspiration of purulent material from the middle ear space is required.

## ▸ 2-1 DIAGNOSTIC ASPIRATION (TYMPANOCENTESIS)

### Indications

Tympanocentesis for culture and sensitivity is indicated in the following instances:

1. Severe or unresponsive (to conventional antimicrobial therapy) AOM present in a child less than 8 weeks of age (neonate) to rule out gram-negative organisms.
2. In patients with AOM with either acquired or congenital immunodeficiency.
3. In patients who develop severe AOM while already taking an appropriate antimicrobial agent.
4. When the child has unusually severe pain, toxicity, or bullous myringitis.

### Preoperative Evaluation

Preoperative evaluation requires a complete pneumatic otoscopic examination. Audiologic evaluation may be difficult to obtain in an acutely ill child and is of limited value before this procedure.

### Operative Technique

1. Local anesthesia is not helpful in the presence of severe acute inflammation. The child must be restrained so that the head is immobile.
2. The external canal is cleared of wax with a cerumen curette and the ear drum is visualized.
3. The tip of a bent 21-gauge spinal needle attached to a 3-cc syringe is inserted through a speculum and into an inferior quadrant of the tympanic membrane (TM) (Fig. 2–1**A**). The syringe is then used to aspirate the fluid (Fig. 2–1**B**).

### Complications

None

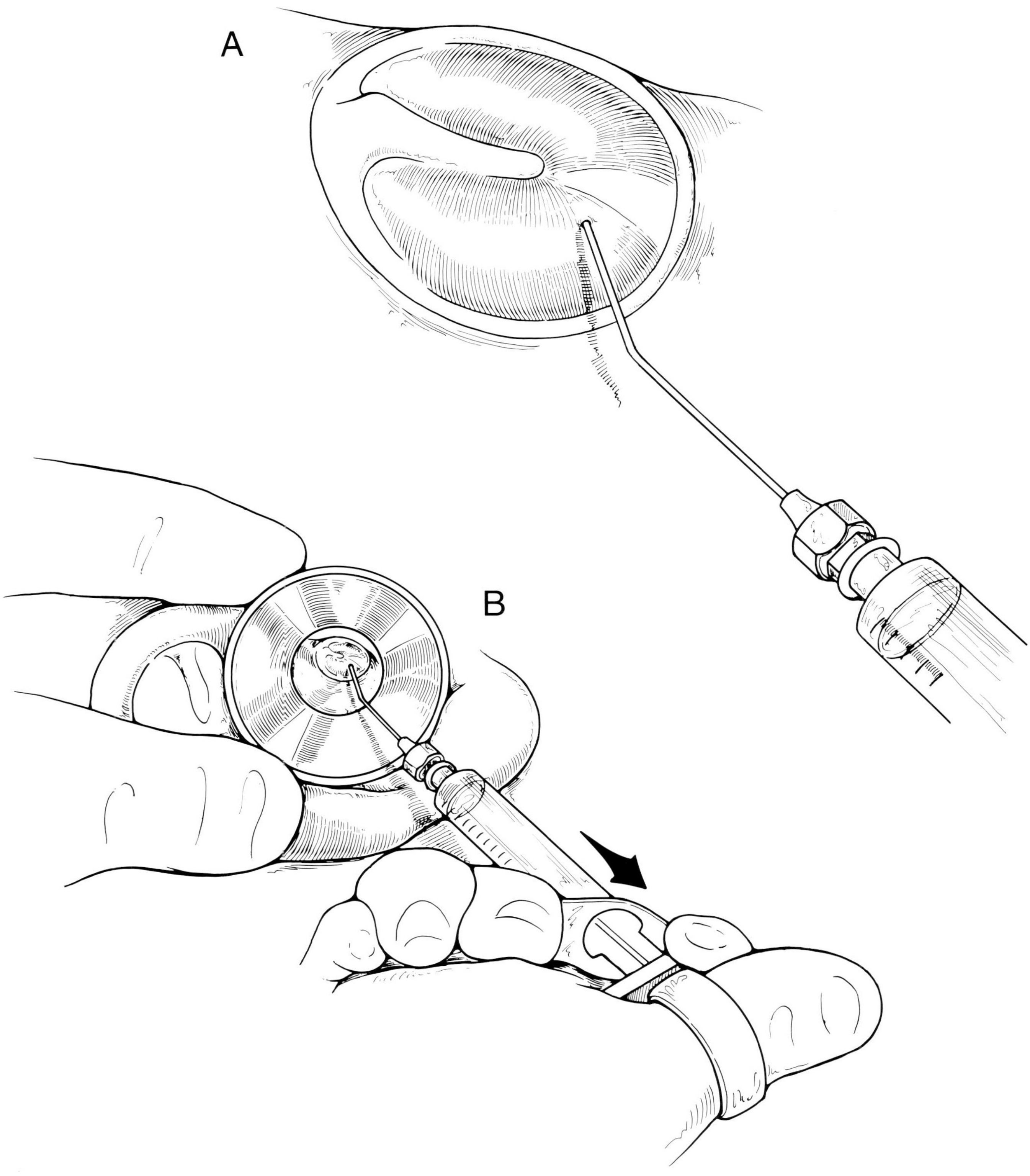


▶ **FIGURE 2-1**

## ▶ 2-2 THERAPEUTIC (WIDE FIELD) MYRINGOTOMY

### Indications

When a patient has facial nerve paralysis, vertigo, or intracranial complications (such as meningitis or cerebritis) caused by AOM, a wide myringotomy for drainage and culture should be performed.

### Preoperative Evaluation

Preoperative evaluation requires a complete pneumatic otoscopic examination. Audiologic evaluation may be difficult to obtain in an acutely ill child and is of limited value before this procedure.

### Operative Technique

1. General anesthesia provides the maximum comfort and surgical exposure for therapeutic myringotomy. However, in some instances, depending upon the child's condition, the procedure may be performed without anesthesia.
2. The ear canal should be cleared of wax to provide visualization.
3. A wide myringotomy should be made from the anterior-inferior quadrant to the posterior-inferior quadrant (Fig. 2–2C).
4. The contents can then be aspirated without difficulty.
5. A tympanostomy tube may be placed at the same time if long-term ventilation is desired (see section 1–1).

### Complications (If Tube is Placed)

1. Purulent otorrhea
2. Early tube extrusion
3. Granuloma
4. Permanent perforation
5. Tympanosclerosis
6. Cholesteatoma

C

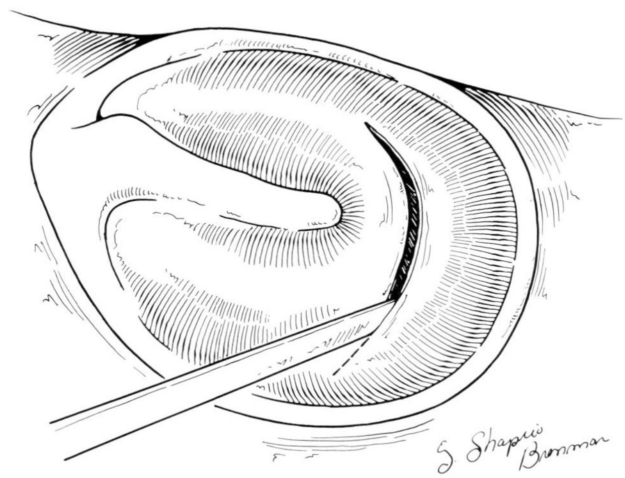

▶ **FIGURE 2-2**

# 3 ▸ Chronic Otitis Media (COM)

The term *chronic otitis media* (COM) describes a permanent perforation of the tympanic membrane (TM) with or without active infection. Cholesteatoma may also be present, associated with a TM perforation or, less frequently, behind an intact TM.

Treatment of COM is surgical and is indicated to accomplish the following:

1. Restore or preserve hearing in the presence of a perforation of the tympanic membrane.
2. Arrest or prevent chronic infection or recurrent acute infection of the middle ear and mastoid.
3. Arrest or prevent destruction of the bony structures of the ear and mastoid.
4. Prevent intracranial complications of otologic infection.
5. Reconstruct the hearing mechanism and mastoid when these have been destroyed by infection or cholesteatoma.

## ▸ 3-1 PAPER PATCH (MYRINGOPLASTY)

### Indications

A small, dry perforation that has not closed spontaneously after at least three months of observation may benefit from closure with a paper patch (Fig. 3–1**A**).

### Preoperative Evaluation

The preoperative evaluation of COM requires a complete otoscopic examination. Most TM perforations are easily seen by otoscopy. Audiologic evaluation should be performed prior to otologic surgery to detect any preexisting sensorineural and/or conductive hearing loss.

### Operative Technique

For most children, this procedure is performed under a general anesthesia.

1. In older, cooperative teenagers, a local anesthetic may be utilized. One percent lidocaine with 1:100,000 epinephrine is injected in the soft tissue of four quadrants of the ear canal just lateral to the edge of the bony ear canal.
2. The edges of the perforation are denuded of epithelium by making linear perforations around the rim with a pick or knife (Fig. 3–1**B**) or cauterizing the edge of the perforation with trichloroacetic acid (Fig. 3–1**C**).
3. If a pick is used, the rim of loose epithelium is removed with a cup forceps (Fig. 3–1**D**).
4. The paper patch is prepared by using a paper hole punch to create disks out of cigarette paper.
5. A cigarette paper patch is placed in contact with the lateral surface of the TM (Fig. 3–1**E–F**).

6. The cigarette paper will separate spontaneously from the TM in 2 to 3 weeks, leaving a healed perforation in the majority of cases.

## Complications

1. Persistent perforation
2. Purulent otorrhea

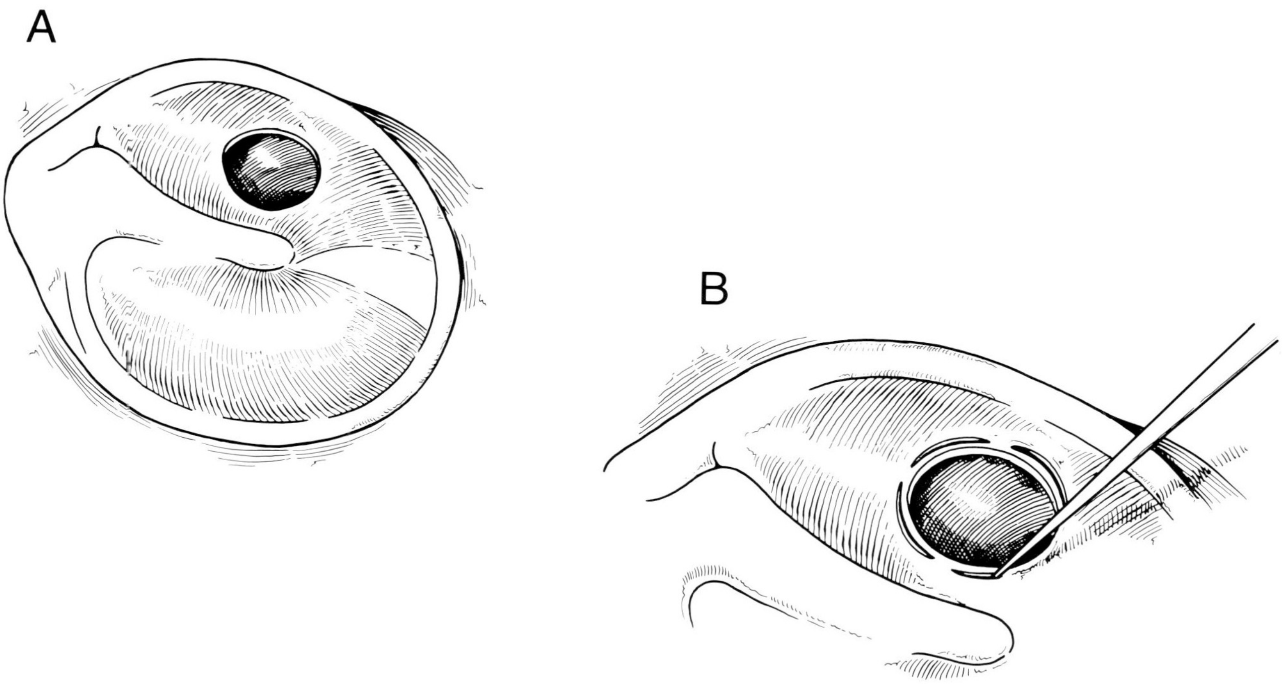


▶ **FIGURE 3-1**

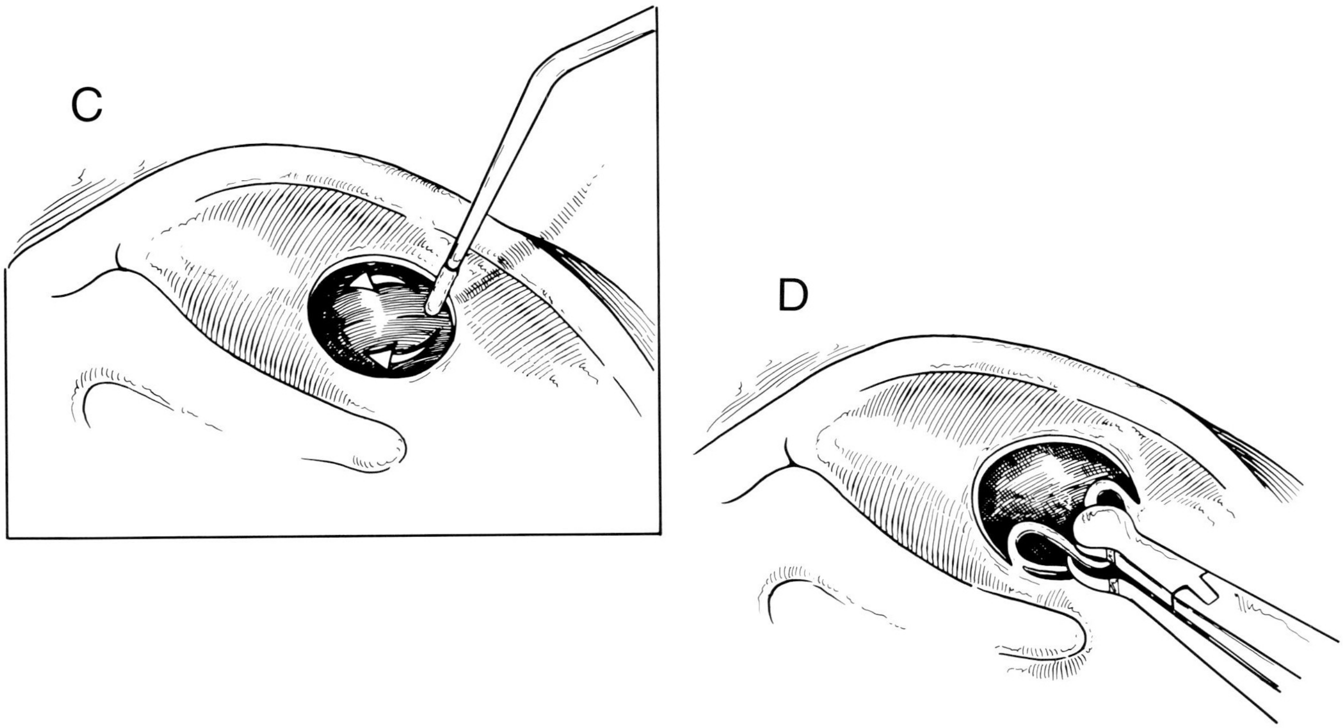


▶ **FIGURE 3-1**

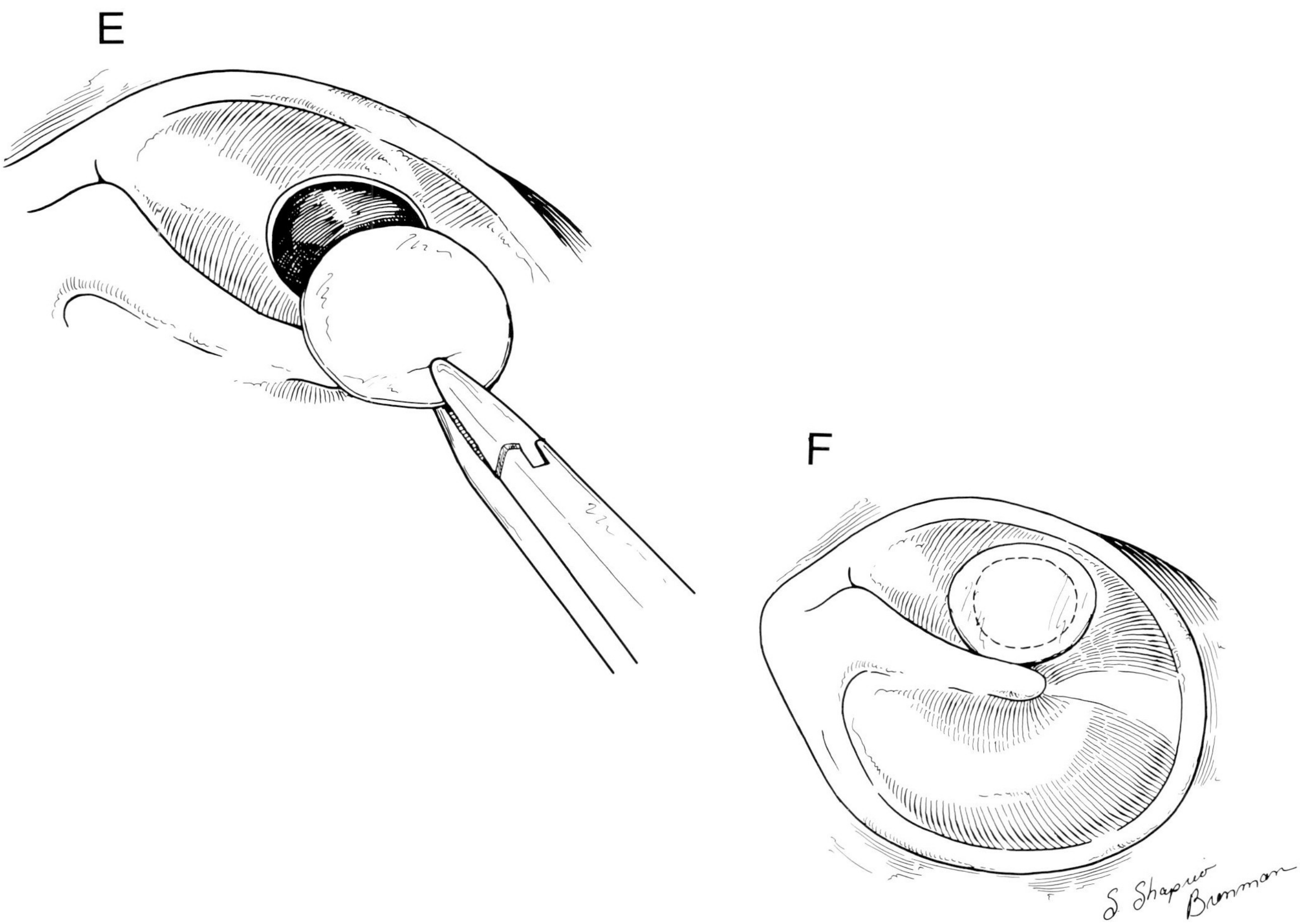


▶ **FIGURE 3-1**

## ▶ 3-2 TYMPANOPLASTY

Tympanoplasty is an operation to close a TM perforation. In a child, tympanoplasty is performed using a postauricular approach and under general anesthesia to obtain complete exposure to the TM and middle ear. Use of an underlay (medial) temporalis fascia graft reestablishes the TM contour and avoids epithelial inclusions that can form between the TM remnant and a lateral graft.

### Indications

Tympanoplasty is indicated to repair a TM perforation that has not spontaneously closed after at least 3 months of observation.

### Preoperative Evaluation

The preoperative evaluation of chronic otitis media requires a complete otoscopic examination and audiologic evaluation. Most TM perforations are easily seen, and the presence of cholesteatoma can be detected by observing white flaky keratin debris in the middle ear space.

Audiometric evaluation should be performed prior to otologic surgery to detect any preexisting sensorineural hearing loss and to assess ossicular function.

### Operative Technique

1. The ear is injected with 1% lidocaine containing 1:100,000 epinephrine in the postauricular crease (Fig. 3–2**A**) and at the edge of the external meatus (Fig. 3–2**B**) prior to scrubbing. Additional solution can be injected at the bony-cartilaginous junction just before the surgery is begun.
2. Pulling the ear laterally, an incision is made at right angles to the skin in the postauricular crease (Fig. 3–2**C**).
3. Dissection of the soft tissue is performed with a knife or cutting cautery toward the external meatus (Fig. 3–2**D**). Care is taken not to transect the skin of the ear canal.
4. The remaining soft tissue and periosteum overlying the mastoid are cut in an angular fashion with the apex pointing to the sinodural angle using a cutting cautery or knife (Fig. 3–2**E**).
5. The periosteum overlying the mastoid is reflected forward, exposing the external meatus by pushing the flap anteriorly with a sponge-covered finger or with a periosteal elevator. It is then held forward with a self-retaining retractor (Fig. 3–2**F**).
6. The periosteum of the external meatus is elevated with a McCabe knife or duck bill elevator to a point just beyond the junction of the thick and thin skin (Fig. 3–2**G**). The elevator is advanced, keeping it against the bone of the ear canal to avoid perforation of the canal skin.
7. The skin of the posterior meatus is transected with a knife at the junction of thick and thin skin (Fig. 3–2**H**). The inferior limb of the incision is extended along the inferior portion of the ear canal with the knife.
8. The canal incision can be adjusted to expose any part of the annulus and leave an attached area for blood supply (Fig. 3–2**I**).

9. The self-retaining retractor is adjusted to reflect the lateral skin of the ear canal forward, exposing the perforation and entire tympanic membrane (Fig. 3–2**J**, **K**).
10. The edges of the perforation are prepared by removing the epithelium with a pick and cup forceps (Fig. 3–2**L**, **M**).
11. Mucosa is scraped from the undersurface of the tympanic membrane remnant with a reverse micro-Tabb knife (Fig. 3–2**N**).
12. The tympanomeatal flap and annulus are elevated and the middle ear is entered (Fig. 3–2**O**). The ossicles are identified and examined for mobility. The condition of the middle ear mucosa and ossicles is noted (Fig. 3–2**P**).
13. The temporalis fascia graft is taken with a knife, scissors, and forceps, leaving a strip of fascia at the inferior border of the temporalis muscle (Fig. 3–2**Q**). The fascia is separated from the underlying muscle and a rectangular graft, of the desired size, is removed (Fig. 3–2**R**).
14. The graft is positioned medial to the malleus and tympanic membrane remnant (Fig. 3–2**S**). Gelfoam is placed medial to the graft to keep it against the TM remnant. This may be made easier by folding the fascia back through the perforation to place Gelfoam under the anterior remnant of the drum (Fig. 3–2**T**).
15. The anterior edge of the graft is then tucked into the perforation beneath the anterior rim of the TM, keeping it lateral to the bed of Gelfoam. The fascia is draped along the posterior ear canal and the tympanomeatal flap is returned to its normal posterior position (Fig. 3–2**U**).
16. Gelfoam moistened with antibiotic ear drops is positioned at the junction of the TM remnant and the graft (Fig. 3–2**V**). The flap is then packed in place with more Gelfoam (Fig. 3–2**W**).
17. The periosteum overlying the mastoid is closed with interrupted 4-0 chromic or Vicryl sutures reapproximating the apex of the incision to avoid posterior canal wall collapse (Fig. 3–2**X**).
18. The postauricular incision is closed with interrupted 4-0 chromic subcuticular sutures. No skin sutures are used (Fig. 3–2**Y**).
19. The remainder of the ear canal is packed with Gelfoam and a standard mastoid dressing is applied (Fig. 3–2**Z**).

## Complications

1. Persistent perforation
2. Hearing loss
3. Vertigo
4. Facial nerve injury
5. Chorda tympani injury
6. Cholesteatoma

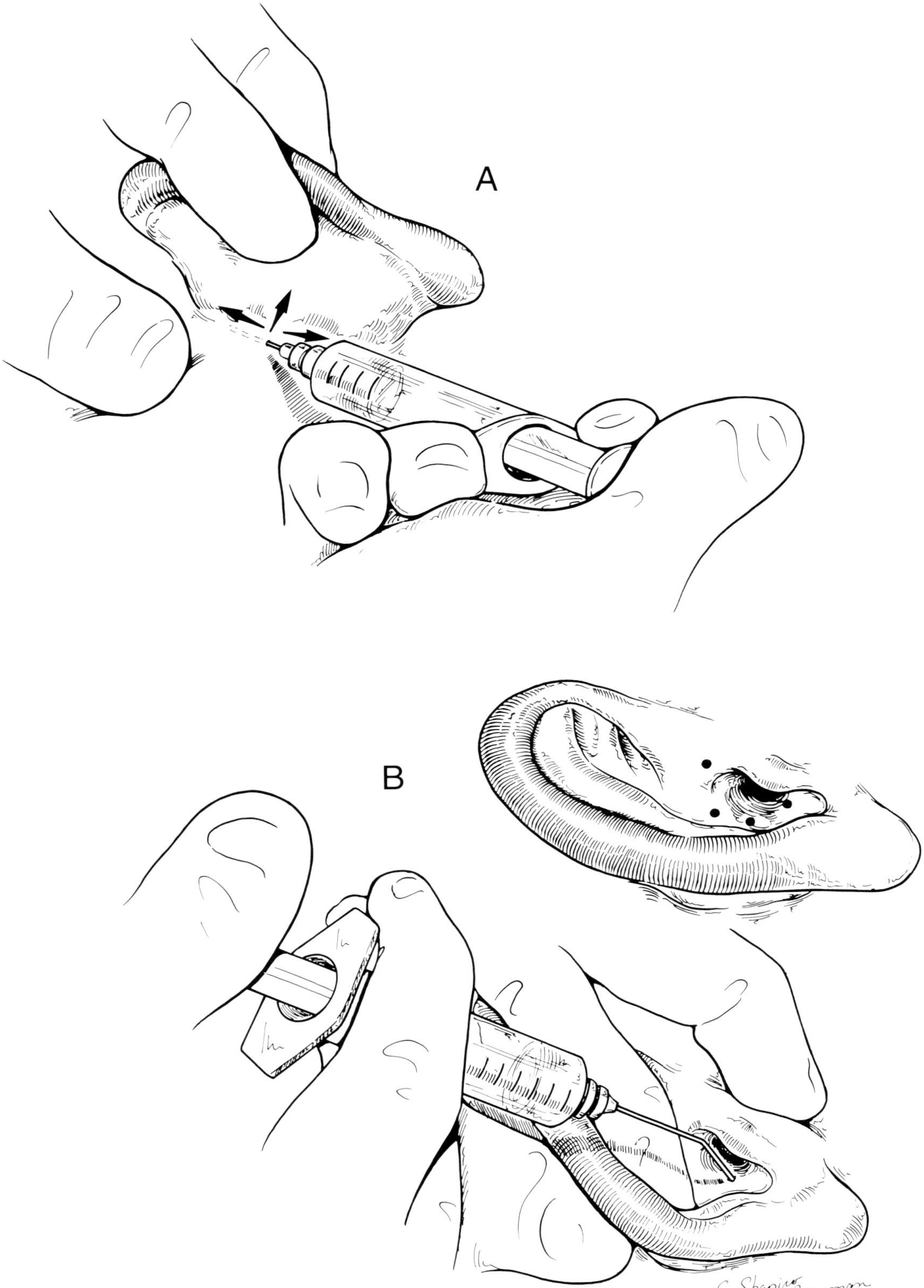


▶ **FIGURE 3-2**

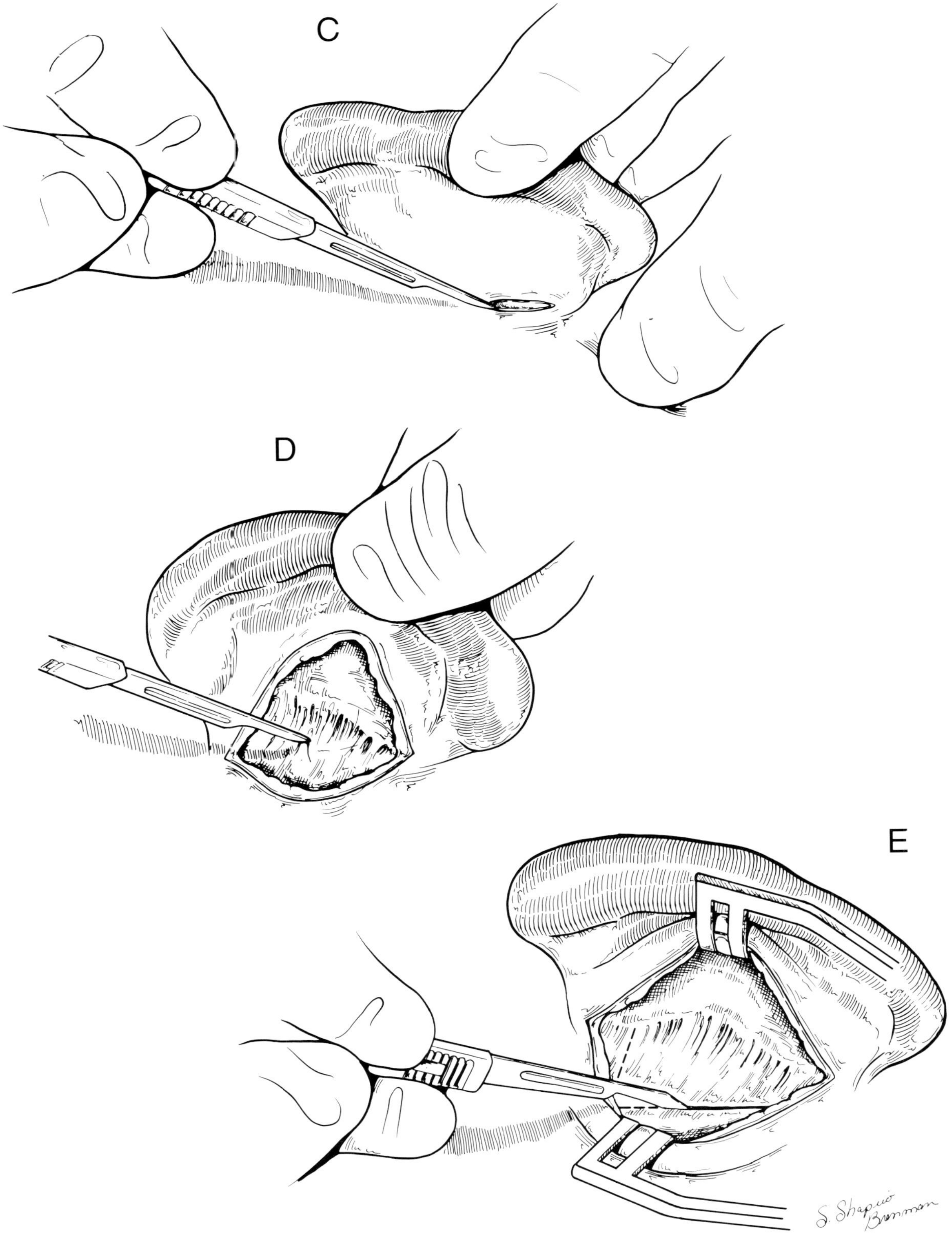


▶ **FIGURE 3-2**

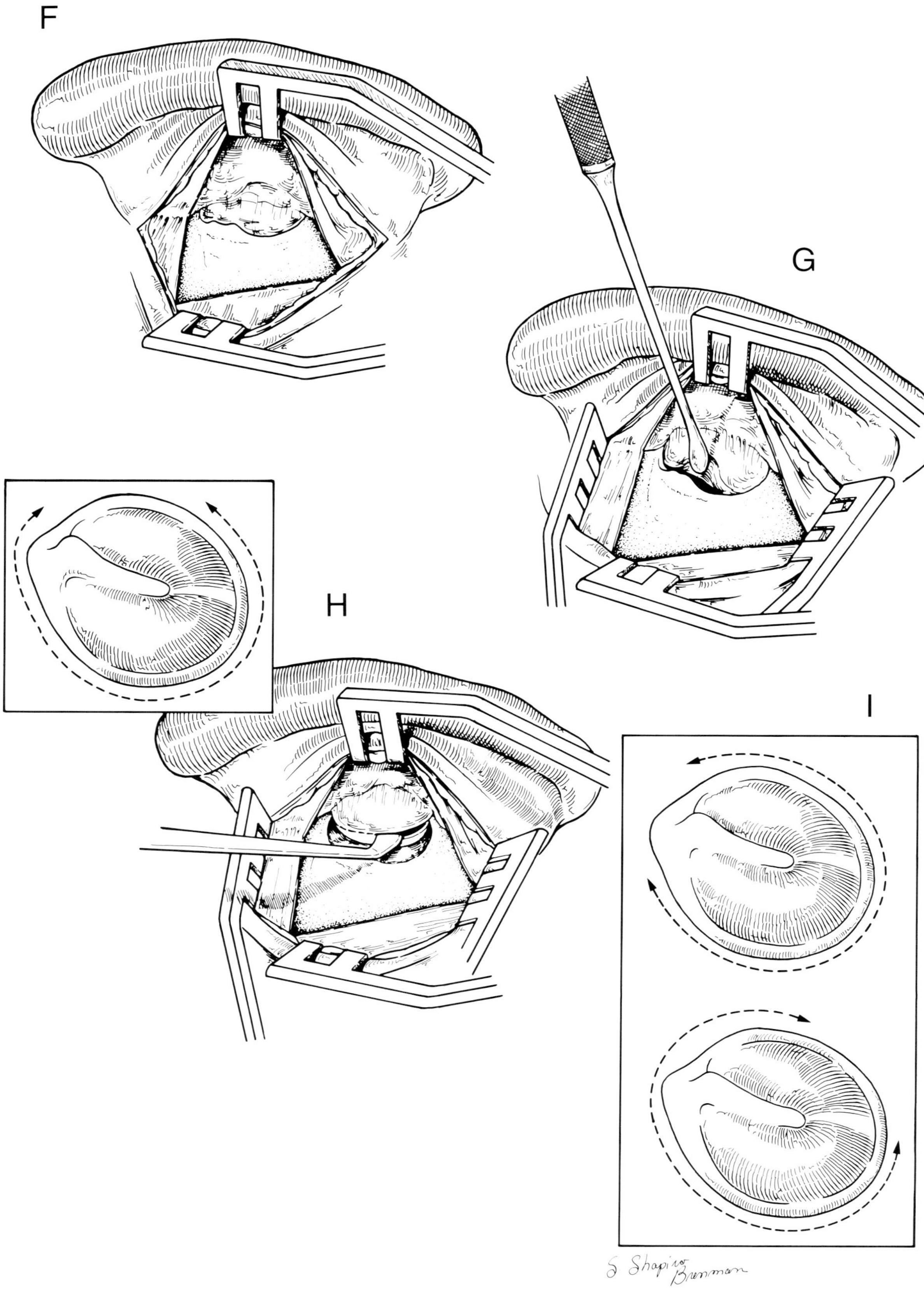


▶ **FIGURE 3-2**

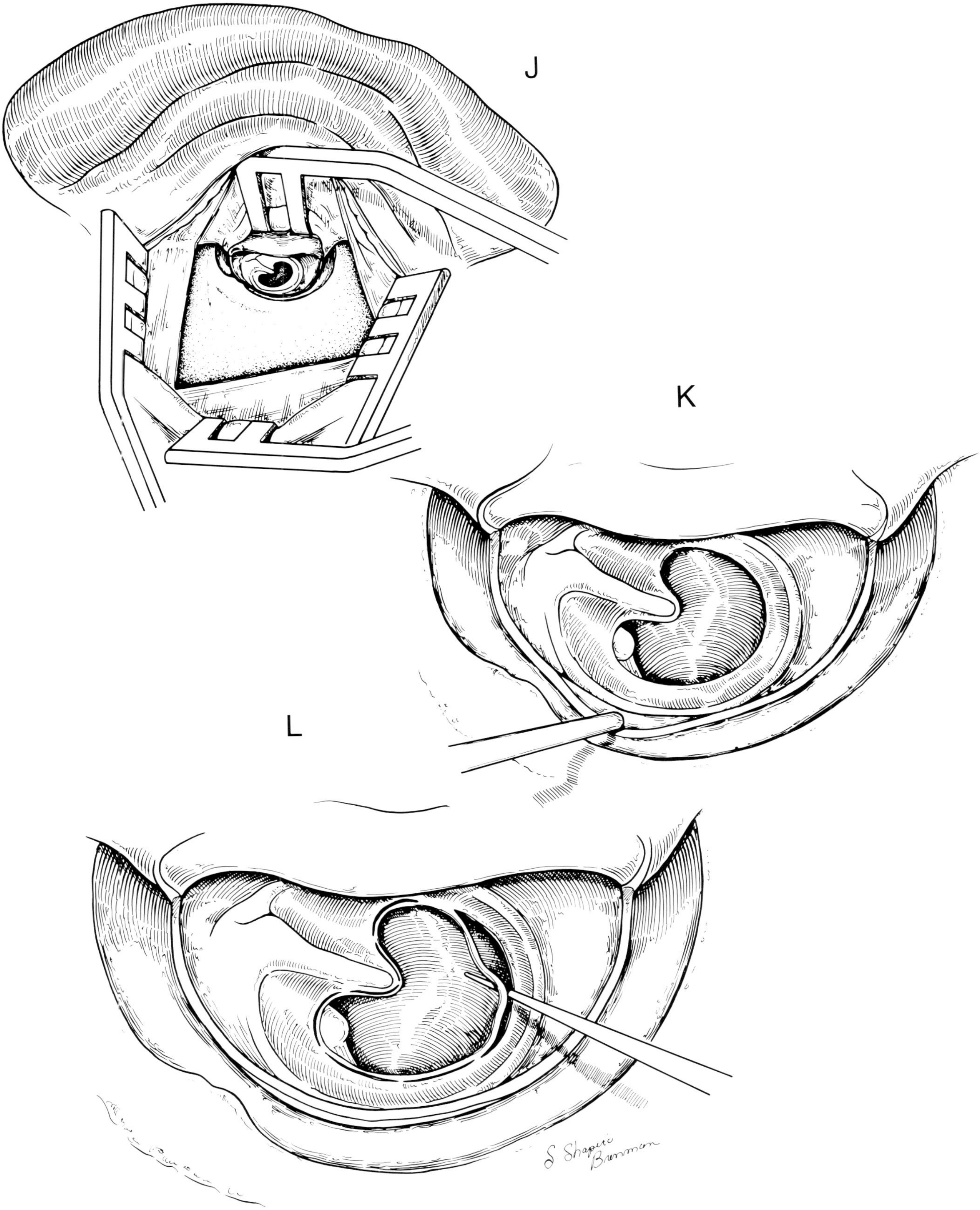


▶ **FIGURE 3-2**

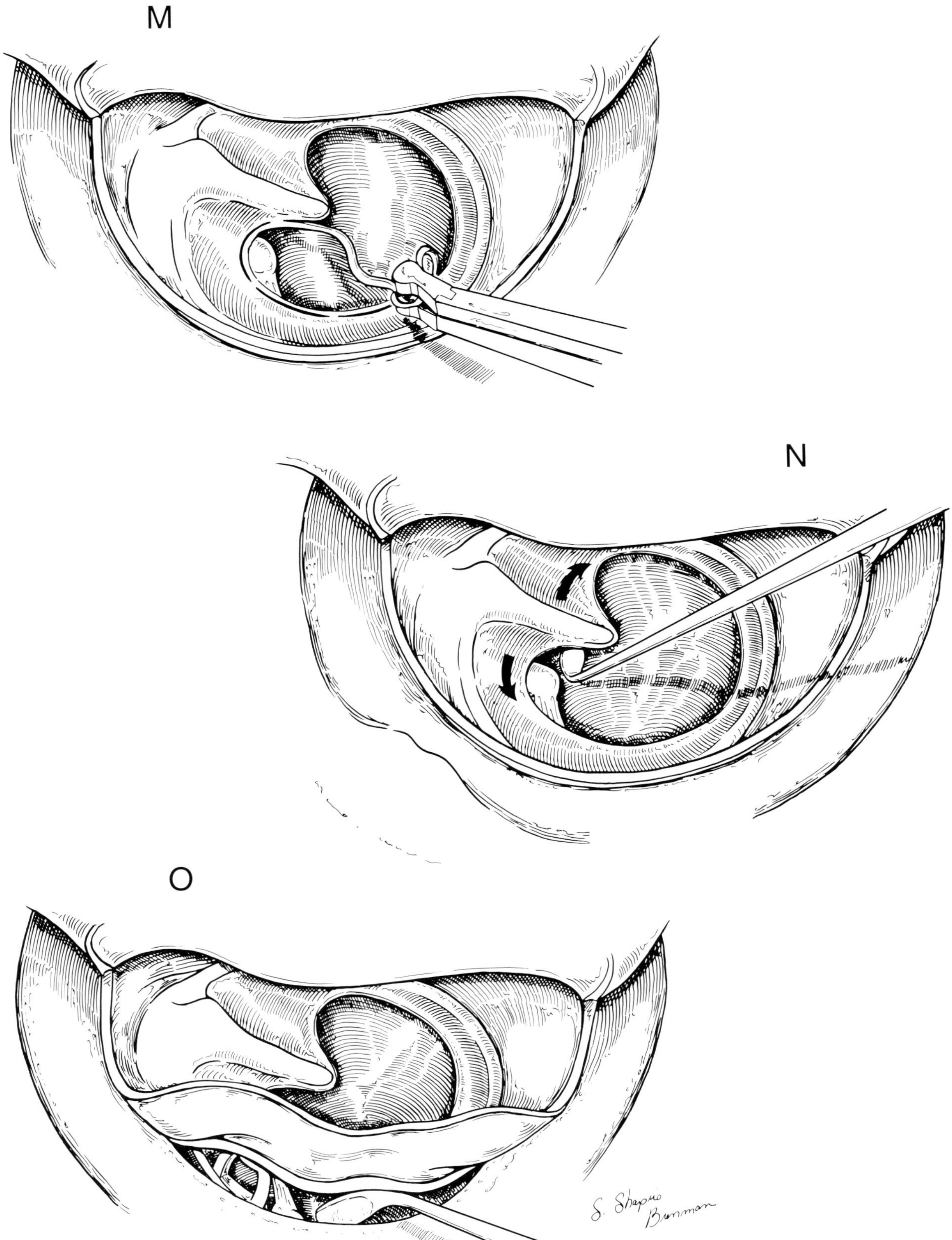


▶ **FIGURE 3-2**

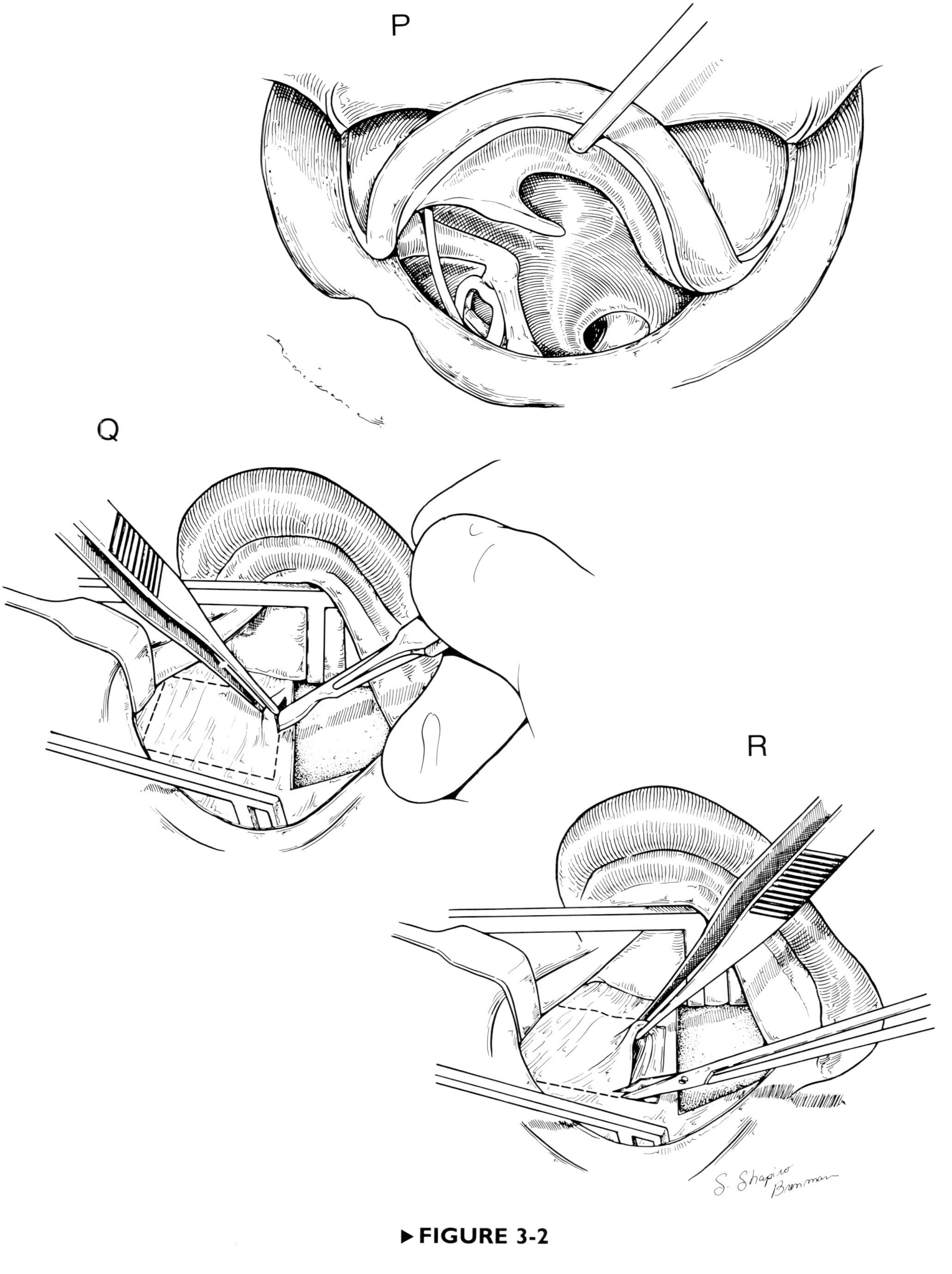


▶ **FIGURE 3-2**

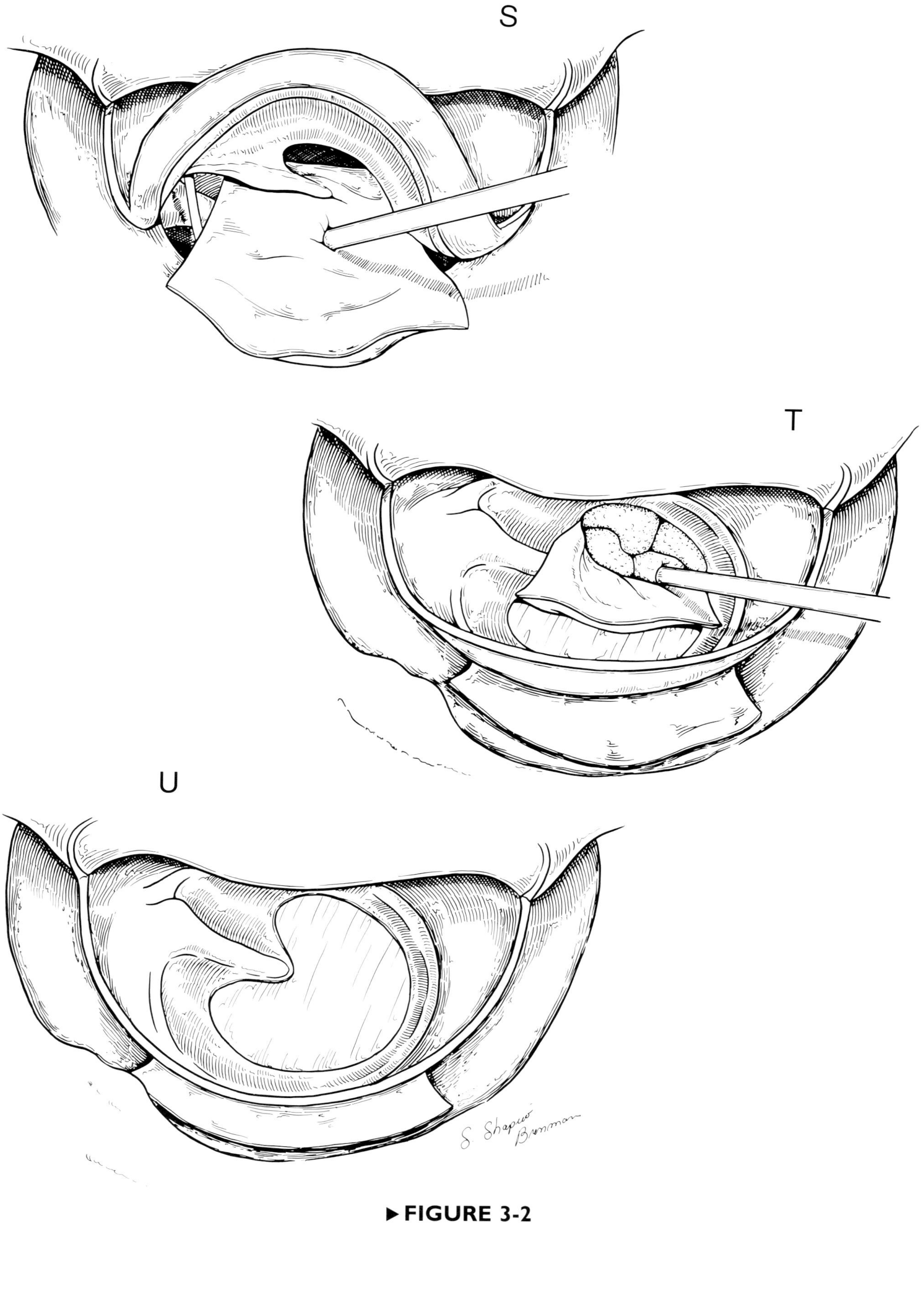


▶ **FIGURE 3-2**

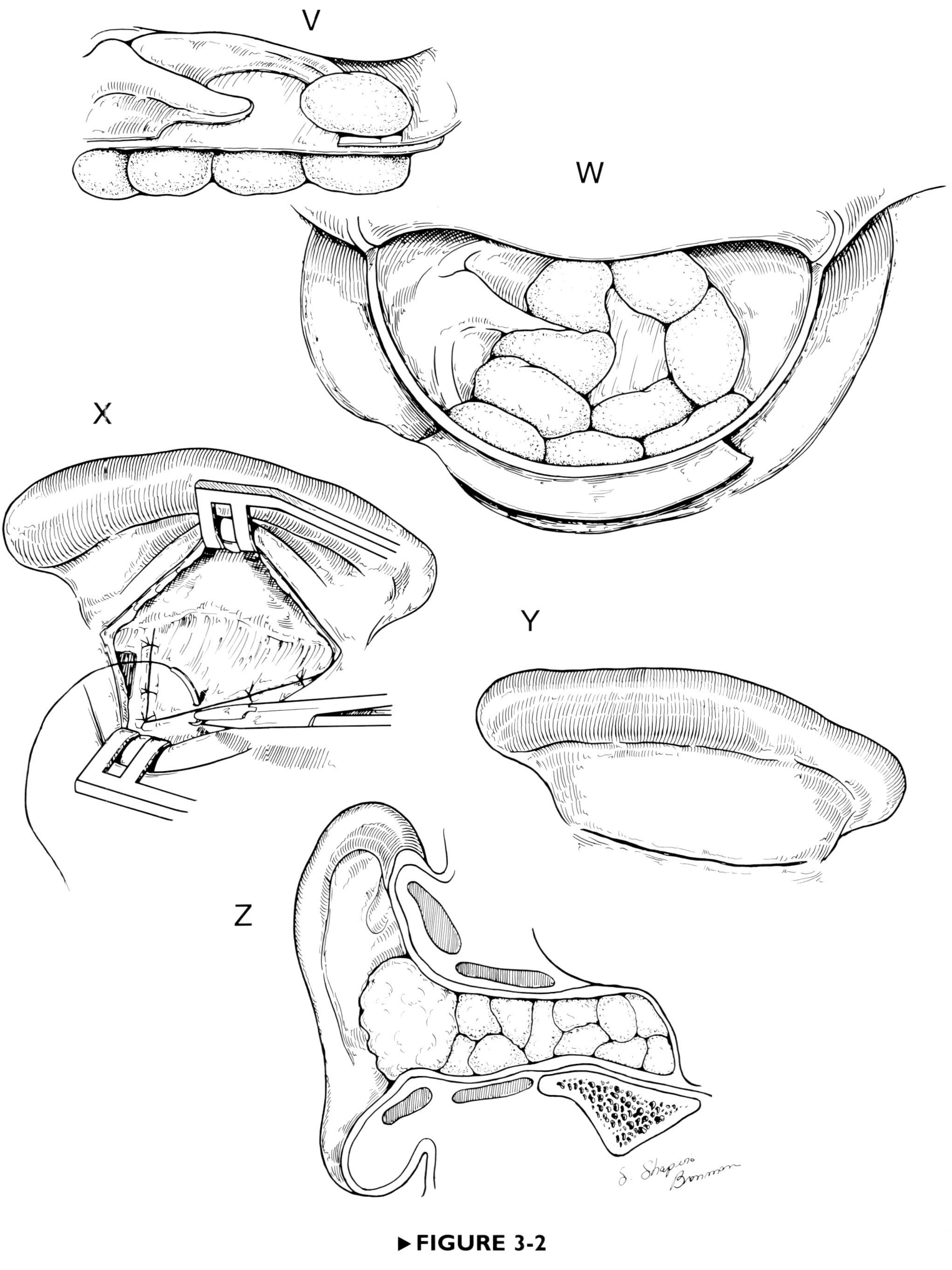


▶ **FIGURE 3-2**

# ▶ 3-3 OSSICULAR RECONSTRUCTION

Traditionally, discontinuities of the ossicular chain have been repaired utilizing carved cortical bone, sculpted incus, or homograft ossicles. Ossicular reconstruction has recently been facilitated by the commercial availability of total ossicular replacement prostheses (TORPs) and partial ossicular replacement prostheses (PORPs). The choice of prosthesis, design, and material depends on the personal preference of the surgeon.

## Indications

Ossicular reconstruction is indicated when the ossicular chain has been interrupted by disease, trauma, or surgery.

## Preoperative Evaluation

A complete otoscopic and audiologic evaluation is required before ossicular reconstruction. Computed tomography (CT) scan may be helpful to document the location and continuity of the ossicles.

## Operative Technique

1. The middle ear is exposed through a canal wall incision as described in section 3–2, Tympanoplasty or section 4–4, Middle Ear Exploration (Fig. 3–3**A**).
2. If the remaining portion of the incus interferes with placement of the PORP, the ossicle must be removed. A portion of the posterior-superior bony annulus and canal wall may be removed with a small cutting bur (Fig. 3–3**B**).
3. The chorda tympani is reflected inferiorly to prevent damage (Fig. 3–3**C**). The incus is separated from the malleus using a small pick or micro-Tabb knife.
4. The remnant of the ossicle is grasped with an alligator forceps and gently removed (Fig. 3–3**D**).
5. When the stapes is mobile and the suprastructure is intact, a PORP is placed between the TM, or TM graft, and the stapes (Fig. 3–3**E**).
6. When the stapes foot plate is mobile but the suprastructure is eroded (Fig. 3–3**F**), a TORP may be placed in a similar fashion between the TM, or TM graft, and the footplate (Fig. 3–3**G**). The TORP may be supported in the middle ear with small pieces of Gelfoam.
7. The prefabricated prosthesis can be cut with a sharp knife to fit the middle ear space.
8. Care must be taken to prevent contact with the surrounding bony ear canal to avoid adhesions and fixation.
9. Depending upon the composition of the prosthesis, a thin piece of conchal or tragal cartilage with attached perichondrium should be used to separate the top of the prosthesis from the TM or graft (Fig. 3–3**E, G**). The cartilage is fixed in place on the prosthesis with a tiny droplet of cyanoacrylate (e.g., Super Glue or Krazy Glue) liquid or gel. The cartilage is placed with the perichondrium against the TM. This helps to prevent extrusion of the prosthesis.

**10.** Some surgeons prefer sculpted homograft ossicles to reconstruct the ossicular chain. Usually, the incus is used and can be shaped with a drill to fit any desired situation (Fig. 3–3H).

**11.** The tympanomeatal flap is replaced and the ear canal packed as described in section 3–2, Tympanoplasty or section 4–4, Middle Ear Exploration.

### Complications

1. Tympanic membrane perforation
2. Hearing loss
3. Vertigo
4. Facial nerve injury
5. Chorda tympani injury
6. Prosthesis displacement

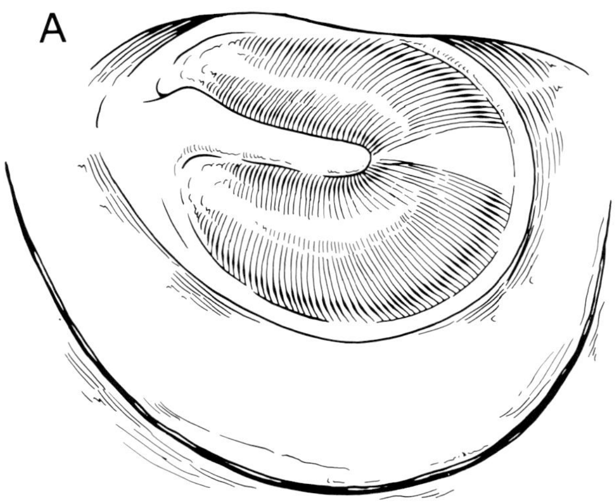


▸ **FIGURE 3-3**

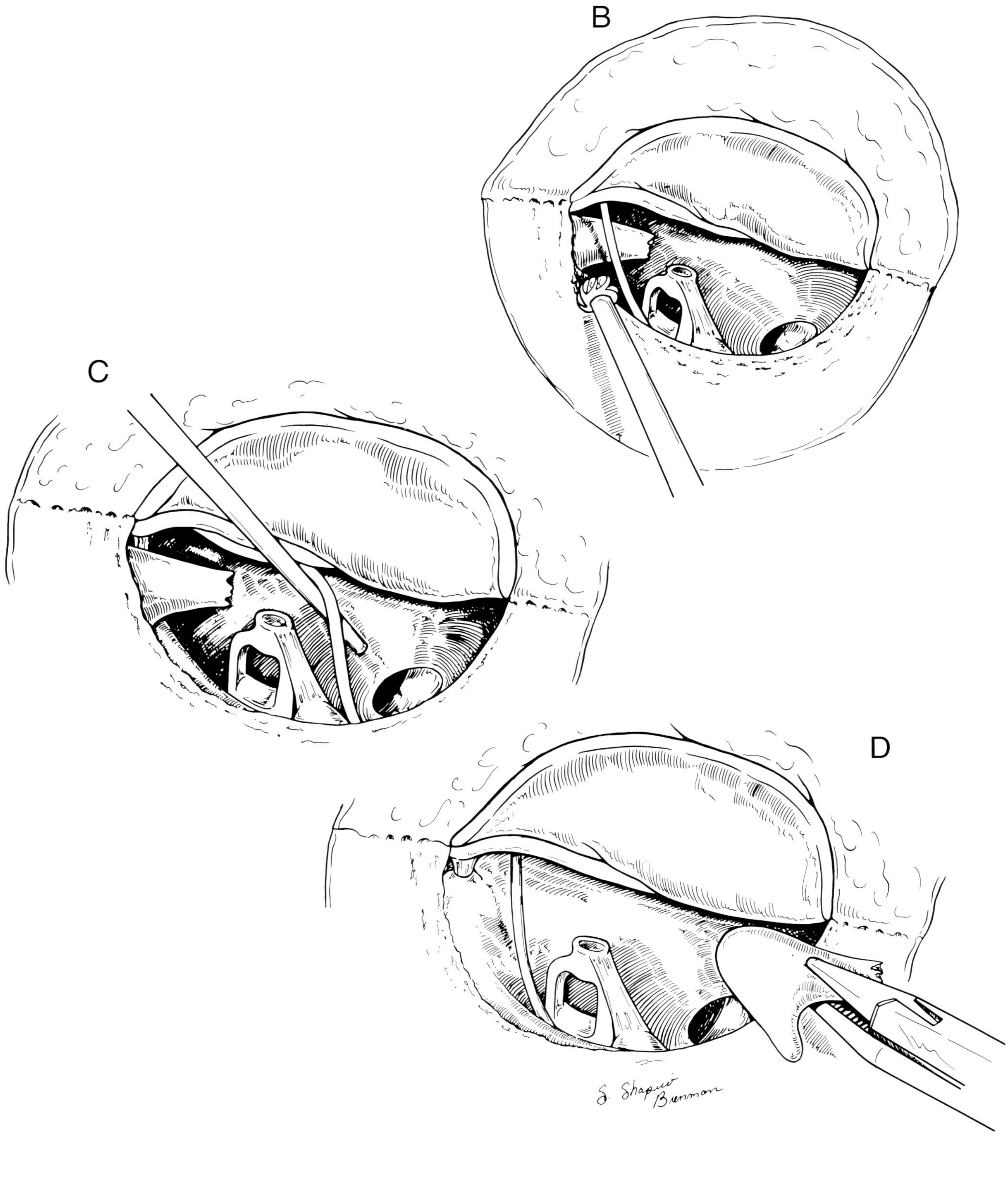


▶ **FIGURE 3-3**

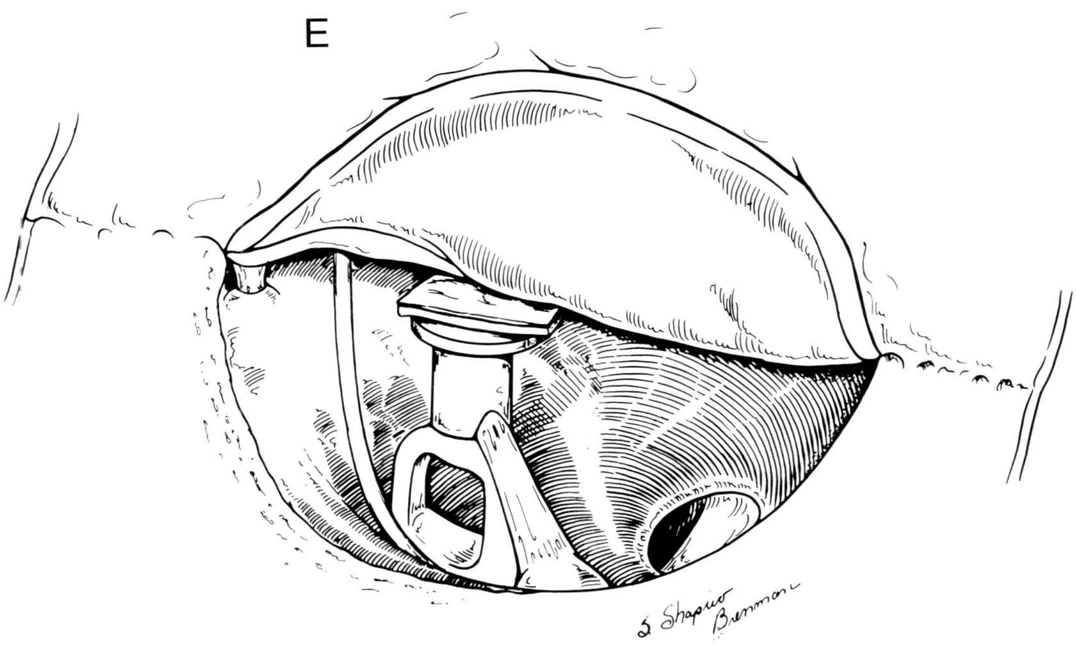


▶ **FIGURE 3-3**

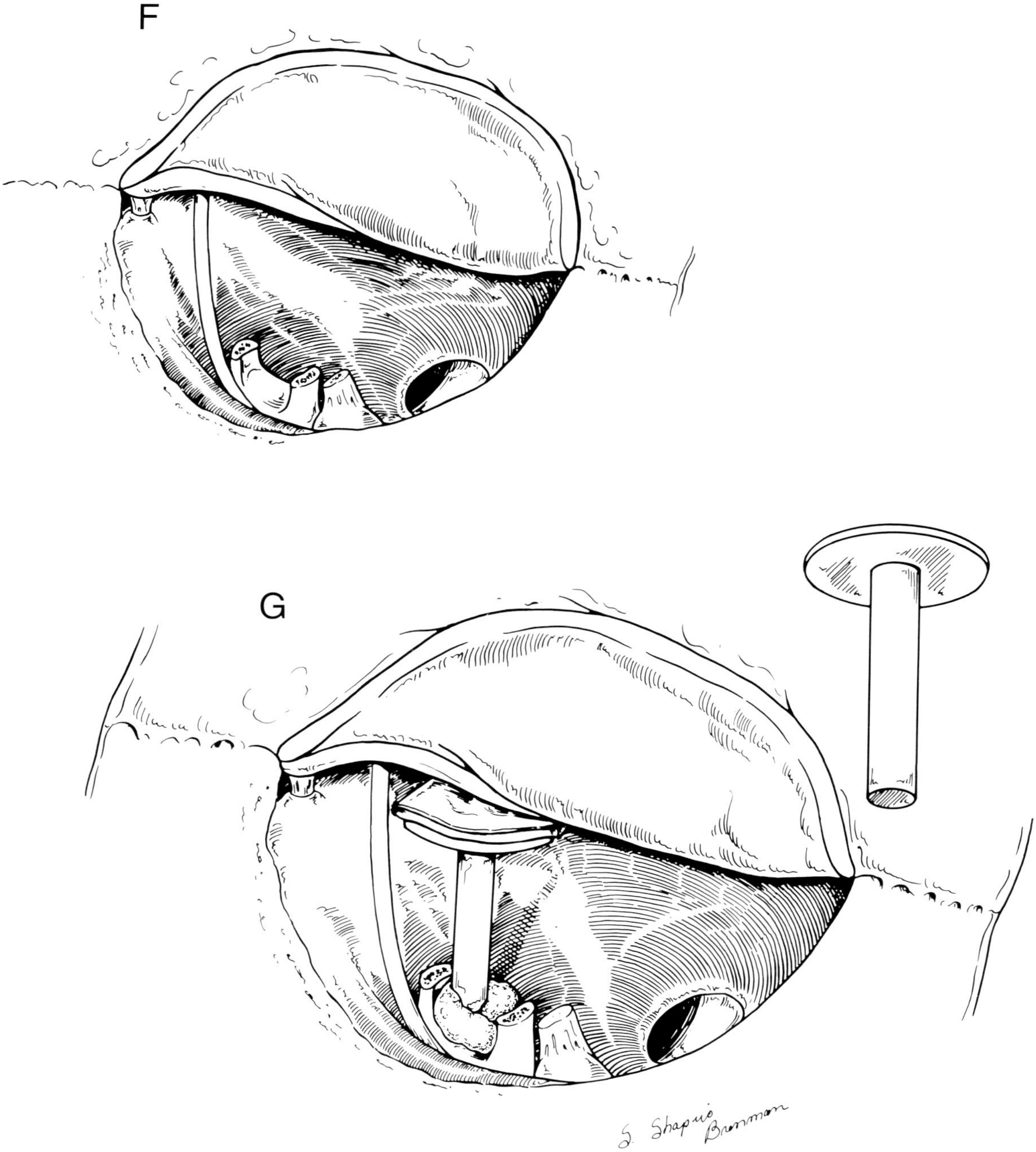


**▶ FIGURE 3-3**

H

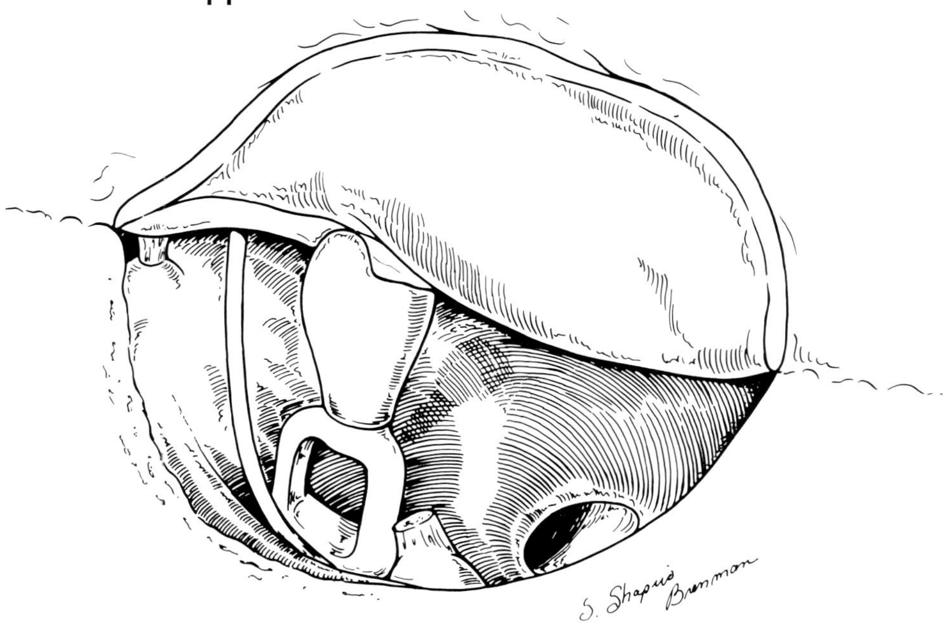


▶ **FIGURE 3-3**

## ▶ 3-4 SIMPLE MASTOIDECTOMY (CORTICAL MASTOIDECTOMY)

The purposes of cortical mastoidectomy are to provide drainage of a mastoid infection; to remove disease such as polypoid mucosa, granulation tissue, and cholesteatoma; and to ensure a route for aeration of the mastoid air cell system via the middle ear.

### Indications

Cortical mastoidectomy is indicated in the treatment of acute coalescent mastoiditis. The operation is also performed if there are complications of acute mastoiditis such as facial nerve paralysis, cerebritis, meningitis, or brain abscess.

### Preoperative Evaluation

The preoperative evaluation of coalescent mastoiditis requires a complete otologic examination. Otorrhea is usually present, and the postauricular crease is often obliterated by edema as the ear stands out from the head. Otoscopy reveals collapse of the posterior-superior canal wall.

Radiographs (especially CT scan) should be obtained to determine the extent of any cholesteatoma, level of the dura, and any other anatomic variant. Audiologic evaluation should be performed prior to otologic surgery to detect any preexisting sensorineural and/or conductive hearing loss. The surgeon may elect to utilize intraoperative facial nerve monitoring.

### Operative Technique

1. Simple mastoidectomy is performed under general anesthesia. A solution of 1% lidocaine containing 1:100,000 epinephrine is injected as is done for tympanoplasty to reduce intraoperative bleeding (see section 3–2).
2. The postauricular incision is made in the standard fashion (Fig. 3–4**A**) (see section 3–2).
3. The subcutaneous tissues of the postauricular area are incised (Fig. 3–4**B**).
4. The periosteal incision is made and may be extended posterosuperiorly from the apex with a cutting cautery if desired (Fig. 3–4**C**). The periosteum is reflected with a periosteal elevator, and self-retaining retractors are placed to expose the mastoid cortex (Fig. 3–4**D**).
5. The mastoid cortex is removed with a large cutting drill in the triangular area posterior to the spine of Henle, called the fossae mastoidea, which overlies the mastoid antrum. The cortex is saucerized to facilitate exposure of deeper areas (Fig. 3–4**E**).
6. After mastoid air cells are opened with a cutting drill, diseased mucosa and granulation tissue are removed with a dissector and cup forceps (Fig. 3–4**F**). The dissection is continued until adequate mastoid drainage is accomplished and the horizontal semicircular canal, head of the malleus, and short process of the incus can be seen (Fig. 3–4**G**).
7. The dissection should be carried inferiorly as far as is necessary to remove diseased cells in the mastoid tip. Disease in the sinodural angle, if present, must be removed.

8. After wide exposure is accomplished, a small Penrose drain is placed in the mastoid cavity and brought out of the inferior portion of the postauricular incision (Fig. 3–4H). The wound is closed with interrupted subcuticular absorbable suture (see section 3–2) (Fig. 3–4I).

### Complications

1. Facial nerve injury
2. Trauma to semicircular canals
3. Dural laceration
4. Sigmoid sinus hemorrhage
5. Ossicular disarticulation

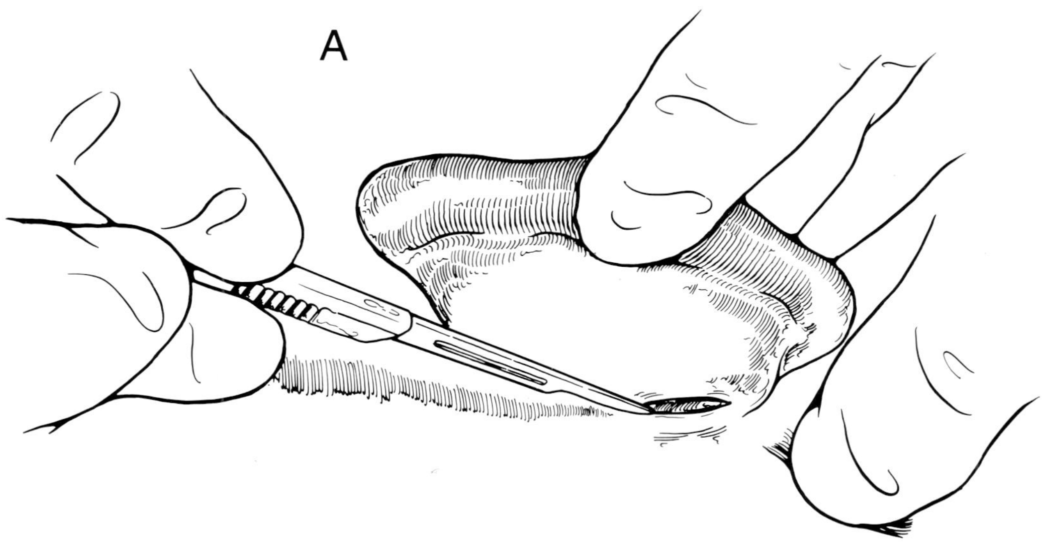


▶ **FIGURE 3-4**

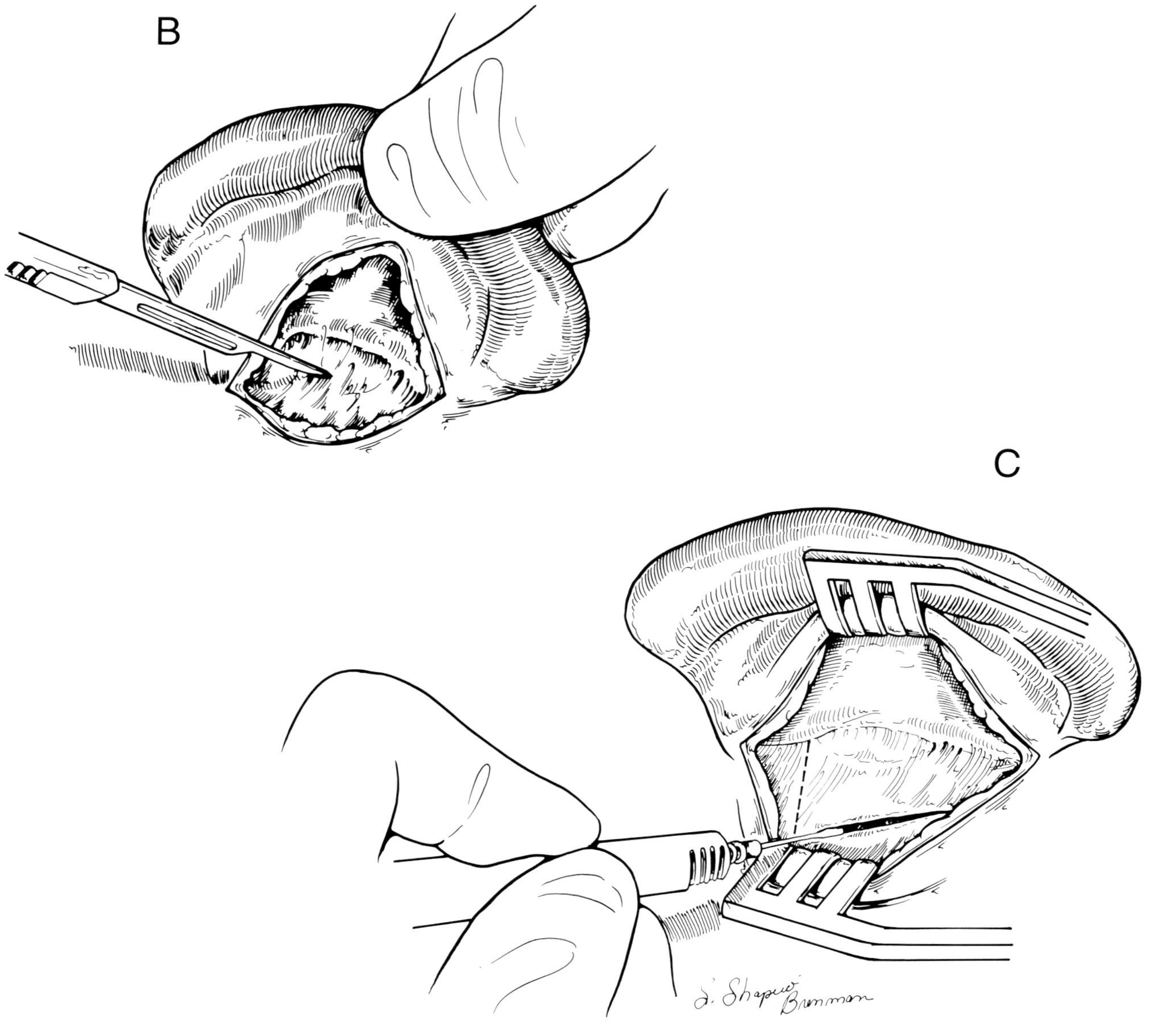


▶ **FIGURE 3-4**

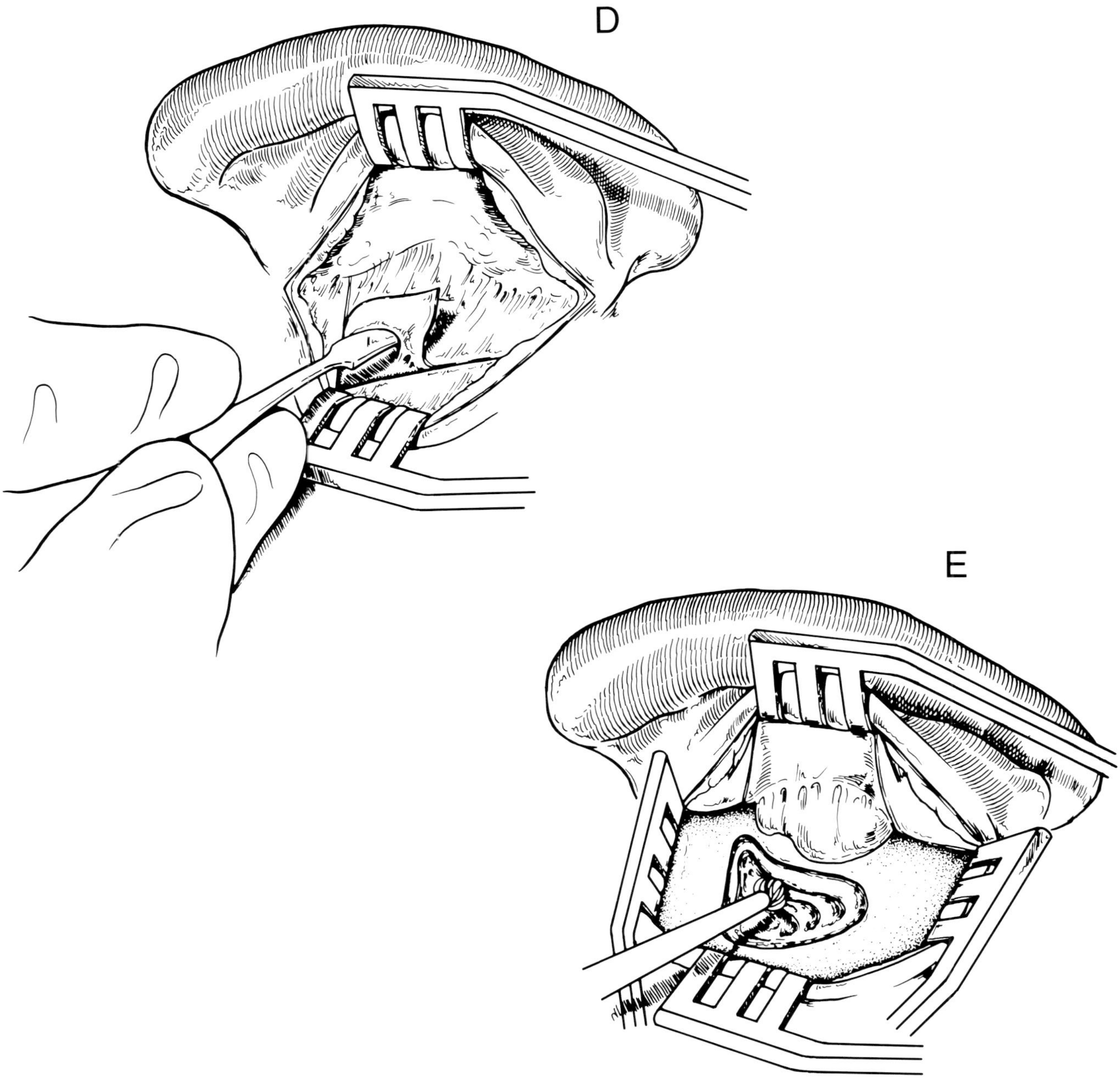


▶ **FIGURE 3-4**

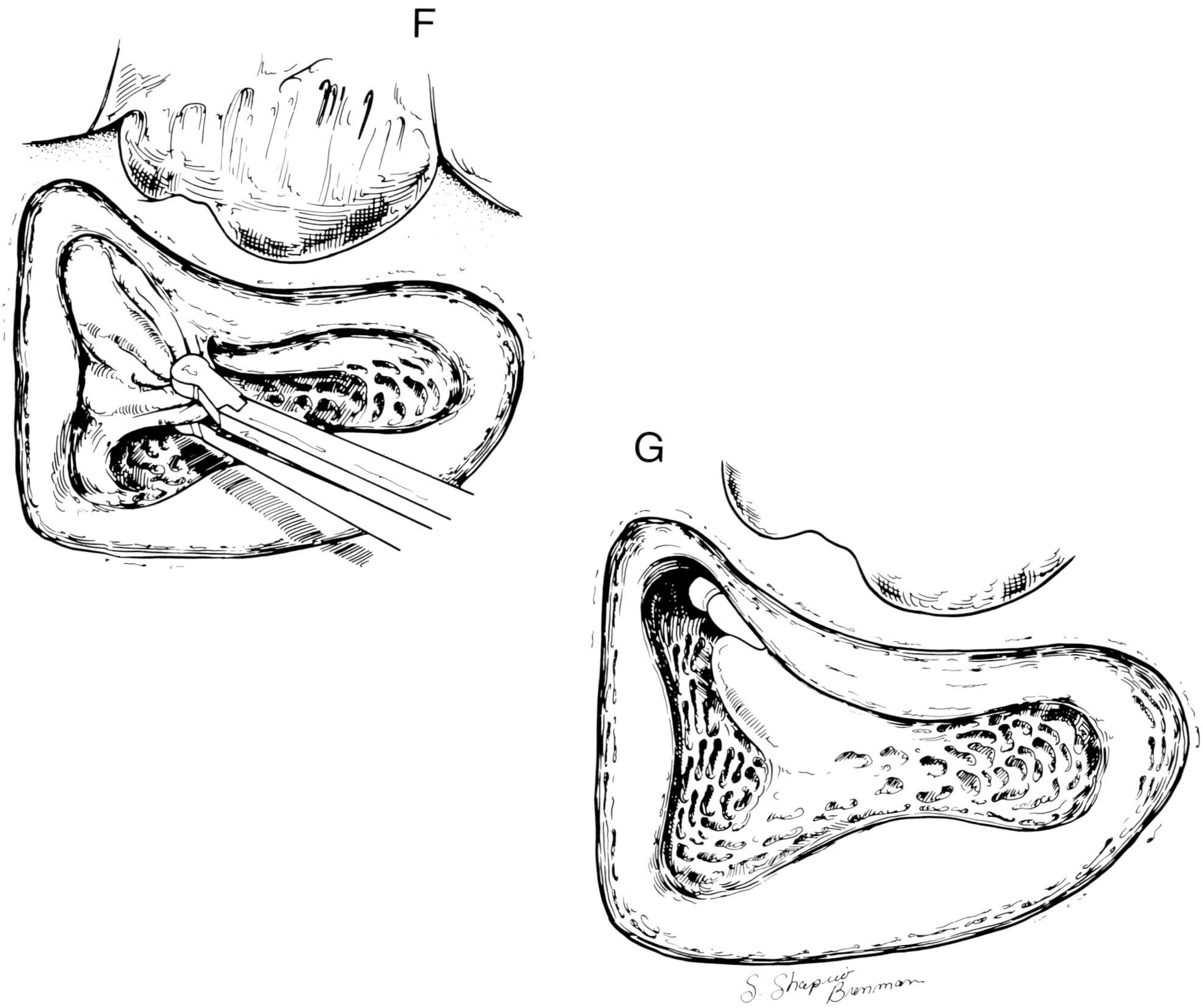


▶ **FIGURE 3-4**

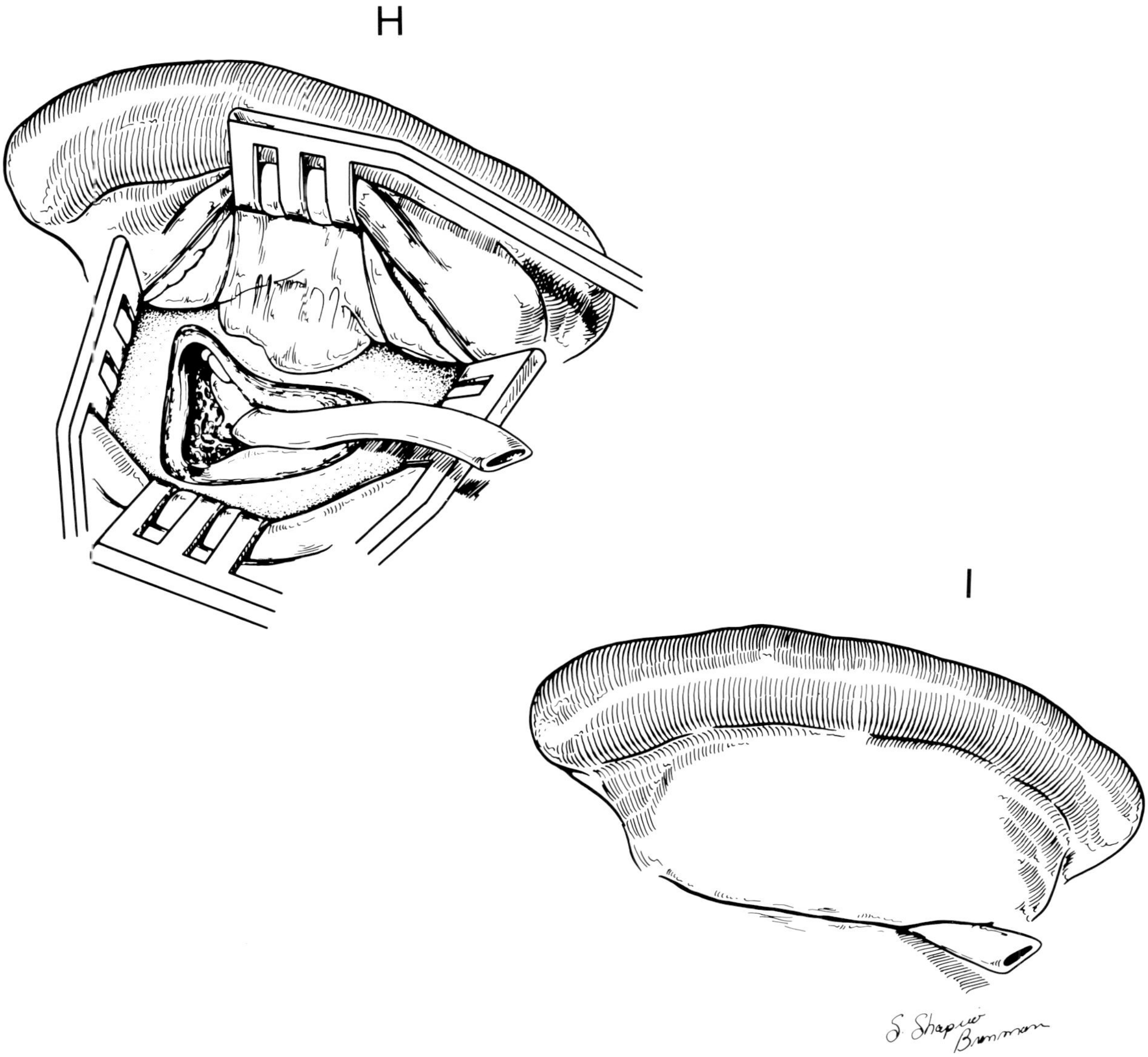


▶ **FIGURE 3-4**

## ▶ 3-5 MODIFIED RADICAL MASTOIDECTOMY

A modified radical mastoidectomy involves removal of the bony bridge between the external auditory canal and the mastoid cavity. The middle ear air space is preserved in this procedure. The goal of the operation is to exteriorize the cholesteatoma to the external auditory canal and to preserve the intact ossicular chain and an aerated middle ear space.

### Indications

Modified radical mastoidectomy is indicated when there is a pars flaccida cholesteatoma that is lateral to the ossicular chain or where removal of the canal wall is necessary to remove a middle ear cholesteatoma.

### Preoperative Evaluation

Preoperative evaluation requires a complete otoscopic examination. The cholesteatoma extending under the TM is usually evident by otoscopy. Often there is a posterior-superior perforation or deep retraction in the posterior-superior quadrant of the pars tensa. Audiologic evaluation should be performed prior to otologic surgery to detect any preexisting sensorineural and/or conductive hearing loss. Radiographs (especially CT scan) should be obtained to determine the extent of the cholesteatoma, level of the dura, and any other anatomic variant. It may not be possible to determine preoperatively if the cholesteatoma has remained lateral to the ossicles. The surgeon may elect to utilize intraoperative facial nerve monitoring.

### Operative Technique

1. The mastoid cortex and the tympanic membrane should be exposed to permit visualization of the cholesteatoma at the level of the TM and in the mastoid area simultaneously. The standard approach for tympanoplasty (section 3–2) and simple mastoidectomy (section 3–4) is used (Fig. 3–5**A**).
2. The mastoid cortex overlying the antrum is removed (Fig. 3–5**B**). The dissection is carried anteriorly to expose the cholesteatoma over the head of the ossicles.
3. The superior bridge of external canal bone may be removed at this time (Fig. 3–5**C**).
4. The cholesteatoma is opened by removing the lateral portion of the matrix. The contents are evacuated to assure that the cholesteatoma is situated lateral to the ossicles (Fig. 3–5**D**).
5. The bony ridge overlying the facial nerve is lowered with a diamond drill to provide adequate exposure of the cholesteatoma (Fig. 3–5**E**).
6. The medial portion of the cholesteatoma matrix (skin) need not be completely removed. It can be left in place where appropriate to line the cavity. This avoids the need for skin grafting (Fig. 3–5**F**).
7. A meatoplasty is performed to enlarge the external ear canal to provide adequate exposure to the mastoid cavity (see section 3–9). The postauricular incision is closed with interrupted absorbable suture in the soft tissue and perichondrium to hold the meatoplasty open.
8. The skin incision is closed with interrupted subcuticular absorbable suture. The mastoid cavity and external meatus are loosely packed with gauze im-

pregnated with antibiotic ointment, and a mastoid dressing is applied. The packing is left in place 10 to 14 days to help ensure a wide meatus.

9. The child is kept on oral antibiotics and antibiotic drops are placed on the packing three times a day as long as it remains in place.

### Complications

1. Recurrent or persistent cholesteatoma
2. Facial nerve injury
3. Trauma to semicircular canals
4. Dural laceration
5. Sigmoid sinus hemorrhage
6. Ossicular disarticulation

A

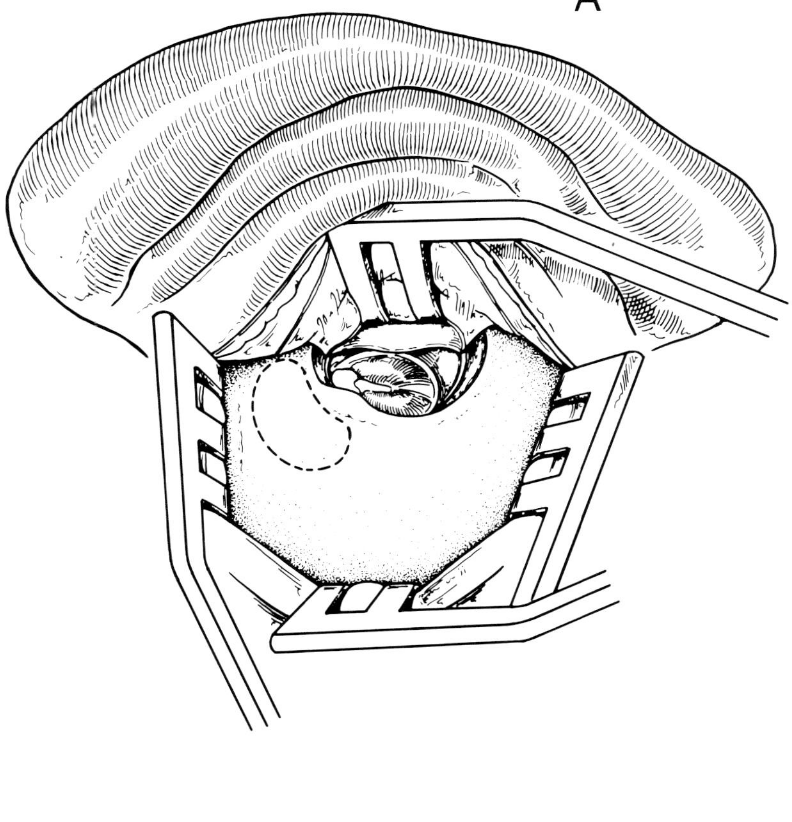

▶ **FIGURE 3-5**

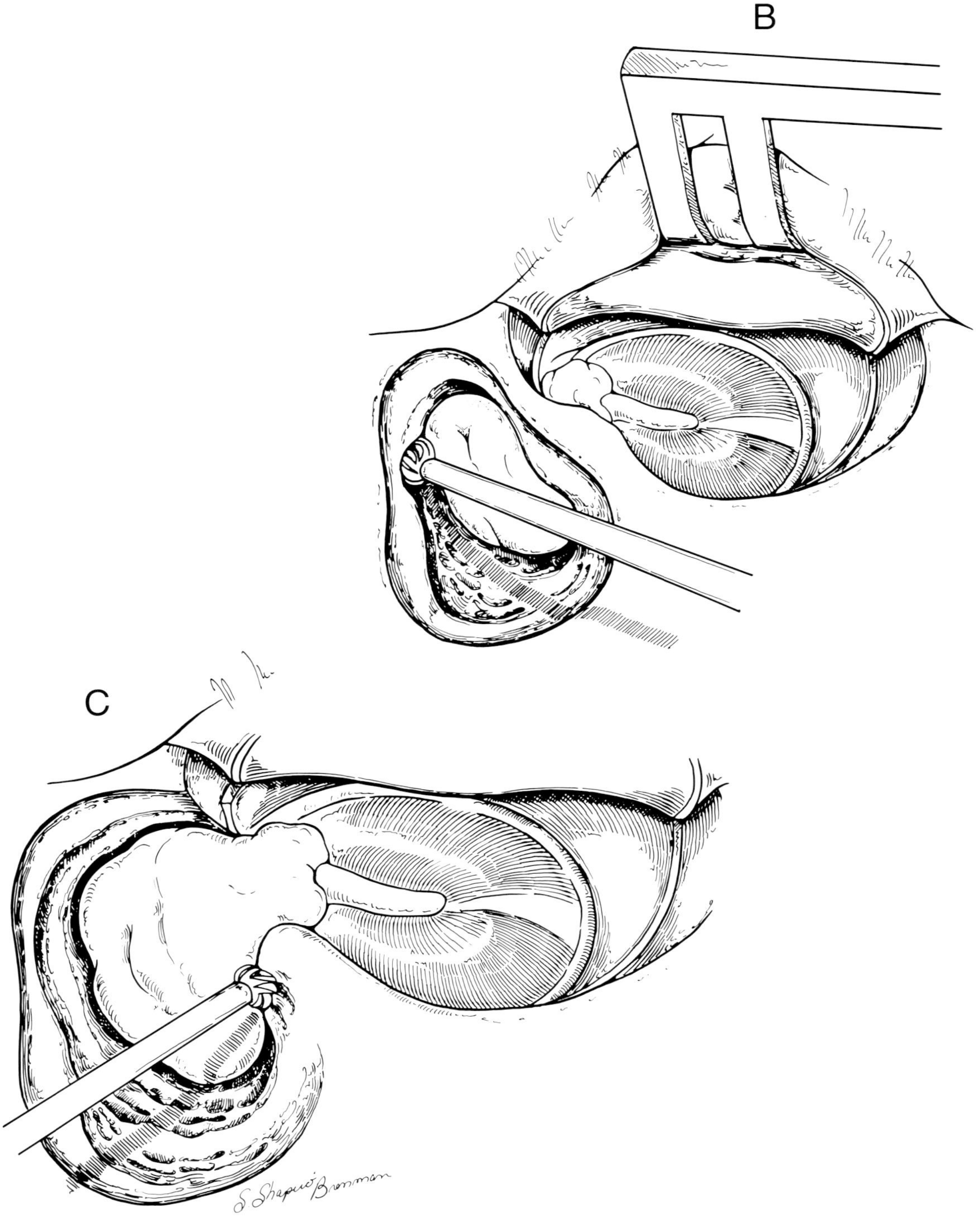


▶ **FIGURE 3-5**

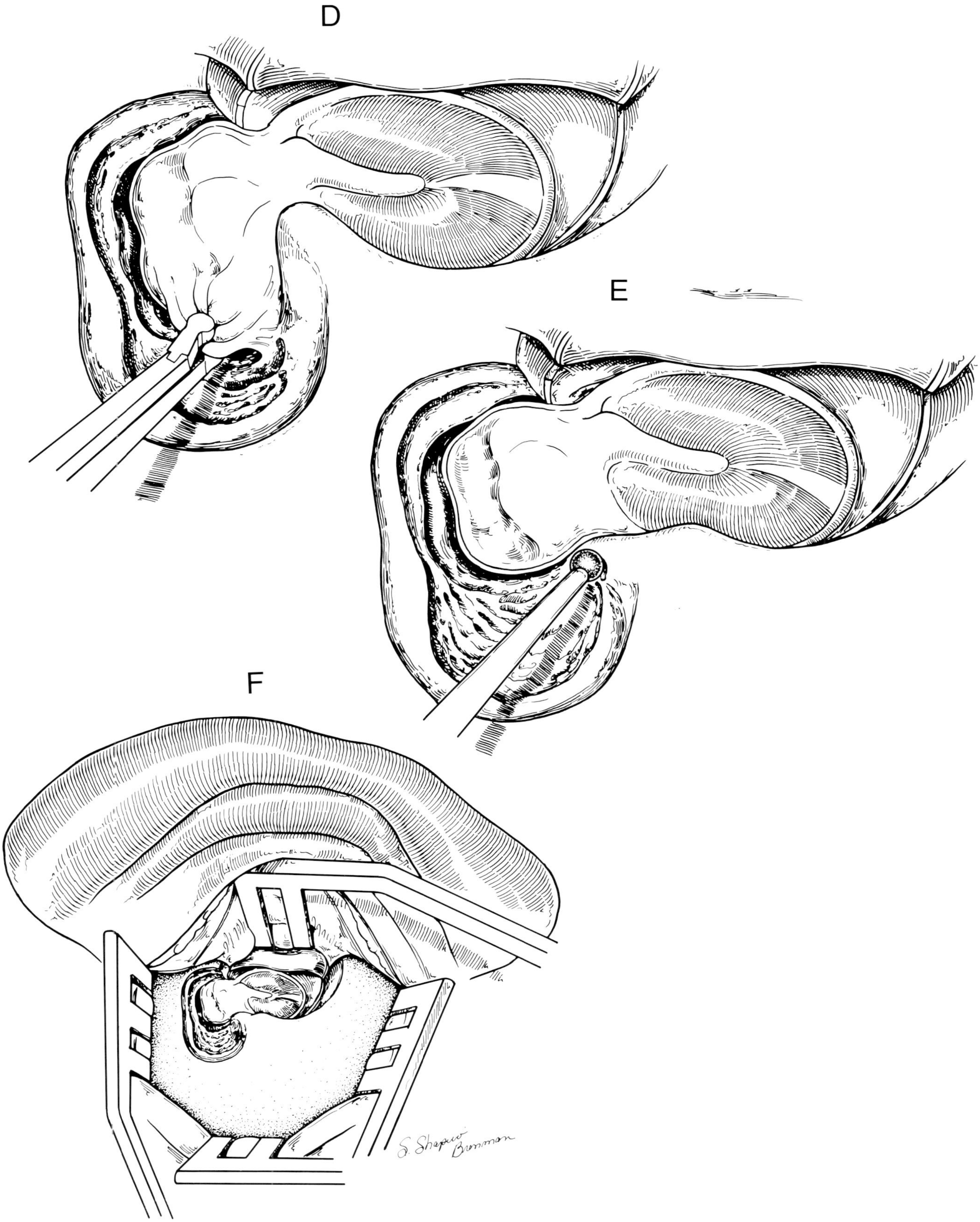


▸ **FIGURE 3-5**

## ▶ 3-6 RADICAL MASTOIDECTOMY

Radical mastoidectomy is a procedure that involves complete exteriorization of the mastoid and middle ear structures. The incus and malleus are removed.

### Indications

A radical mastoidectomy is indicated when cholesteatoma has extended medial to the middle ear ossicles, making complete removal of cholesteatoma impossible.

### Preoperative Evaluation

Preoperative evaluation requires a complete otoscopic examination. Otoscopy usually reveals a posterior-superior perforation or deep retraction in the posterior-superior quadrant of the pars tensa. Cholesteatoma often can be seen in the middle ear extending under the TM. Audiologic evaluation should be performed prior to otologic surgery to detect any preexisting sensorineural and/or conductive hearing loss. Radiographs (especially CT scan) should be obtained to determine the extent of the cholesteatoma, level of the dura, and any other anatomic variant. The surgeon may elect to utilize intraoperative facial nerve monitoring.

### Operative Technique

1. The standard postauricular exposure for tympanoplasty (section 3–2) and simple mastoidectomy exposure (section 3–4) is used (Fig. 3–6**A**).
2. The mastoid is opened, exposing the antrum and attic (Fig. 3–6**B**). The bone of the superior portion of the external meatus is removed with a drill. The cholesteatoma is removed by blunt and sharp dissection to visualize the ossicles and the horizontal semicircular canal (Fig. 3–6**C**).
3. The incus is removed with a forceps after disarticulating the incudostapedial joint and incudomalleolar joint with a knife (Fig. 3–6**D**). The malleus is then removed with a forceps after cutting the tensor tympani tendon with a scissors (Fig. 3–6**E**). The chorda tympani nerve is usually sacrificed.
4. The facial ridge is further lowered with a diamond drill to provide complete communication between the middle ear and mastoid cavity (Fig. 3–6**F**).
5. The surfaces of the mastoid cavity are smoothed with a diamond bur to avoid trapping of cholesteatoma. Flat areas of cholesteatoma matrix may be left in place. This promotes rapid relining of the cavity by squamous epithelium (Fig. 3–6**G**).
6. The remaining tympanic membrane is excised. In the classic radical mastoid operation, the fibrous annulus is removed and the eustachian tube occluded with tissue. However, if there is a possibility of later tympanomastoid reconstruction when the chronic disease is under control, the fibrous annulus and the eustachian tube should be left intact to facilitate the reconstruction.
7. A meatoplasty is performed as described in section 3–9.
8. The mastoid cavity and external meatus are loosely packed with gauze impregnated with antibiotic ointment and a mastoid dressing is applied. The packing is left in place 10 to 14 days to help ensure a wide meatus.
9. The child is kept on oral antibiotics, and antibiotic drops are placed on the packing as long as it remains in place.

### Complications

1. Recurrent or persistent cholesteatoma
2. Facial nerve injury
3. Trauma to semicircular canals
4. Dural laceration
5. Sigmoid sinus hemorrhage
6. Ossicular disarticulation

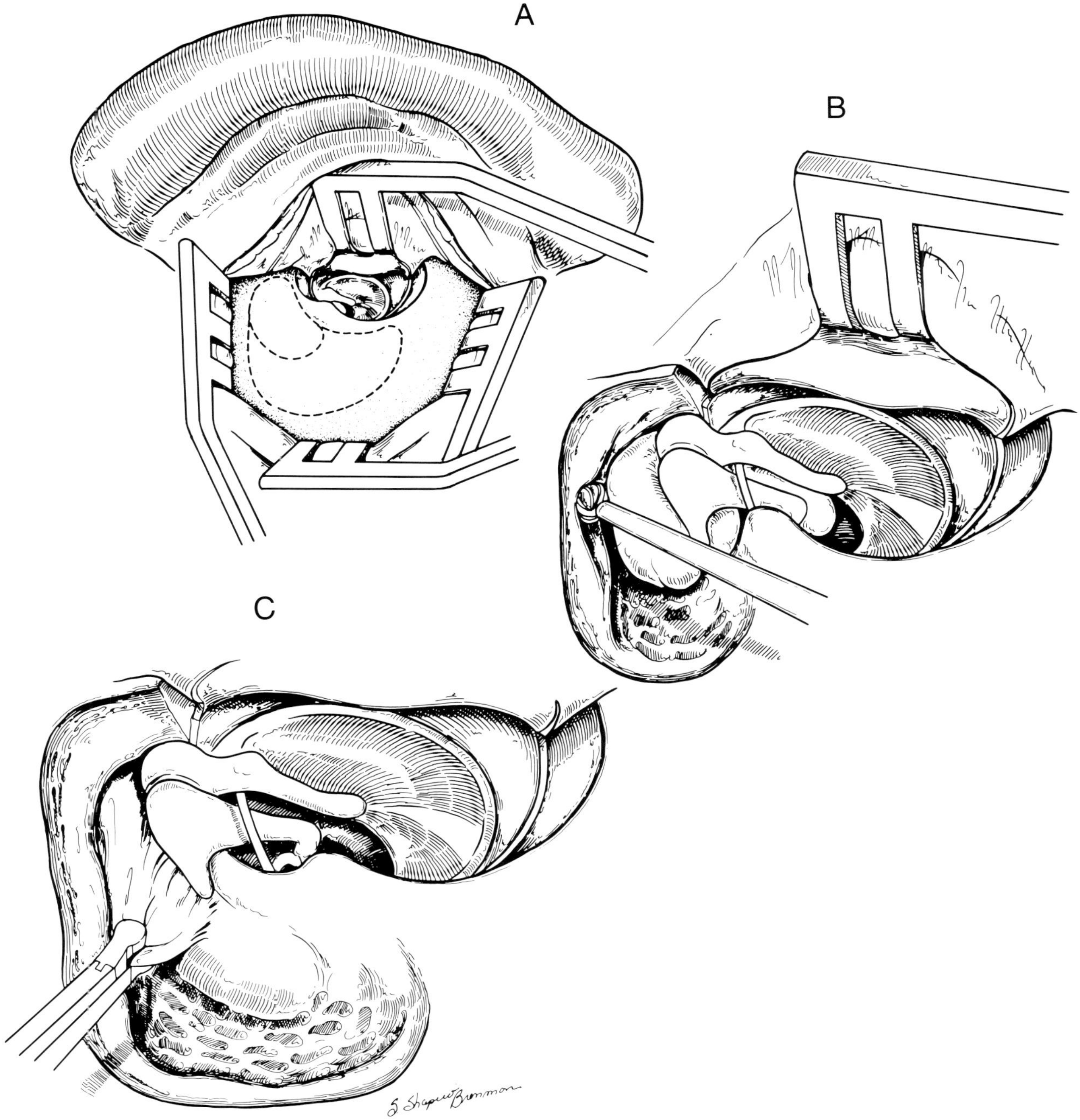


▶ **FIGURE 3-6**

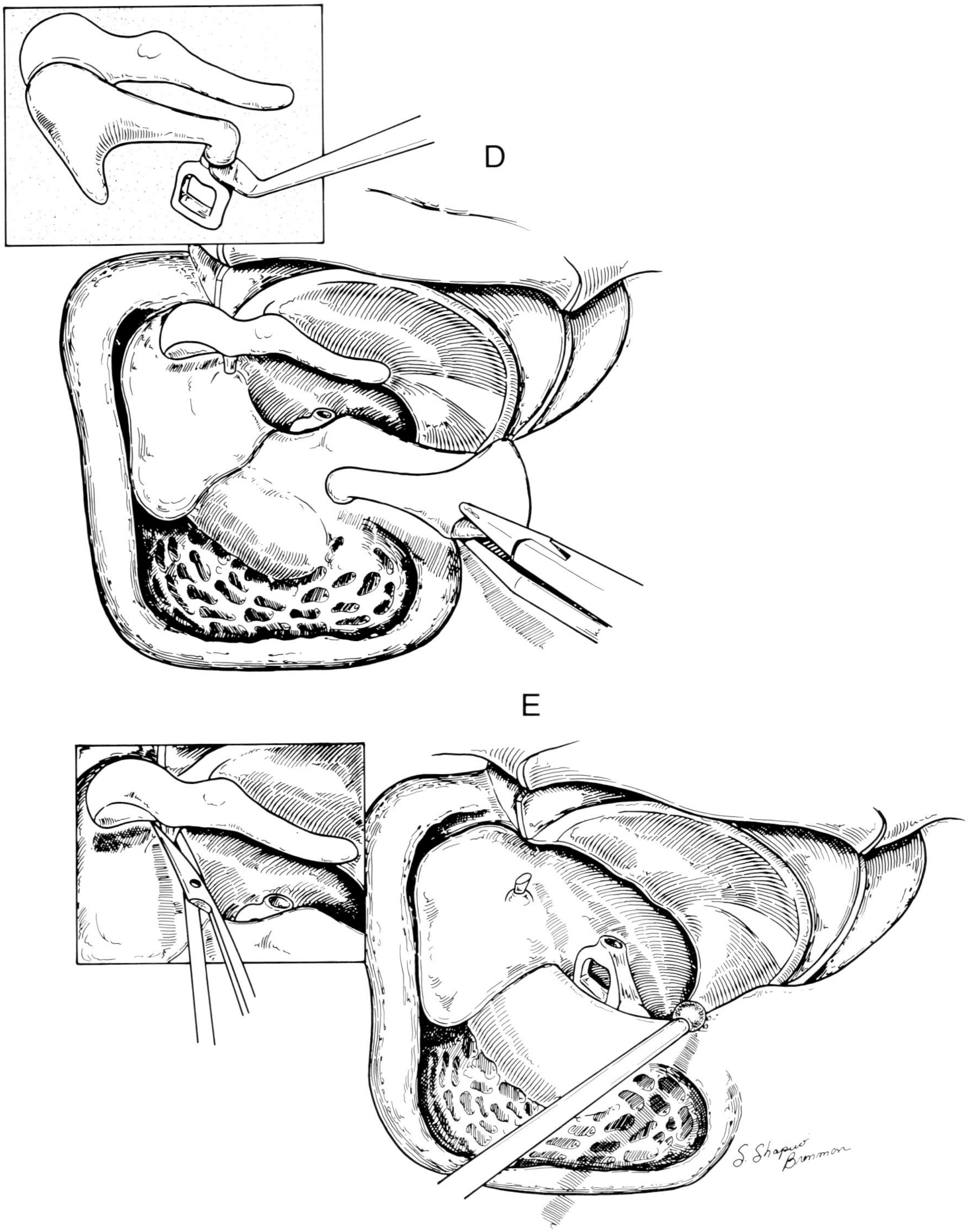


▶ **FIGURE 3-6**

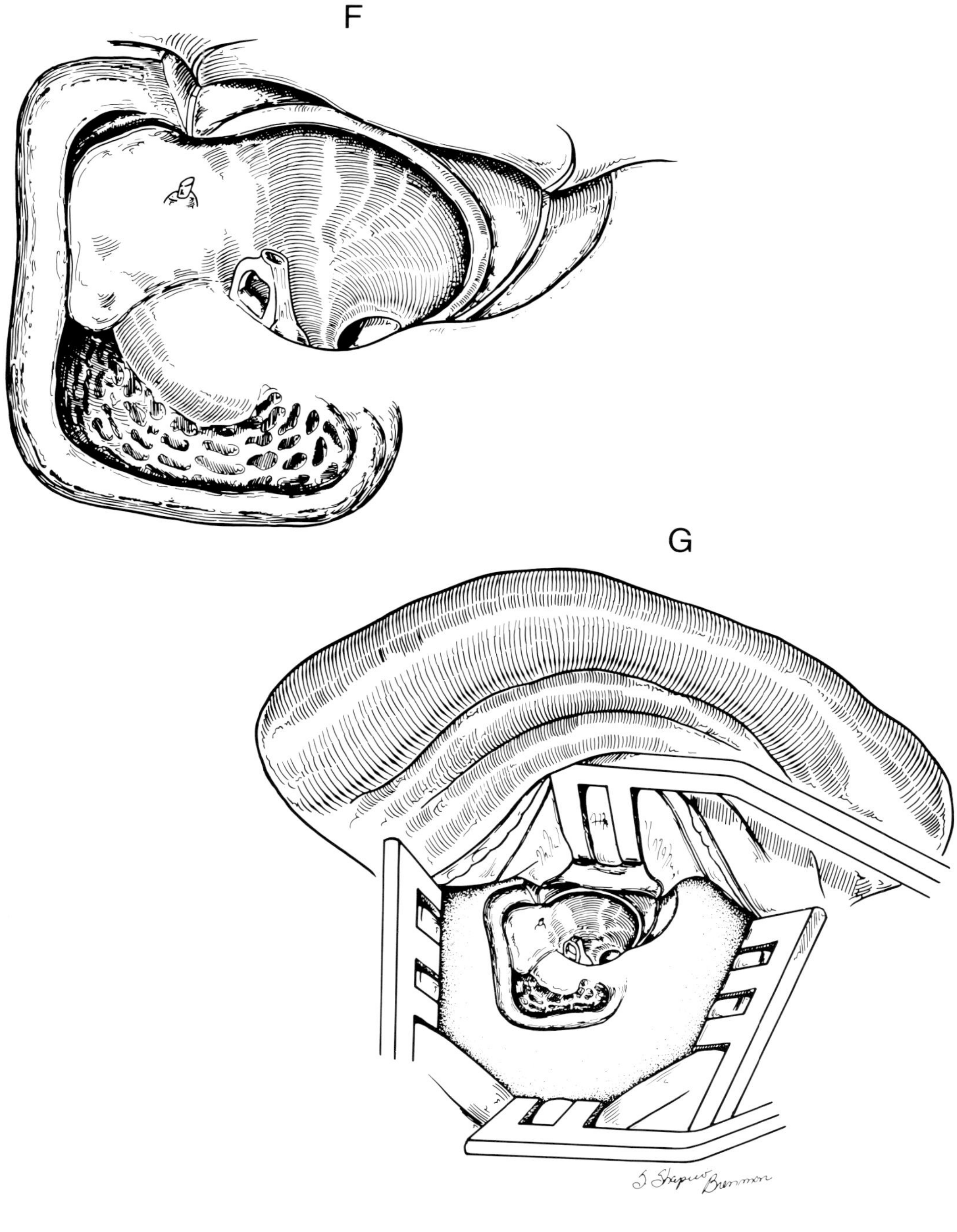


▶ **FIGURE 3-6**

## ▶ 3-7 INTACT CANAL WALL TYMPANOPLASTY AND MASTOIDECTOMY

Intact canal wall tympanoplasty and mastoidectomy is a procedure that can be used to remove cholesteatoma while preserving the middle ear space, ossicles, and the aeration between the middle ear and the mastoid.

### Indications

Intact canal tympanoplasty and mastoidectomy is indicated when cholesteatoma can be completely excised from the middle ear and facial recess without removal of the bony canal wall.

### Preoperative Evaluation

Preoperative evaluation requires a complete otoscopic examination. Otoscopy usually reveals a posterior superior perforation or deep retraction in the posterior superior quadrant of the pars tensa. Cholesteatoma may be seen in the middle ear extending under the TM. Audiologic evaluation should be performed prior to otologic surgery to detect any preexisting sensorineural and/or conductive hearing loss. Radiographs (especially CT scan) should be obtained to determine the extent of the cholesteatoma, level of the dura, and any other anatomic variant. The surgeon may elect to utilize intraoperative facial nerve monitoring.

### Operative Technique

1. The standard postauricular tympanoplasty and mastoidectomy approach is used (see sections 3–2 and 3–5).
2. A cortical mastoidectomy is performed exposing the horizontal semicircular canal and the heads of the ossicles in the attic as in performing a simple mastoidectomy (Fig. 3–7**A**).
3. The posterior canal is thinned with a cutting bur to approximately 1 mm thickness by drilling on the mastoid side of the canal (Fig. 3–7**B**).
4. The bone of the canal wall is removed from the angle between the facial nerve and the chorda tympani nerve using a diamond bur (Fig. 3–7**C**). The bridge of bone inferior to the short process of the incus may also be removed as needed.
5. The region of the stapes and round window niche can be visualized through the facial recess and from the ear canal, facilitating removal of middle ear disease (Fig. 3–7**D**).
6. The postauricular incision is closed with absorbable sutures in the same fashion as described for tympanoplasty (see section 3–2).
7. Reexploration of the tympanomastoid space may be needed 6 to 12 months later to detect residual or recurrent cholesteatoma.

### Complications

1. Recurrent or persistent cholesteatoma
2. Facial nerve injury
3. Trauma to semicircular canals
4. Dural laceration
5. Ossicular disarticulation

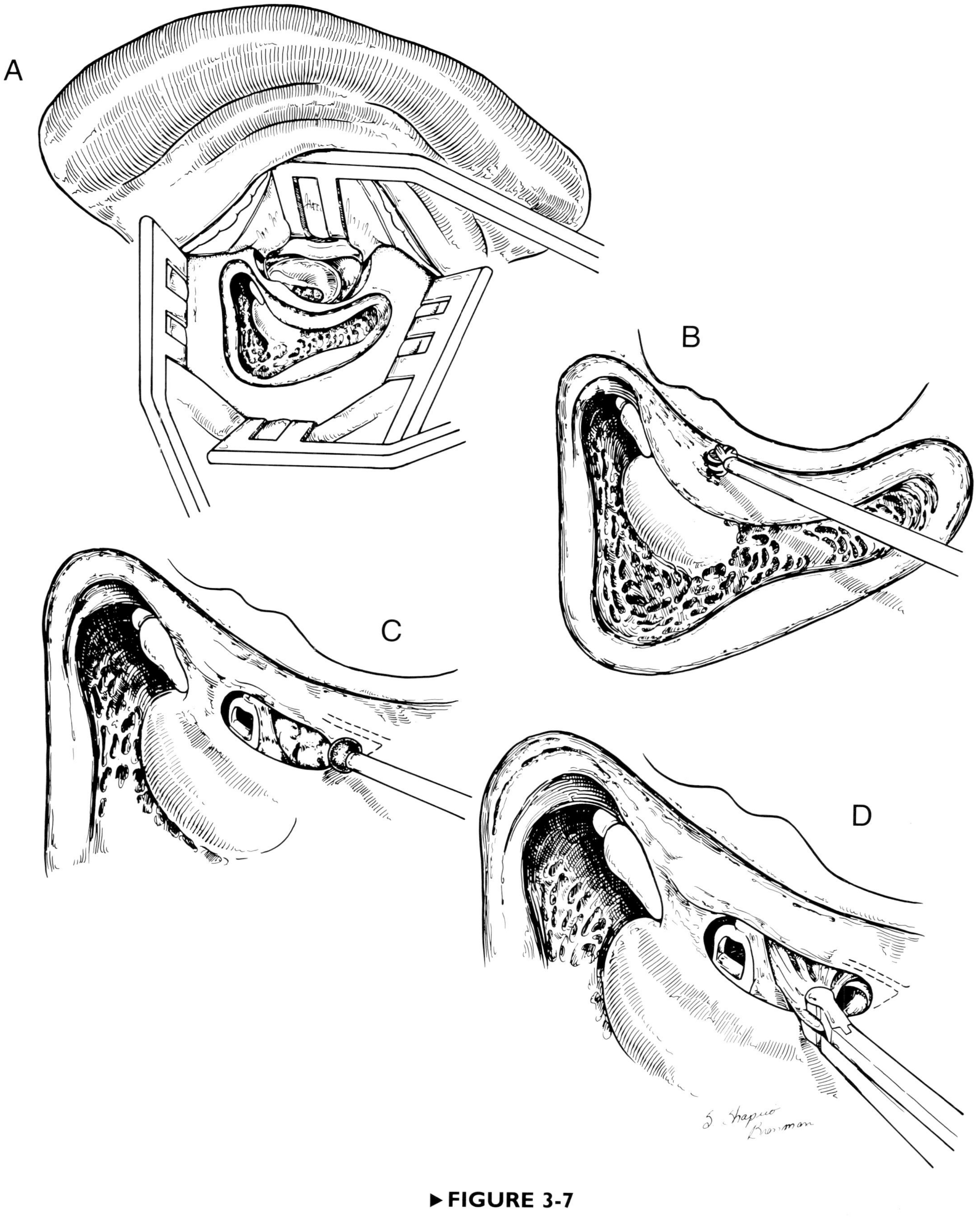


▶ **FIGURE 3-7**

## ▶ 3-8 MASTOIDPLASTY

Mastoidplasty (mastoid reconstruction) is a procedure to reconstruct the bony posterior canal wall in a patient who has had a radical or modified radical mastoidectomy. This re-creates the original separation between the mastoid cavity and the external ear canal.

### Indications

Mastoidplasty is indicated when the cholesteatoma can be removed from the middle ear and mastoid only after removal of the posterior canal wall (see section 3–5 or section 3–6).

Mastoidplasty is also indicated in patients who have chronically infected and draining radical mastoid cavities. If the eustachian tube is functioning, tympanoplasty is also possible. Mastoidplasty can only be done if complete removal of cholesteatoma is assured.

### Preoperative Evaluation

Preoperative evaluation requires a complete otoscopic examination. Audiometric evaluation should be performed prior to otologic surgery to detect any preexisting sensorineural and/or conductive hearing loss. Radiographs (especially CT scan) should be obtained to determine the extent of the cholesteatoma, level of the dura, and any other anatomic variant. The surgeon may elect to utilize intraoperative facial nerve monitoring.

### Operative Technique

1. Middle ear and mastoid exposure is obtained by using the standard postauricular approach (see section 3–2 or section 3–4).
2. A cortical mastoidectomy is performed exposing the cholesteatoma. The posterior canal wall is removed to whatever extent is required to remove disease (Fig. 3–8**A**).
3. A 2-mm thick sheet of Proplast or conchal cartilage is positioned to reconstruct the defect in the bony canal (Fig. 3–8**B**).
4. A sheet of thick fascia (anterior temporalis) is placed over the implant or cartilage (Fig. 3–8**C**).
5. A larger piece of thin fascia (posterior temporalis) is then placed medial to the tympanic membrane remnant anteriorly and draped over the implant or cartilage laterally to create a new middle ear space as in a standard tympanoplasty (Fig. 3–8**D**). The fascia is then draped laterally over the mastoid (Fig. 3–8**E**, **F**).
6. The TM fascia graft is held in place with Gelfoam in the middle ear and in the external meatus. The Gelfoam is soaked in antibiotic-containing otic drops as described for tympanoplasty.
7. The postauricular incision is closed in the standard fashion (see section 3–2). The external meatus is packed with antibiotic-impregnated gauze for 10 to 14 days. The child is kept on oral antibiotics, and antibiotic drops are placed on the packing three times a day as long as it remains in place.
8. Reexploration of the mastoid and middle ear is required in 6 to 12 months to be certain that no residual or recurrent cholesteatoma is present. Small pearls of cholesteatoma can be removed at this time and ossicular reconstruction performed as permitted.

### Complications

1. Recurrent or persistent cholesteatoma
2. Facial nerve injury
3. Trauma to semicircular canals
4. Dural laceration
5. Sigmoid sinus hemorrhage
6. Ossicular disarticulation

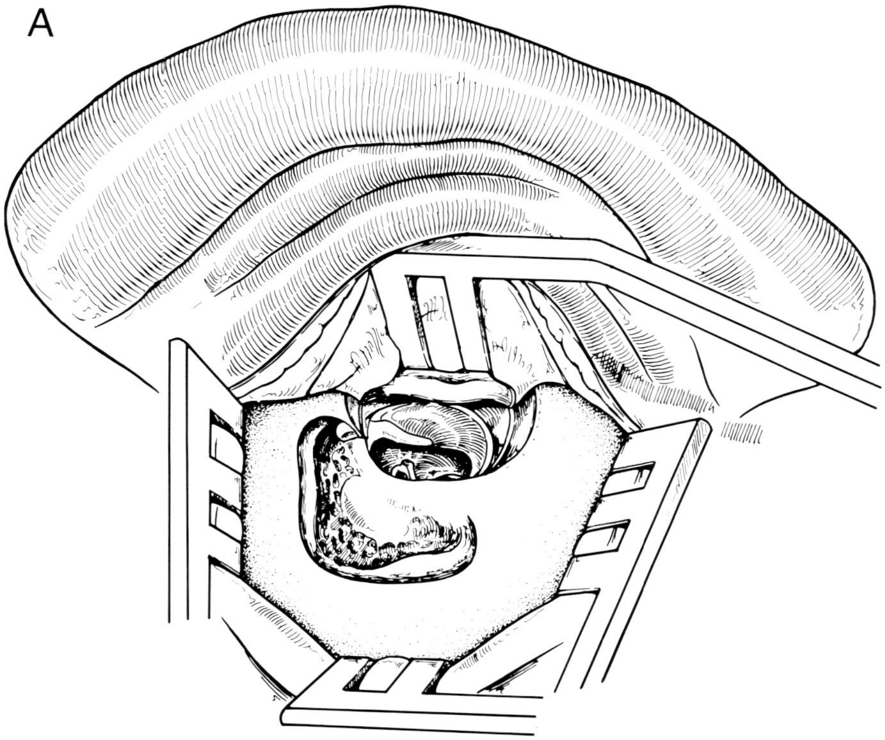


▶ **FIGURE 3-8**

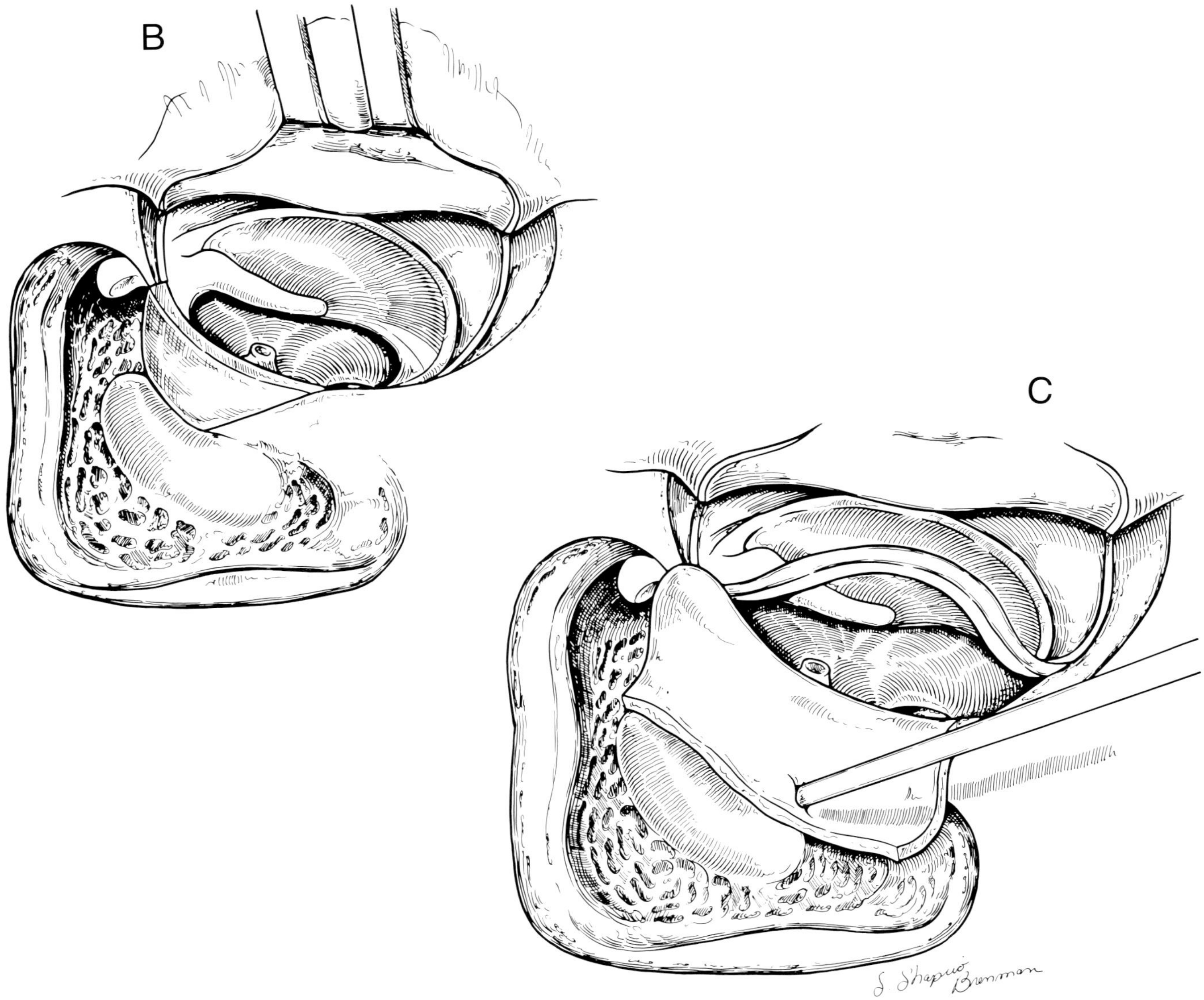


▶**FIGURE 3-8**

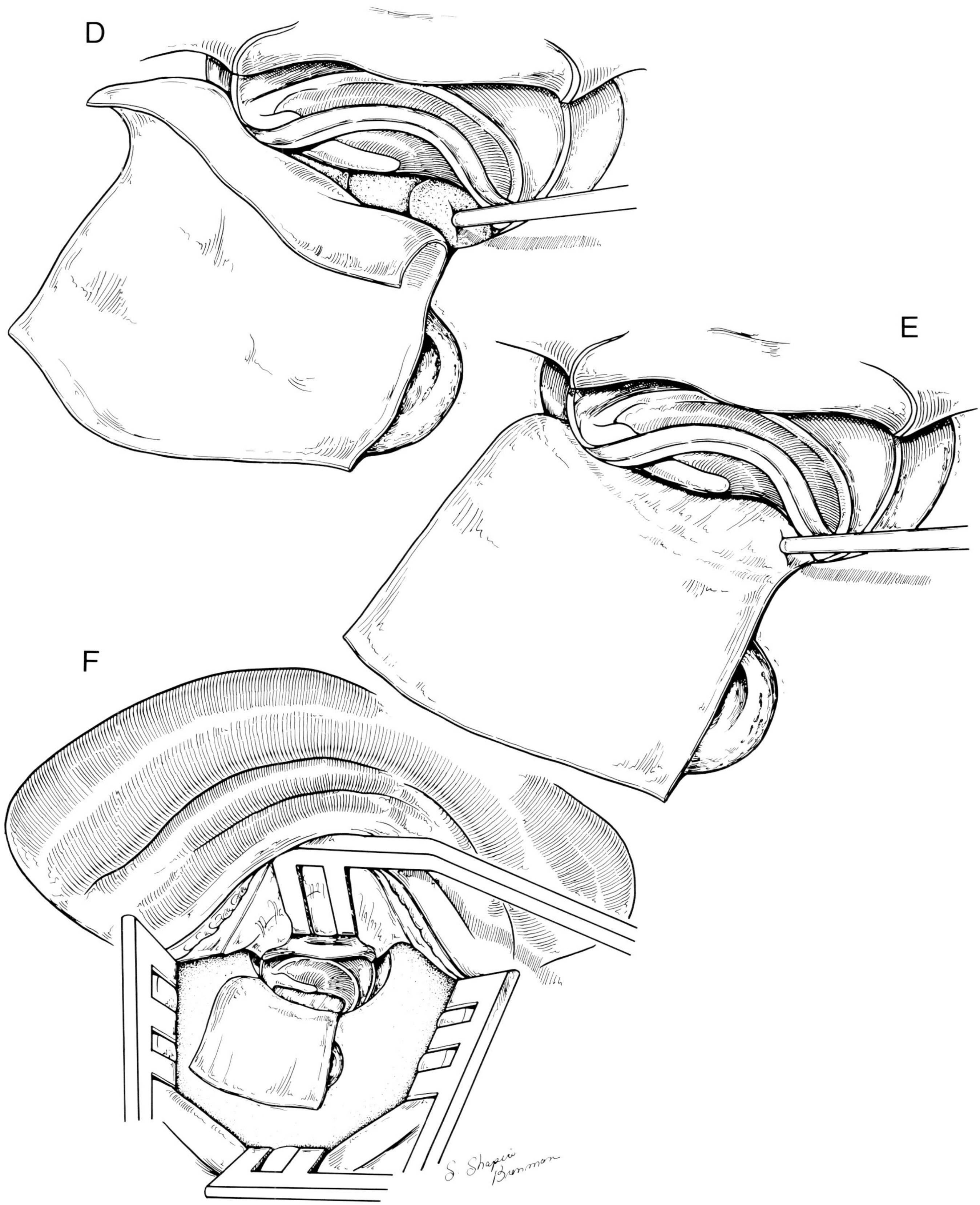


▶ **FIGURE 3-8**

## ▶ 3-9 MEATOPLASTY

A meatoplasty is performed to widen the ear canal. This permits egress of wax and desquamated skin as well as providing access for mastoid cleansing.

### Indications

Meatoplasty is indicated when there is an open mastoid cavity and access to the entire mastoid bowl is desired (e.g., after section 3–5, Modified Mastoidectomy or after section 3–6, Radical Mastoidectomy).

### Preoperative Evaluation

This procedure is usually performed in conjunction with a modified or radical mastoidectomy. No additional preoperative evaluation is required for meatoplasty.

### Operative Technique

1. After the tympanomastoid portion of the operation is completed through a postauricular incision (Fig. 3–9**A**), an incision is made through the superior portion of the ear canal from the external meatal incision and extended superiorly between the helix and tragus (Fig. 3–9**B**).
2. The incision is extended to the periosteum. A self-retaining retractor is temporarily placed to assess the size of the meatus (Fig. 3–9**C**).
3. The soft tissue (postauricular fibrous tissue and periosteum) is removed from the back of the external meatus with a knife (Fig. 3–9**D**).
4. A crescent-shaped incision is made through the conchal cartilage adjacent to the external meatus (Fig. 3–9**E**). Care is taken to cut through cartilage, but to avoid perforating the skin anteriorly.
5. The crescent of cartilage is removed by dissection with a scissors (Fig. 3–9**F**).
6. The patency of the meatoplasty is gauged by grasping the perichondrium of the remaining concha and pulling it back to the position it will have after closure of the postauricular incision.
7. If the meatus is not large enough to permit access to the entire mastoid cavity, additional soft tissue and cartilage are removed around the meatus until adequate exposure of the mastoid is accomplished.
8. The perichondrium of the remaining concha is sutured posteriorly to the periosteum of the mastoid with 3-0 chromic suture (Fig. 3–9**G**) to maintain the opening of the meatus (Fig. 3–9**H**).
9. The postauricular incision is closed with 3-0 interrupted subcuticular absorbable suture as in tympanoplasty (see section 3–2 Tympanoplasty).
10. The mastoid cavity is packed loosely, but completely, and the meatus is packed firmly with gauze impregnated with antibiotic ointment. The skin incision of the meatoplasty may be partially closed with interrupted subcuticular absorbable suture (Fig. 3–9**I**).
11. A mastoid dressing is applied.
12. The child is kept on oral antibiotics and antibiotic drops are placed on the packing three times a day as long as it remains in place, usually 3 weeks.

### Complications

1. Meatal stenosis

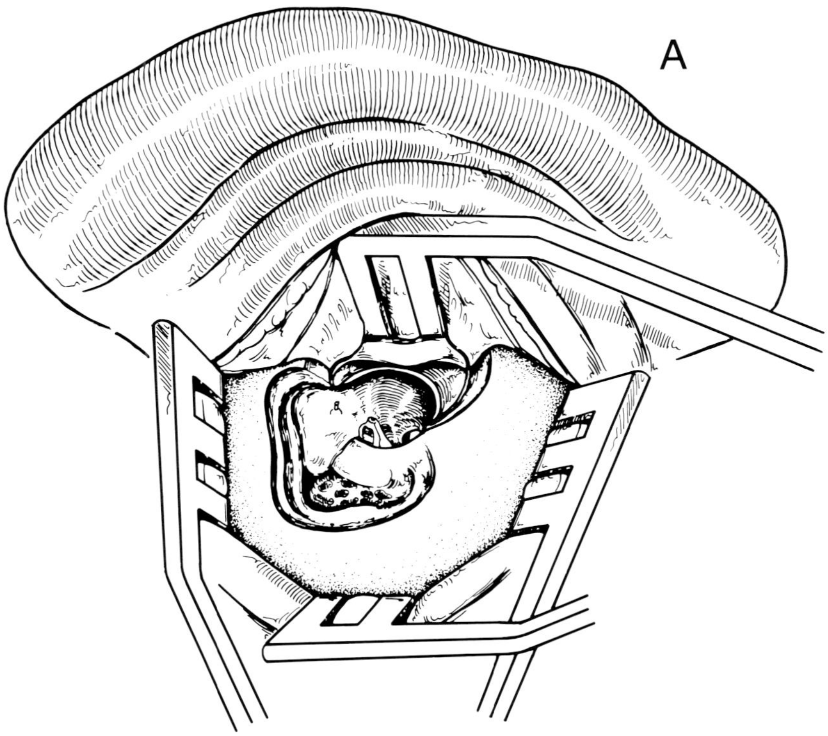


▶ **FIGURE 3-9**

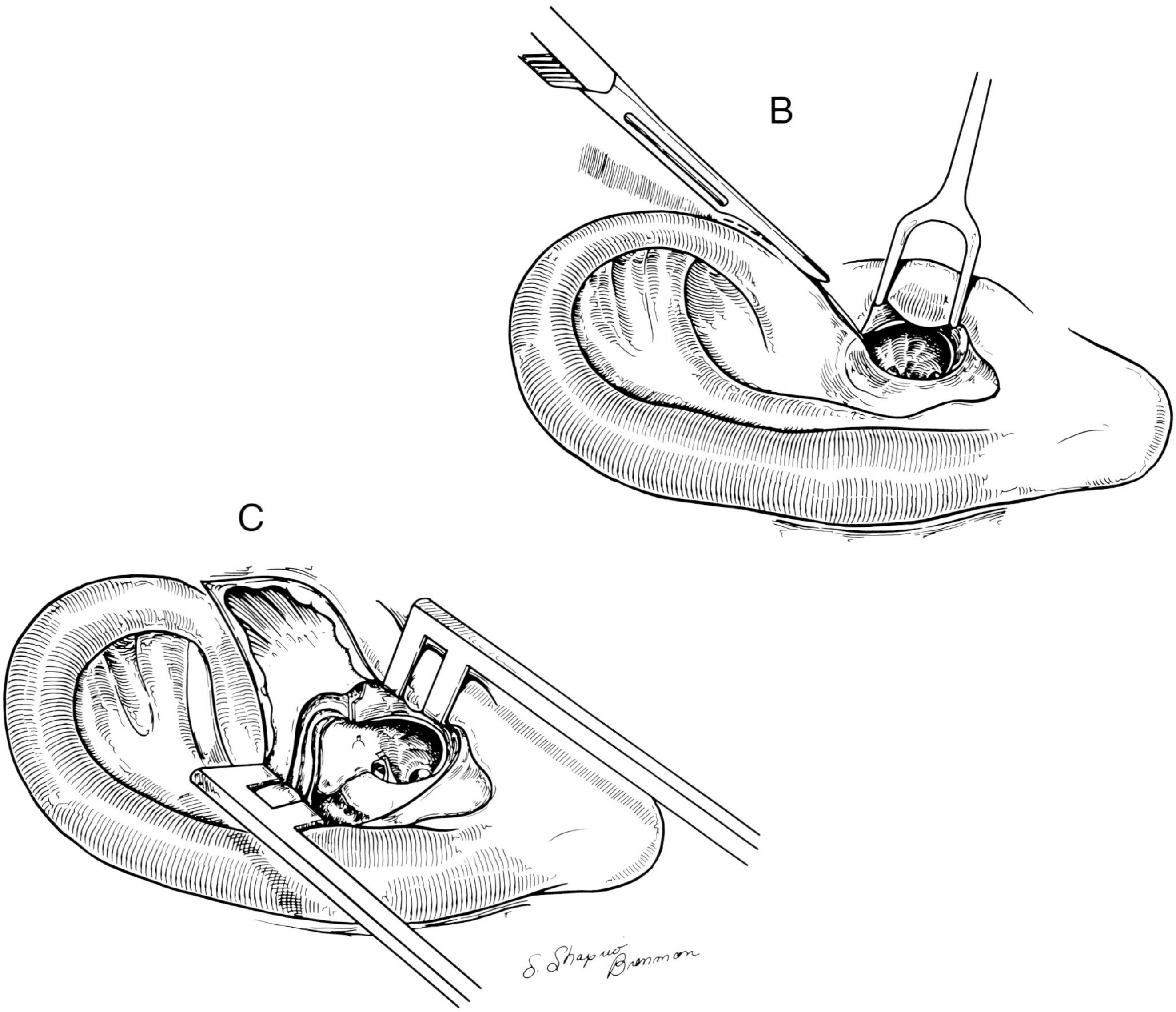


▶ **FIGURE 3-9**

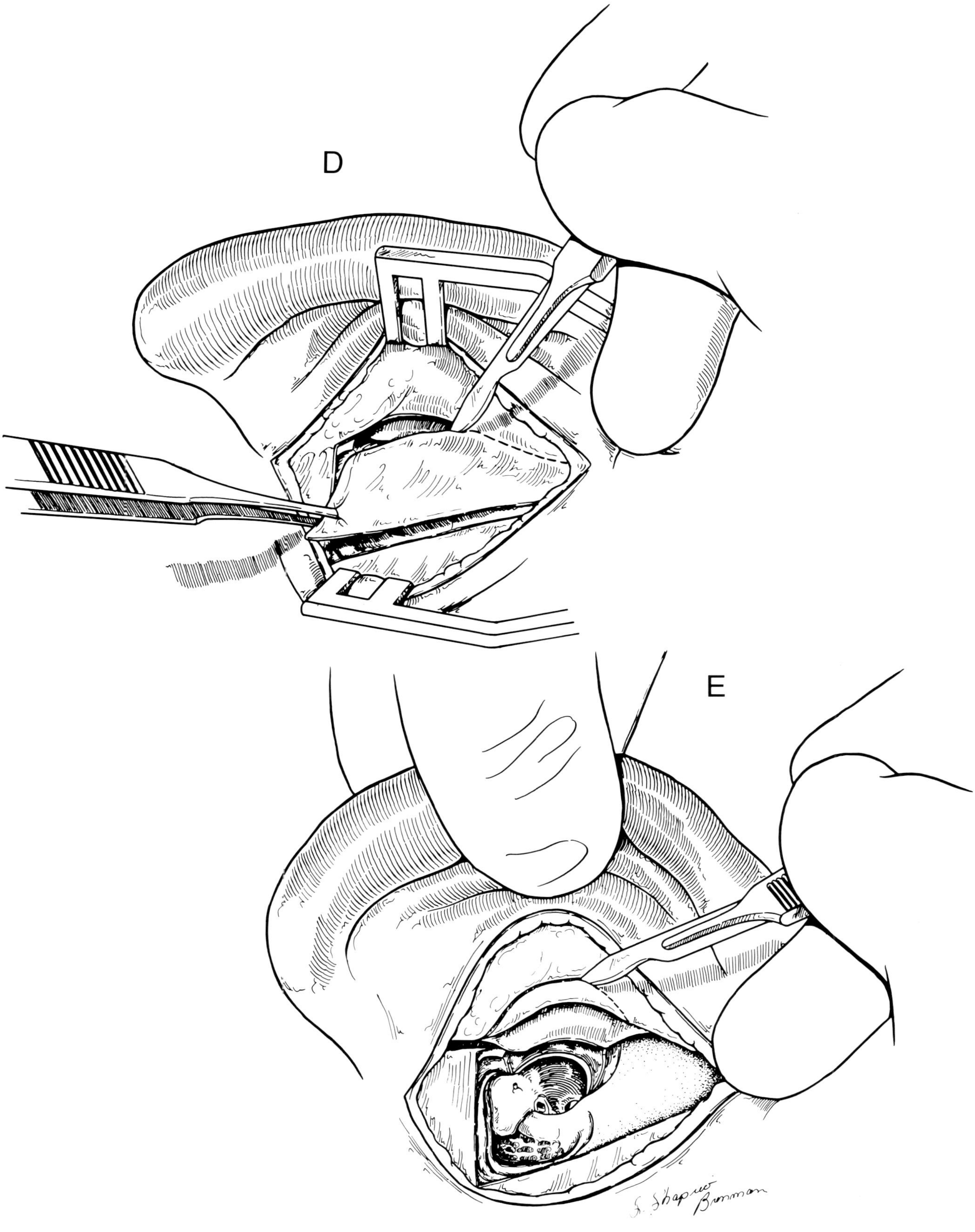


▶ **FIGURE 3-9**

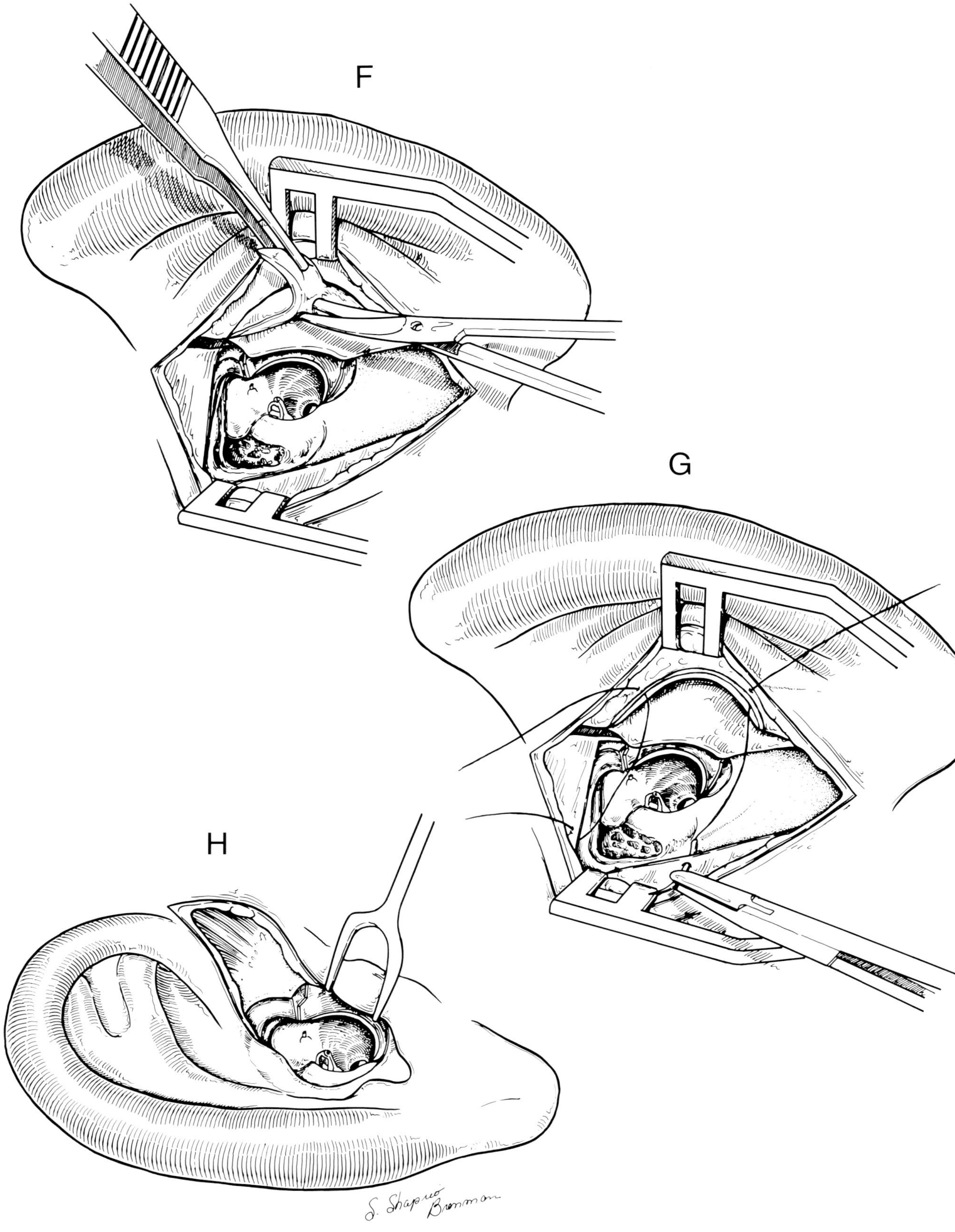


▶ **FIGURE 3-9**

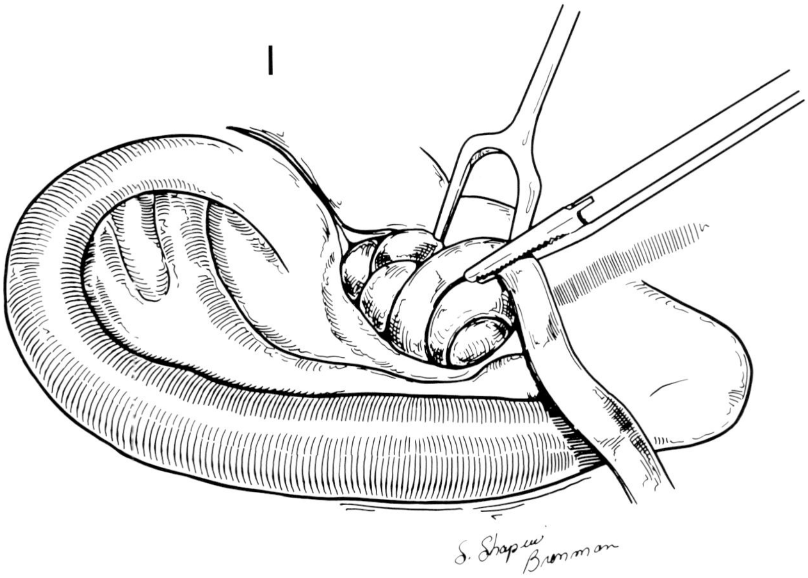


▶ **FIGURE 3-9**

# 4 ▸ Congenital Malformations of the Ear

Congenital malformations of the auricle, external ear canal, tympanic membrane, middle ear cleft, and ossicles may occur as isolated entities or in association with other deformities.

## ▸ 4-1 Preauricular Tags

Preauricular tags are congenital malformations associated with incomplete migration and/or coalescence of the auricular hillocks. These are usually anterior to the tragus, and they may be single or multiple (Fig. 4–1**A**). They vary in shape but most often consist of skin and subcutaneous tissue. Occasionally, there is cartilage in the base of the tag.

### Indications

Removal of the preauricular tags is performed for cosmetic purposes.

### Preoperative Evaluation

No special preoperative evaluation is required, except to recognize that any congenital outer ear anomaly may be associated with the presence of another ear (e.g., ossicular) malformation.

### Operative Technique

1. A general anesthetic is usually required. Local infiltration of the base of the preauricular tag with 1% lidocaine containing 1:100,000 epinephrine will decrease bleeding.
2. An elliptical skin incision is made in the lines of the facial creases in front of the ear (Fig. 4–1B).
3. The tag can be grasped with a toothed forceps and placed on gentle traction while dissecting the underlying cartilage and subcutaneous tissue with sharp scissors (Fig. 4–1C).
4. The subcutaneous stalk and cartilage are cut free with sharp scissors (Fig. 4–1D).
5. Hemostasis should be obtained with needlepoint cautery.
6. The wound is closed in two layers. The skin is closed with interrupted subcuticular absorbable suture, thus avoiding the need to remove skin sutures (Fig. 4–1E, F).

### Complications

None

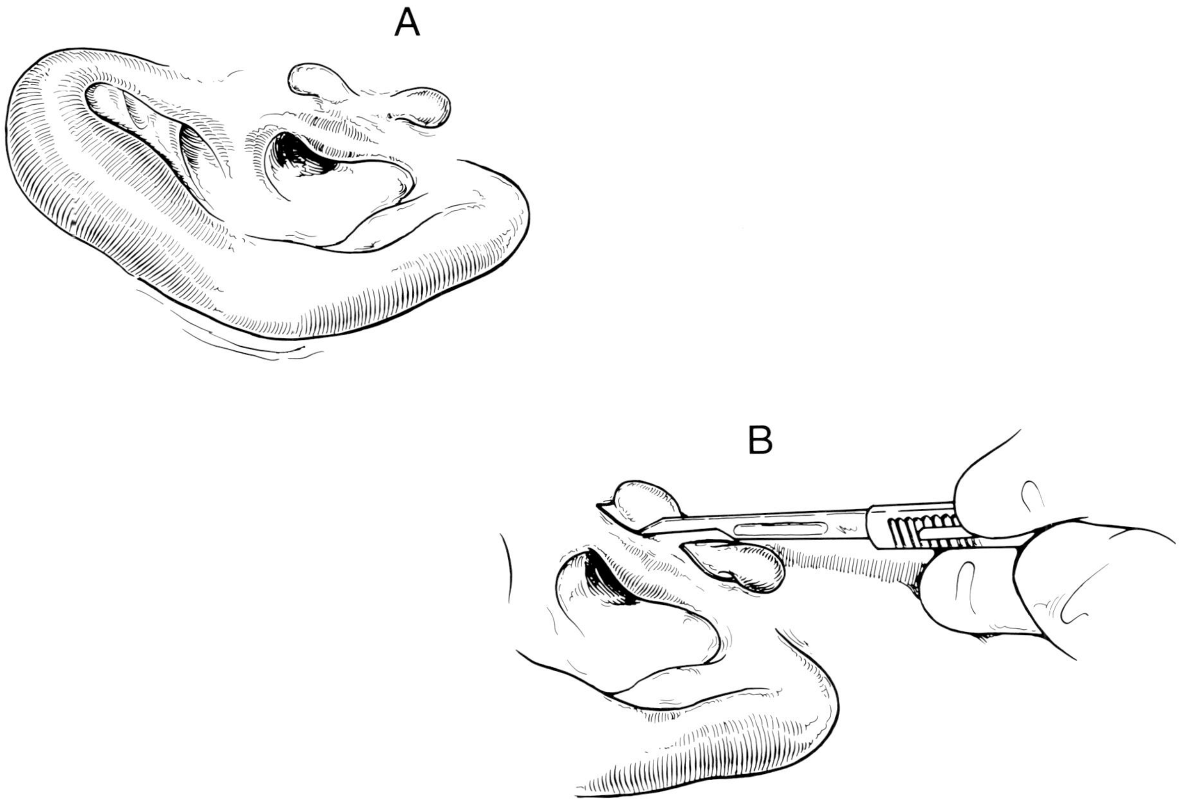


▶ **FIGURE 4-1**

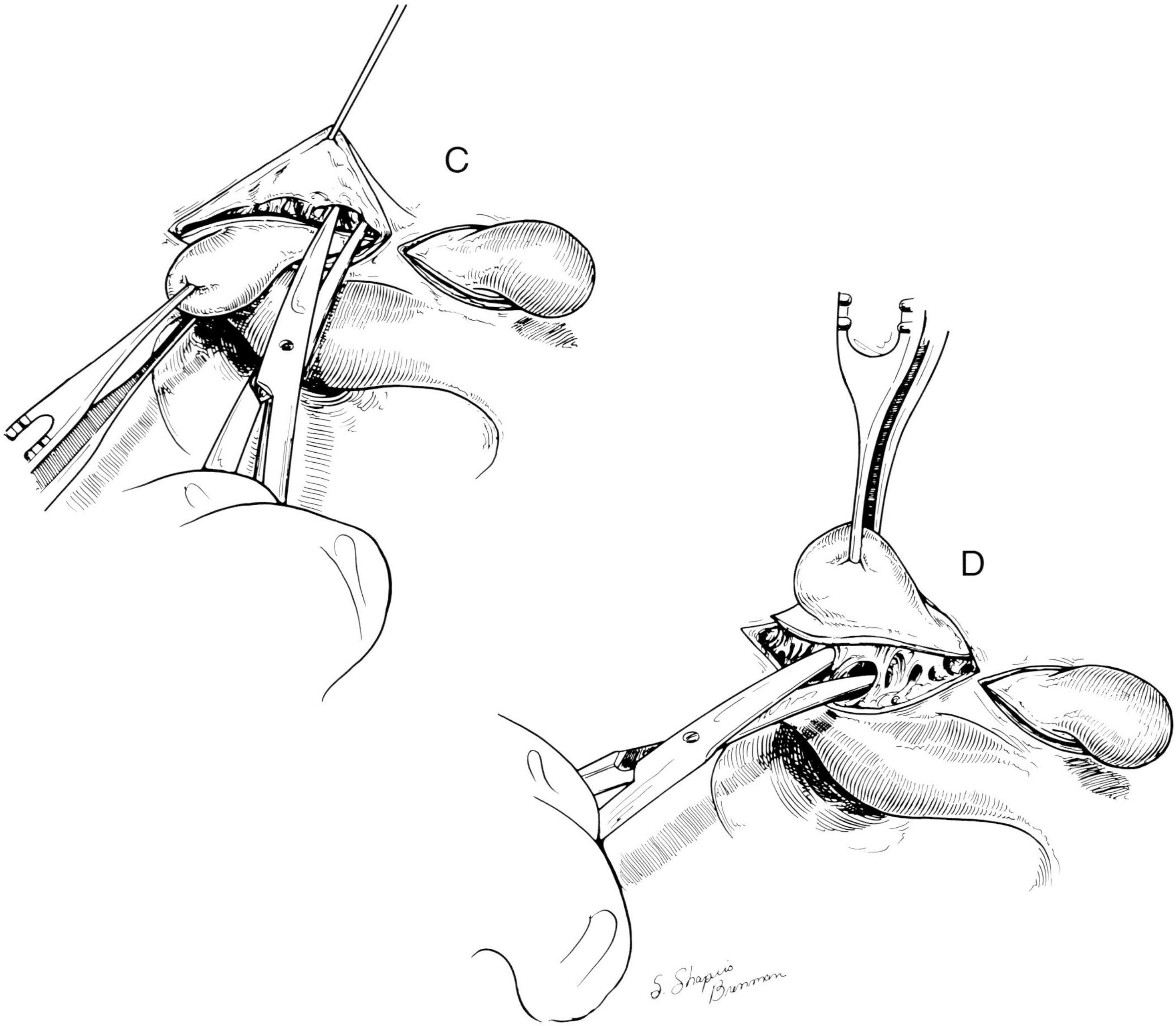


▶ **FIGURE 4-1**

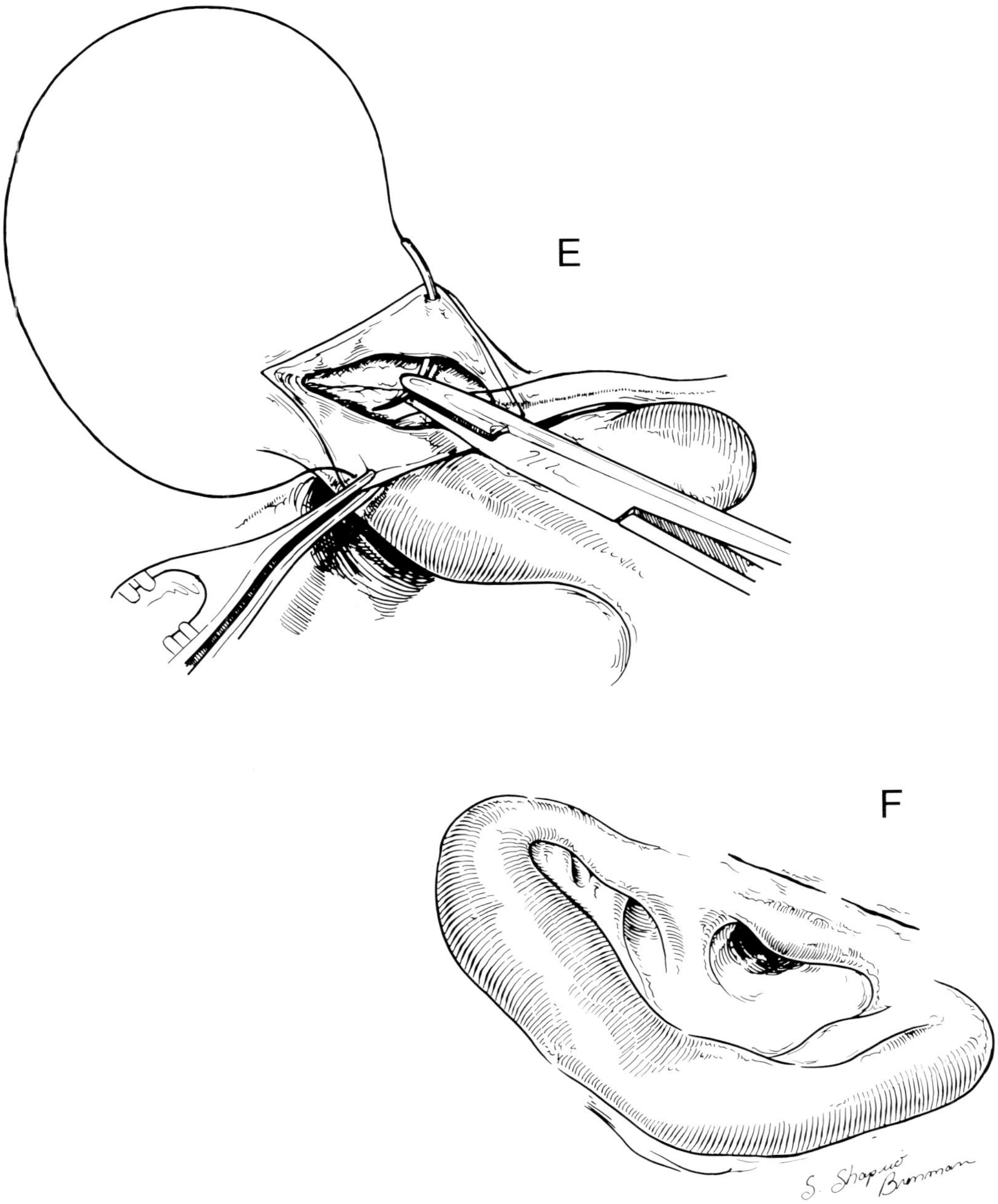


▶ **FIGURE 4-1**

## ▶ 4-2 PREAURICULAR SINUSES

Preauricular sinuses occur as a result of the trapping of epithelium between the developing ear hillocks. They usually present as a pit in the area just superior and anterior to the tragus. The lesions often arborize in the subcutaneous tissues and may attach to the helical cartilage.

### Indications

Asymptomatic sinus tracts require no treatment. Excision is necessary if these skin-lined tracts become infected or form an obvious cyst.

### Preoperative Evaluation

No special preoperative evaluation is required except to recognize that any congenital outer ear anomaly may be associated with the presence of another ear (e.g., ossicular) malformation.

### Operative Technique

1. Preauricular sinuses are removed under a general anesthetic with local infiltration of 1% lidocaine with 1:100,000 epinephrine for hemostasis.
2. An elliptical incision is made in the skin line in the preauricular area (Fig. 4–2A).
3. Skin flaps are elevated anteriorly and posteriorly (Fig. 4–2B).
4. Using blunt and sharp dissection, the subcutaneous tracts are followed (Fig. 4–2C). A lacrimal probe may be helpful to determine the direction and degree of arborization and the depth of the tract(s).
5. If the tract attaches to cartilage and cannot be easily separated from the perichondrium, an ellipse of helical cartilage should also be excised (Fig. 4–2D).
6. The wound is closed in two layers after hemostasis is obtained. The skin is closed with interrupted buried absorbable suture, avoiding the need to remove sutures (Fig. 4–2E). Steri-strips are often helpful to keep the skin edges approximated.

### Complications

1. Recurrence secondary to incomplete excision

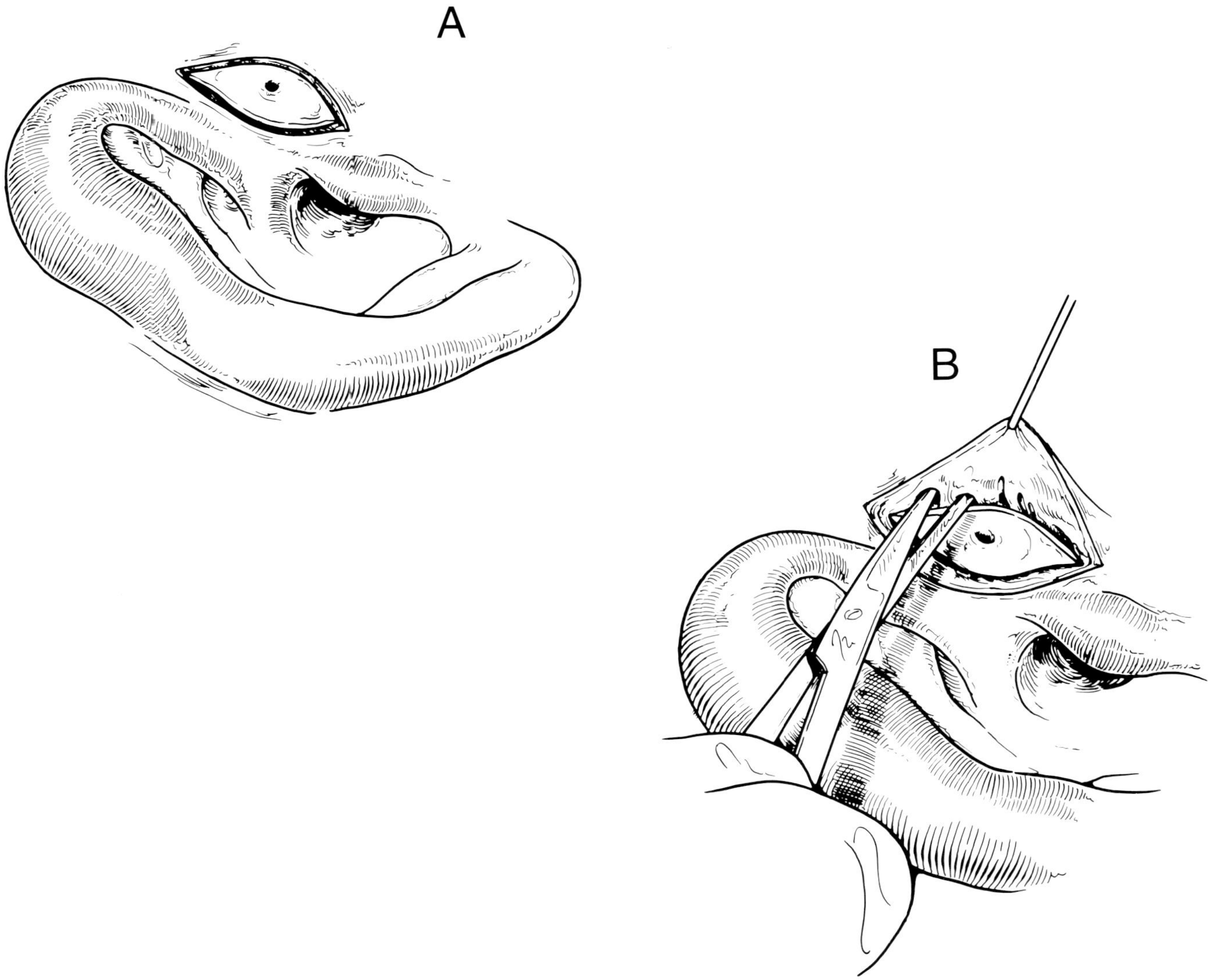


▶ **FIGURE 4-2**

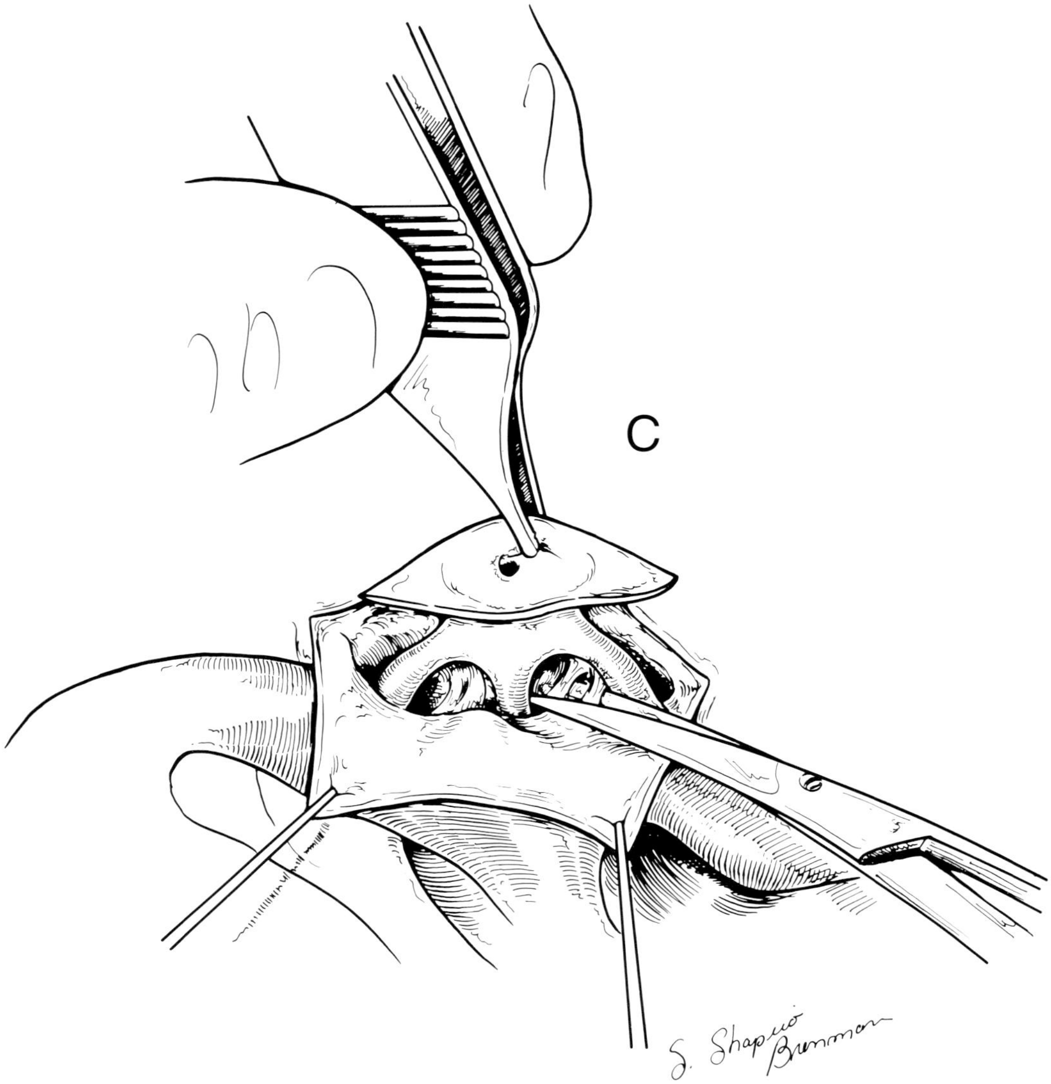


▶ **FIGURE 4-2**

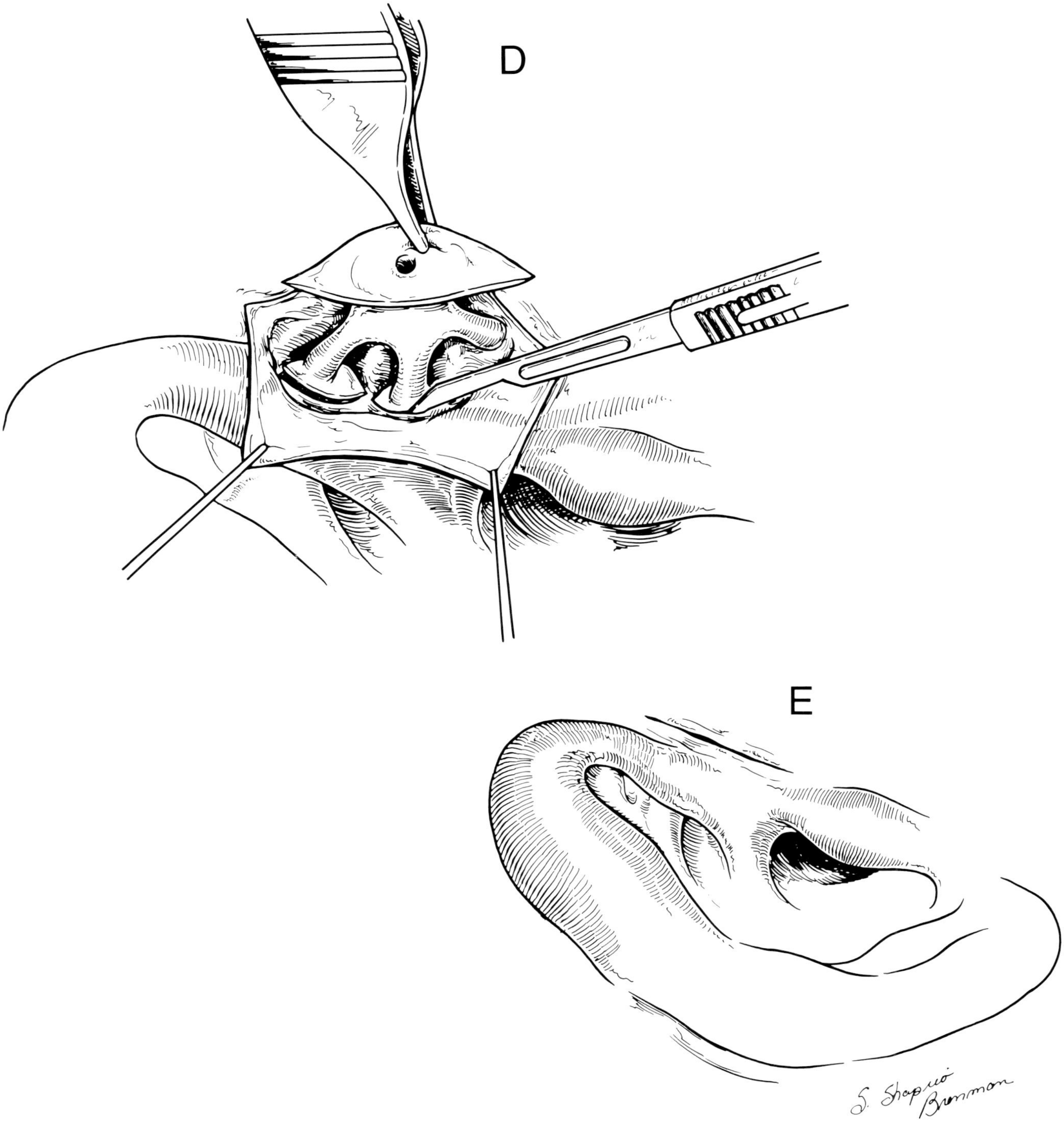


▶ **FIGURE 4-2**

## ▶ 4-3 OTOPLASTY (PROMINOTIA)

Protruding ear (prominotia) is a relatively common deformity that varies greatly in degree of severity (Fig. 4–3**A**). It is usually caused by a combination of the absence of the antihelical fold and a large conchal cartilage.

### Indications

The indication for surgery is the desire of the child and parents to restore normal anatomy. The procedure is best performed between ages 4 and 5, when the child can cooperate with postoperative care and before the child is subjected to teasing by school-age peers.

### Preoperative Evaluation

A complete examination of the ear and external canal is mandatory to determine the components of the deformity. Preoperative photographs are necessary to document the preoperative condition and to compare to the results after surgery.

### Operative Technique

1. General anesthesia is utilized for all children having otoplasty.
2. The desired degree of correction is determined by manipulating the auricle to create the missing fold in the antihelix and by depressing the concha against the mastoid bone.
3. The posterior surface of the auricle is injected with 1% lidocaine with 1:100,000 epinephrine to aid in hemostasis. The line of injection is the full length of the ear and is halfway between the postauricular fold and the edge of the helix (Fig. 4–3**B**).
4. An incision is made along the line of injection down to the perichondrium (Fig. 4–3**C**).
5. Skin flaps are elevated on both sides of the incision.
6. If the cartilage is thick, it is necessary to weaken the tissue to allow proper folding. (If cartilage is thin and pliable, skip to step 8, Fig. 4–3**G**.) A small incision is made through the cartilage and an elevator is used to elevate the perichondrium of the anterior surface of the cartilage along the line of the desired antihelical fold (Fig. 4–3**D, E**).
7. A thin, narrow rasp is then used to score the cartilage and break the spring of the anterior surface (Fig. 4–3**F**).
8. Twenty-five-gauge needles are passed through the cartilage from the anterior surface of the ear to guide the mattress sutures (Fig. 4–3**G**). The points of insertion (indicated by small circles) should be at least 5 mm from the top of the proposed antihelical fold so that the sutures will create a rounded, and not a sharp, fold.
9. Methylene blue is placed on the bevel of the needles, and they are withdrawn to mark the cartilage (Fig. 4–3**H**).
10. Horizontal mattress sutures with 4-0 white mersaline are placed at the methylene blue marks to re-create the antihelical fold (Fig. 4–3**I**). The suture should go through the cartilage and anterior and posterior perichondrium. Care is taken to avoid perforation of the lateral (anterior) skin surface of the ear while placing the sutures.

11. The sutures are tied just tight enough to create the desired effect of a rounded fold (Fig. 4–3J).

12. If it is felt that the concha is prominent, one or two sutures of 3-0 Vicryl can be placed between the concha and the mastoid periosteum to rotate the ear posteriorly against the mastoid cortex (Fig. 4–3K).

13. Enough excess skin to permit closure of the incision with minimal tension is removed. Slits are cut in the skin of the posterior flap to the edge of the lateral flap (Fig. 4–3L). The skin between the cuts is removed with a sharp scissors (Fig. 4–3M).

14. The incision is then closed with 5-0 interrupted subcuticular absorbable sutures (Fig. 4–3N). No drain is used.

15. The effect of the sutures to create the desired result is demonstrated in Figure 4–3O.

16. Cotton soaked in saline is applied to the anterior surface of the auricle conforming to the auricular folds (Fig. 4–3P).

17. A bulky mastoid dressing is used to apply gentle pressure. The dressing is removed 12 hours later to examine the ear. Another loose dressing is placed for 24 hours. An elastic headband is used to keep the ear in place. It is used day and night for 2 weeks, and then just at night for another 2 weeks.

## Complications

1. Incomplete correction of deformity
2. Chondritis
3. Unnatural appearance of auricle
4. Narrowing of external auditory canal

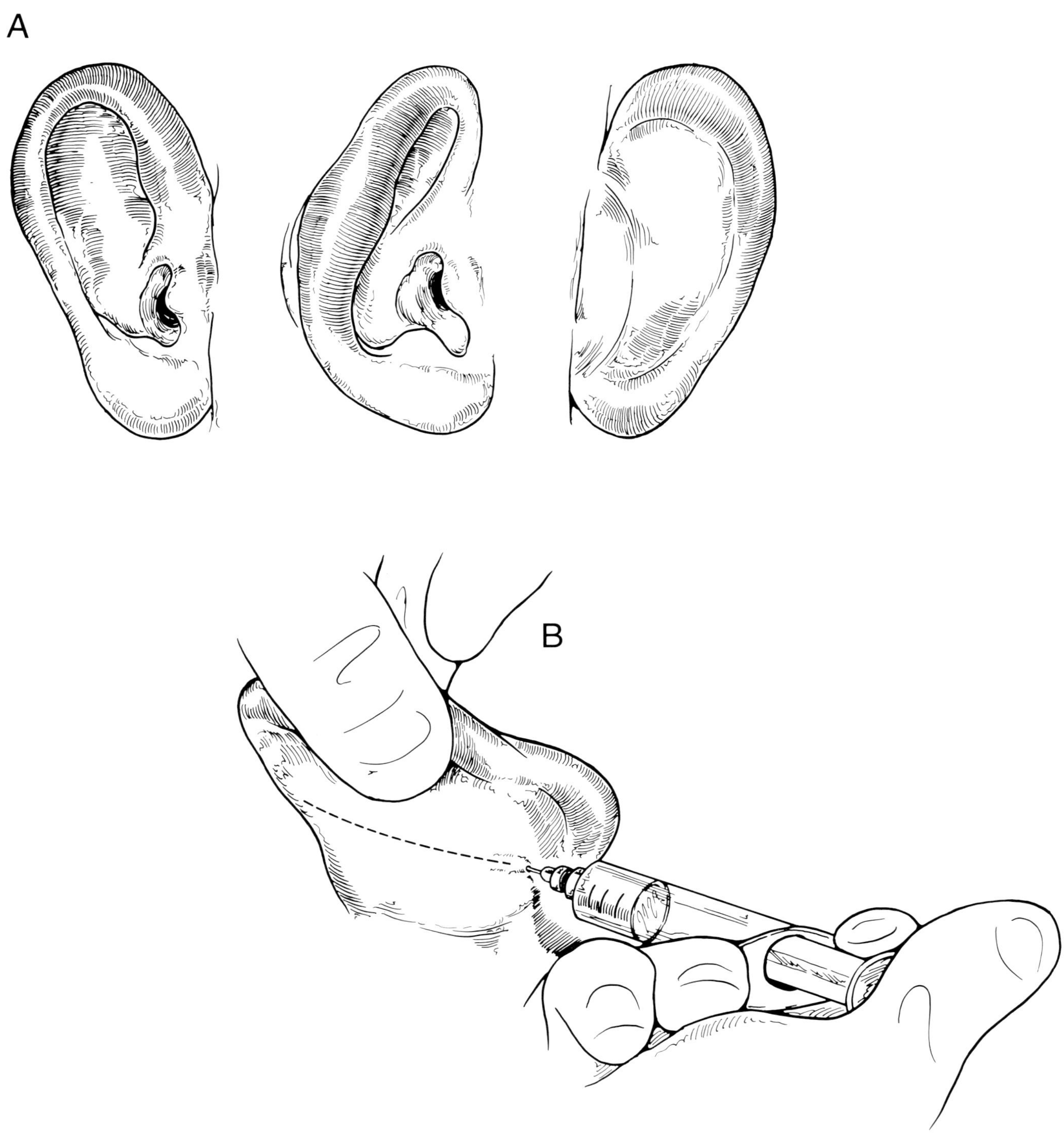


▶ **FIGURE 4-3**

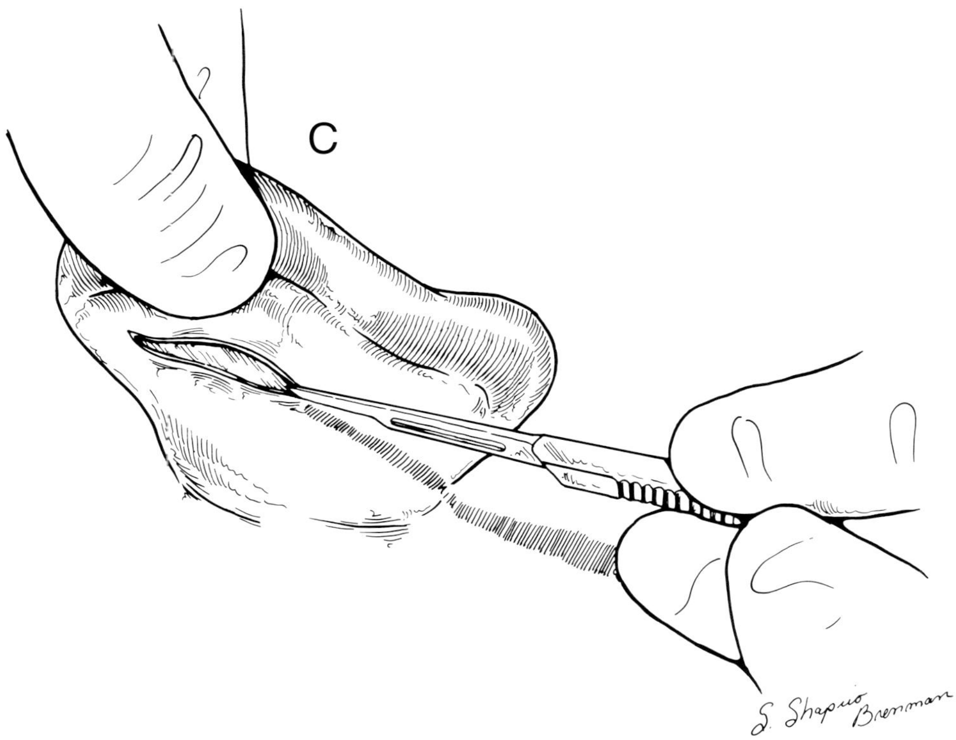


▶ **FIGURE 4-3**

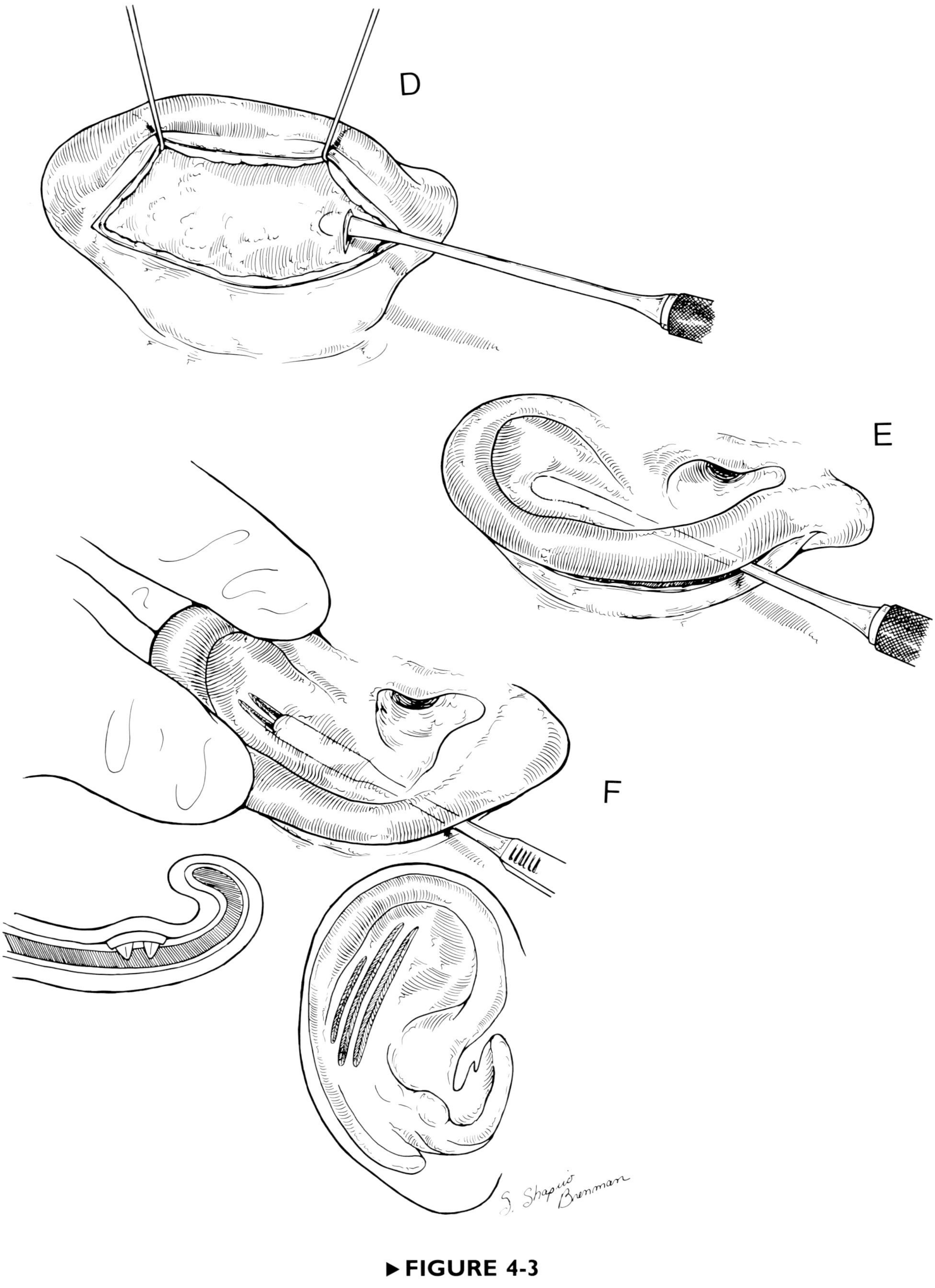


▶ **FIGURE 4-3**

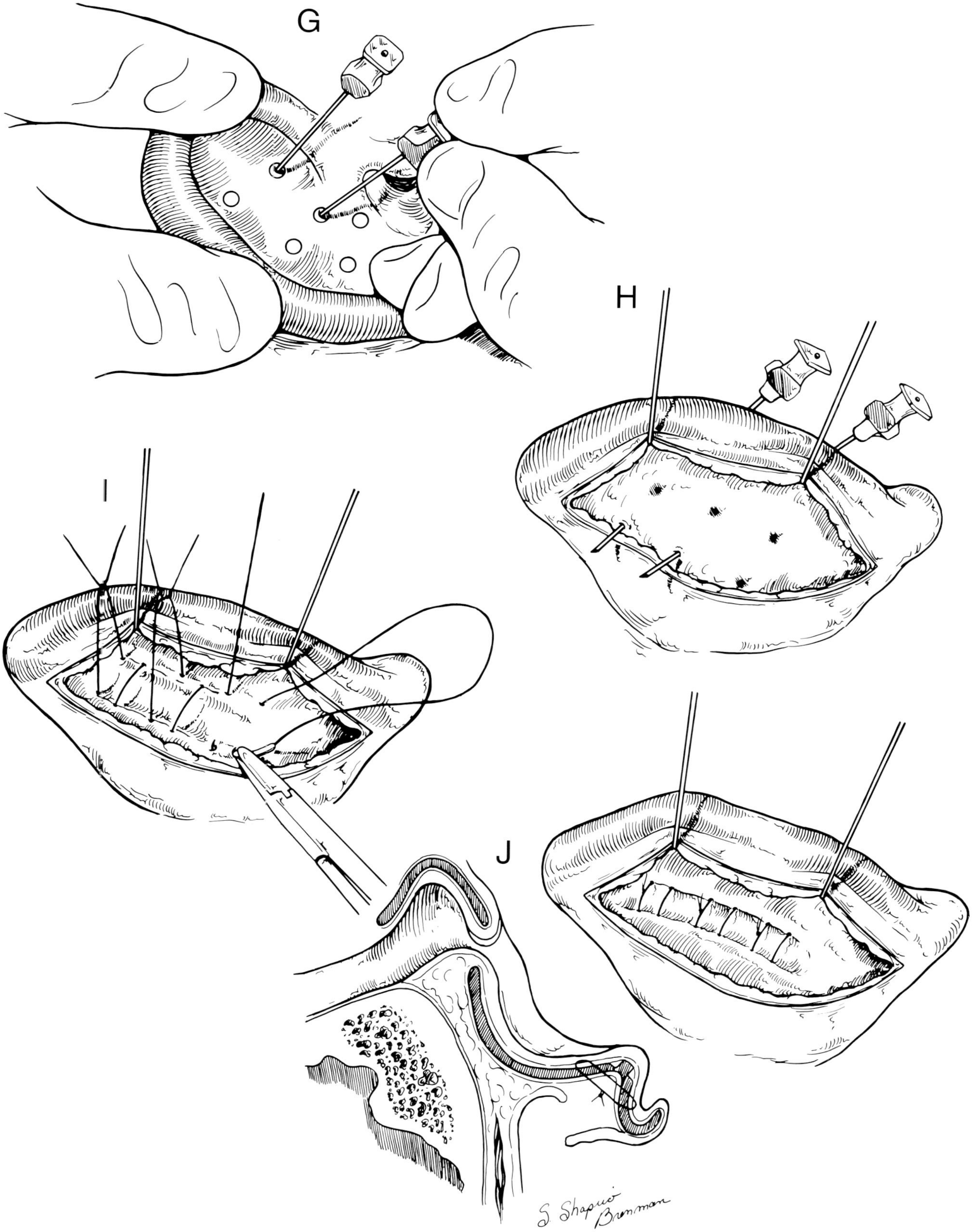


▶ **FIGURE 4-3**

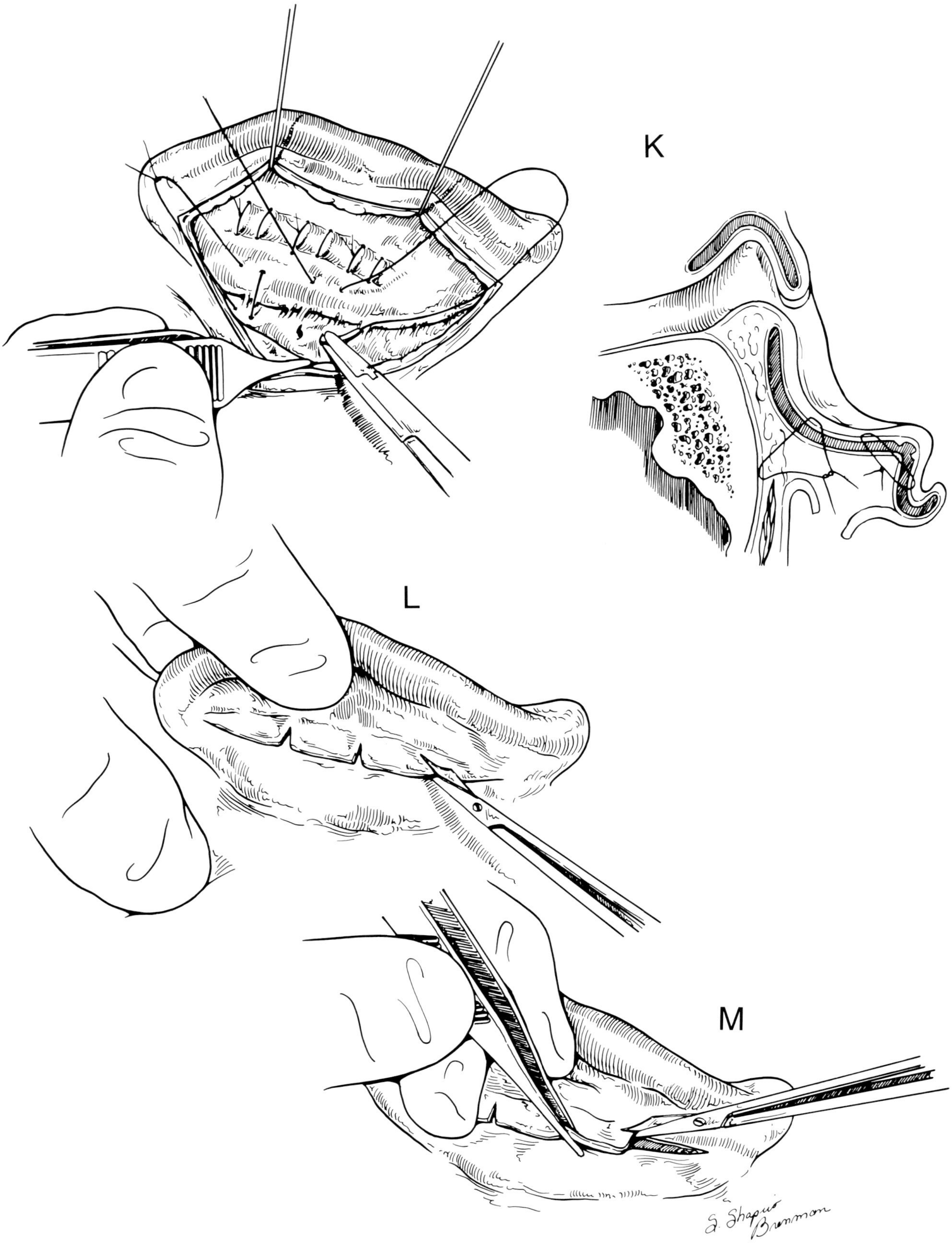


▶ **FIGURE 4-3**

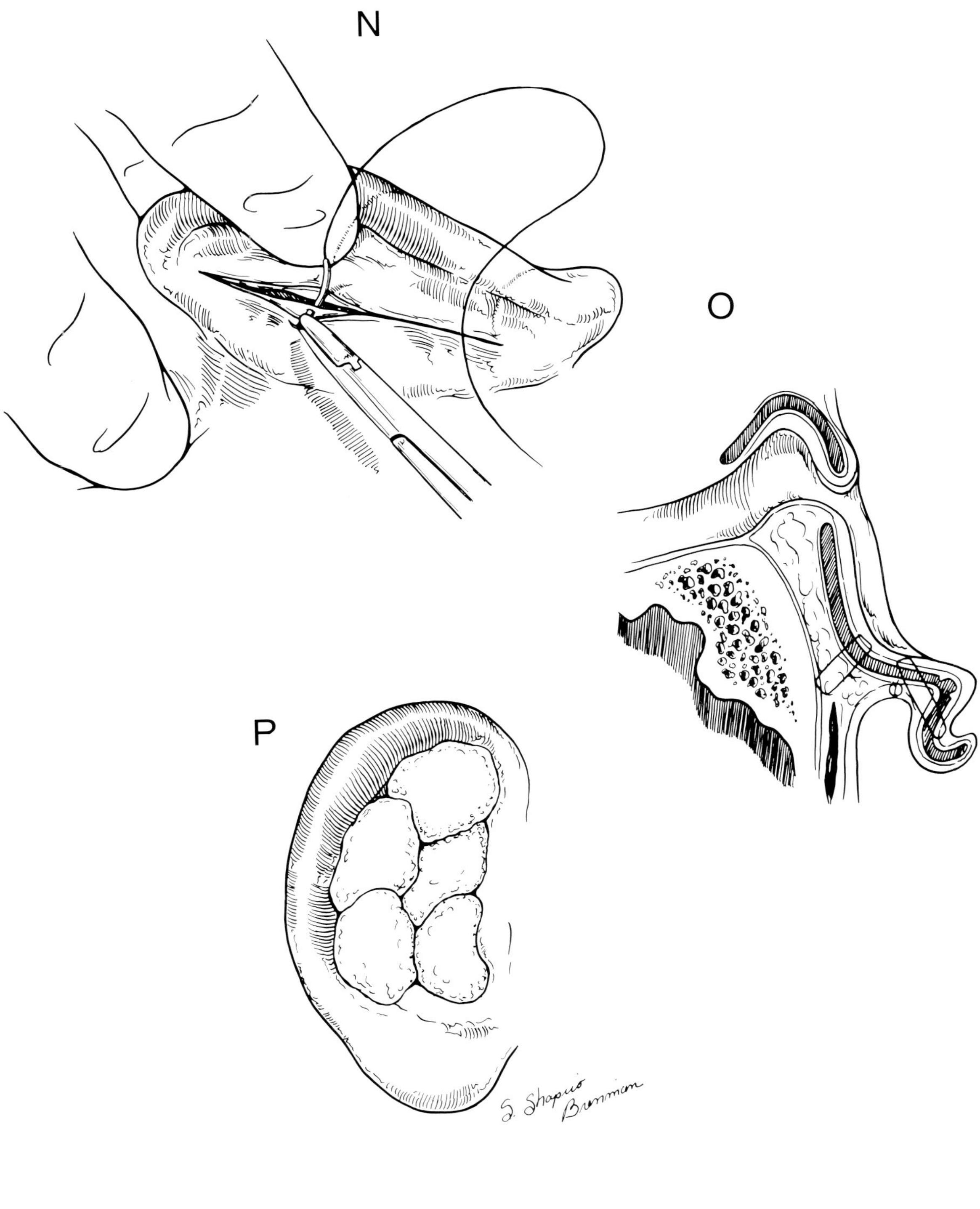


▶ **FIGURE 4-3**

## ▶ 4-4 MIDDLE EAR EXPLORATION—EXPLORATORY TYMPANOTOMY

Middle ear exploration is performed to examine the contents and condition of the middle ear. Middle ear exploration should permit adequate visualization of the ossicular chain to assess mobility, as well as inspection of the region of the oval and round windows.

### Indications

Middle ear exploration is indicated to determine the causes of and to correct a conductive hearing deficit, to biopsy or remove middle ear masses such as congenital cholesteatoma, or to identify and repair a perilymph fistula.

### Preoperative Evaluation

The preoperative evaluation of conditions affecting the middle ear includes pneumatic otoscopy, complete audiometry, and radiographs of the middle ear. This usually involves computed tomography (CT). Magnetic resonance imaging (MRI) is rarely helpful in the evaluation of the middle ear.

### Operative Technique

Middle ear exploration in children is best performed under general anesthesia. Adequate middle ear exposure may be possible in older children using a transcanal approach, but most often a postauricular approach as described for tympanoplasty (see section 3–2) provides better exposure (especially anteriorly).

1. If the transcanal approach is selected, local anesthetic (1% lidocaine with 1:100,000 epinephrine) (see "dots," Fig. 4–4**A**) is injected in the soft tissue of the posterior cartilaginous ear canal just lateral to the bony canal (Fig. 4–4**A**).
2. If a postauricular incision is used, the approach is identical to that used to enter the middle ear for tympanoplasty (see section 3–2).
3. An incision is made with a knife from a spot above the short process of the malleus to the posterior-inferior portion of the ear canal. The flap outlined should be approximately 5 mm wide in the midportion of the incision (Fig. 4–4**B**). The superior or inferior limb of the incision can be extended to provide access to the anterior-superior or inferior quadrants, respectively.
4. The flap is released by elevating the periosteum with a knife until the fibrous annulus of the tympanic membrane is identified (Fig. 4–4**C**).
5. The annulus is elevated with a knife or sulcus elevator along the full extent of the incision, and the middle ear is entered (Fig. 4–4**D**).
6. The tympanomeatal flap can then be folded anteriorly to expose the contents of the middle ear (Fig. 4–4**E**).
7. Bone of the posterior-superior canal wall may be removed with a curette or drill for full exposure of the stapes footplate, if necessary. Care is taken to avoid trauma to the chorda tympani nerve (Fig. 4–4**E**).
8. If anterior-superior exposure is desired for excision of a congenital cholesteatoma, an incision is made in the periosteum along the full length of the posterior surface of the malleus with a micro-Tabb knife by scraping against the bone (Fig. 4–4**F**).

9. The periosteum is then released from the malleus by dissection with a micro-Tabb knife until the anterior-superior quadrant is visualized (Fig. 4–4G).
10. If needed, the tympanic membrane can be released from its attachment to the malleus at the umbo by cutting the fibrous bands with a small Bellucci scissors.
11. When the middle ear surgery is complete, the tympanomeatal flap is replaced, and a single large piece of Gelfoam is placed across the incision line (Fig. 4–4H).

## Complications

1. Ossiclar disruption
2. Chorda tympani trauma
3. Perforation of the tympanic membrane

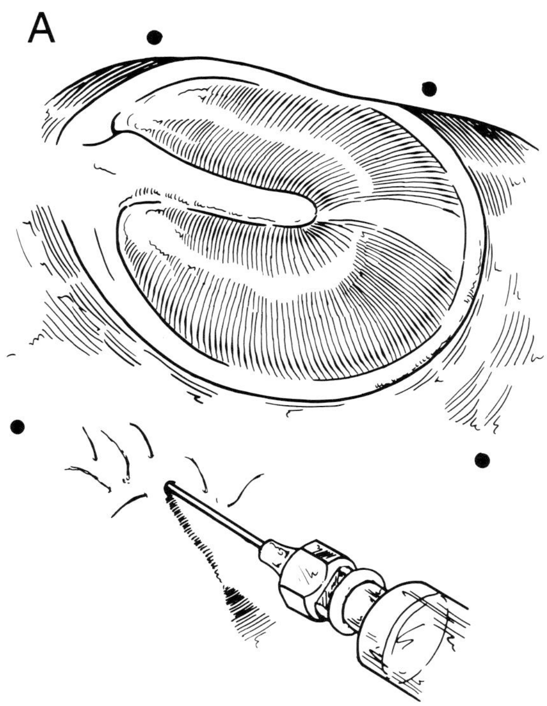


▶ **FIGURE 4-4**

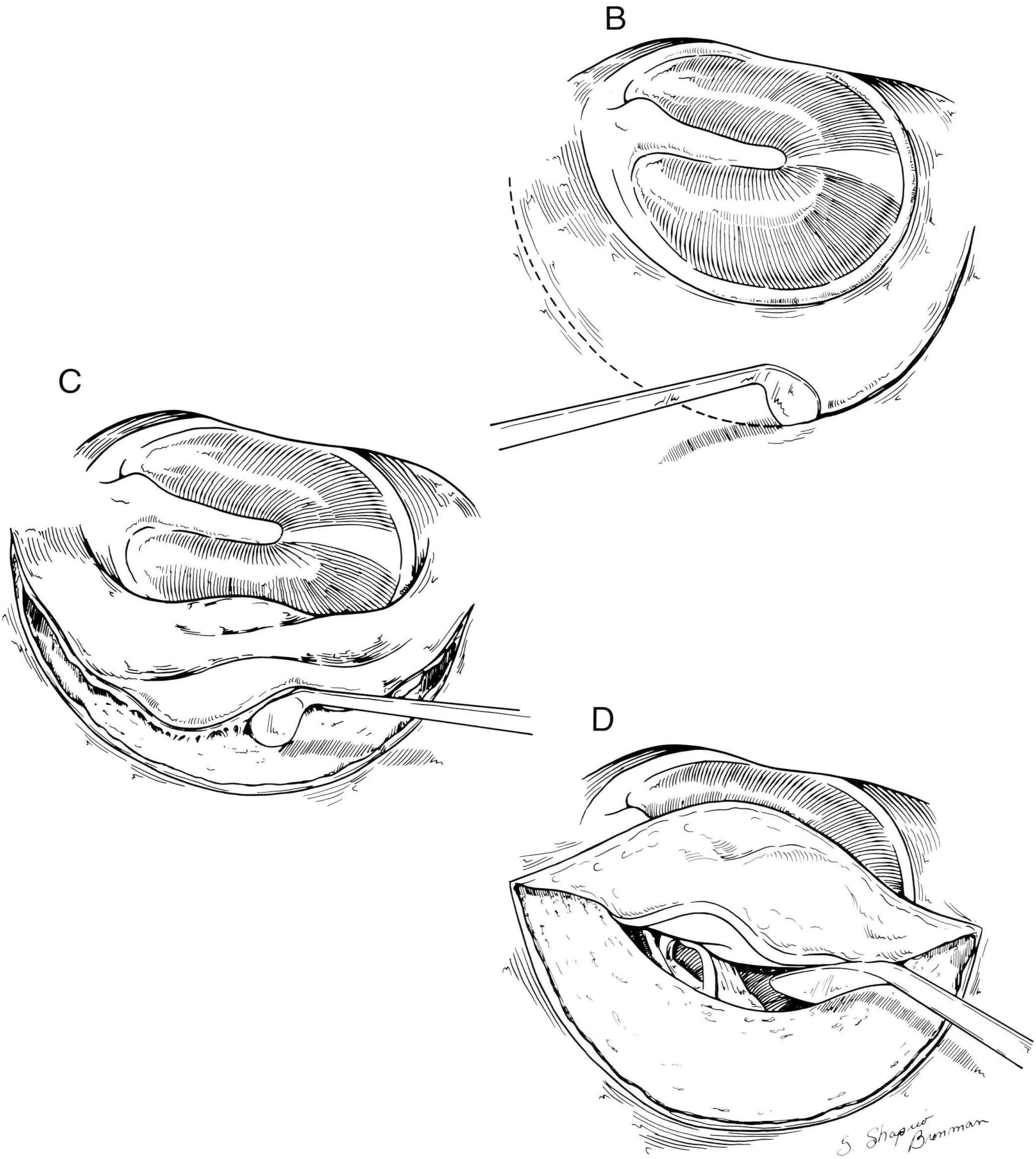


▶ **FIGURE 4-4**

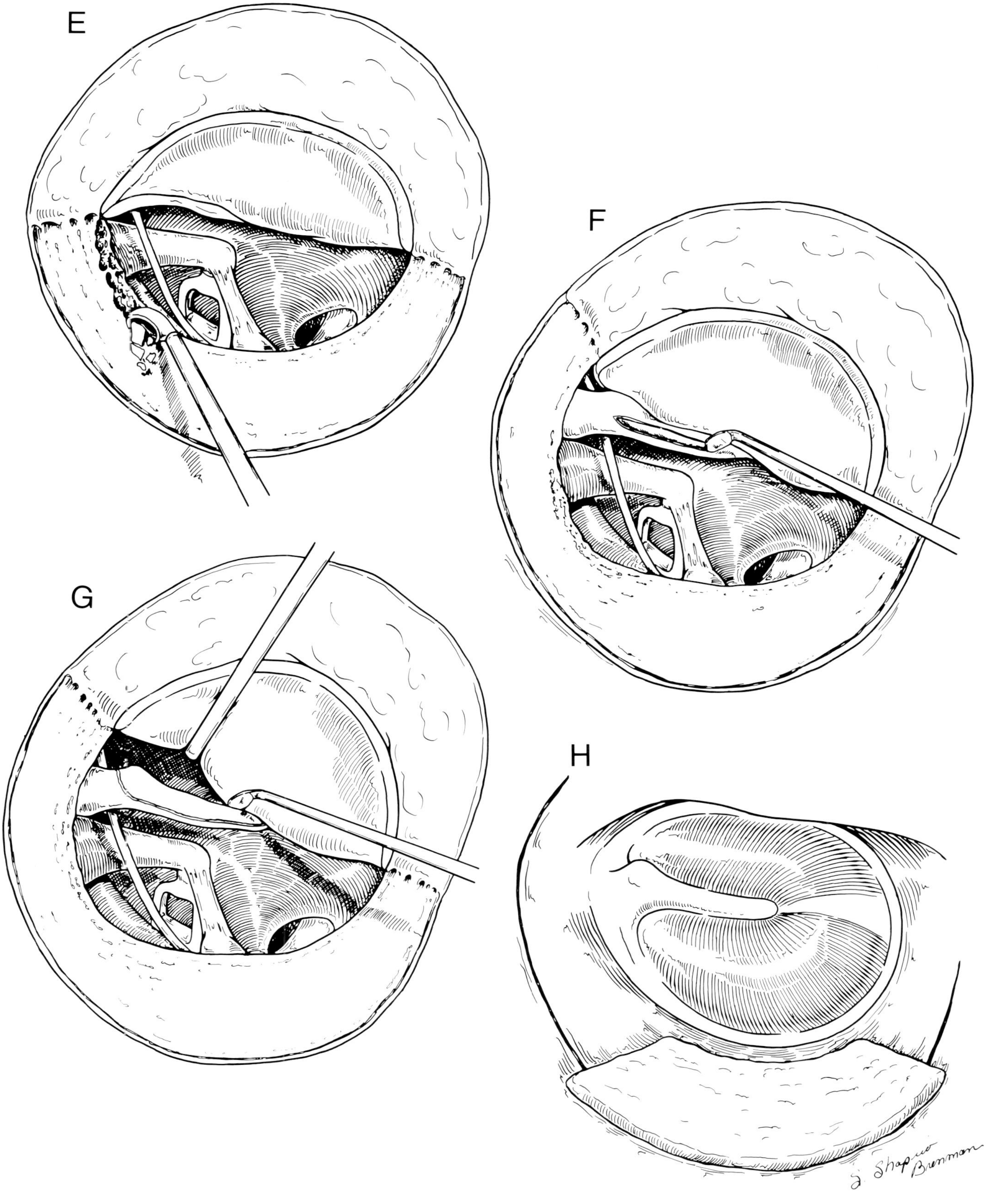


▶ **FIGURE 4-4**

## ▶ 4-5 ATRESIA AND ASSOCIATED OSSICULAR ANOMALIES

Atresia of the ear varies in its severity and may include a combination of external and middle ear anomalies. When only one ear is involved, surgical reconstruction for hearing improvement is deferred until the child is a teenager and can participate in the decision to have the procedure. When both ears are affected, the functional deficit is usually so severe, even with hearing aid amplification, that reconstruction is desirable.

### Indications

Atresia reconstruction is indicated for bilateral atresia and is best performed between the ages of 3 and 5 years when the child can cooperate with postoperative care.

### Preoperative Evaluation

The preoperative evaluation requires CT of the temporal bone to determine the extent of mastoid pneumatization and to define the structures of the external canal, middle ear, and inner ear. Complete audiometry is also required to be certain that there is no sensorineural hearing loss. This may require brainstem auditory testing.

Successful surgical reconstruction to establish an external meatus and improve hearing depends upon adequate development of the mastoid bone so that there is sufficient space to create an external meatus and a middle ear cavity in which to reconstruct the sound conduction mechanism (Fig. 4–5**A**). This, of course, assumes that the inner ear functions normally. The ear that appears to provide the best anatomy for reconstruction is operated upon first. The decision to operate on the second ear must take into account the functional and anatomic result obtained on the first ear. The surgeon may elect to utilize intraoperative facial nerve monitoring.

### Operative Technique

1. General anesthesia is required to correct aural atresia. The postauricular area and the region where the external meatus is to be created are injected with 1% lidocaine containing 1:100,000 epinephrine (Fig. 4–5**B**).
2. The vestigial auricle is almost always overlying or anterior to the site for the external canal. A Z-plasty incision is made, which permits the auricle to be rotated posteriorly. This also creates a pedicle flap to partially line the newly created external meatus (Fig. 4–5**C**). If the external ear is nearly fully developed, the external meatus is created by removing the plug of skin and soft tissue overlying the proposed site of the external meatus (Fig. 4–5**D**). If the auricle is well formed, a standard postauricular incision as for tympanoplasty is performed (see section 3–2).
3. After the Z-plasty flaps are elevated, the periosteum of the mastoid is incised and reflected with a self-retaining retractor, exposing the mastoid and temporal line (Fig. 4–5**E**).
4. A cutting bur is used to create a new bony external meatus that is as large as possible, allowing for postoperative contraction. The dissection should be directed anteriorly along the temporal line to approach the attic. This protects the region of the facial nerve and permits limited mastoid dissection. The head of the malleus and body of the incus are the first middle ear structures usually seen (Fig. 4–5**F**).

5. Bone of the tympanic plate is then thinned with cutting and diamond burs to release the malleus-incus complex and expose the middle ear.
6. The final release of the thinned bony plate is done with a curette to avoid sensorineural hearing loss from drilling on the ossicles (Fig. 4–5G). The ossicular reconstruction will depend on the condition of the ossicular chain. Often, only release of the fused malleus-incus complex from its bony attachment is required.
7. A ledge of bone (pseudoannulus) is created with a small drill around the rim of the bony external meatus at the level of the middle ear (Fig. 4–5H).
8. A temporalis fascia graft is taken as described in tympanoplasty (see section 3–2). The anterior edge is cut to create a flap that will be tucked under the anterior ledge of the canal to reduce lateralization (Fig. 4–5I). The graft is then draped over the ossicles and onto the external meatus (Fig. 4–5J).
9. The previously created pedicle flap is rotated into the posterior superior portion of the external meatus and sewn in place with 5-0 interrupted nylon suture (Fig. 4–5K, L). Any additional widening of the external meatus is accomplished by removing skin and soft tissue with a knife and scissors.
10. A split thickness 13/1,000 inch is taken from the upper thigh (above the swimsuit line) with a dermatome.
11. The skin graft is notched to allow the edges to overlap the fascia when the graft is placed in the canal (Fig. 4–5L).
12. The skin graft is placed in the canal with the cut edges overlapping each other on the surface of the fascial graft. After the flaps are rotated, any exposed areas of bone or soft tissue should be covered with additional strips of split thickness skin graft. The skin graft is tacked to the edge of the meatus with 6-0 mild chromic suture (Fig. 4–5L).
13. A thin Silastic disk is placed on the skin overlying the site of the new tympanic membrane to hold it in place, and the remainder of the external meatus is packed with Gelfoam in the medial one third and antibiotic ointment-impregnated gauze in the outer two thirds (Fig. 4–5M, N).
14. The remaining skin incisions are closed with 4-0 interrupted nylon suture and a standard mastoid dressing is applied.
15. The packing is left in place for 3 weeks. The child is kept on oral antibiotics and an antibiotic containing otic drops that are administered three times a day for the entire time the packing is in place or longer, as judged by the surgeon.
16. The packing is removed under general anesthesia. Granulation tissue is removed and overlapping nonviable skin is trimmed with a Bellucci scissors.

## Complications

1. External canal stenosis
2. Poor hearing result
3. Vertigo
4. Facial nerve injury
5. Sensorineural hearing loss

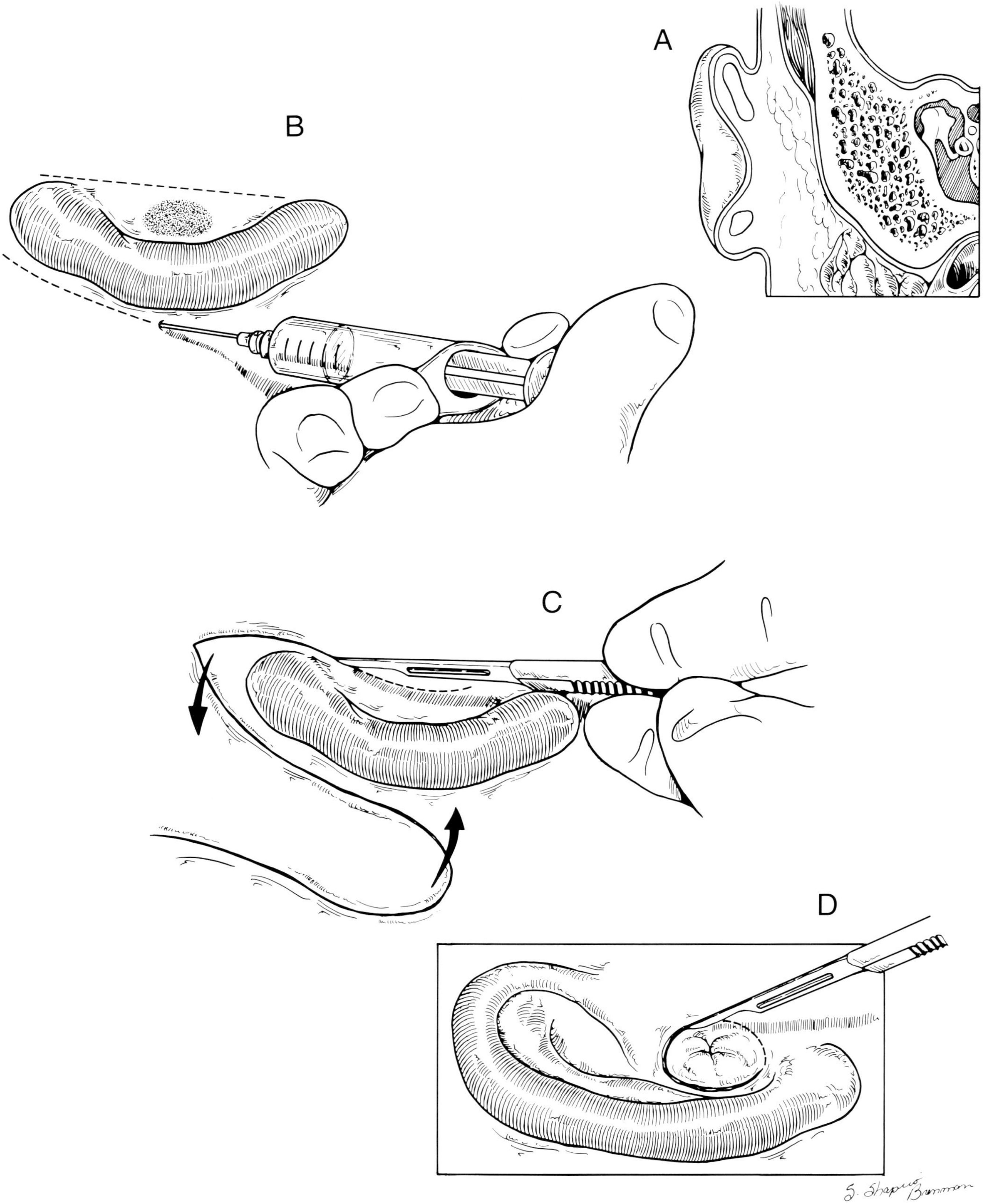


▶ **FIGURE 4-5**

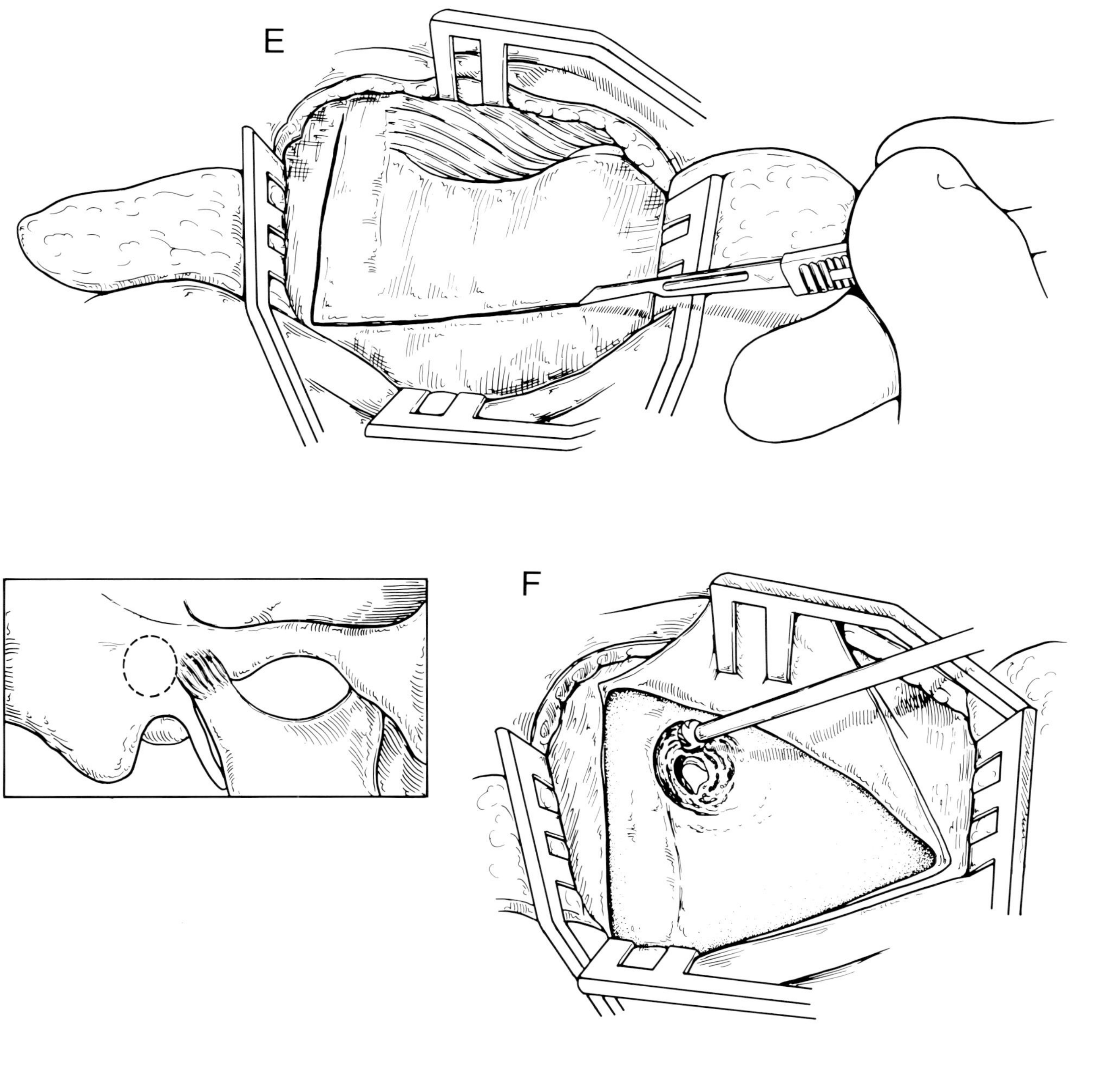


▶ **FIGURE 4-5**

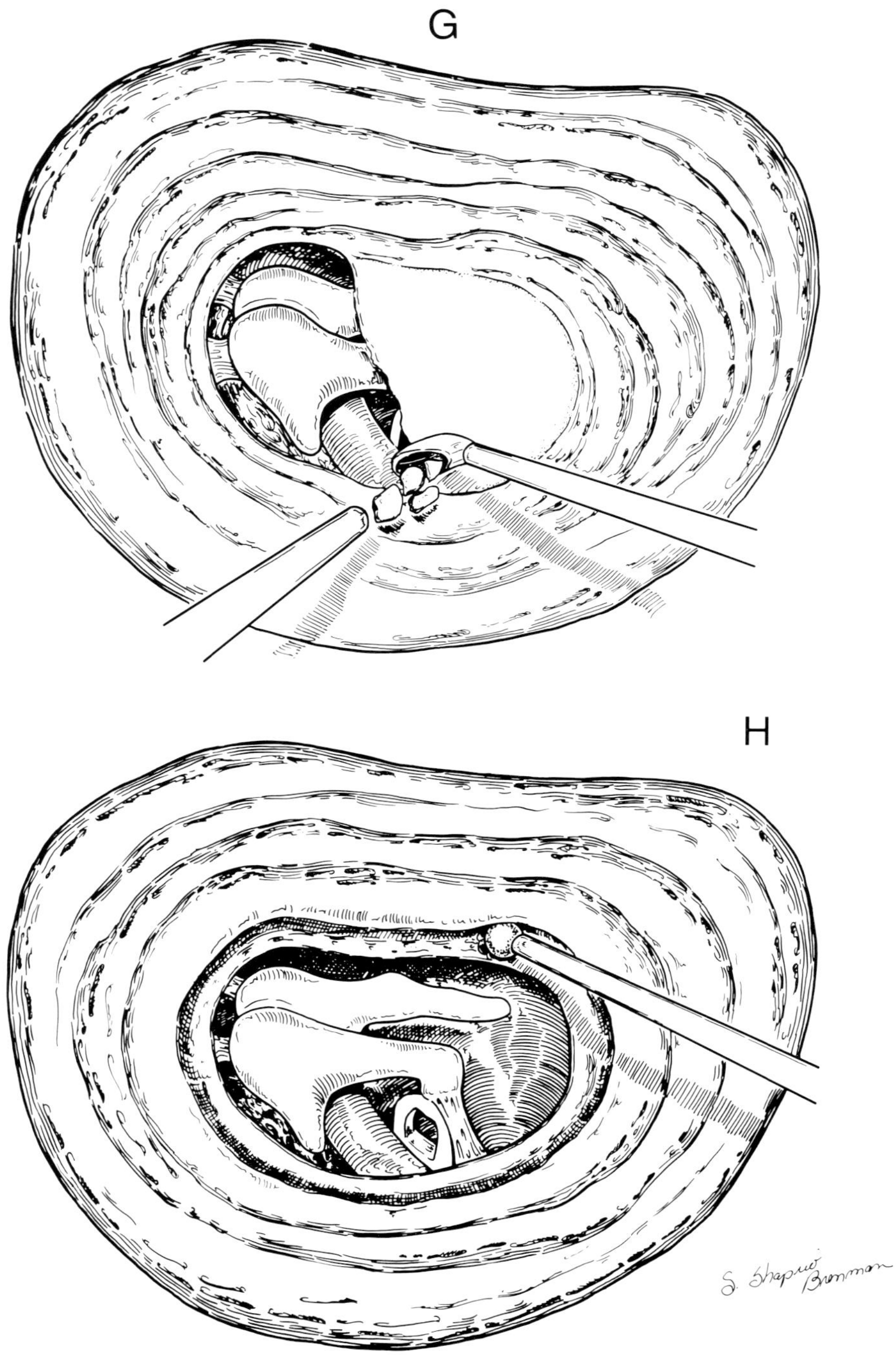


▶ **FIGURE 4-5**

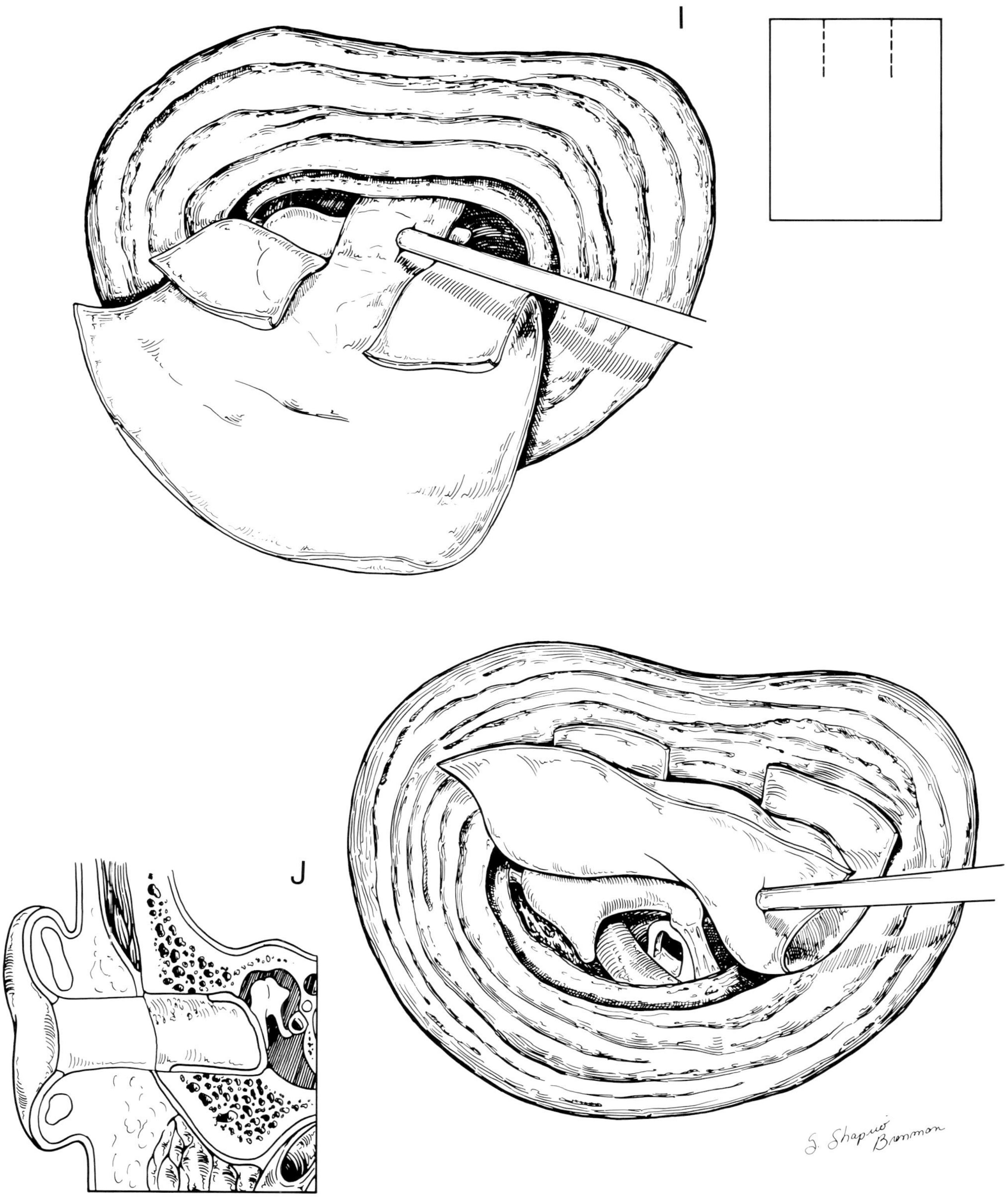


▶ **FIGURE 4-5**

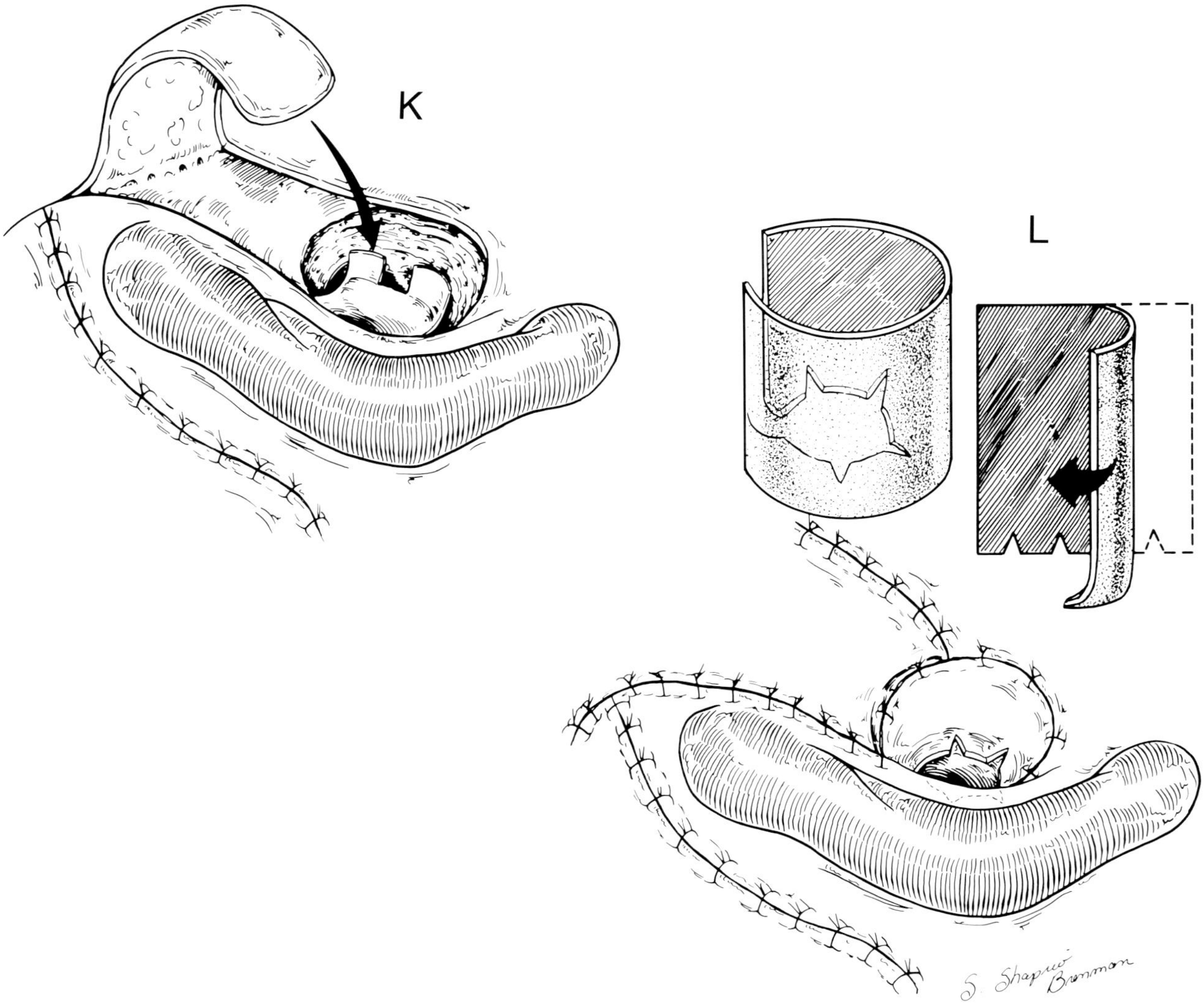


▶ **FIGURE 4-5**

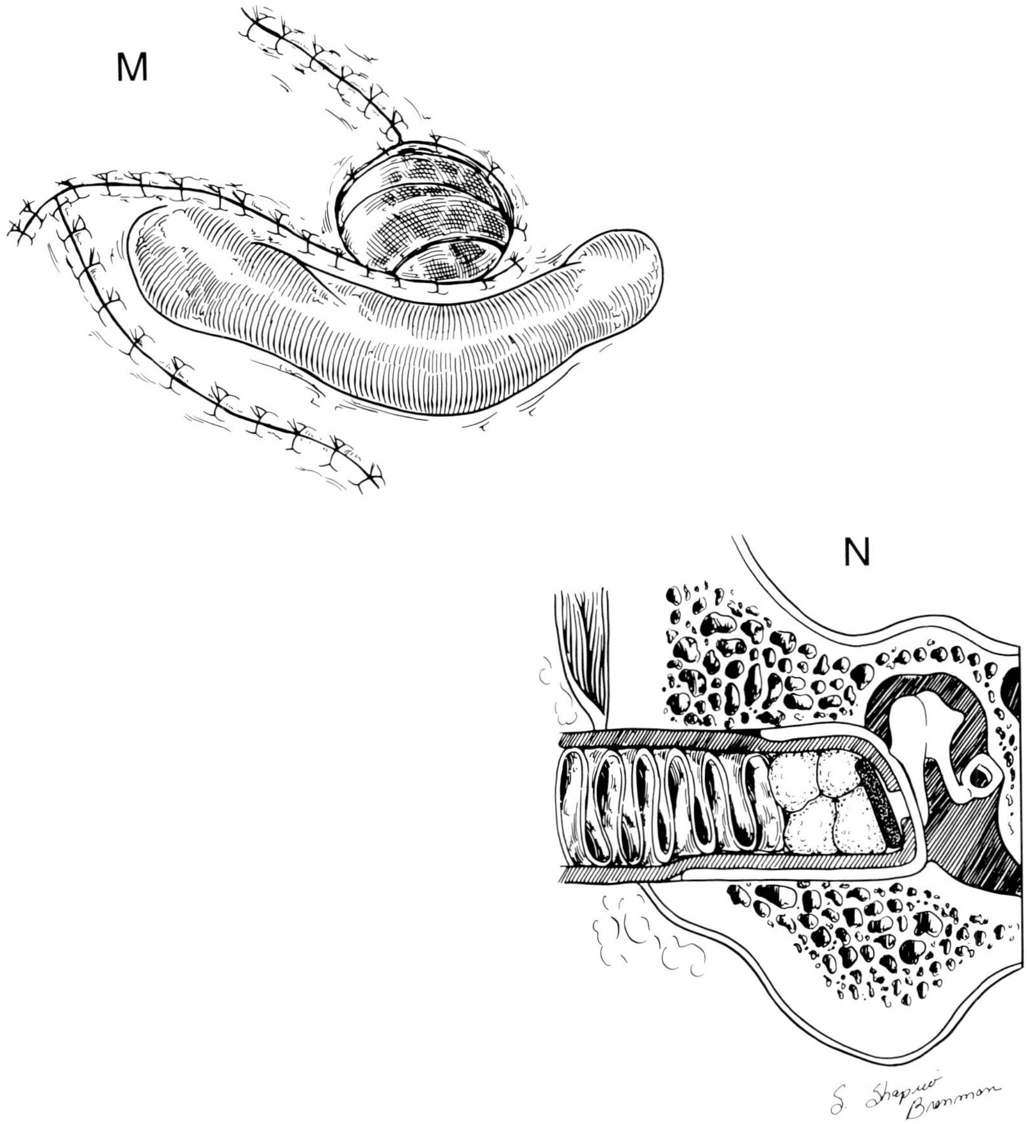


▶ **FIGURE 4-5**

## ▶ 4-6 STAPES SURGERY (STAPEDOTOMY/ STAPEDECTOMY AND STAPES MOBILIZATION)

Abnormalities of the stapes are uncommon in children.

### Indications

Stapes surgery is indicated to correct a moderate-to-severe conductive hearing loss secondary to stapes fixation. Stapes fixation in children may be congenital or a result of tympanosclerosis or otosclerosis.

### Preoperative Evaluation

The preoperative evaluation includes otoscopic examination and complete audiometry and radiographic evaluation. Computed tomography (CT) is helpful to demonstrate the detail of the stapes and surrounding structures in congenital middle ear malformations and to rule out other causes for the hearing loss.

### Stapes Mobilization, Stapedotomy—Operative Technique

1. General anesthesia is used for this procedure in young children. Local infiltration with 1% lidocaine with 1:100,000 epinephrine is injected in the postauricular crease and external meatus to decrease bleeding as described for tympanoplasty (see section 3–2).
2. A standard postauricular exposure, as used for tympanoplasty (section 3–2), provides maximum exposure. Older children with a large external meatus may permit a transcanal approach as described for middle ear exploration (see section 4–4) (Fig. 4–6**A**).
3. After the middle ear is exposed, bone is removed from the canal wall posterior-superiorly with a drill or curette to expose the stapes and surrounding area (Fig. 4–6**B**). Care should be taken to preserve the chorda tympani nerve, if possible (Fig. 4–6**C**).
4. If the stapes is fixed, an attempt to mobilize it is made. A small pick is placed on the head of the stapes, and the ossicle is gently rocked and pushed medially. If the stapes footplate becomes mobile, the procedure is terminated.
5. If the stapes cannot be mobilized, the distance from the long process of the incus to the footplate is measured with a measuring instrument (Fig. 4–6**D**).
6. The incudostapedial joint is divided with a micro-Tabb knife (Fig. 4–6**E**), and the stapedius tendon is cut with scissors (Fig. 4–6**F**).
7. The suprastructure of the stapes is removed after fracturing the crura with a knife (Fig. 4–6**G, H**).
8. A hole is made in the footplate with a sharp pick, microdrill, or laser and enlarged with a small hook, if necessary. The hole should be just large enough to accommodate the piston of a wire Teflon prosthesis (Fig. 4–6**I**).
9. A wire Teflon piston is placed in the opening of the footplate, and the wire hook is looped over the long process of the incus (Fig. 4–6**J**).
10. The wire hook is secured by closing it around the incus with a crimper or alligator forceps (Fig. 4–6**K**).
11. Small pieces of fascia are placed around the prosthesis to help seal the oval window (Fig. 4–6**L**).

When the stapes is deformed and must be removed, or if a large piece of the footplate comes out of the oval window niche during removal of the stapes suprastructure (Fig. 4–6M), a formal stapedectomy (see below) is performed and a connective tissue closure of the oval window is used.

## Stapedectomy—Operative Technique

1. A perichondrial graft is taken from the tip of the tragus. If desired, it may be flattened with a Gelfoam or fascia press.
2. The entire or remaining portions of the footplate are removed with a small hook (Fig. 4–6N).
3. The boat-shaped perichondrial tissue fits well into the oval window (Fig. 4–6O).
4. A wire or wire Teflon prosthesis is then placed on the graft and positioned in the center of the oval window (Fig. 4–6P).
5. The wire is crimped around the incus, and Gelfoam is placed around the prosthesis (Fig. 4–6Q).
6. The tympanomeatal flap is then replaced and the canal packed with Gelfoam soaked in antibiotic drops. If a postauricular incision was used, it is closed with subcutaneous absorbable suture.

## Complications

1. Poor hearing result
2. Chorda tympani injury
3. Facial nerve injury
4. Tympanic membrane perforation
5. Vertigo

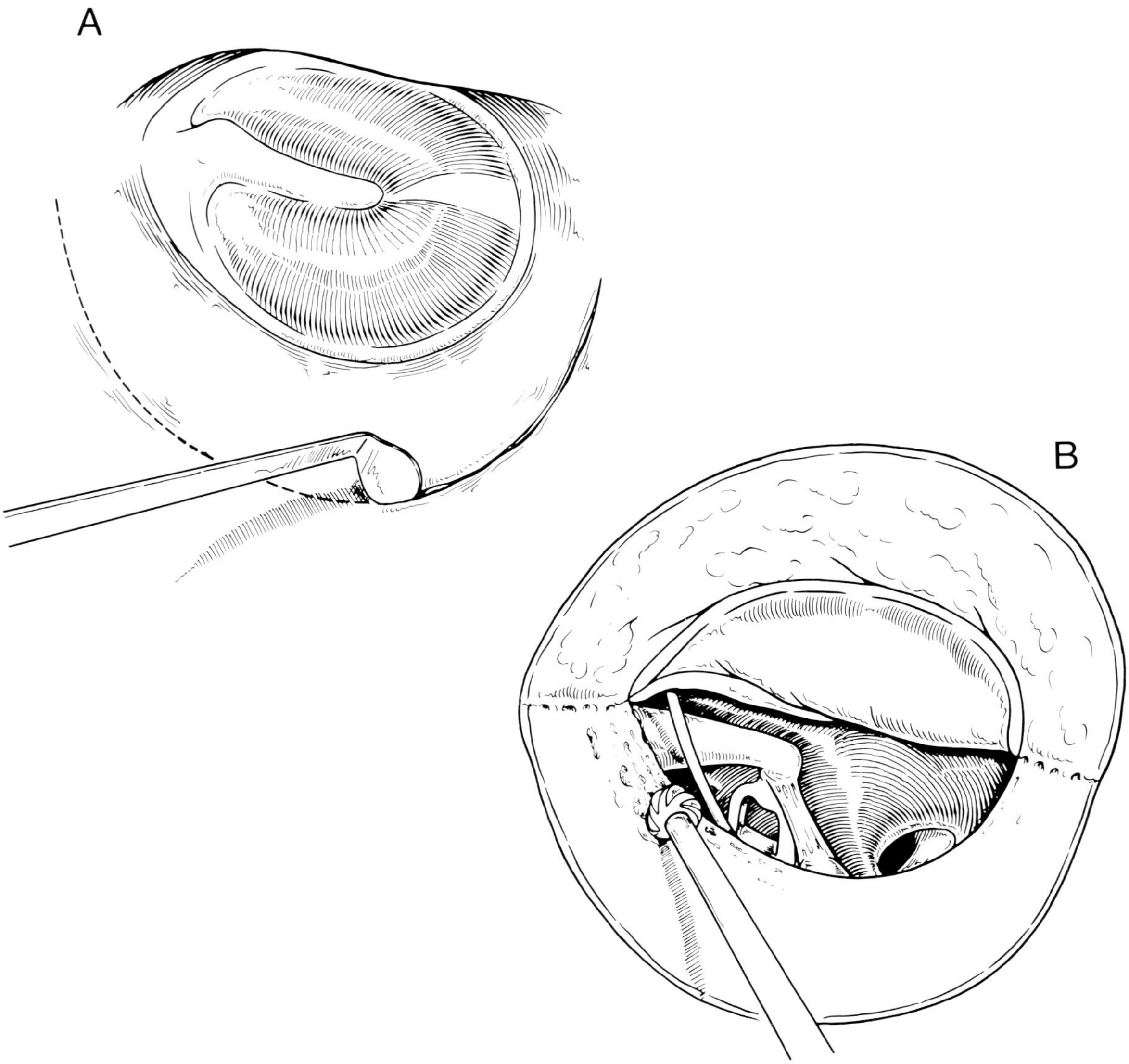


▶ **FIGURE 4-6**

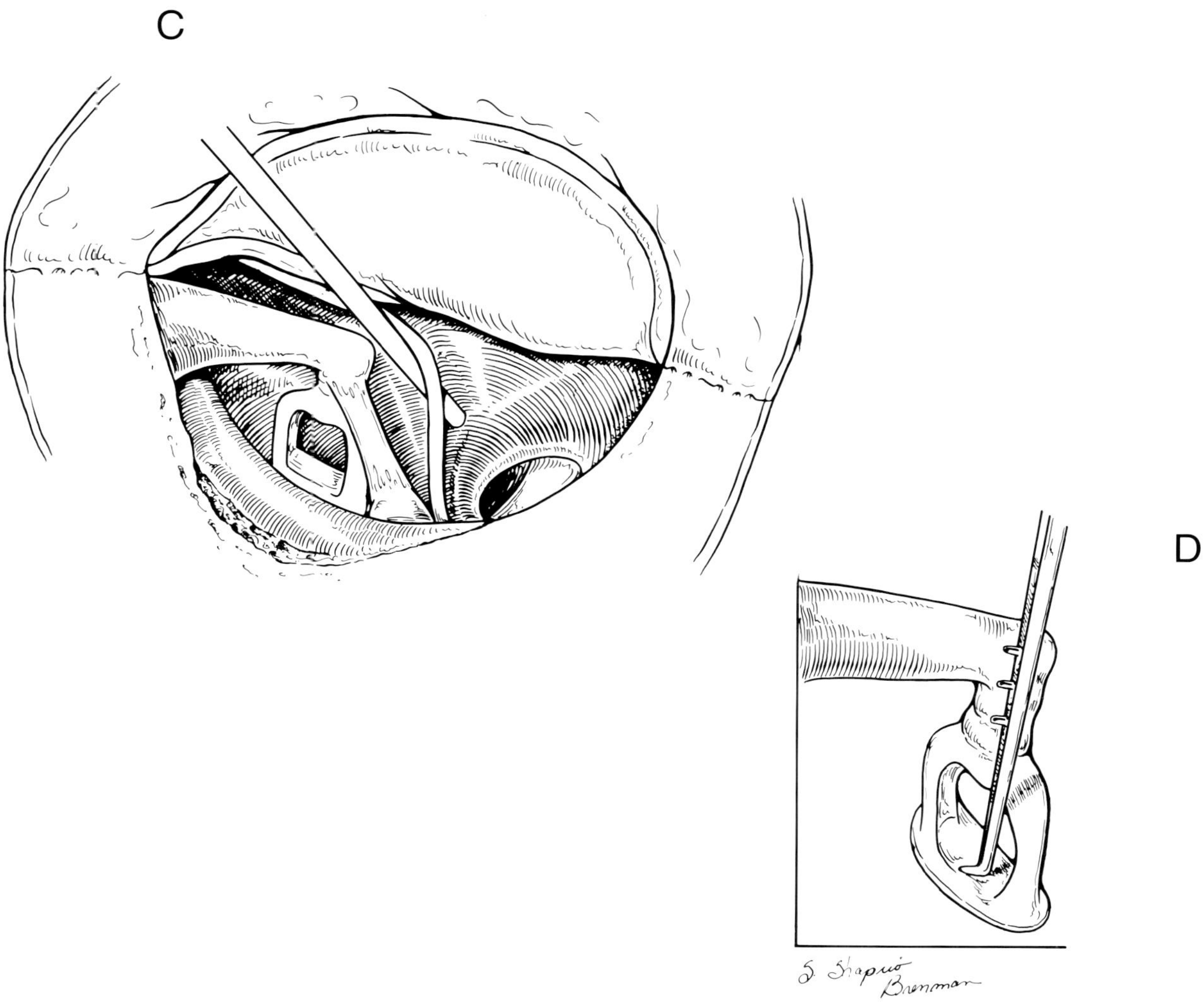


▶ **FIGURE 4-6**

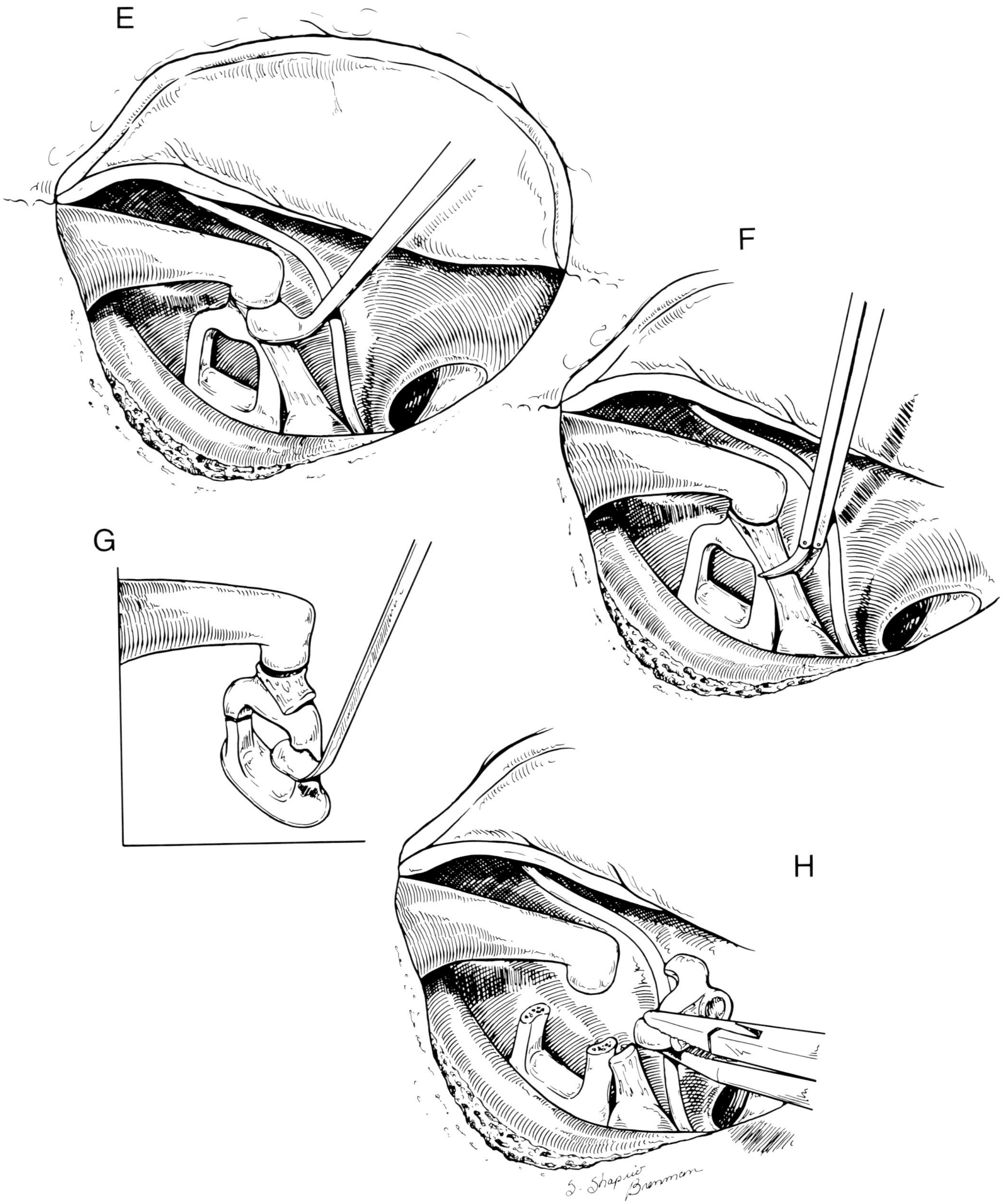


▶ **FIGURE 4-6**

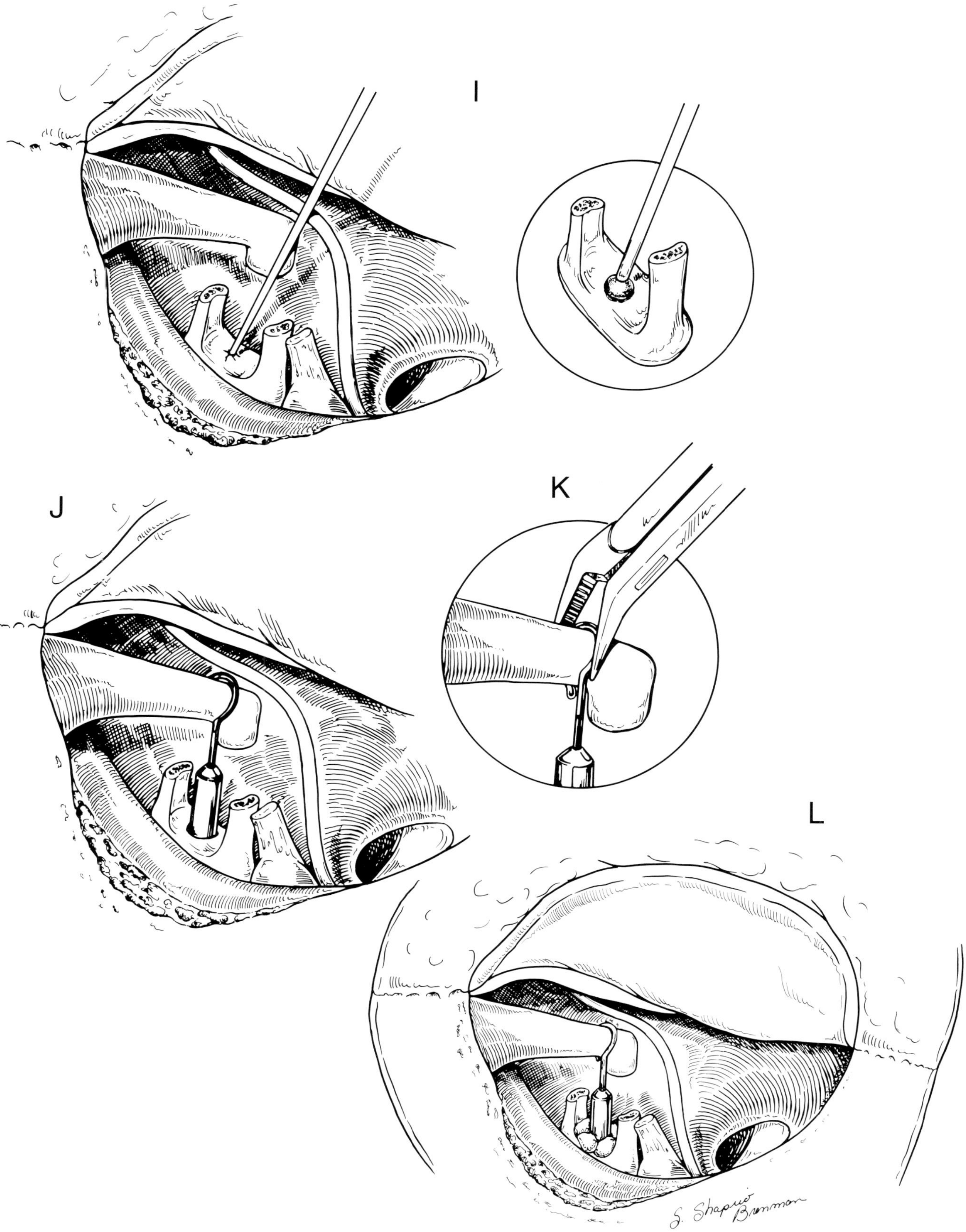


▶ **FIGURE 4-6**

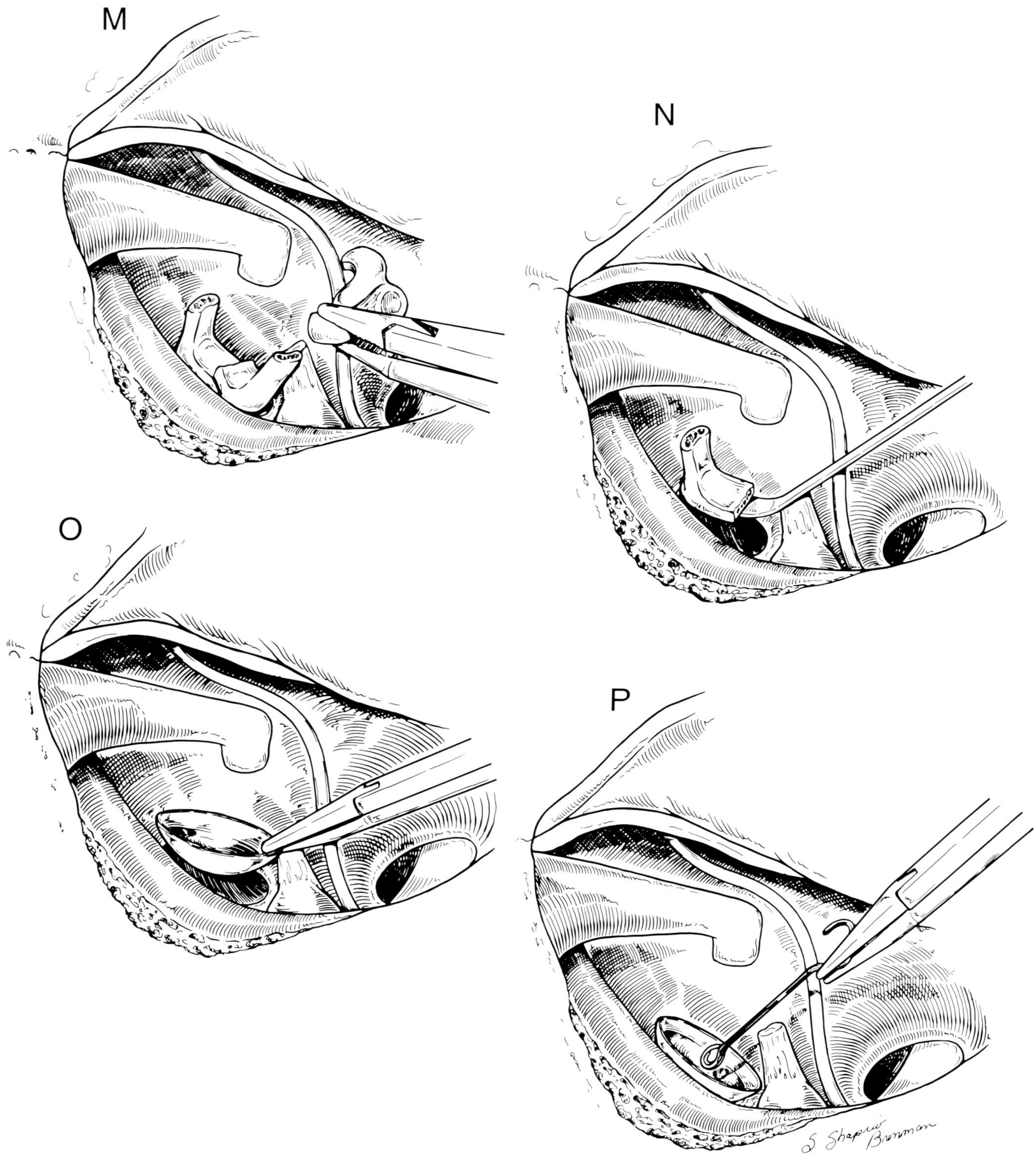


▶ **FIGURE 4-6**

Q

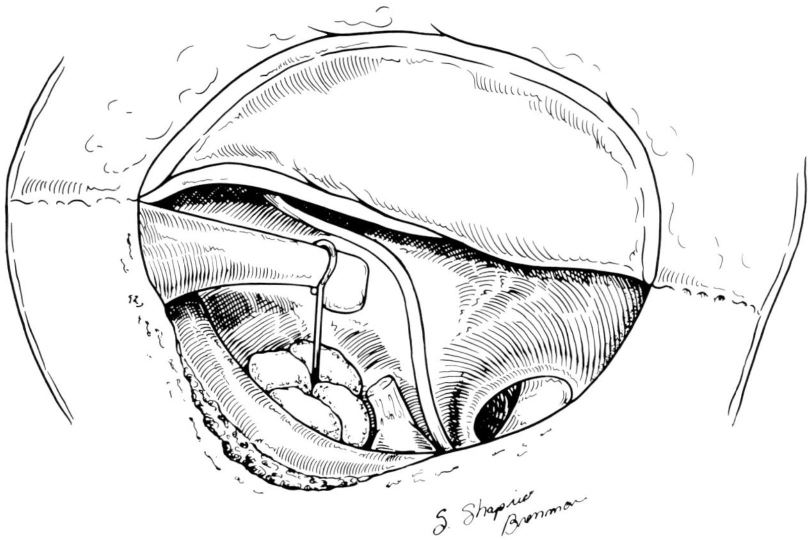

▶ **FIGURE 4-6**

# 5 ▶ Facial Nerve Surgery

## ▶ 5-1 FACIAL NERVE DECOMPRESSION (TYMPANIC AND MASTOID SEGMENTS)

Facial nerve decompression is a procedure to open the bony facial nerve canal to decrease pressure on the facial nerve. Facial nerve decompression is performed rarely in children because idiopathic facial nerve paralysis (Bell's palsy) frequently resolves spontaneously and traumatic facial paralysis is uncommon.

### Indications

Facial nerve decompression is indicated in the treatment of complete traumatic paralysis when nerve excitability testing indicates a poor prognosis for spontaneous recovery. Facial nerve injury medial to the geniculate ganglion may require total facial decompression, which is not described in this atlas.

### Preoperative Evaluation

Pneumatic otoscopy and complete audiometry are prerequisites to this procedure. Computed tomography (CT) scan of the temporal bone is needed to define any fractures. Electroneurography (ENOG) testing is used to determine the degree of degeneration and need for surgery. Magnetic resonance imaging (MRI) may be helpful to locate the site of facial nerve involvement. The surgeon may elect to utilize intraoperative facial nerve monitoring.

### Operative Technique

1. Facial nerve decompression is performed utilizing general anesthesia. The postauricular area and external meatus are injected with 1% lidocaine with 1:100,000 epinephrine as described for tympanoplasty (see section 3–2) and simple mastoidectomy (see section 3–4).
2. A wide simple mastoidectomy is performed with a cutting bur (see section 3–4). Superiorly, mastoid bone is removed until the dura is identified. Posteriorly, drilling is performed to outline the sigmoid sinus and continued inferiorly down to the digastric ridge at the mastoid tip. The posterior wall of the bony meatus is also thinned (Fig. 5–1**A**).
3. A wide exposure of the mastoid cortex is necessary, and elevation of a generous tympanomeatal flap (see section 3–2) is helpful to visualize the middle ear and gauge the depth of the facial nerve. This also makes it easy to disarticulate the incudostapedial joint, if needed, to avoid damaging the inner ear when touching an intact ossicular chain with the drill.
4. The facial nerve is located by thinning the bone over the nerve with a medium-sized diamond bur (Fig. 5–1**B**). The nerve is followed and exposed without entering the bony covering, down to the stylomastoid foramen (Fig. 5–1**C**).
5. Care should be taken always to drill parallel to the course of the nerve. To avoid heat injury to the nerve, drilling is performed for short periods, and copious irrigation is used.

6. A small diamond bur is then used to develop a groove on each side of the nerve, leaving a thin covering of bone over the nerve (Fig. 5–1D).
7. The thin bone is cracked and removed by elevating the fragments with a micro-Tabb knife throughout its length (Fig. 5–1E). If bony fragments are sticking into the nerve or compressing the nerve at the site of a fracture, these are completely removed.
8. The nerve sheath is carefully slit with the tip of a blade taking care not to injure the blood supply of the nerve. A small blunt hook can be used to elevate the sheath as it is slit and to guide the blade (Fig. 5–1F).
9. The postauricular incision is closed as described for tympanoplasty (see section 3–2).

### Complications

1. Facial nerve injury
2. Trauma to semicircular canals
3. Dural laceration
4. Sigmoid sinus hemorrhage
5. Ossicular disarticulation

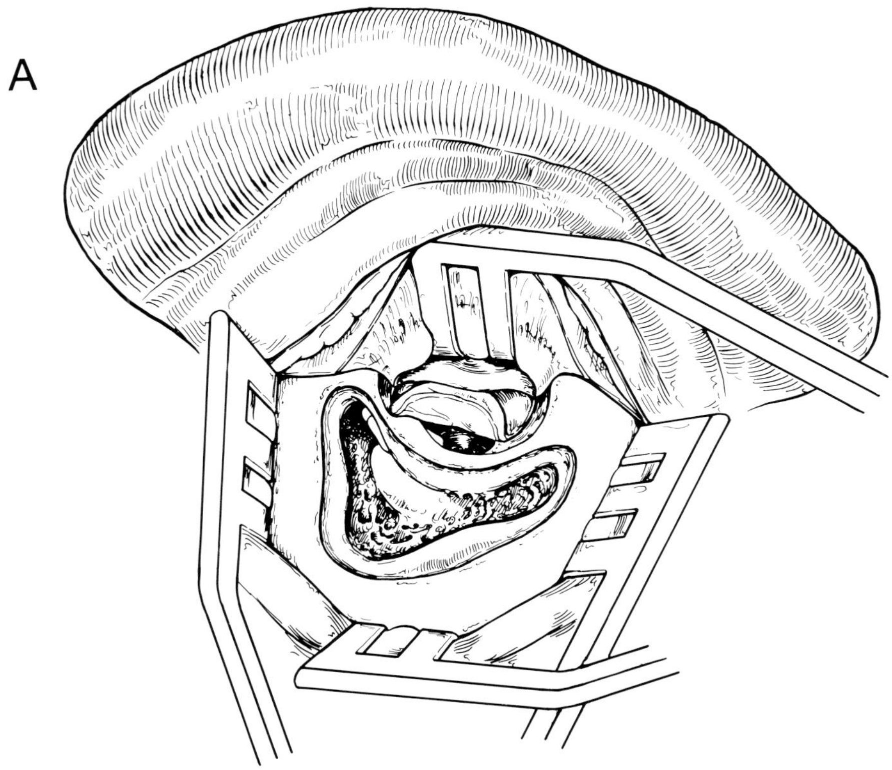


▶ **FIGURE 5-1**

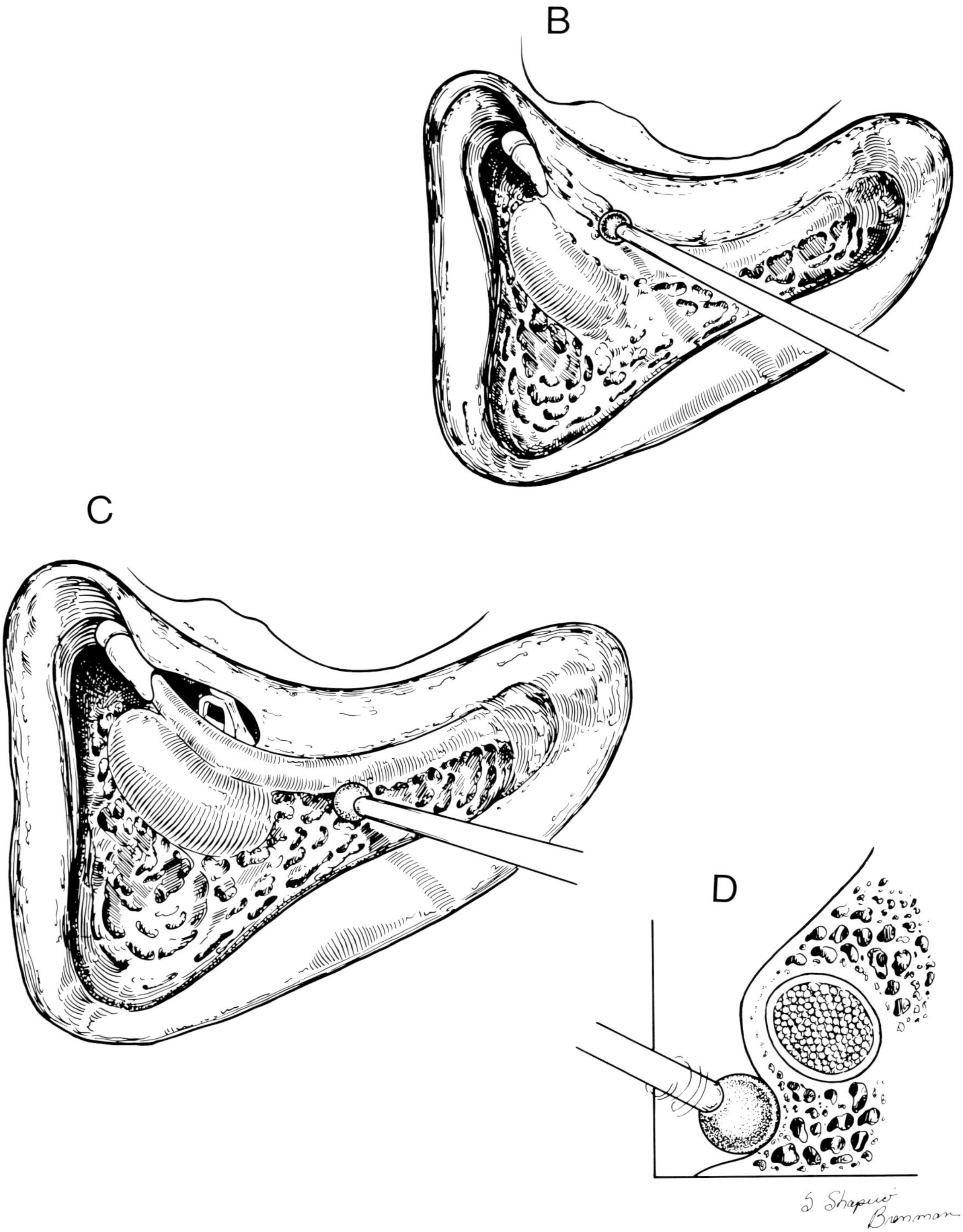


▶ **FIGURE 5-1**

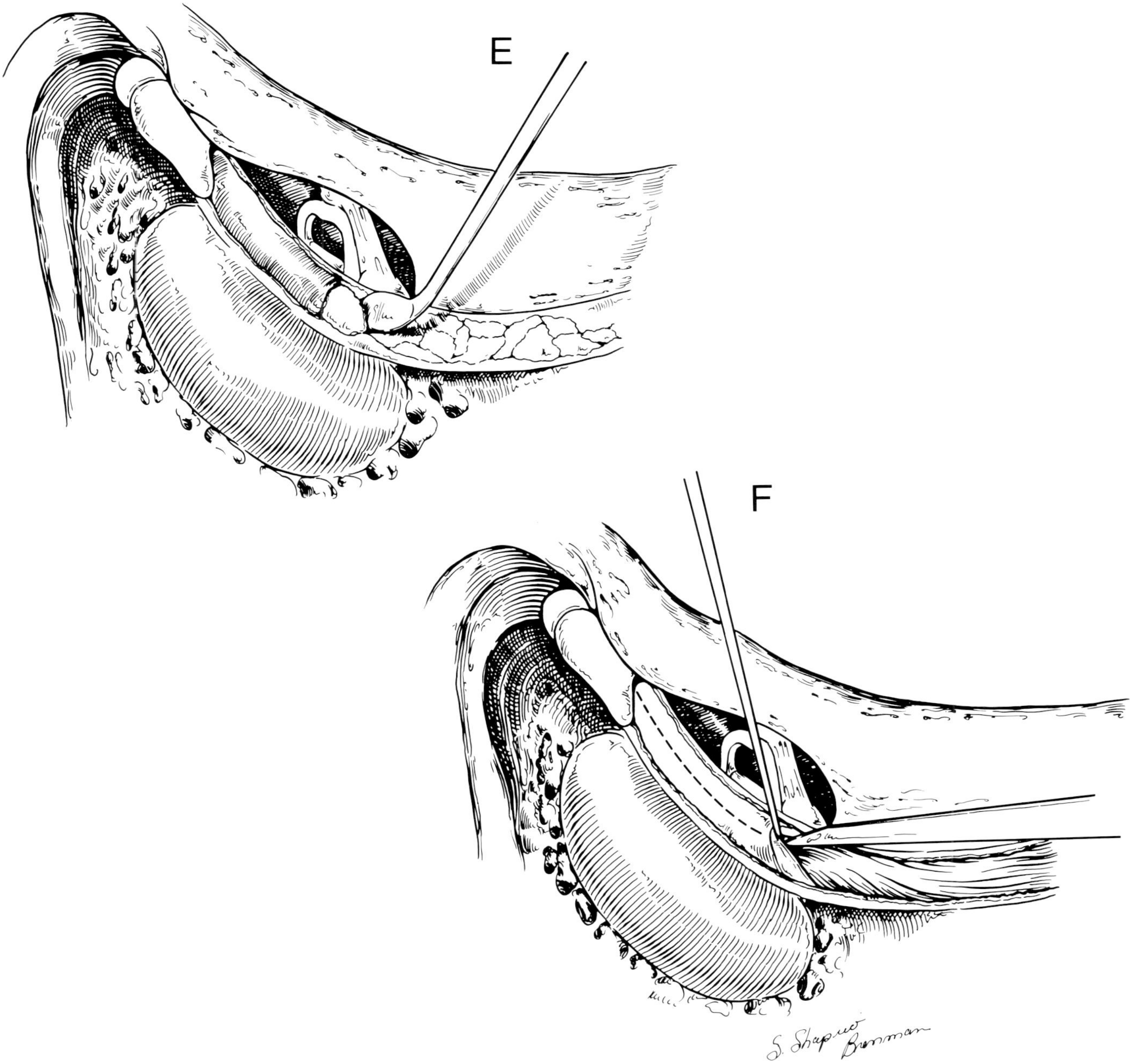


▶ **FIGURE 5-1**

## ▶ 5-2 FACIAL NERVE GRAFTING

Facial nerve grafting is a technique to restore continuity to a severely crushed or severed facial nerve after temporal bone trauma.

### Indications

Facial nerve grafting is indicated when a transsected or severely crushed facial nerve is encountered when performing facial nerve exploration or decompression.

### Preoperative Evaluation

Pneumatic otoscopy and complete audiometry are prerequisites to this procedure. CT scan of the temporal bone is needed to define any fractures. Nerve excitability tests are used to determine the degree of degeneration and need for surgery. The surgeon may elect to utilize intraoperative facial nerve monitoring.

### Operative Technique

1. Facial nerve decompression is performed (see section 5–1).
2. The remaining segments of the nerve are decompressed and the sheath slit as previously described, taking care not to further injure the perineural blood supply (Fig. 5–2**A**). The ragged nerve end is cut cleanly with a 52 Beaver blade (Fig. 5–2**B**). If a segment of nerve has been crushed, it is removed in a similar fashion.
3. A segment of greater auricular nerve is taken through a separate incision in the neck (Fig. 5–2**C**).
4. A single 9-0 monofilament fascicular suture is placed on each side to orient and stabilize the segment of greater auricular nerve between the cut segments of the facial nerve (Fig. 5–2**D, E**).
5. The grafted nerve is covered with wet Gelfilm (Fig. 5–2**F**) and the postauricular incision is closed as in tympanoplasty (see section 3–2).

### Complications

1. Facial nerve injury
2. Trauma to semicircular canals
3. Dural laceration
4. Sigmoid sinus hemorrhage
5. Ossicular disarticulation

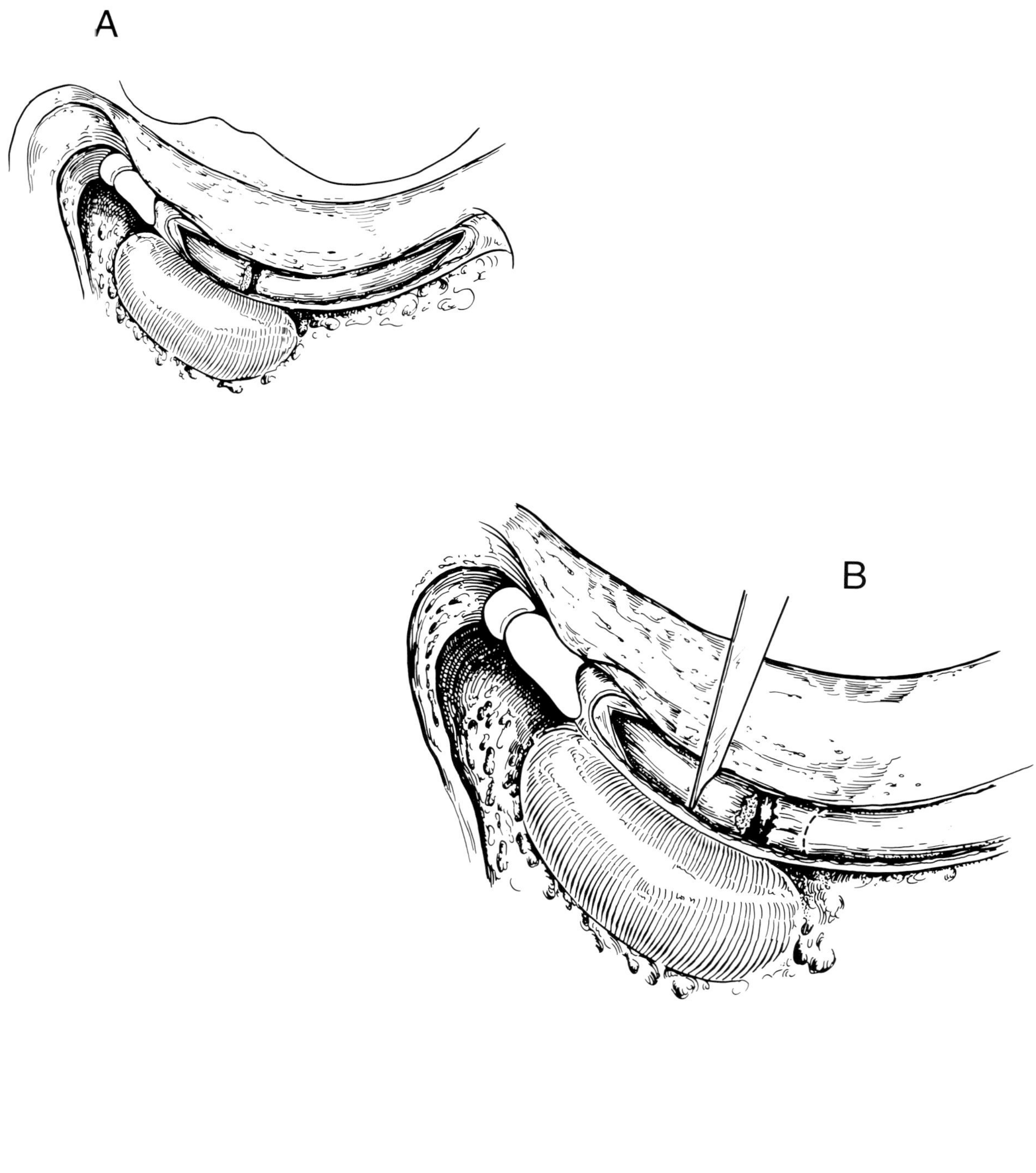


▶ **FIGURE 5-2**

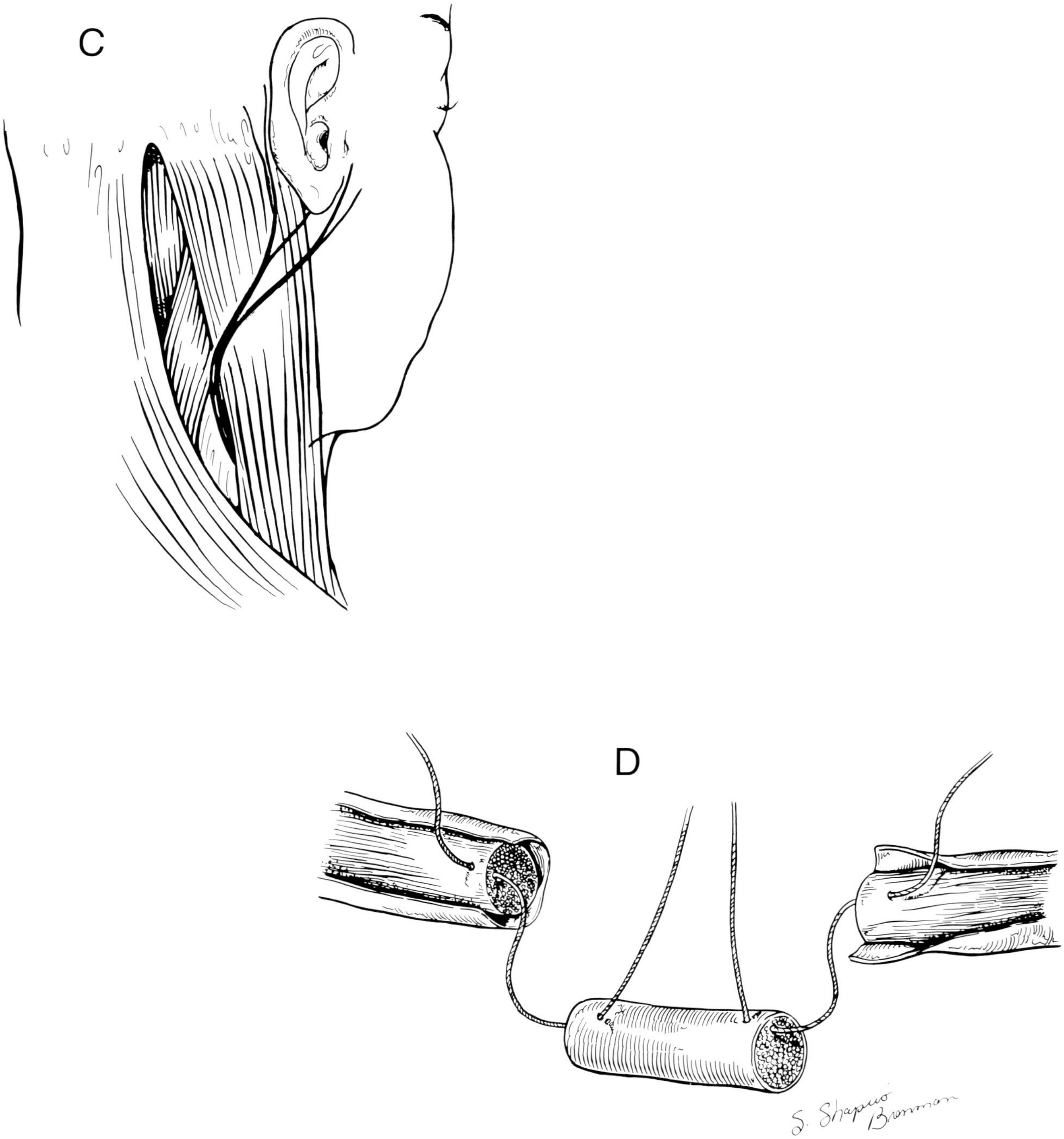


▸ **FIGURE 5-2**

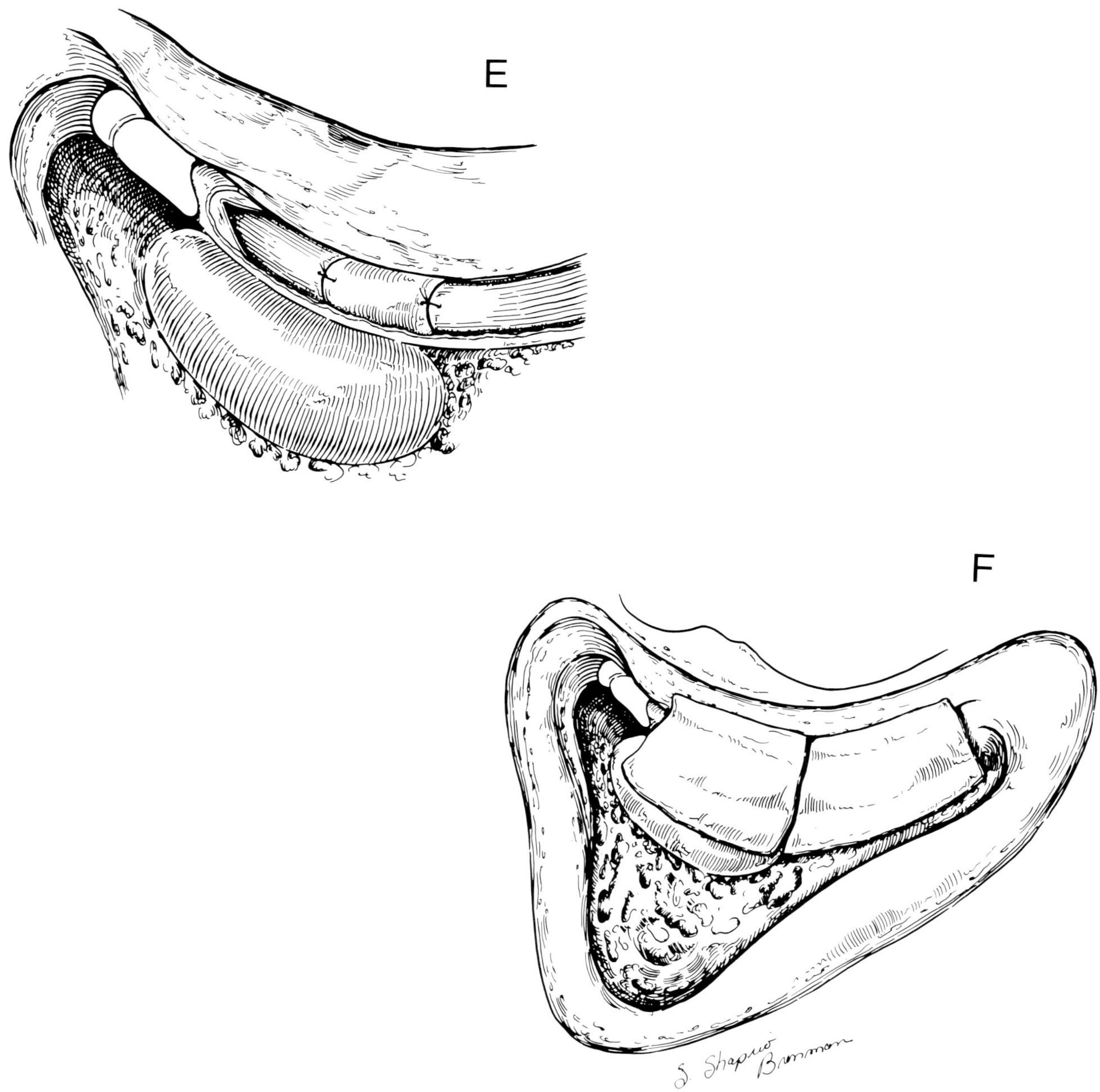


▶ **FIGURE 5-2**

# 6 ▸ Ear Trauma

## ▸ 6-1 HEMATOMA OR SEROMA ASPIRATION

External ear trauma occurs frequently in children because of its prominent and unprotected position and the reflex tendency of head turning to avoid direct facial injury. Blunt trauma may occur during contact sports, such as wrestling, or when children fall. Blunt trauma can lead to separation of the perichondrium from the anterior surface of the auricular cartilage. A hematoma or seroma may fill the space causing a deformity of the ear.

### Indications

Surgical removal of the seroma or hematoma collection is indicated to avoid permanent auricular deformity.

### Preoperative Evaluation

Preoperative evaluation consists of noting the presence of a seroma or hematoma. Associated injuries to the inner and middle ear and the rest of the head must be ruled out.

### Operative Technique (Aspiration)

1. No anesthetic is necessary.
2. After the skin is cleansed with an iodine-containing solution, the tip of a 16- or 18-gauge needle on a 10-cc syringe is placed into the most fluctuant area of the collection (Fig. 6–1**A**).
3. Using gentle pressure with the fingers of the opposite hand, the collection is "milked" to the needle as the fluid is aspirated (Fig. 6–1**A**).
4. After the fluid is aspirated, the area should be firmly compressed by digital pressure for several minutes to prevent immediate reaccumulation of the fluid.
5. A contoured pressure dressing should be created by fitting wet cotton pledgets (soaked with collodion, tincture of benzoin, or saline) to the curves of the auricle and applying a standard mastoid dressing (Fig. 6–1**B**).
6. Antistaphylococcal antibiotics are prescribed for 10 days to prevent chondritis.

### Complications

1. Reaccumulation of hematoma/seroma
2. Chondritis
3. Perichondritis

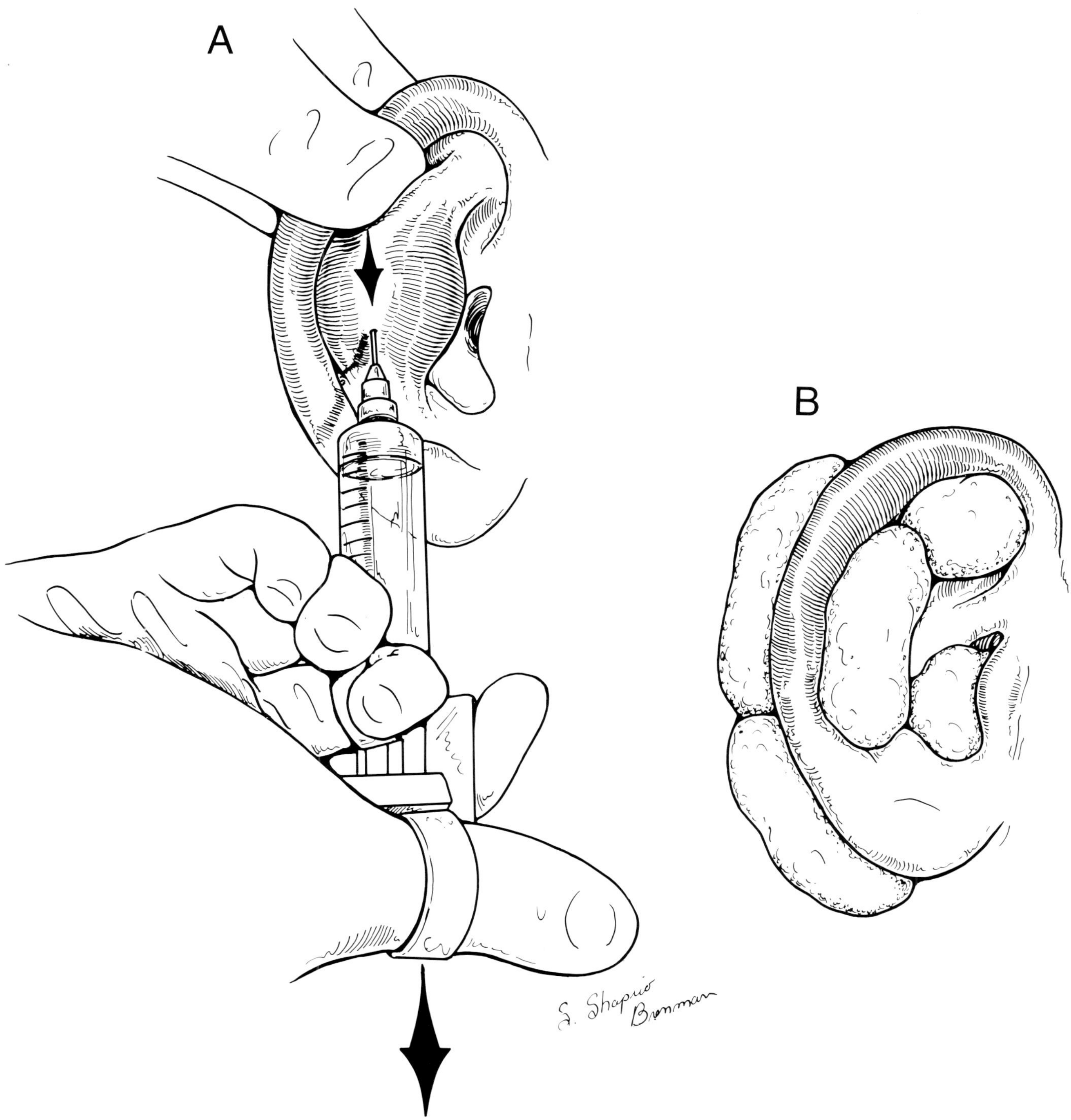


▶**FIGURE 6-1**

## ▶ 6-2 INCISIONAL EVACUATION OF HEMATOMA

### Indications

When a hematoma or seroma is present more than 72 hours, or has recurred after aspiration, incisional evacuation is best (Fig. 6–2A).

### Preoperative Evaluation

Preoperative evaluation consists of noting the presence of a seroma or hematoma. Associated injuries to the inner and middle ear and the rest of the head must be ruled out.

### Operative Technique

1. This procedure usually requires a general anesthetic for children.
2. An incision is made along the lateral margin of the hematoma (Fig. 6–2B).
3. The hematoma is removed thoroughly with a suction (Fig. 6–2C). If necessary, gentle curettage with a small, sharp mastoid curette will remove any fibrogranulomatous material that may have formed.
4. The skin perichondrial flap is replaced, and the skin incision is loosely closed with interrupted 6-0 mild chromic sutures. This allows a pathway for drainage of any additional fluid between the sutures. These sutures dissolve and do not need to be removed (Fig. 6–2D).
5. The perichondrial flap is held in position with 4-0 monofilament sutures (tied over cotton pledgets or rolls) to obliterate the dead space, immobilize the perichondrium, and to apply precise pressure (Fig. 6–2E). These can be removed in 7 to 10 days.
6. Antistaphylococcal antibiotics are prescribed for 10 days to prevent chondritis.

### Complications

1. Reaccumulation of hematoma/seroma
2. Chondritis
3. Perichondritis

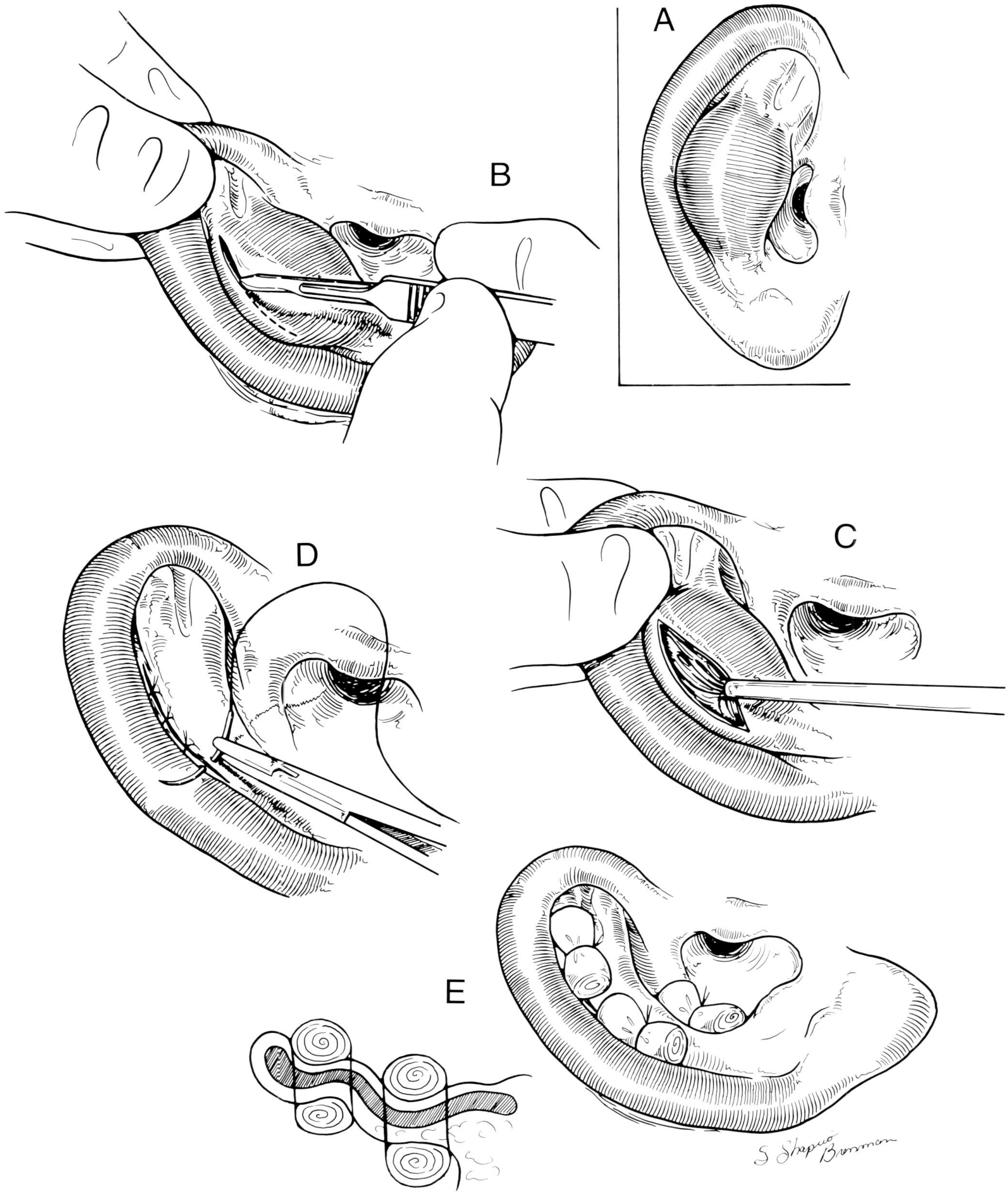


▶ **FIGURE 6-2**

## ▶ 6-3 LACERATIONS

Lacerations of the auricle are frequent in children (Fig. 6–3**A**). Most often they are simple skin lacerations that can be closed easily in a conventional fashion using good, basic plastic surgical technique (see section 45–1). Through-and-through lacerations should be repaired in a way that preserves the contours of the helix and everts the skin to avoid an unsightly notch.

### Indications

Any through-and-through laceration of the auricle must be closed.

### Preoperative Evaluation

The ear must be examined carefully to detect any embedded debris. Associated injuries must also be ruled out.

### Operative Technique

1. Closure of through-and-through lacerations in children is usually accomplished best under general anesthesia using local infiltration with 1% lidocaine and 1:100,000 epinephrine for hemostasis.
2. The wound is carefully debrided of any foreign material.
3. The helical curve is reestablished with a single 6-0 nylon skin suture (Fig. 6–3**B**).
4. The cartilage contour is reestablished by reapproximating only the posterior perichondrium only with 5-0 chromic sutures (Fig. 6–3**C**). Intercartilaginous sutures are rarely required to approximate cartilage.
5. The posterior surface is closed with 5-0 or 6-0 nylon skin sutures (Fig. 6–3**D**).
6. The anterior surface is closed with 5-0 or 6-0 nylon skin suture only (Fig. 6–3**E**).
7. No dressing for the wound is required.

### Complications

1. Poor cosmetic result
2. Chondritis

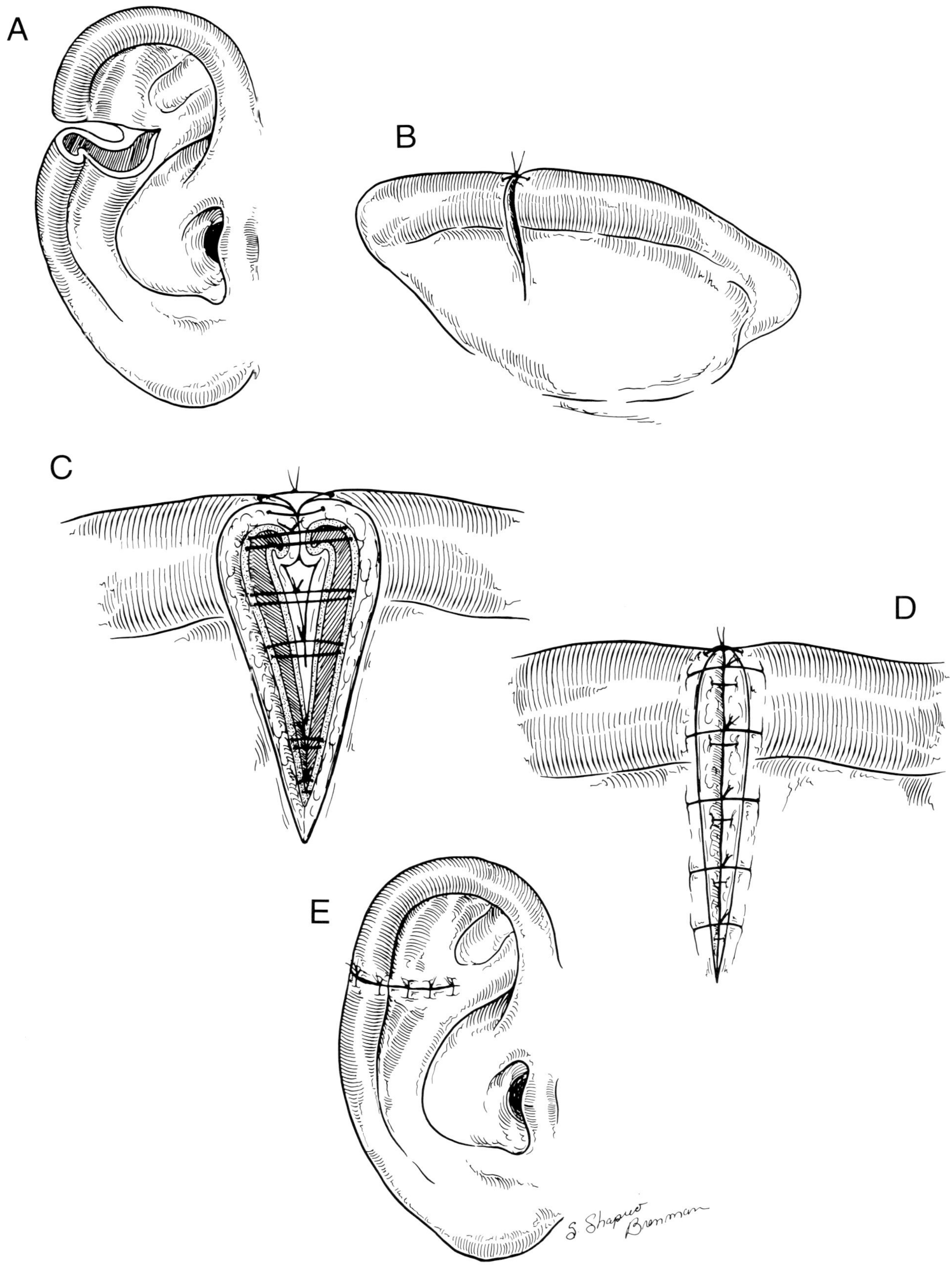


▶ **FIGURE 6-3**

## ▶ 6-4 BURNS AND FROSTBITE

The auricle is often exposed to injury by heat or cold because of its unprotected position and its pedicled blood supply from the scalp.

First- and second-degree burns require only protection from mechanical trauma and antibiotic ointments to prevent infection. Blebs should not be broken unless they become infected. Areas of full-thickness skin loss should be protected and infection prevented by use of systemic and topical antibiotics until the granulating surface can be covered with a split-thickness skin graft.

### Indications

Areas of full-thickness burn or freeze of the ear should be excised to avoid infection and chondritis. Complete demarcation of the dead tissue may take several days. The procedure should be delayed until the full extent of the injury is known because this will determine the extent of the surgical resection.

Chondritis and chondronecrosis often occur several weeks after the acute thermal injury. When it is evident, the involved cartilage must be removed to avoid loss of the entire auricle.

### Operative Technique

1. The debridement of burns and frostbite injuries of the ear is best performed under a general anesthetic.
2. The skin overlying the necrotic cartilage and surrounding any drainage tract is excised with a 5-mm margin of tissue (Fig. 6–4**A, B**).
3. The surrounding skin and perichondrium is elevated with a periosteal elevator exposing the underlying necrotic cartilage below (Fig. 6–4**C**).
4. A wide excision of full-thickness cartilage is performed to the depth of the subcutaneous tissue on the opposite side of the ear. Cartilage should be removed until a normal edge is present (Fig. 6–4**D**).
5. The defect is permitted to granulate and epithelize (Fig. 6–4**E**).
6. Light mesh dressings, changed daily, will keep the surface clean.

### Complications

1. Chondritis
2. Auricular deformity
3. Perichondritis

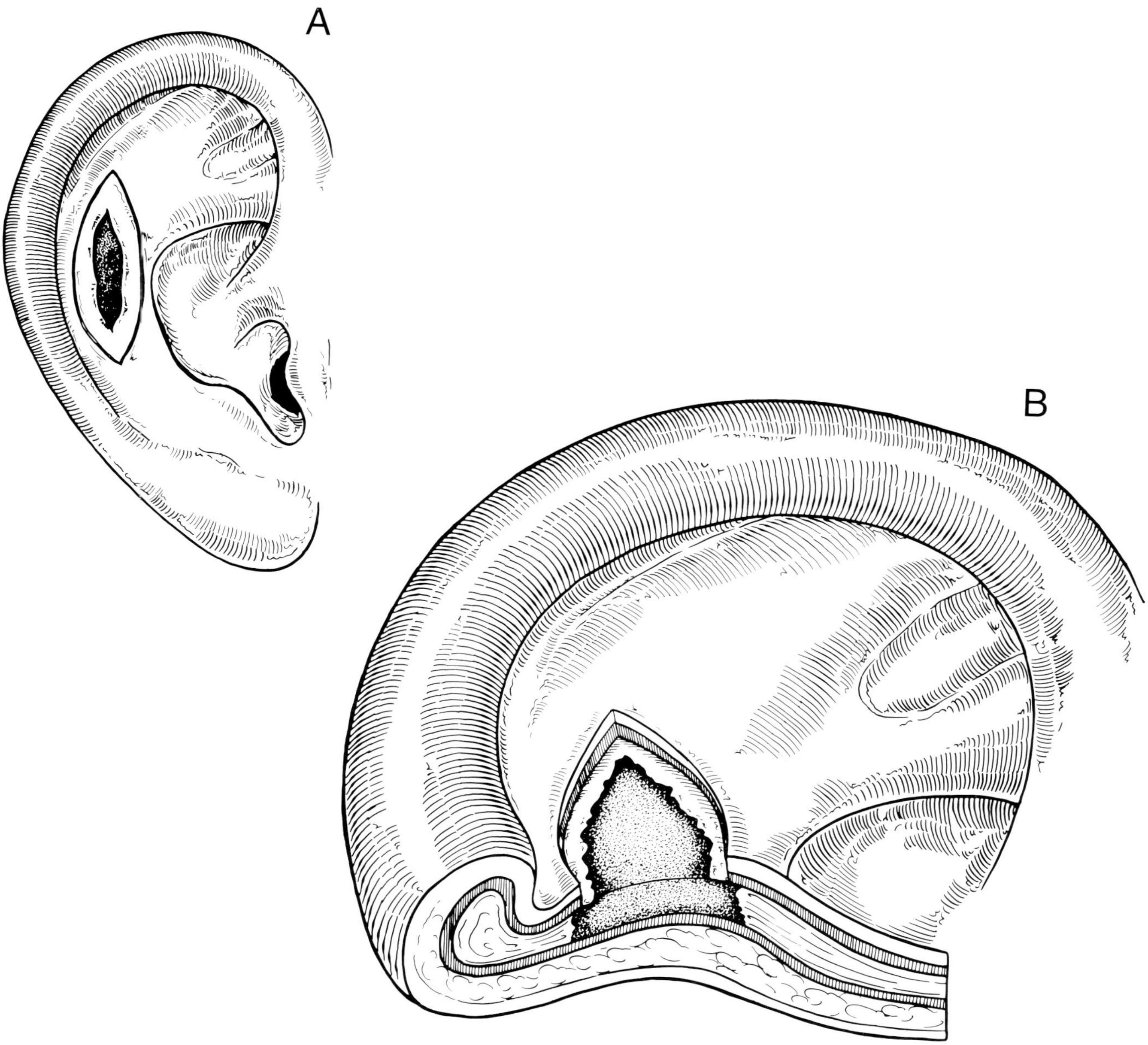


▶ **FIGURE 6-4**

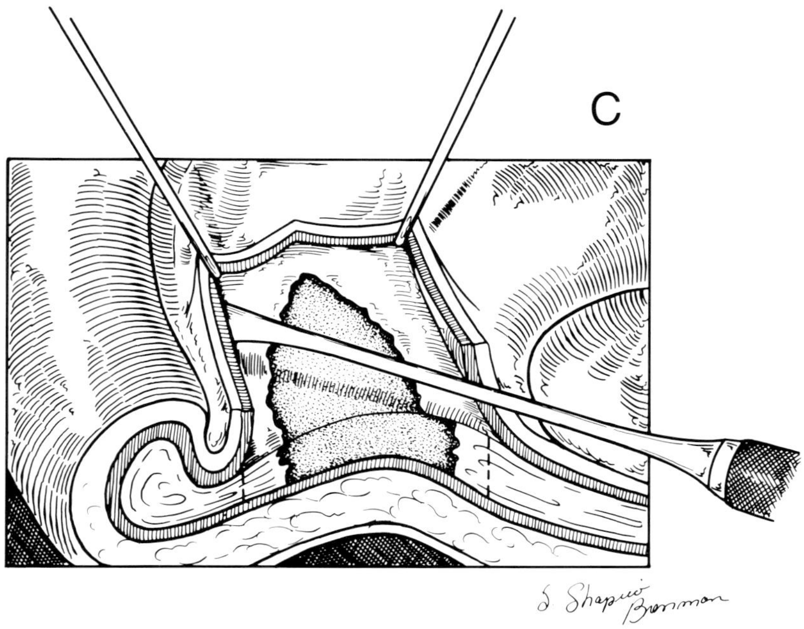

▸ **FIGURE 6-4**

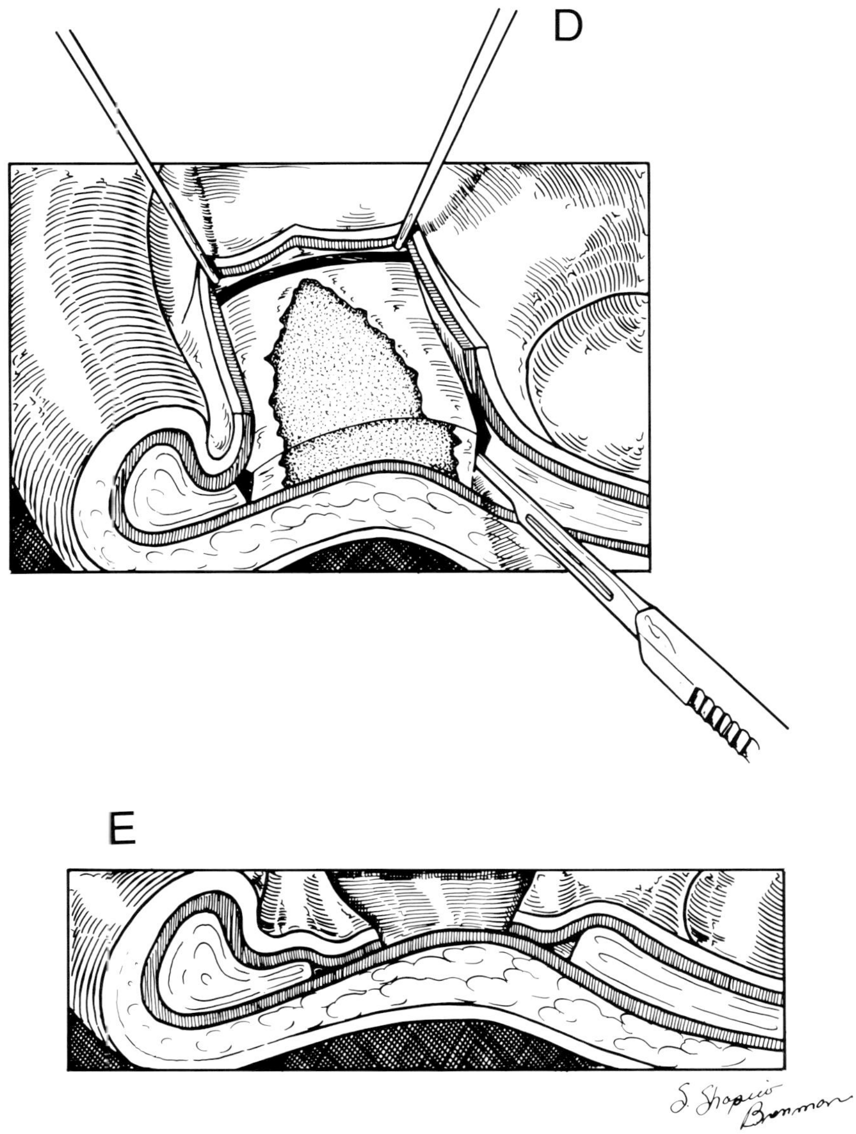


▶ **FIGURE 6-4**

# 7 ▶ Foreign Bodies in the Ear Canal

Foreign bodies in the ear canal are common in children. The most commonly found materials are stones, erasers, paper, and vegetables, such as peas, beans, and corn. Foreign bodies should be removed as soon as possible to avoid infection. No anesthesia is required if the child is cooperative. General anesthesia is indicated in uncooperative children and when the foreign body cannot be removed without pain or damage to the tympanic membrane or ear canal.

## ▶ 7-1 REMOVAL OF FOREIGN BODIES FROM THE EAR CANAL

### Indications

The presence of a foreign body in the ear canal.

### Preoperative Evaluation

An attempt is made to visualize the tympanic membrane distal to the foreign body. This is especially important if one wishes to flush the foreign body out with water. An audiogram may be obtained to determine if there has been damage to the tympanic membrane, ossicles, or inner ear as a result of the foreign body.

### Operative Technique

A large speculum is placed in the outer aspect of the ear canal to visualize the foreign body.

#### Smooth Objects

1. Smooth foreign bodies in the ear canal that do not completely occlude the lumen should be removed with a curette, loop, or blunt ear hook.
2. The loop or hook is gently passed along the ear canal. With gentle pressure, the object is rolled to the external meatus (Fig. 7–1**A**).

#### Sharp-Edged Objects

1. Sharp-edged foreign bodies are most easily and comfortably removed with a small otologic forceps.
2. Rapid removal is important because the sharp edges may scratch the ear canal and make continued patient cooperation impossible.
3. The leading edge should be grasped firmly with a toothed forceps and withdrawn rapidly (Fig. 7–1**B**).

#### Occluding Foreign Bodies

1. Foreign bodies occluding or nearly occluding the ear canal should be irrigated out.
2. The most effective instrument is a 20-cc syringe with a flexible intravenous catheter tip that can be directed to produce a thin, powerful stream of water.
3. Body temperature water is injected along the posterior wall of the ear canal providing a pressure head of water against the drum that forces the foreign body out of the meatus (Fig. 7–1**C**).

### Complications

1. Tympanic membrane perforation
2. Laceration of external canal

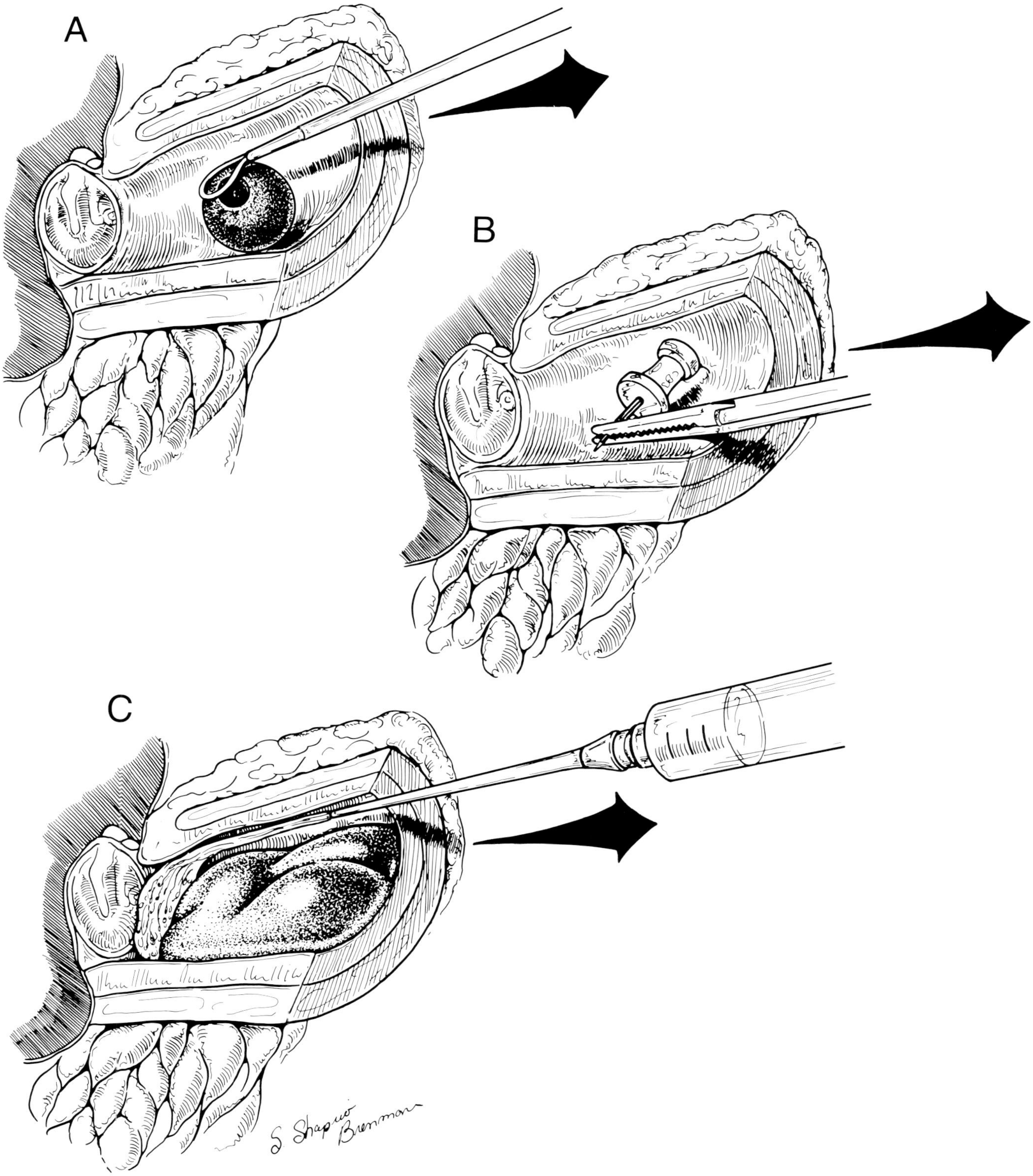


▶ **FIGURE 7-1**

# 8 ▶ Perilymph Fistula Repair

## ▶ 8-1 PERILYMPH FISTULA REPAIR

Perilymph fistula is a leak of fluid from the inner ear into the middle ear. It usually occurs in children following severe head trauma or barotrauma. Spontaneous fistulas do occur and most often happen suddenly during physical stress. Intermittent vertigo and fluctuating hearing loss are characteristics of perilymph fistulas but both are not always present. Recurrent meningitis may result from a perilymph fistula that allows cerebrospinal fluid (CSF) to enter the middle ear space. The location of the leak is usually at the round or oval window areas. However, congenital fissures or traumatic injuries may also be the site of the leak.

### Indications

Middle ear exploration and repair of perilymph fistula is indicated if a perilymph fistula is suggested as the cause of vertigo and/or hearing loss, or recurrent meningitis.

### Preoperative Evaluation

The preoperative evaluation of a child with a suspected perilymph fistula includes an audiogram to document the hearing loss. Computed tomography (CT) may demonstrate inner pathology, such as Mondini's deformity, or middle ear pathology, such as a dislocated incus, especially following severe trauma. However, these studies are rarely positive. Electronystagmography may be helpful to document the nystagmus that may accompany the perilymph fistula.

### Operative Technique

1. General anesthesia and local infiltration with 1% lidocaine with 1:100,000 epinephrine is used as described for tympanoplasty (see section 3–2). A standard postauricular incision for maximum exposure is also employed. In older children, with a large ear canal, a transcanal approach can be used as described for middle ear exploration (see section 4–4).
2. The middle ear space is exposed by incising and elevating a tympanomeatal flap (Fig. 8–1**A**).
3. Bone is removed with a curette or drill in the posterior-superior portion of the ear canal to provide visualization of the entire stapes footplate (Fig. 8–1B). Care is taken to avoid traumatizing the chorda tympani nerve.
4. Sufficient bone is removed to permit complete visualization of the oval and round window areas (Fig. 8–1C). The middle ear is examined and the fistula, if present, is located. The region of the oval window and round window should be dried with gentle suction and watched for accumulation of fluid for up to 20 minutes. Having the anesthesiologist maintain a full inhalation for several seconds may increase the pressure in the subarachroid space and increase the flow of fluid out of the fistula.

5. If the fistula is small, the mucosa surrounding the edges of the fistula of the round and/or oval window is removed with a pick and small hook (Fig. 8–1D).
6. The defect and surrounding denuded bone is covered with connective tissue, (e.g., fascia or perichondrium) (Fig. 8–1E). Fascia may be obtained from the temporalis muscle and perichondrium is easily obtained from the tragus or conchal cartilage. The connective tissue graft is held firmly in place with Gelfoam pledgets (Fig. 8–1F).
7. The tympanomeatal flap is then replaced and is held in place with a single piece of Gelfoam (see section 4–4, Middle Ear Exploration).

If a large or complex defect occurs in the stapes footplate, removal of the mucosal edge of the fistula may be difficult, and covering the defect with connective tissue may not be sufficient to close the leak (Fig. 8–1G). Stapedectomy (see section 4–6) is then required. A piece of "boat-shaped" perichondrium is obtained from the tip of the tragus.

1. The suprastructure of the stapes should be removed by disarticulating the incudostapedial joint (Fig. 8–1G) and cutting the stapedius tendon (Fig. 8–1H).
2. The crura should be removed with a forceps exposing the remaining footplate (Fig. 8–1I).
3. The footplate fragments and mucosal adhesions are removed with a hook (Fig. 8–1J).
4. The previously obtained perichondrial "boat" graft is placed over the open oval window (Fig. 8–1K).
5. A wire or wire Teflon prosthesis is then positioned between the incus and the connective tissue graft overlying the oval window if the ear has auditory function (Fig. 8–1L).
6. The wire is secured by closing it around the incus with a crimper or alligator forceps. Several small pieces of connective tissue are then placed around the wire to hold it in place (Fig. 8–1M).
7. The tympanomeatal flap is then replaced and the postauricular incision is closed as described for tympanoplasty (see section 3–2).

## Complications

1. Recurrent fistula
2. Trauma to chorda tympani
3. Facial nerve injury
4. Tympanic membrane perforation
5. Sensorineural hearing loss
6. Vertigo

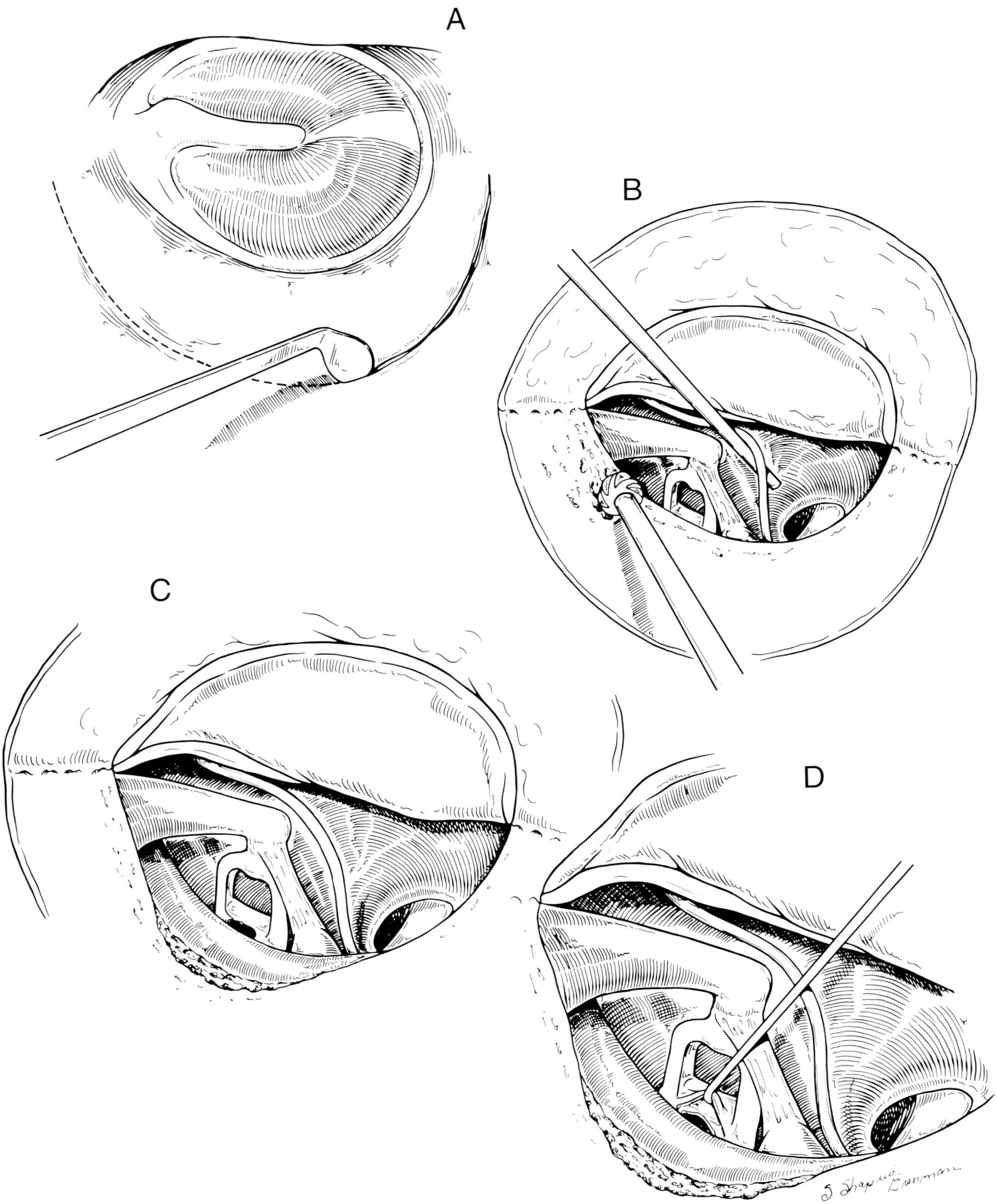


▶ **FIGURE 8-1**

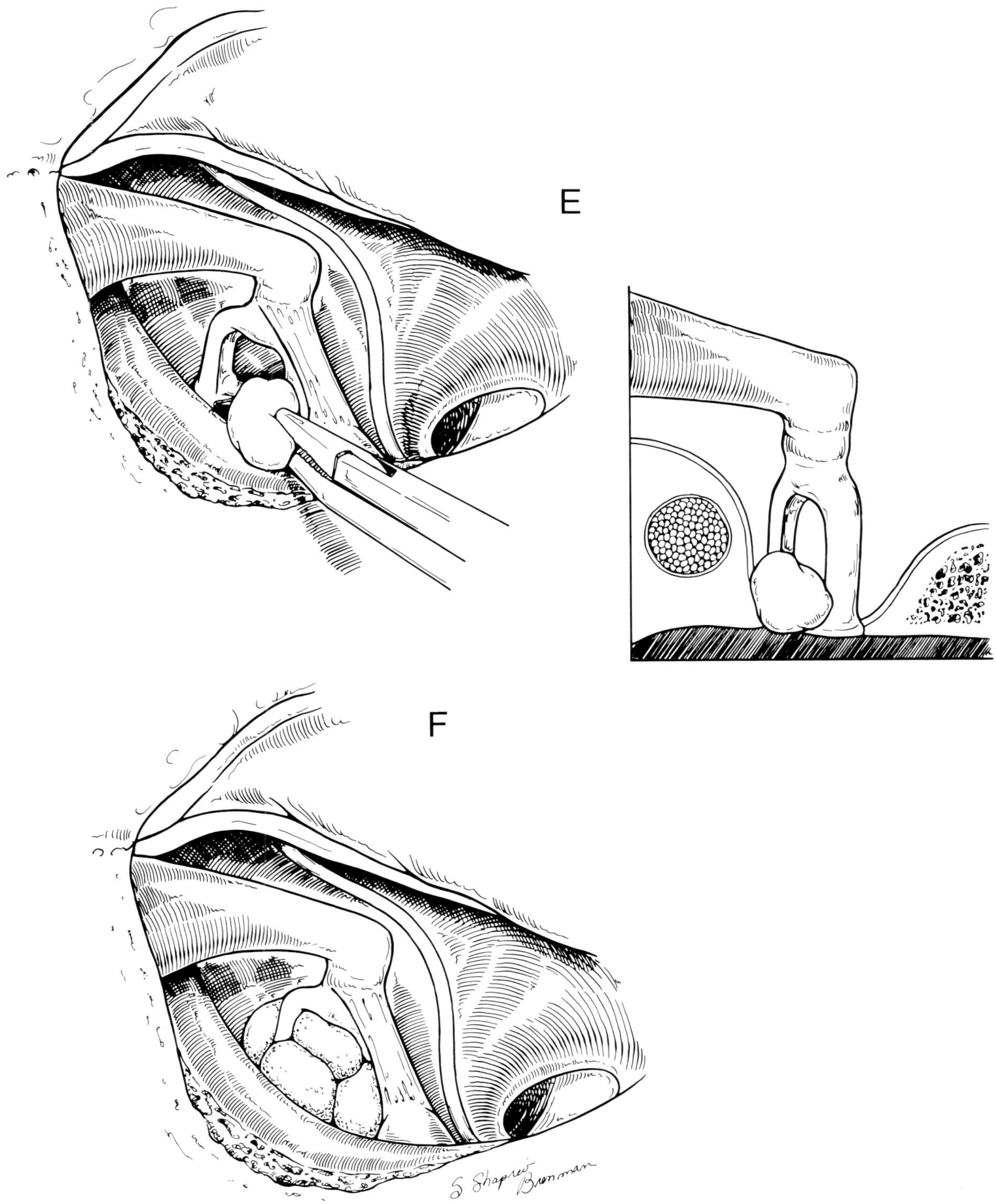


▸ **FIGURE 8-1**

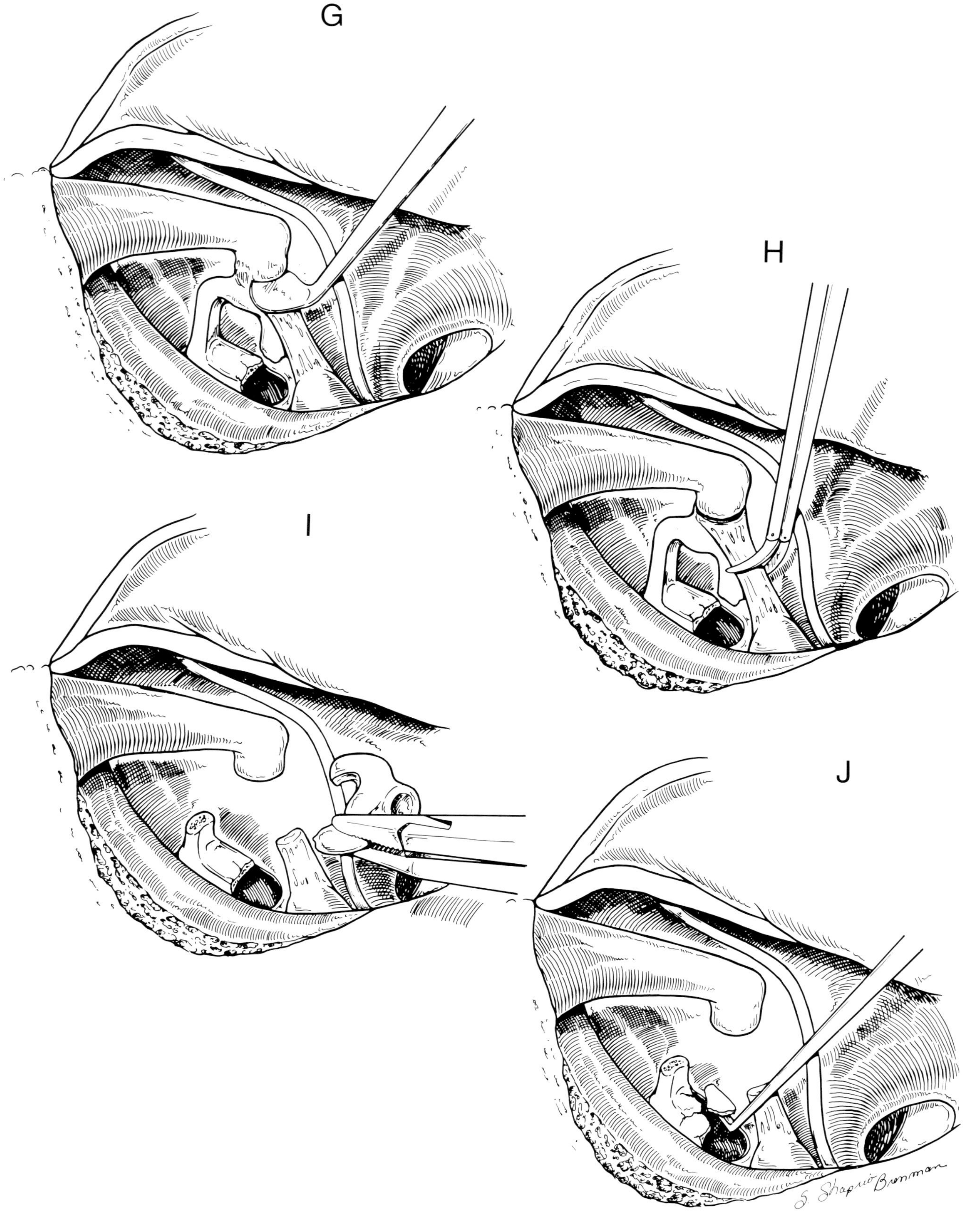


▶ **FIGURE 8-1**

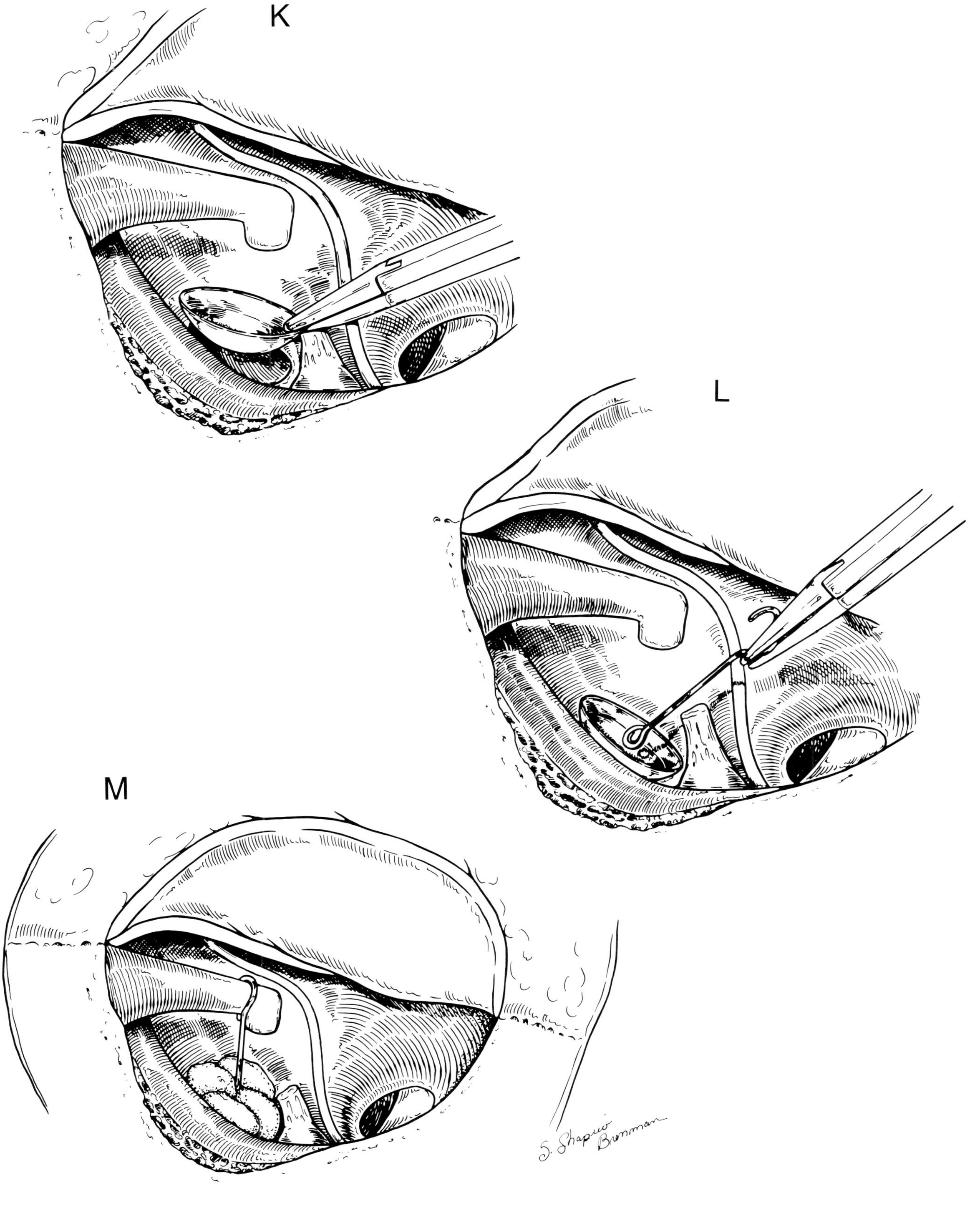


▶ **FIGURE 8-1**

# 9 ▶ Osteoma of the Ear Canal

Osteomas occur in the bony external meatus and are usually seen in teenagers who are cold-water swimmers or surfers. They are often multiple and bilateral. They appear as rounded, broad masses covered by thin skin.

## ▶ 9-1 EXCISION OF OSTEOMA OF THE EAR CANAL

### Indications

Removal of osteomas is indicated if they are large enough to occlude the external canal so that wax accumulates and sound transmission is hampered. Recurrent bouts of otitis externa from moisture and wax trapped behind the osteomas is another indication for removal.

### Preoperative Evaluation

Otoscopy will usually show a narrowed external auditory canal. Computed tomography (CT) should be performed to determine the medial extent of the osteoma if it cannot be determined by inspection. A complete audiologic assessment is performed prior to the procedure.

### Operative Technique

1. Any external canal infection or retained debris should be treated preoperatively by a 10-day course of antibiotic-containing ear drops.
2. Osteomas are most often removed under general anesthesia. The ear canal and postauricular area are injected with 1% lidocaine with 1:100,000 epinephrine as described for tympanoplasty (see section 3–2).
3. A standard postauricular incision as in tympanoplasty (see section 3–2) is used to expose the ear canal lateral to the osteomas (Fig. 9–1**A**).
4. An "H" incision is made on the dome of the osteoma. The lateral skin and periosteal flap is elevated (Fig. 9–1**B**).
5. The remaining medial skin and periosteal flap is elevated as far as is possible exposing the osteoma (Fig. 9–1**C**).
6. The center of the osteoma is removed with a cutting bur (Fig. 9–1**D, E**).
7. The bone of the dome is then thinned with a diamond bur from within the excavated osteoma leaving only a thin superior rim (Fig. 9–1**F**).
8. The periosteum and skin overlying the osteoma can be protected as the thin shell of bone is removed with a curette (Fig. 9–1**G**).
9. This should be done gradually until the osteoma is removed and the tympanic membrane can be seen.
10. The skin flaps are then replaced to cover the exposed bone. Excess overlapping skin should be trimmed as needed (Fig. 9–1**H**).
11. The ear canal is packed with Gelfoam soaked in antibiotic otic drops and the postauricular incision is closed in the standard fashion as for tympanoplasty (see section 3–2).

## Complications

1. Recurrence of osteoma
2. Tympanic membrane perforation
3. Canal stenosis

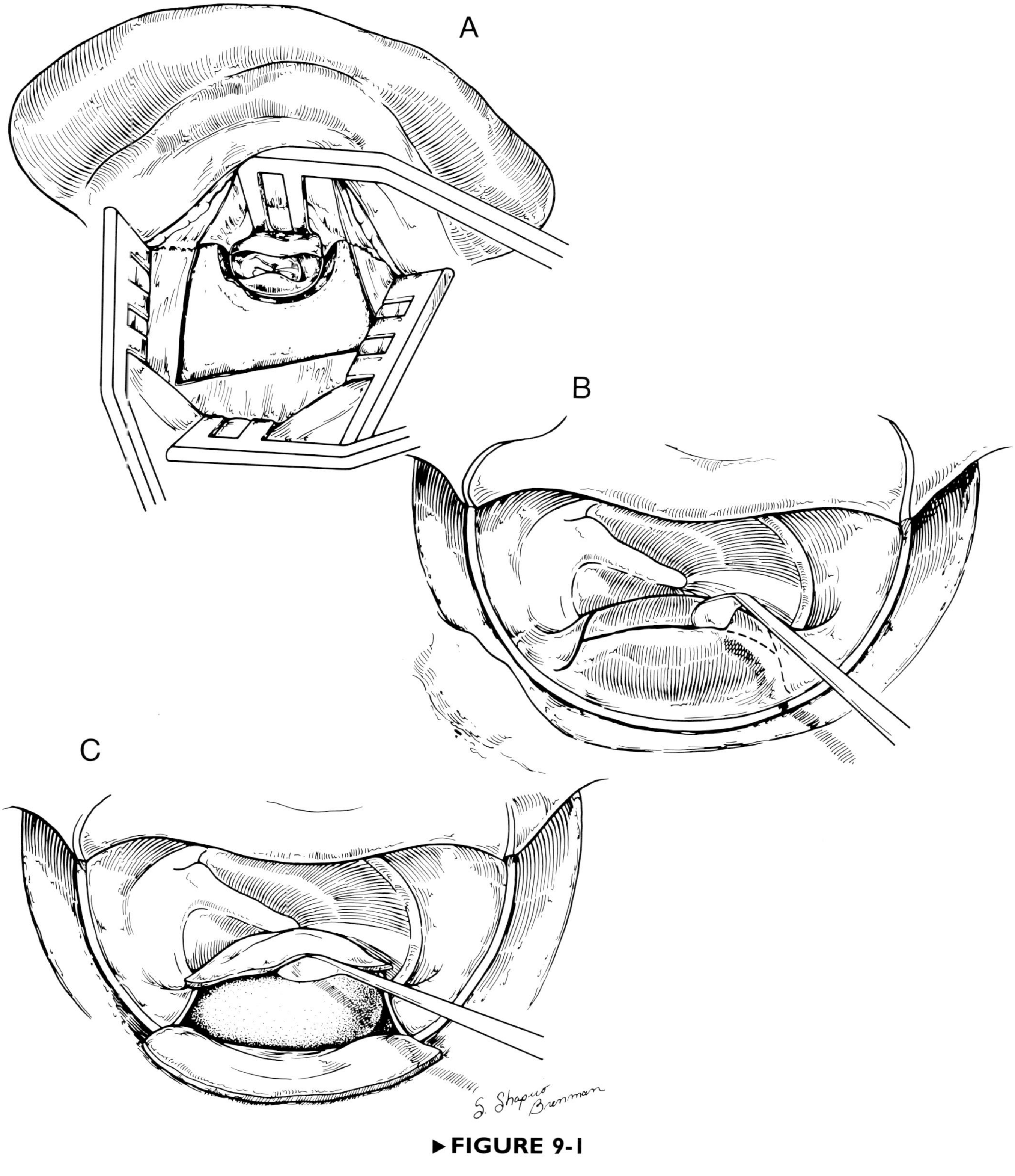


▶ **FIGURE 9-1**

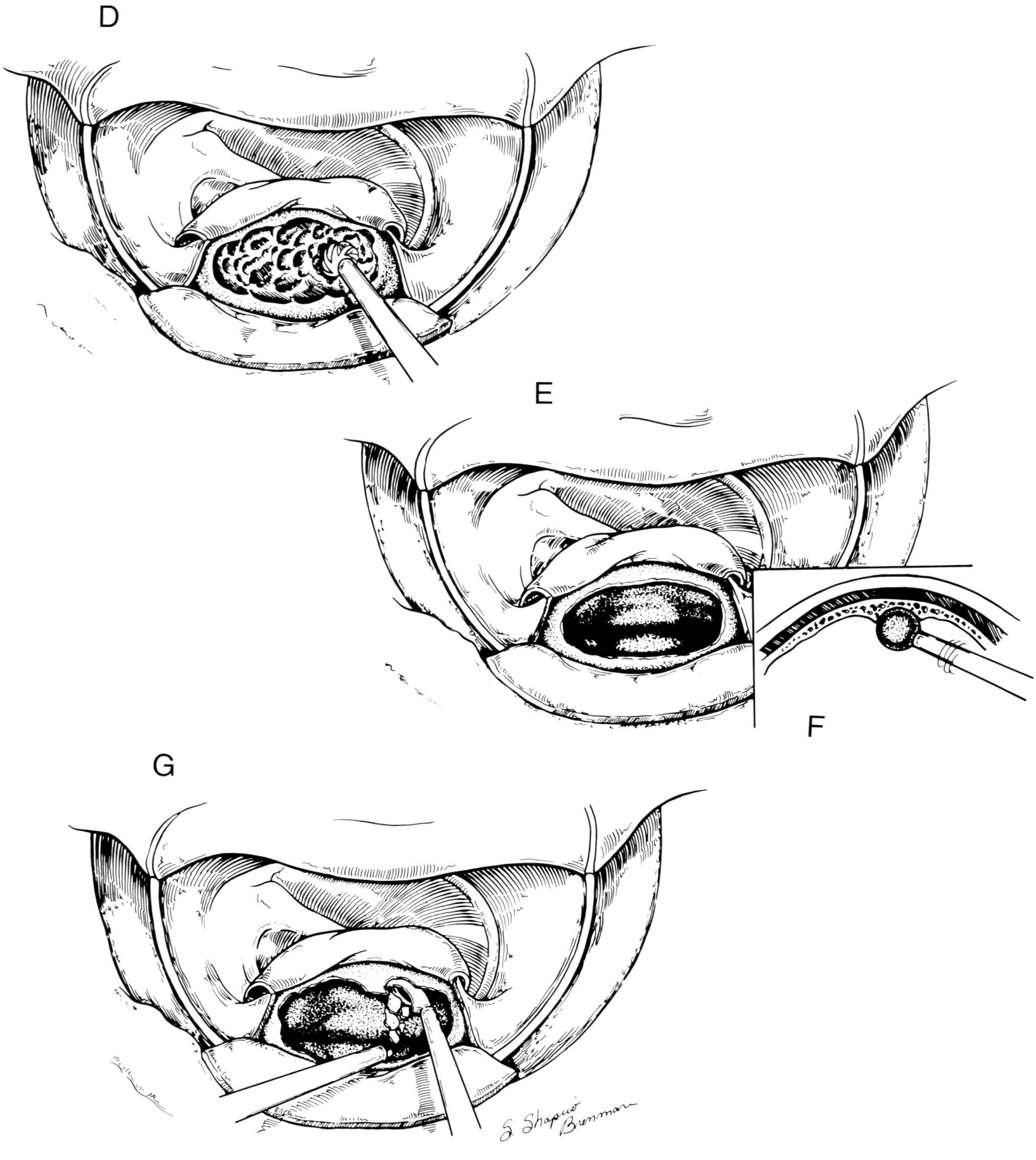


▶ **FIGURE 9-1**

H

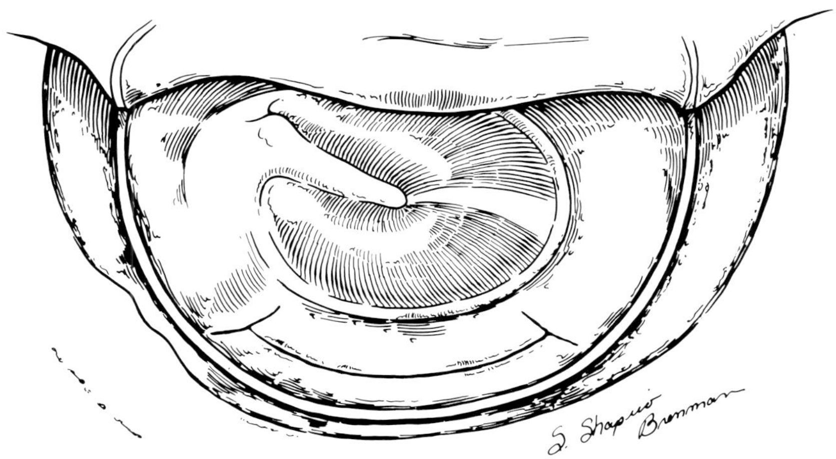

▶ **FIGURE 9-1**

# 10 ▶ Cochlear Implantation (Bruce Gantz, M.D.)

Cochlear implantation is a procedure in which a device is implanted into the cochlea to transform received sound into electrical energy to stimulate the cochlea. This procedure is in a constant state of development and will improve with advances in technology. Implantation in children has advanced beyond the experimental stage to taking its place among the methods available for rehabilitation of profoundly hearing-impaired children.

## ▶ 10-1 COCHLEAR IMPLANTATION

### Indications

Cochlear implantation is indicated in children aged 2 years or older who are bilaterally, profoundly deaf, and unable to understand speech with an appropriate hearing aid. The devices are being used in both pre- and postlingually deafened children.

### Preoperative Evaluation

Computed tomography (CT) of the temporal bone with views of the cochlea are obtained to determine the anatomy of the temporal bone and patency of the cochlea.

A complete multidisciplinary cochlear implant team evaluation is required to determine the auditory status, as well as the psychosocial suitability of the child and family for implantation. The surgeon may elect to utilize intraoperative facial nerve monitoring.

### Operative Technique

1. Cochlear implantation in children is performed under general anesthesia without muscle paralysis to permit facial nerve monitoring. Intravenous broad spectrum antibiotics are given intraoperatively.
2. The patient is positioned lying flat on his/her back with the head turned to the opposite side.
3. The hair is shaved to approximately 6 cm behind the hairline (Fig. 10–1**A**).
4. After prepping, placing facial nerve monitoring electrodes, and draping the patient, the incision line is drawn with a marking pencil. A wide strip of tissue attachment (4–5 cm) is maintained superior and posterior to the helix to provide adequate blood supply to the skin flap through branches of the superficial temporal artery. The skin is injected with 1% lidocaine with 1:100,000 epinephrine for hemostasis (Fig. 10–1**B**).
5. The incision is made through the scalp and subcutaneous tissue to the level of the temporalis fascia. A skin and subcutaneous tissue flap is elevated anteriorly by sharp dissection with a knife to the level of the external meatus exposing the temporalis fascia and mastoid periosteum. Hemostasis is obtained by cauterization (Fig. 10–1**C**).
6. The skin flap is wrapped with a wet sponge and reflected forward.

7. A rectangular flap $2\frac{1}{2}$ to 3 cm wide is made by cutting through periosteum with a bovie along the temporalis line superiorly. The lower incision is 0.5 cm inferior to the lower edge of the external meatus, and the limbs are connected posteriorly (Fig. 10–1**D**).
8. The periosteal flap is elevated anteriorly with a periosteal elevator (Fig. 10–1**E**).
9. An incision is made with the cautery through the temporalis muscle to bone and through the mastoid periosteum (Fig. 10–1**F**).
10. A subtemporalis-subperiosteal flap is developed posteriorly with the periosteal elevator. The flap is used to hold the implant in place, prevent extrusion (as well as skin breakdown), and to ensure that the implant is not in contact with the skin suture line (Fig. 10–1**G**).
11. A self-retaining retractor is positioned to expose the mastoid area. A mastoidectomy is performed with a cutting bur while maintaining a small overhang of mastoid cortex bone in the region of the tegmen (Fig. 10–1**H**).
12. The antrum is opened and the horizontal semicircular canal and short process of the incus are identified (Fig. 10–1**I**). The posterior wall of the bony external meatus is then thinned with a cutting bur.
13. A seat for the electronics of the implant is made by removing a flat portion of the posterior-superior mastoid cortex and skull bone (Fig. 10–1**J**). Hemostasis of the bone is obtained with bone wax. Sufficient bone is removed to accommodate a portion of the inner coil of the electronics package in the skull (Fig. 10–1**K**).
14. Two holes, approximately 0.5 cm apart, are drilled through the overhang of bone with a small cutting bur (Fig. 10–1**L**).
15. A small diamond bur is used to carefully open the facial recess, permitting visualization of the stapes and round window niche, which is inferior to the oval window. The chorda tympani nerve is preserved, if possible (Fig. 10–1**M**). Care is taken *not* to remove all bone over the facial nerve.
16. Mucosa is removed from the bone of the round window niche with a small hook.
17. The bony overhang is removed with a 1-mm diamond bur to expose the round window membrane (Fig. 10–1**N**).
18. A cochleostomy is made with a 0.8-mm diamond bur anterior and inferior to the round window membrane annulus. The bone is gradually removed until the blue-appearing inner portion can be seen. Small bone fragments may be removed with a pick or rasp (Fig. 10–1**O**).
19. Before handling the cochlear implant, the surgical field is irrigated and suctioned clean. The surgeon's gloves are washed with saline and the monopolar cautery is removed from the field. Bipolar cautery is used throughout the remainder of the operation to avoid damage to the implant.
20. The electrodes of the implant are advanced through the cochleostomy by gentle manipulation with a claw or smooth alligator forceps, and by rotating the electrode (clockwise for the left ear and counterclockwise for the right ear) (Fig. 10–1**P**). Care is taken *not* to damage or kink the electrode array.
21. In a Nucleus implant, the last 10 electrodes in the implant are nonfunctioning and may be manipulated more safely (Fig. 10–1**Q**).

22. After advancing as many electrodes as possible (without using force) through the cochleostomy, the implant is secured with a 4-0 nylon suture passed through the perforations in the mastoid bone near the tegmen and tied in place (Fig. 10–1**R**).
23. A strip of temporalis fascia and muscle are taken from the region of the temporalis incision. A portion is placed around the electrode and tucked into the cochleostomy with a pick (Fig. 10–1**R**). A second piece is positioned between the facial ridge and the implant in the opened facial recess, elevating the implant from the facial nerve.
24. The electronics package is placed securely in the mastoid-skull seat (Fig. 10–1**S**) with the posterior portion under the temporalis periosteal flap (Fig. 10–1**T**).
25. A $\frac{1}{4}$-inch Penrose drain is placed in the mastoid and brought out of the inferior portion of the wound. The implant site is then closed by suturing the temporalis incision, mastoid periosteal incision, and the quadrangular flap as closely approximated as possible with 3-0 Vicryl suture (Fig. 10–1**U**).
26. If the quadrangular flap is not desired to help secure the implant, it is draped into the mastoid to reinforce the posterior canal and enhance its blood supply.
27. The incision is closed with 4-0 interrupted undyed Vicryl in the subcutaneous soft tissue and 4-0 running, interlocking nylon in the skin (Fig. 10–1**V**).
28. The external magnet is placed over the implant to test the electrodes to assure function of the implant (Fig. 10–1**V**).
29. The relationship of the external magnet to the underlying implant is shown in Figure 10–1**W**.
30. A mastoid pressure dressing is applied.
31. The drain is removed on the first or second postoperative day, depending on the amount of drainage. The patient is given broad spectrum antibiotics for 10 to 14 days. The skin sutures are removed in 7 to 10 days.

## Complications

1. Skin flap tissue loss
2. Electrode not placed properly
3. Facial nerve paralysis
4. Implant damage
5. Vertigo

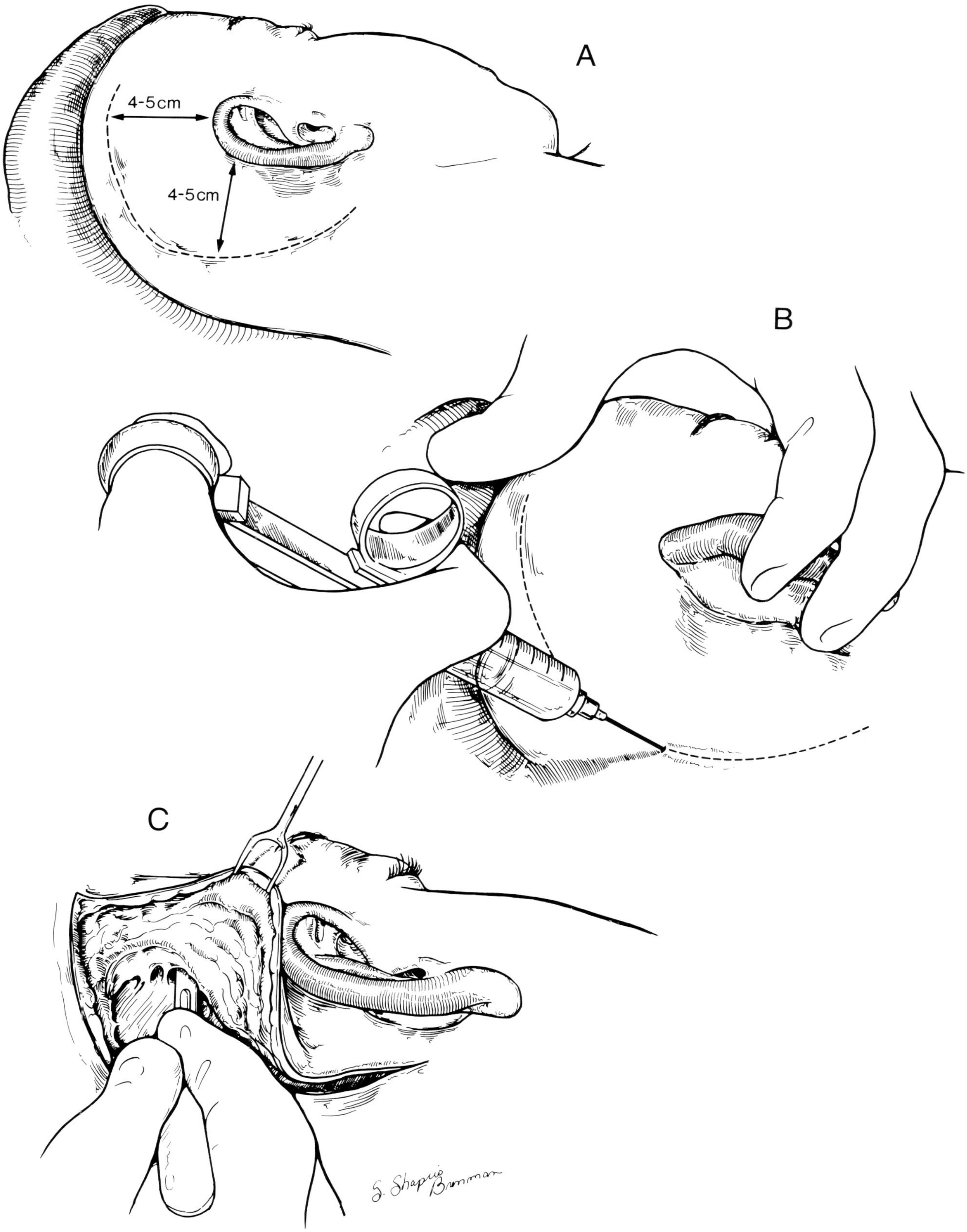


▶ **FIGURE 10-1**

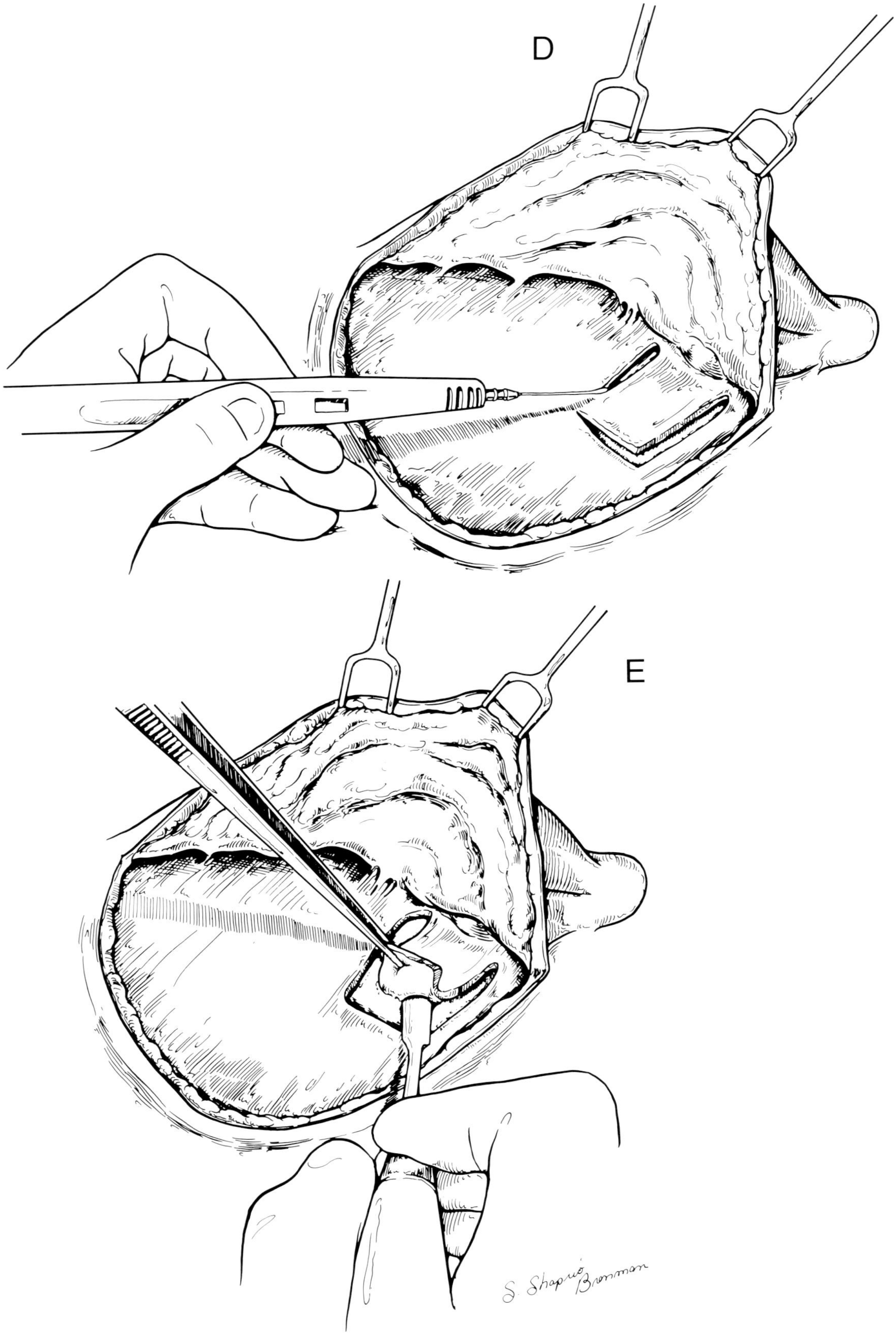


▶ **FIGURE 10-1**

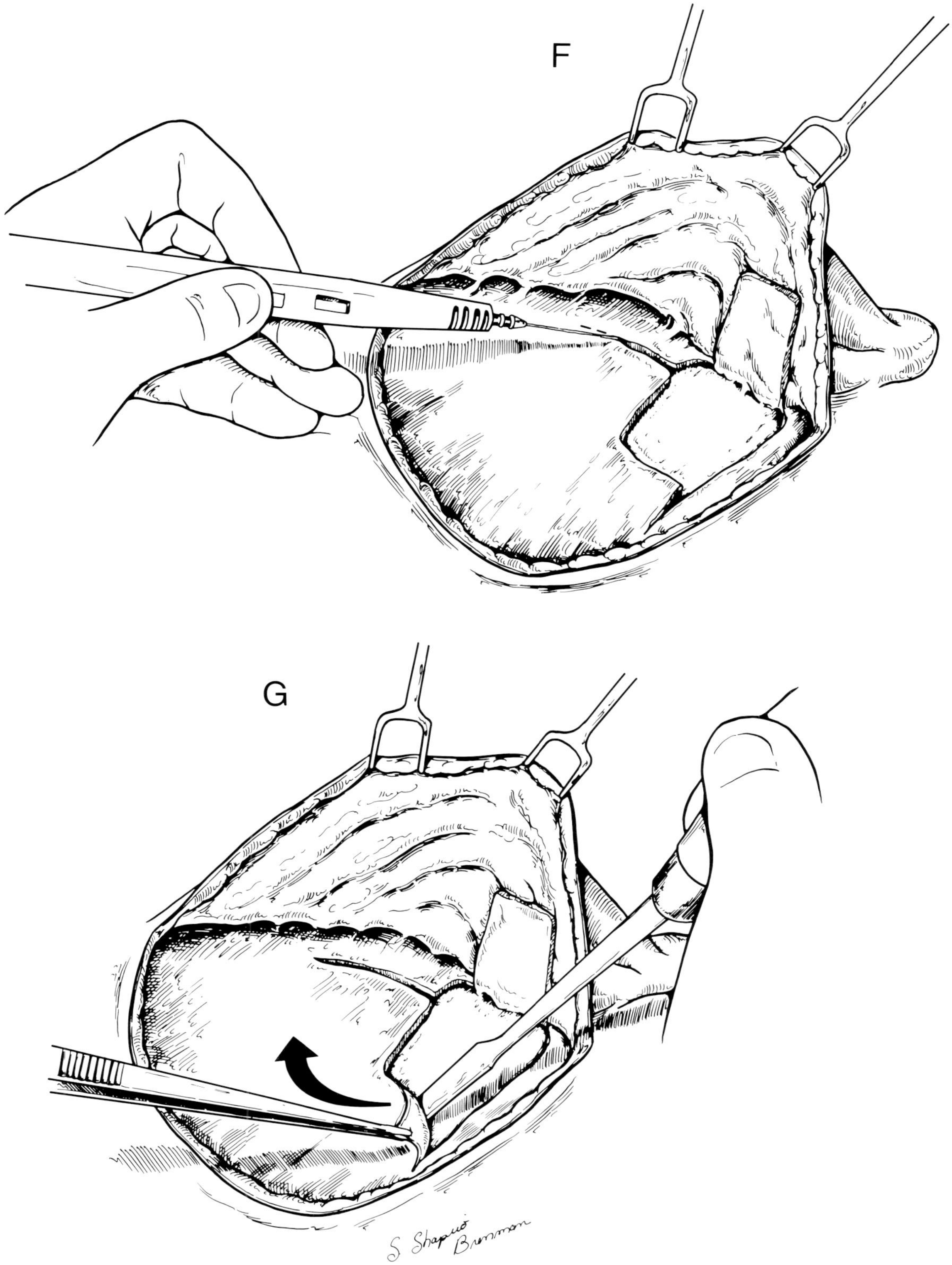


▶**FIGURE 10-1**

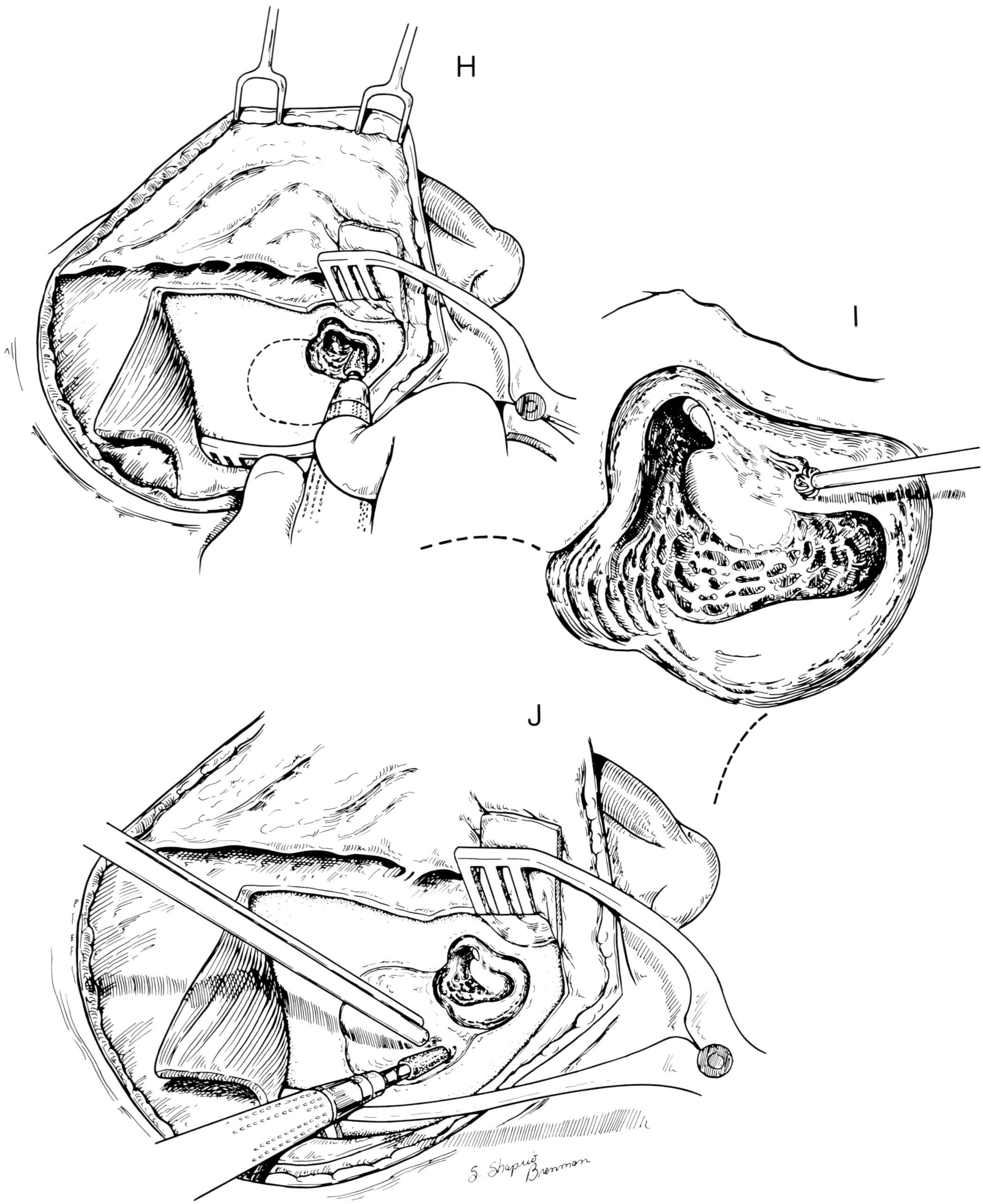


▶ **FIGURE 10-1**

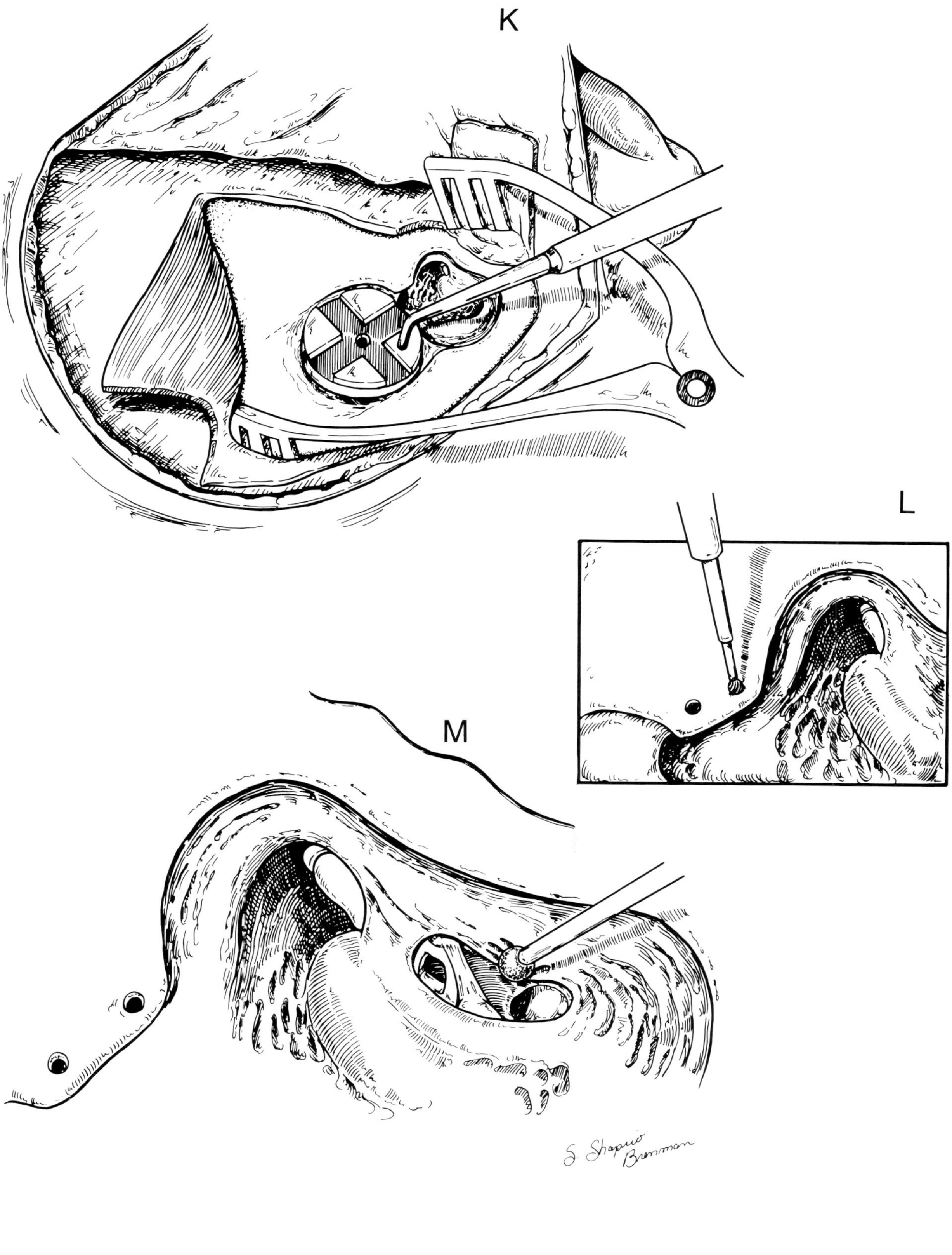


▸ **FIGURE 10-1**

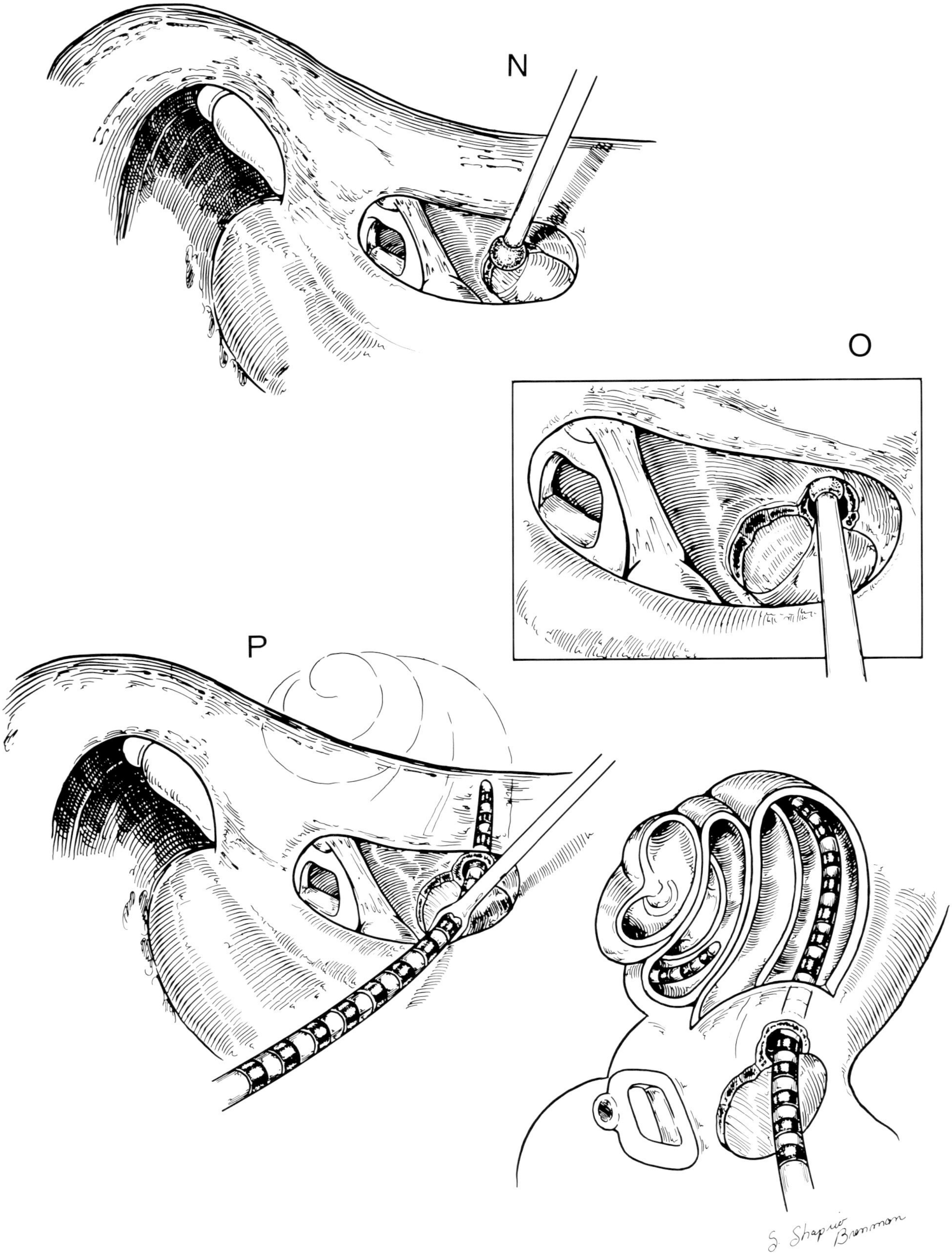


▶ **FIGURE 10-1**

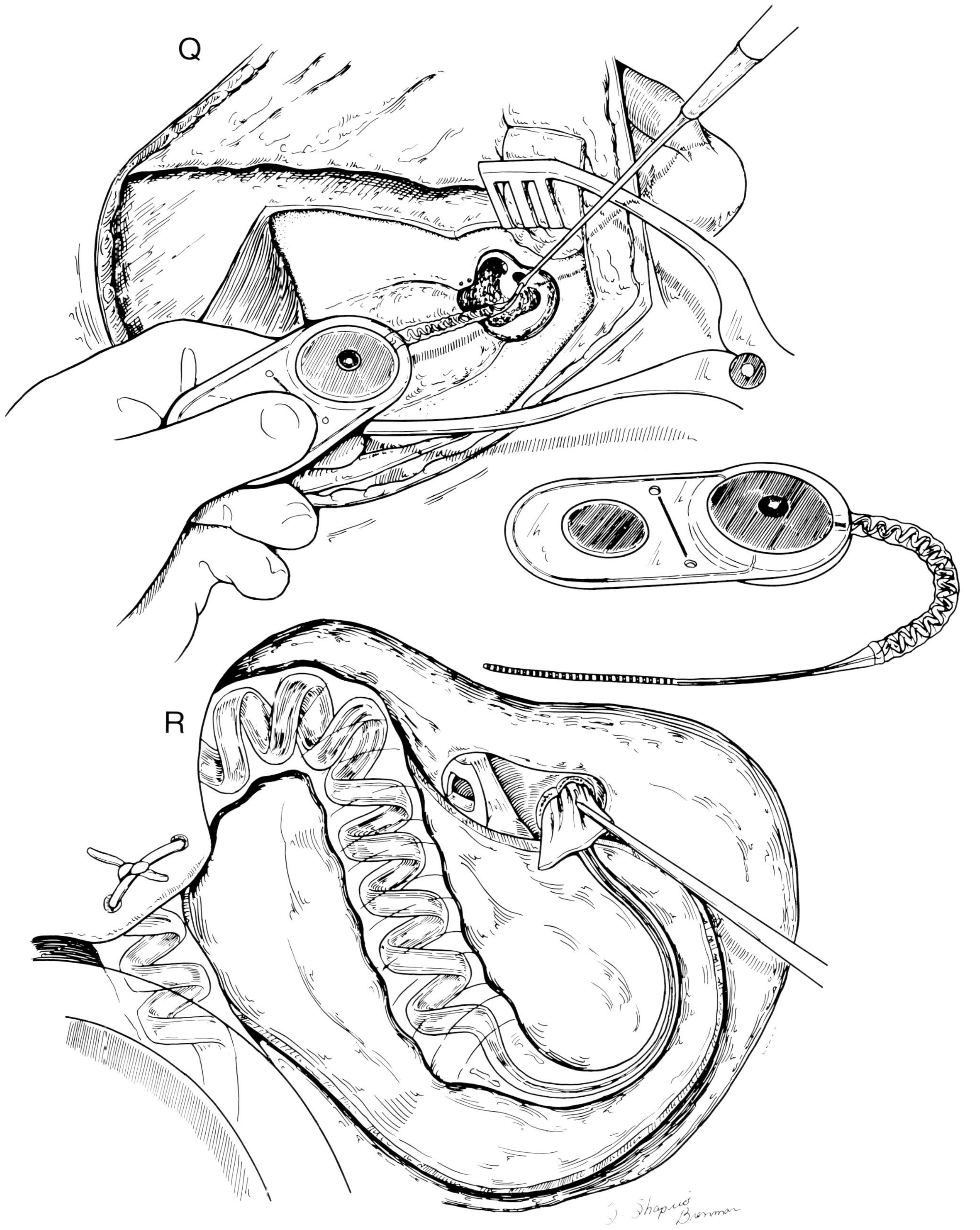


▶ **FIGURE 10-1**

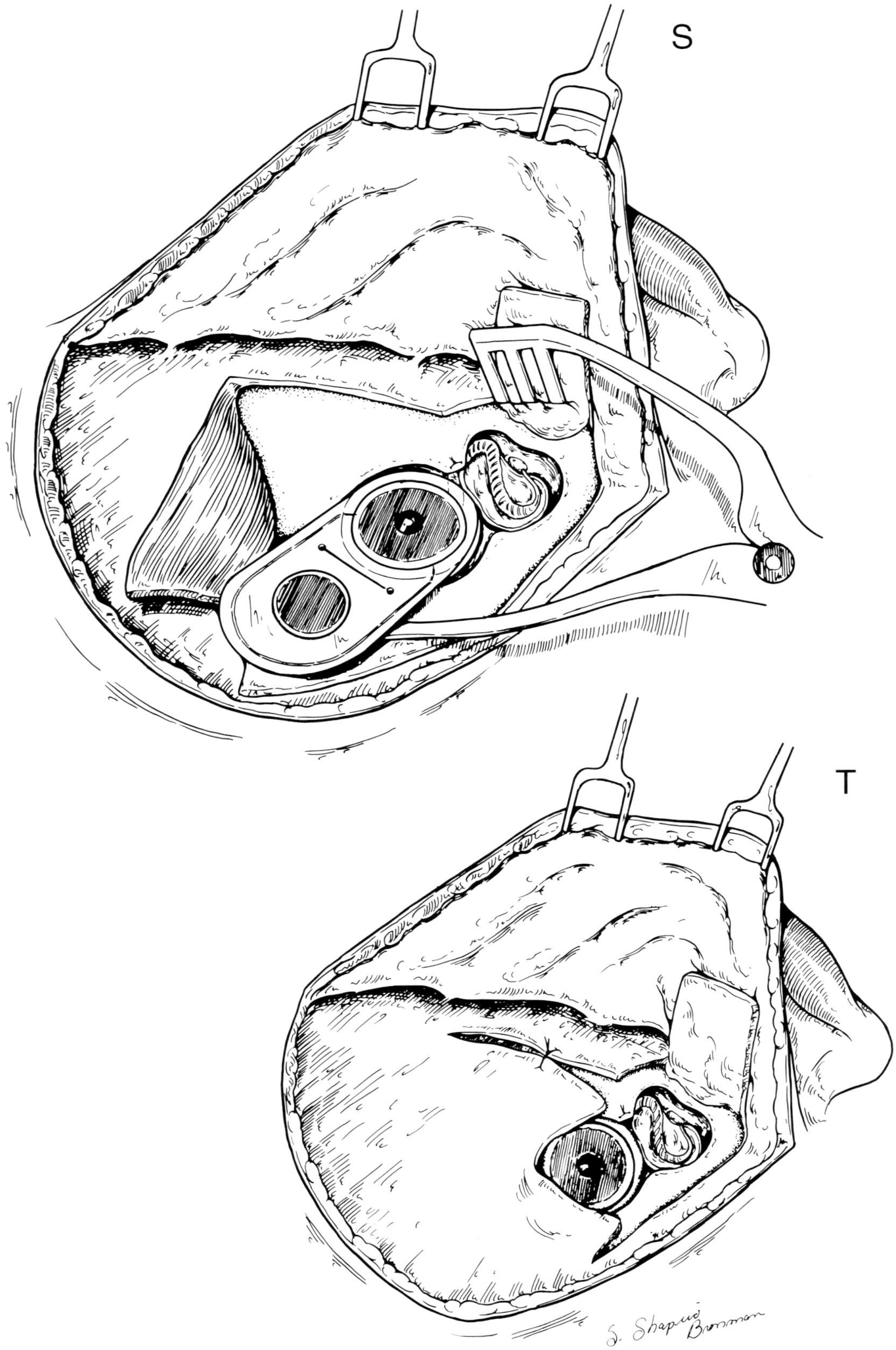


▶ **FIGURE 10-1**

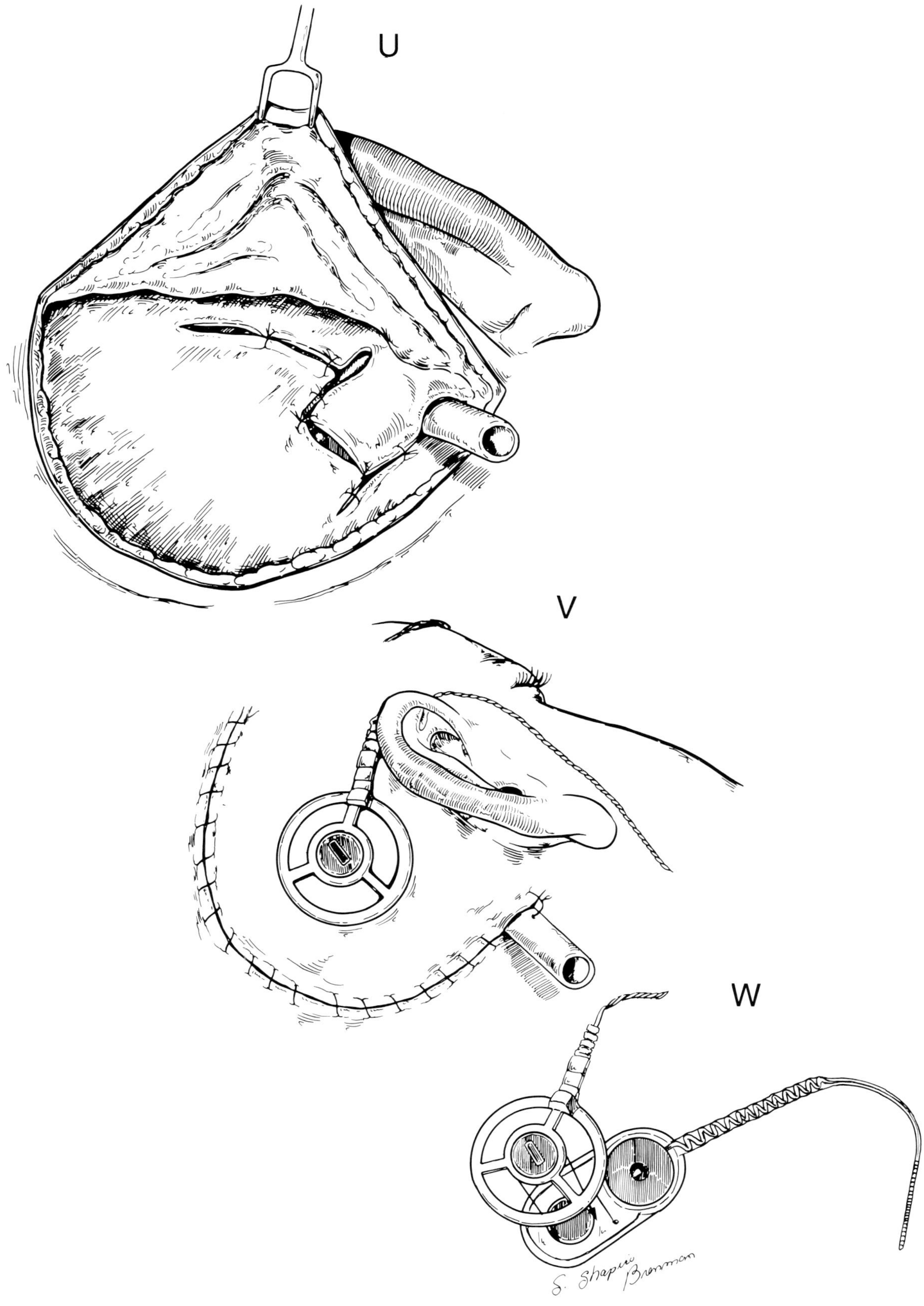


▶ **FIGURE 10-1**

# PART II

# The Nose

▼▼▼

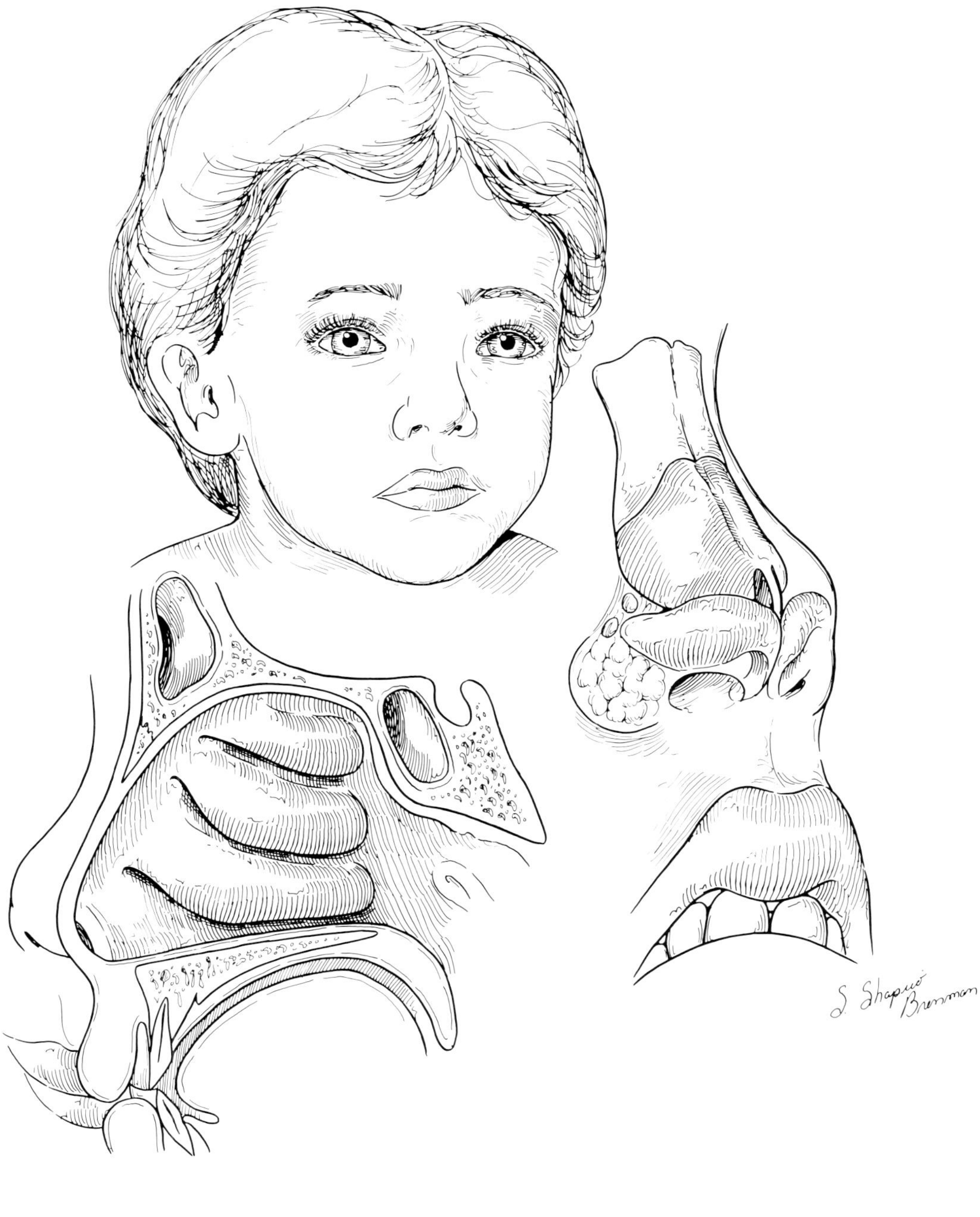

# 11 ▶ Intranasal Trauma/Epistaxis

## ▶ 11-1 EVACUATION OF SEPTAL HEMATOMA AND ABSCESS

Septal hematomas may develop following blunt nasal trauma. The septum is often fractured, but not displaced. Blood collects between the perichondrium and cartilage on one or both sides of the nose. A septal abscess can result from a hematoma that is not promptly drained.

### Indications

Hematomas and abscesses must be drained expeditiously to prevent septal cartilage necrosis with loss of nasal support and a resultant saddle nose deformity.

### Preoperative Evaluation

Preoperative evaluation consists of a thorough intranasal examination, recognition of the abscess or hematoma, and evaluation for associated facial and cranial trauma.

### Operative Technique

1. General anesthesia is recommended in children to accomplish complete evacuation of the hematoma.
2. An incision is made at the caudal edge of the fluctuance (Fig. 11–1**A**).
3. The contents of the hematoma or abscess are removed by suction and, if necessary, gentle curettage (Fig. 11–1**B**).
4. A cut rubber band drain is placed in the cavity and brought out of the bottom of the incision. The incision is closed loosely with one 5-0 chromic suture (Fig. 11–1**C**).
5. The nose is then packed with Gelfoam or gauze to approximate the perichondrial flap to the cartilage. Antibiotic impregnated gauze may be used in older children, but biodegradable material is easier to remove in the young child (Fig. 11–1**D**). Both the drain and the packing are removed in 2 days.
6. Ten days of oral antistaphylococcal antimicrobial treatment are indicated when treating a child with septal abscess or hematoma.

### Complications

1. Saddle nose deformity
2. Septal perforation
3. Reaccumulation of hematoma/abscess

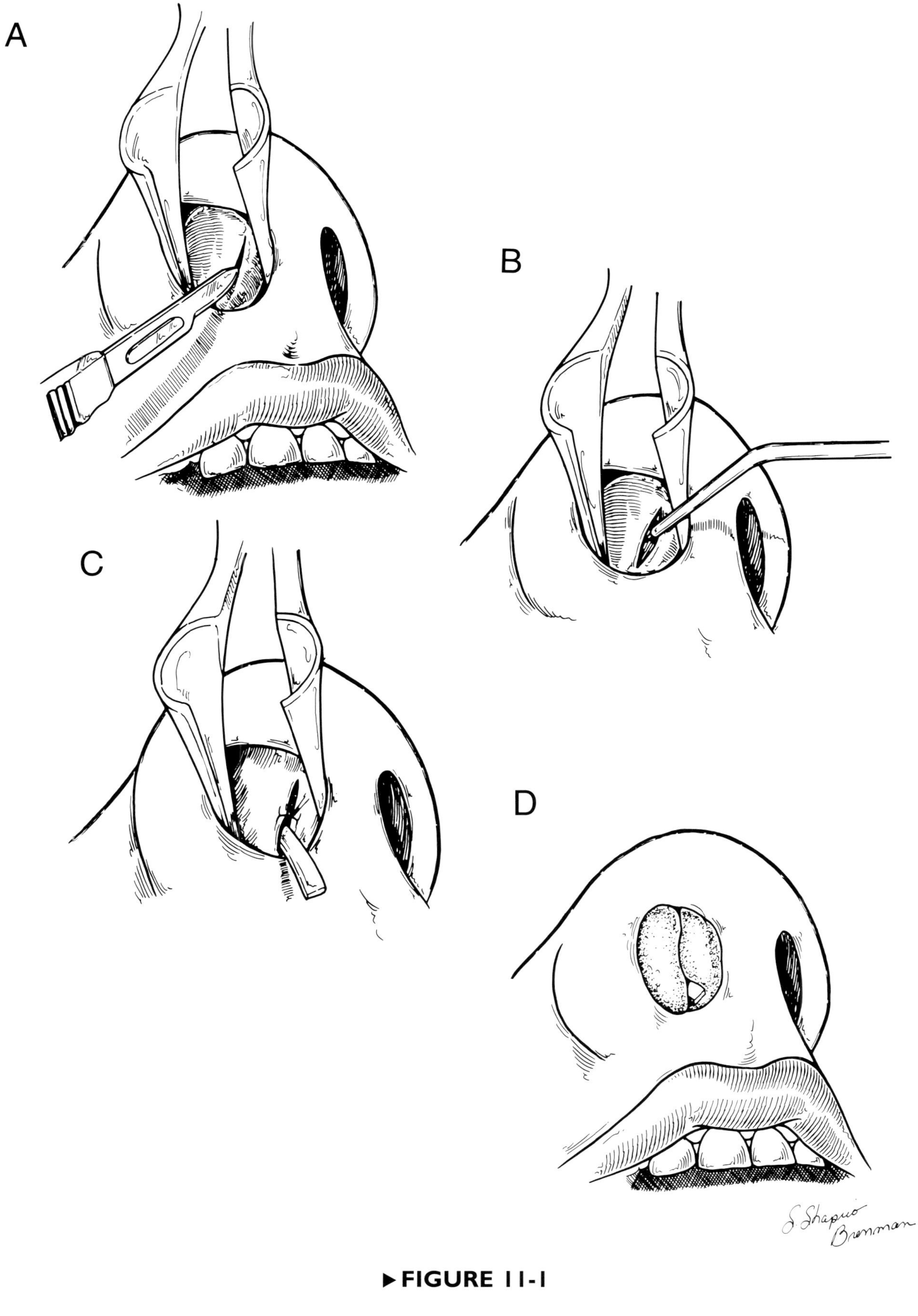


▶ **FIGURE 11-1**

## ▶ 11-2 NASAL CAUTERY

Epistaxis is a common problem of childhood and adolescence. Most episodes stop spontaneously or with gentle pressure. However, recurrent epistaxis can be debilitating by its frequency and/or severity. In those instances, surgical intervention is required.

### Indications

Cauterization is indicated in those cases of recurrent epistaxis that do not respond to conservative methods of humidification and topical ointments.

### Preoperative Evaluation

The preoperative evaluation of a patient with recurrent epistaxis must include a thorough examination of the nose and nasopharynx. This is essential to identify hemangiomas, neoplasms, septal deflections, or foreign bodies that may be the cause of the epistaxis. A complete coagulation profile is obtained to rule out the presence of a coagulopathy. Radiographic examination of the sinuses and pharynx may be done. While plain films can demonstrate large masses, computed tomography (CT) affords the best radiographic view of the nose and sinuses.

### Operative Technique

1. Nasal septal cauterization in children is most effectively accomplished utilizing general anesthesia.
2. The nose should be cleared of all debris and clots before cotton pledgets soaked in 4% cocaine are applied to the bleeding area (alternately, any combination of a topical vasoconstrictor and local anesthetic may be used). This provides a dry field for cautery. If there is no active bleeding, this step may be unnecessary.
3. The septal blood vessels feeding the bleeding area are cauterized individually with a protected suction or needlepoint cautery, or Hyfrecator (Fig. 11–2A).
4. Cauterization of only the feeding vessels provides the best control of epistaxis, allows rapid healing, and avoids a large mucosal burn that may result in atrophic mucosa or a septal perforation.
5. Care must be taken not to cauterize extensively on both sides of the septum. This may result in damage to the underlying perichondrium. Loss of both perichondrial layers can lead to cartilage necrosis and septal perforation.
6. Antibiotic ointment should be applied to the cauterized area twice daily until the site has healed, usually 7 to 10 days.

### Complications

1. Continuing epistaxis
2. Septal perforation

A

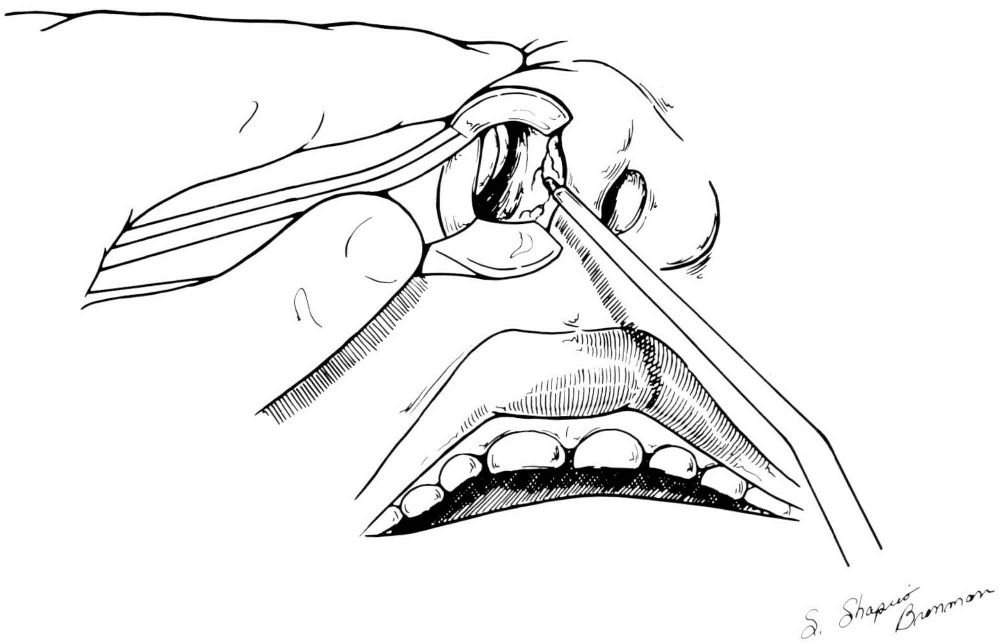

▶ **FIGURE 11-2**

## ▶ 11-3 ANTERIOR PACKING

### Indications

When active epistaxis is not controlled by measures such as gentle pressure or silver nitrate cautery, nasal packing may be required. The source of the bleeding is usually from the superior septal vessels or the lateral wall of the nose. Both sides of the nose should be packed for maximum control and stabilization of nasal structures.

### Preoperative Evaluation

No further preoperative evaluation is needed (see section 11–2, Nasal Cautery).

### Operative Technique

1. Because bleeding is uncontrolled, packing the nose is urgent and performed utilizing a topical anesthetic.
2. Mucoid debris and blood clots should be cleared from both sides of the nose with a suction.
3. The nasal mucosa should be anesthetized and vasoconstricted with 4% cocaine soaked neurosurgical pledgets (alternately, any combination of a topical vasoconstrictor and local anesthetic may be used). Three $\frac{1}{2}''$ × 3″ pledgets on each side of the nose are usually sufficient.
4. A $\frac{1}{4}''$ × 72″ gauze strip is impregnated with antibiotic ointment by rubbing the ointment into the gauze.
5. The nasal cavity is then packed by grasping the gauze with a bayonet forceps and placing it deep in the nose (Fig. 11–3**A**).
6. The packing is pushed down against the floor of the nose (Fig. 11–3**B**).
7. Each side of the nose is packed in a similar fashion, layering the packing from the floor of the nose toward the top of the nasal cavity. The final portion of packing is placed anteriorly (Fig. 11–3**C**).
8. Alternately, commercially available expanding sponge packs may be used instead of gauze packing to control anterior hemorrhage.
9. The packing is kept in place by taping the nose across the nostrils. It is removed after 72 hours (Fig. 11–3**D**).
10. Antistaphylococcal antibiotics are administered for 7 to 10 days to prevent the occurrence of toxic shock syndrome, which has been associated with nasal packing.

### Complications

1. Continuation of bleeding
2. Mucosal abrasion

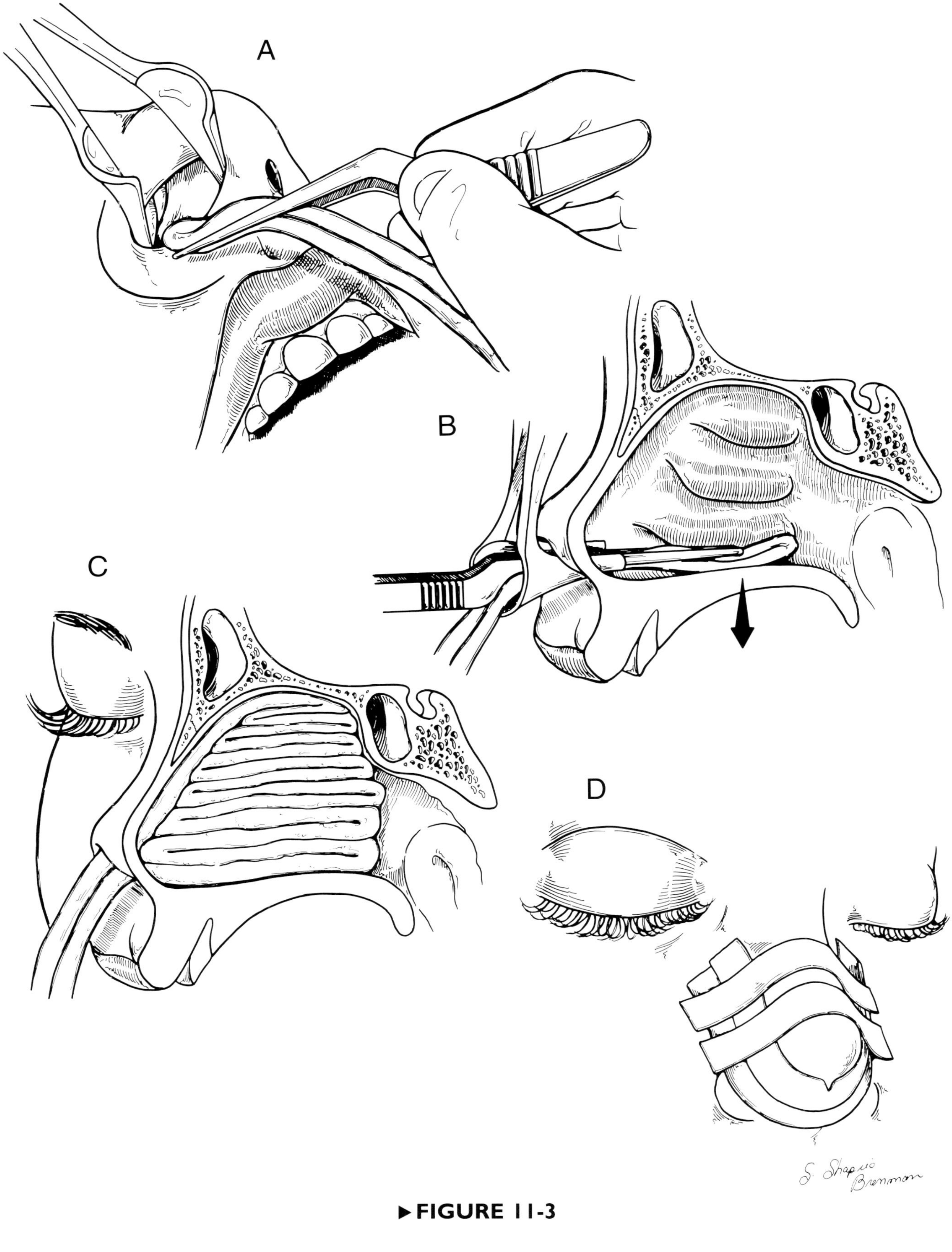


▶ **FIGURE 11-3**

## ▶ 11-4 POSTERIOR PACKING

The purpose of a posterior pack is to provide a wall at the posterior choana against which packing can be placed. It also provides some pressure at the choana, posterior nasal cavity, and nasopharynx.

### Indications

When an anterior pack is insufficient to control bleeding, a posterior pack should be used. Posterior packs are rarely required in children.

### Preoperative Evaluation

No further preoperative evaluation is needed (see section 11–2, Nasal Cautery).

### Operative Technique

1. Placement of a posterior pack in a child may require a general anesthetic. However, teenagers may be able to tolerate the procedure with only topical intranasal 4% cocaine (alternately, any combination of a topical vasoconstrictor and local anesthetic may be used).
2. The nose is cleared of mucus and blood with a Frazier suction.
3. The nasal mucosa is anesthetized and vasoconstricted with 4% cocaine-soaked neurosurgical pledgets (alternately, any combination of a topical vasoconstrictor and local anesthetic may be used). Three $\frac{1}{2}'' \times 3''$ pledgets on each side is usually sufficient.
4. A 2 to 3-cm length of clear plastic suction tubing is passed over a 12- or 14-gauge Foley catheter that has a 30-cc balloon (Fig. 11–4**A**).
5. The tip of the Foley extending beyond the balloon should be cut off to minimize gagging when the catheter is in position (Fig. 11–4**A**).
6. The integrity of the balloon should be tested by filling it with 30 cc of water.
7. With the balloon deflated, the catheter should be advanced into the side of the nose that is bleeding until the tip is visible in the oropharynx (Fig. 11–4B). Only one catheter is needed because one balloon will occlude the entire nasopharynx.
8. After 15 to 20 cc of water are introduced into the balloon, the catheter is withdrawn until it is seated in the posterior choana (Fig. 11–4C).
9. A bilateral anterior pack is then applied as previously described with gauze impregnated with antibiotic ointment (see section 11–3, Anterior Packing).
10. The piece of suction tubing is positioned against the pack inside the nostril and clamped in place while gentle traction is applied to the Foley (Fig. 11–4D). This is done to avoid alar necrosis.
11. The pack is left in place 3 to 5 days. The patient is placed on a broad spectrum antistaphylococcal antimicrobial given intravenously. Intravenous hydration may be necessary since oral intake is difficult with a posterior pack in place.
12. The child should be monitored in an intensive care unit because a posterior pack may cause hypoxia and hypercapnia. Supplemental oxygen should be administered.

### Complications

1. Hypoxia/hypercapnia
2. Altered mental state
3. Cardiac arrhythmia
4. Continued bleeding

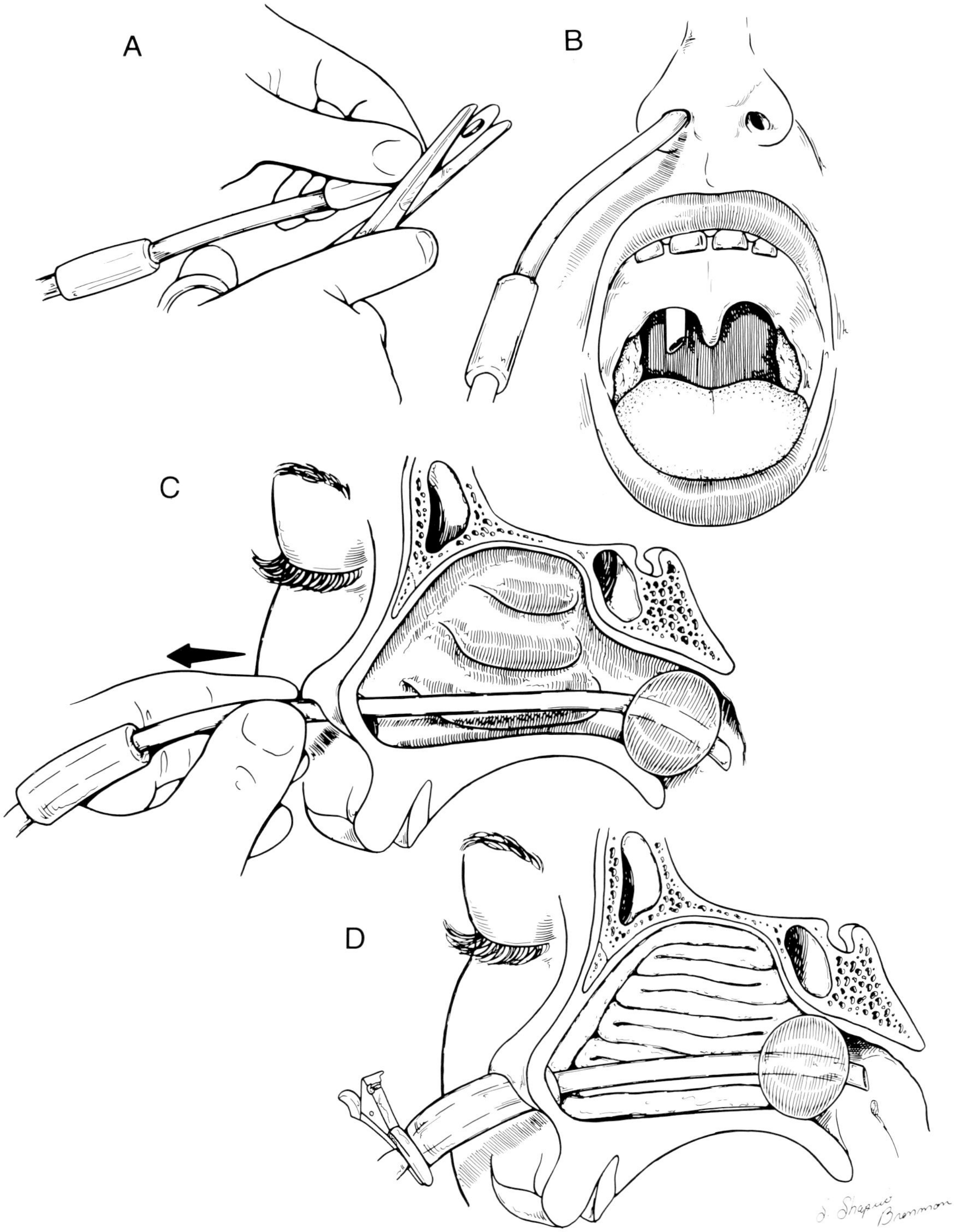


▶ **FIGURE 11-4**

# ▶ 11-5 LIGATION OF INTERNAL MAXILLARY ARTERY

## Indications

Ligation of the internal maxillary artery is indicated in patients with posterior epistaxis who have not responded to, or will not tolerate, anterior/posterior packing. Access to the internal maxillary artery is obtained through the maxillary sinus (Fig. 11–5J). Ligation of the internal maxillary artery is often done in conjunction with ligation of the ethmoid arteries.

## Preoperative Evaluation

Bilateral carotid angiography should be performed prior to the procedure. This is to ensure that the source of the bleeding is from the external carotid system. Sinus radiography, especially computed tomography (CT), should be obtained to define the maxillary sinus anatomy.

## Operative Technique

1. The procedure is performed utilizing a general anesthetic.
2. The gingival buccal groove is injected with 1% lidocaine with 1:100,000 epinephrine for hemostasis (Fig. 11–5**A**).
3. An incision is made with a cutting cautery through the mucosa and the periosteum of the anterior wall of the maxilla from the lateral incisor tooth back to the lateral wall of the maxillary sinus (Fig. 11–5**B**).
4. The periosteum is elevated superiorly to the level of the infraorbital nerve (Fig. 11–5**C, D**).
5. The maxillary sinus is opened in the canine fossa with a chisel (Fig. 11–5**D**).
6. The anterior and lateral wall of the maxillary sinus is removed with a bone rongeur. The mucosa is removed with a forceps to open the sinus widely (Fig. 11–5**E**).
7. Self-retaining retractors are placed, and an operating microscope is used to visualize the posterior wall of the sinus.
8. The mucosa of the posterior wall is cauterized with a suction cautery to minimize bleeding (Fig. 11–5**F**). The mucosa is peeled aside with an elevator and removed with a cup forceps (Fig. 11–5**G**).
9. The posterior wall of the maxillary sinus is then cracked with the elevator and the bone pieces removed with the elevator and cup forceps. The posterior periosteum is kept intact (Fig. 11–5**H**).
10. The periosteum is cauterized in a cruciate fashion with a suction cautery to minimize bleeding and cut along the line of cauterization with a sickle knife (Fig. 11–5**I**). This permits direct access to the pterygomaxillary space (Fig. 11–5**J**).
11. The periosteal flaps are laid aside. The internal maxillary artery can then be seen pulsating in the fat (Fig. 11–5**J, K**). The artery is exposed and cleansed of fat with a small forceps and a blunt hook (Fig. 11–5**L**).
12. The main trunk and branches are clipped with vascular clips (Fig. 11–5**M**).
13. The gingival buccal incision is closed loosely with three or four interrupted 4-0 chromic sutures (Fig. 11–5**N**).

**14.** The nasal cavity is usually left unpacked or very lightly packed with antibiotic-impregnated gauze.

**15.** Antibiotics are administered for 7 to 10 days, especially if nasal packing is used.

## Complications

1. Numbness of the lip
2. Laceration of the internal maxillary artery

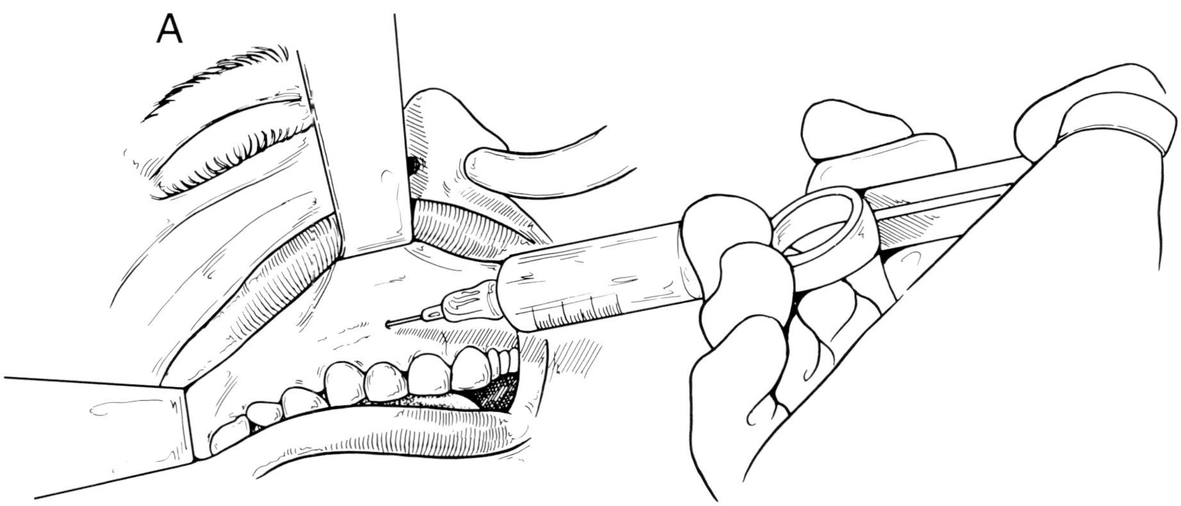

▶ **FIGURE 11-5**

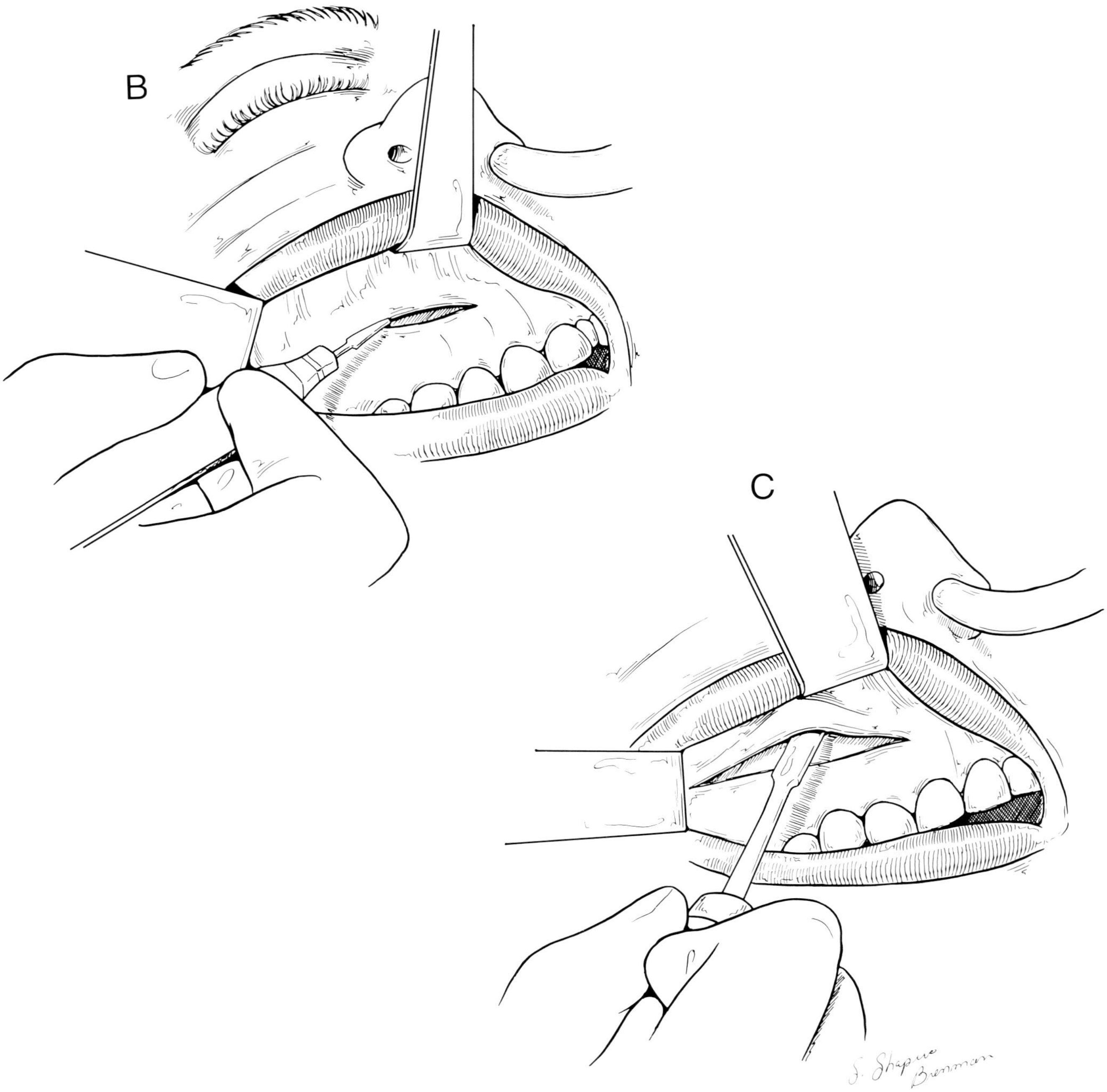


▶ **FIGURE 11-5**

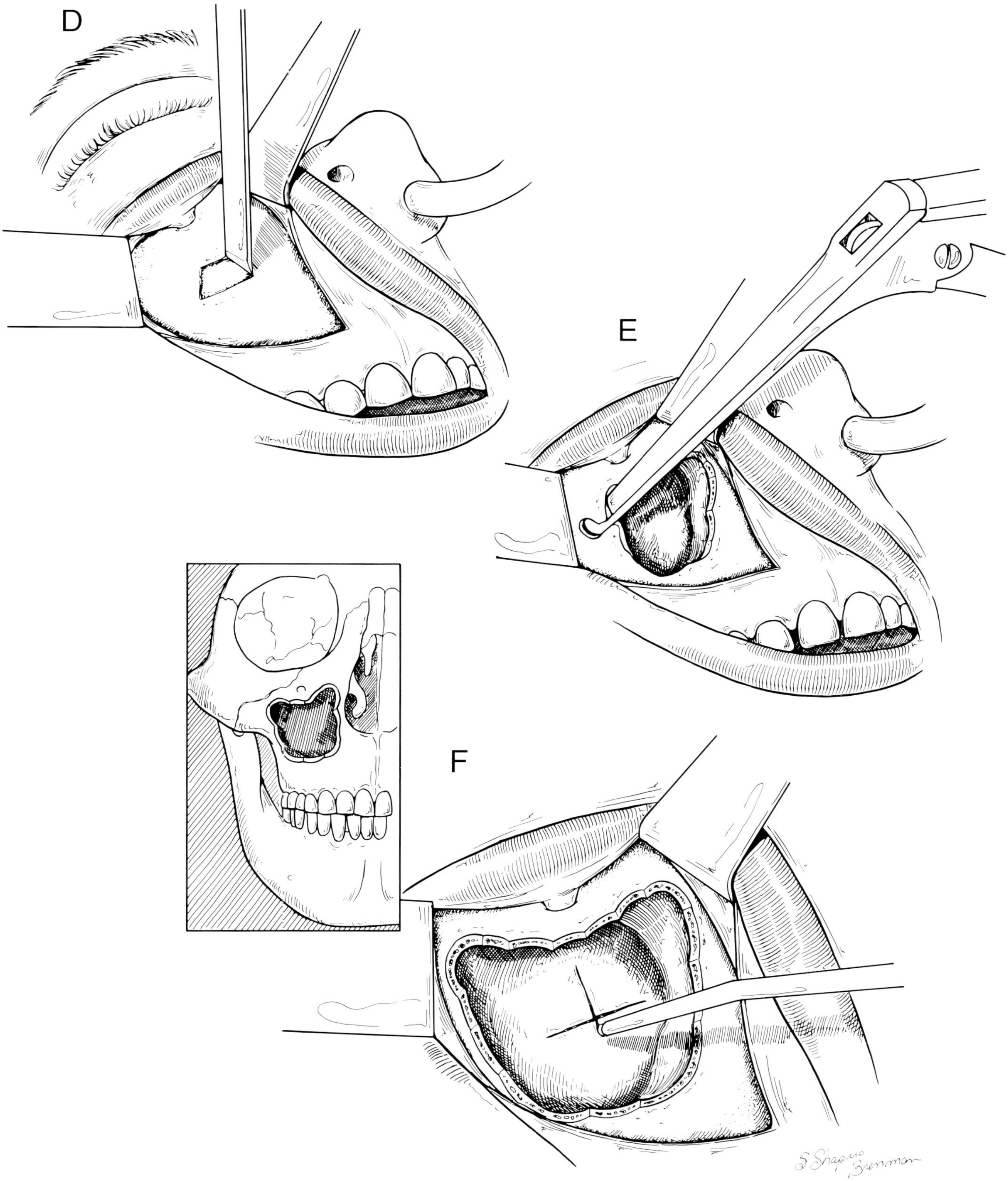


▶**FIGURE 11-5**

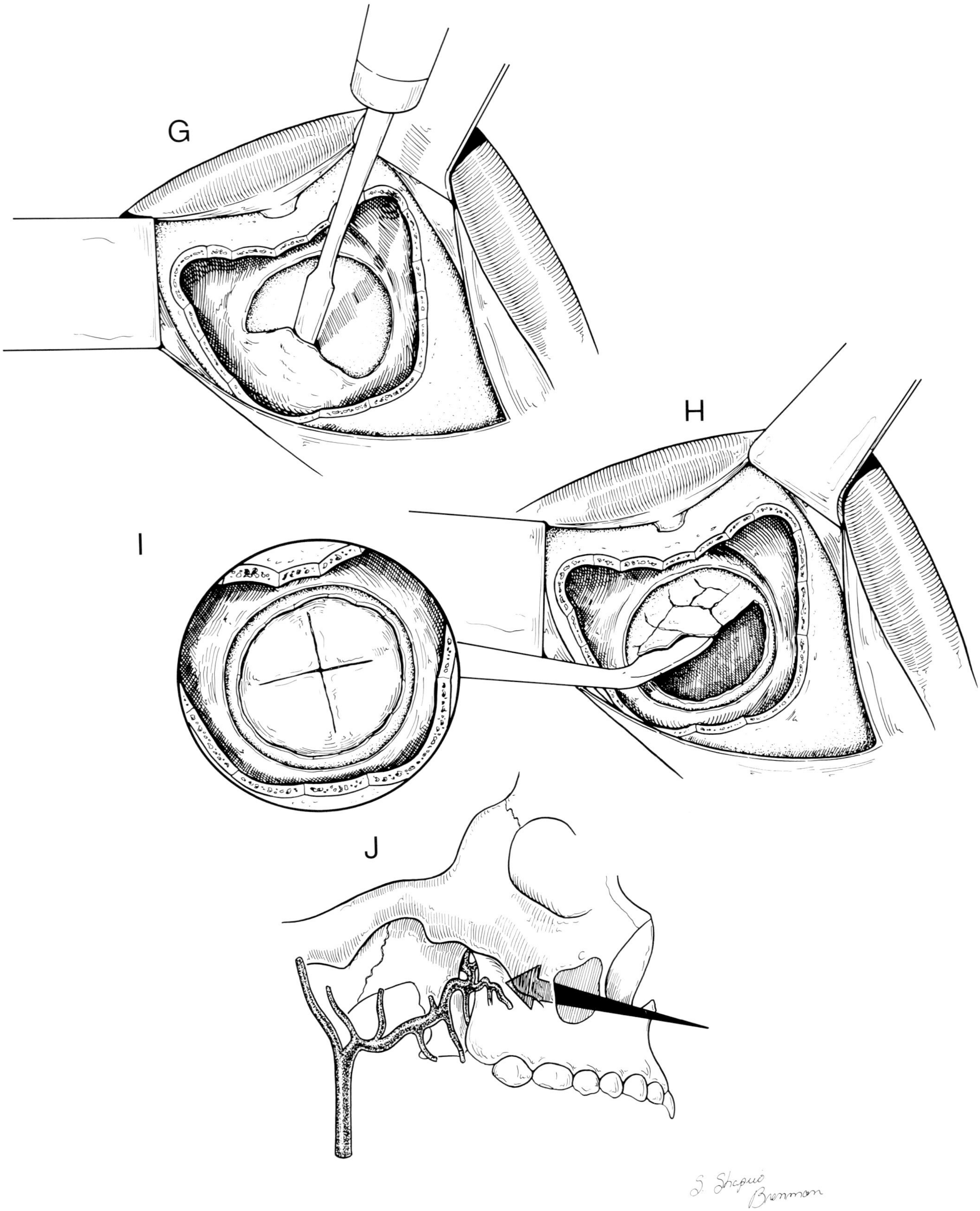


▶**FIGURE 11-5**

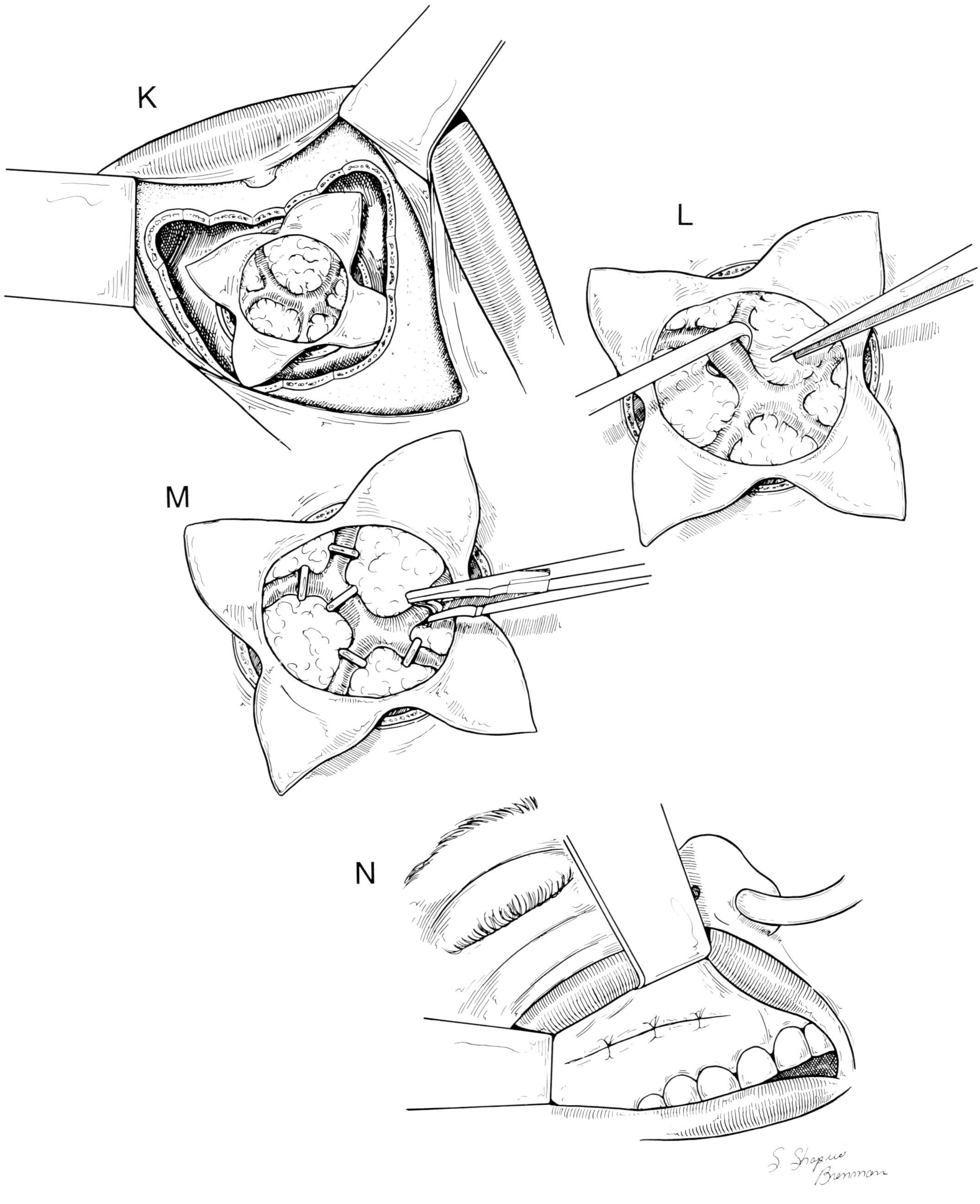


▶ **FIGURE 11-5**

# ▶ 11-6 LIGATION OF ETHMOID ARTERIES

On rare occasions, in older children and teenagers, nasal bleeding may not be controlled with anterior and posterior packing. This can become a life-threatening problem. In this case, ligation of the blood vessels supplying the nasal cavity on the bleeding side should be carried out. Ligation of the anterior and posterior ethmoid arteries is most often performed in conjunction with ligation of the internal maxillary artery (see section 11–5, Ligation of Internal Maxillary Artery).

## Indications

Ligation of the ethmoid arteries is required in cases of epistaxis that do not cease with nasal packing.

## Preoperative Evaluation

Bilateral carotid angiography should be performed prior to the procedure. This is to ensure that the source of the bleeding is from the internal carotid system. Sinus radiography (especially CT) should be obtained to define the nasal and sinus anatomy.

## Operative Technique

1. Anterior and posterior ethmoid artery ligation is carried out under general anesthesia. The area of the proposed incision is injected with 1% lidocaine with 1:100,000 epinephrine.
2. A curvilinear incision is made one half of the distance between the medial canthus and the dorsum of the nose. The incision is carried down through the lateral nasal periosteum to bone (Fig. 11–6**A**).
3. The periosteum is elevated medially with a Freer elevator until the frontoethmoidal suture is identified. Care is taken to avoid damage to the lacrimal sac at the inferior aspect of the surgical field. The ethmoidal vessels pass from the orbit to the nose through this suture line (Fig. 11–6**B**).
4. The frontoethmoidal suture line is followed until the anterior ethmoid artery is identified (Fig. 11–6**C**).
5. The artery is then ligated with two small vascular clips (Fig. 11–6**D**). The vessel is divided between the clips.
6. The frontoethmoidal suture is then followed further back until the posterior ethmoid artery is identified and clipped in a similar fashion (Fig. 11–6**E**). Care is taken to avoid the optic nerve, which lies approximately 1 cm posterior to the posterior ethmoid artery.
7. The incision is closed with 3-0 interrupted chromic sutures in the periosteum and 4-0 interrupted subcuticular chromic sutures in the skin. No drain is required.

## Complications

1. Continued bleeding
2. Intraorbital hemorrhage
3. Optic nerve damage

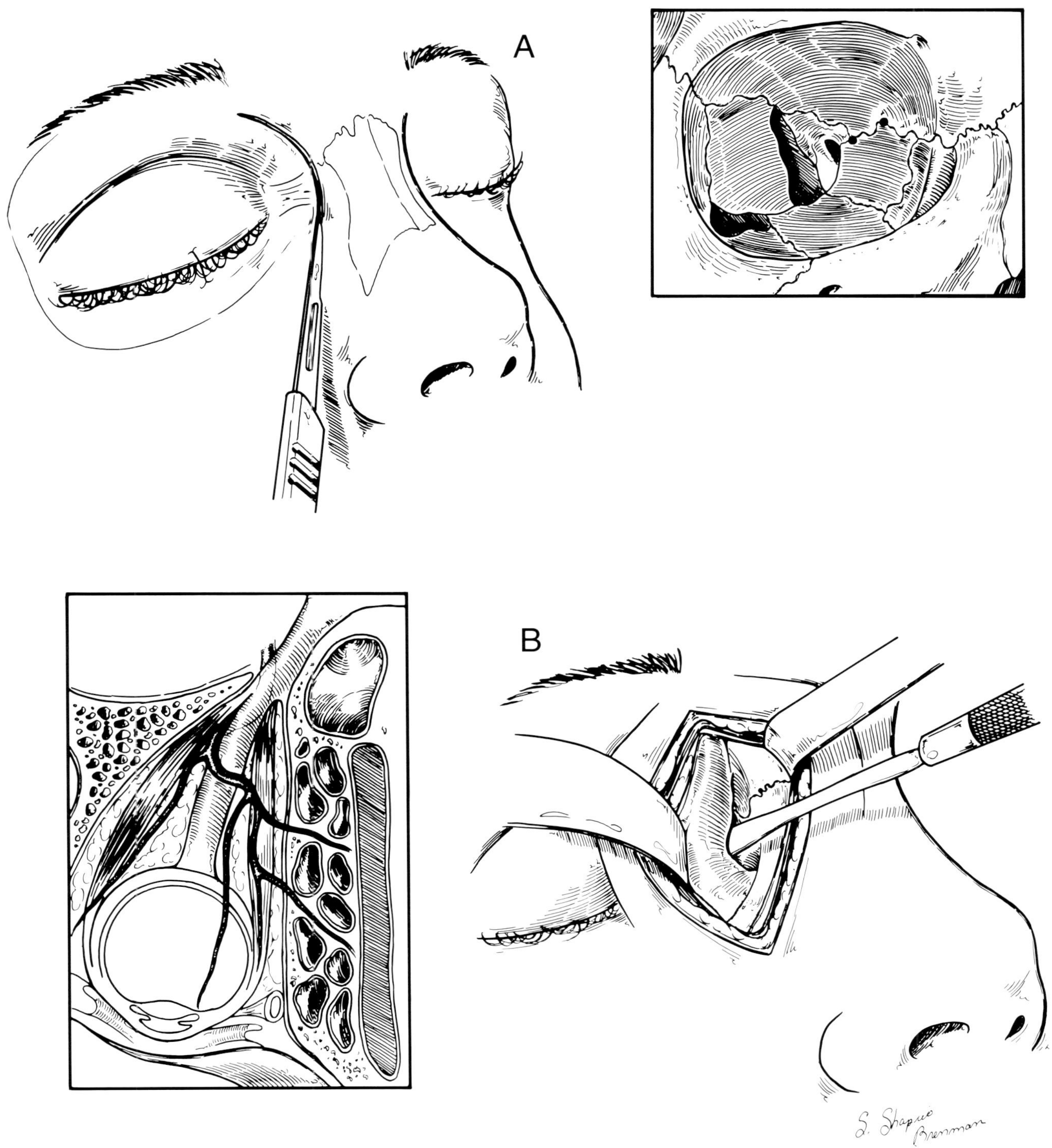


▶ **FIGURE 11-6**

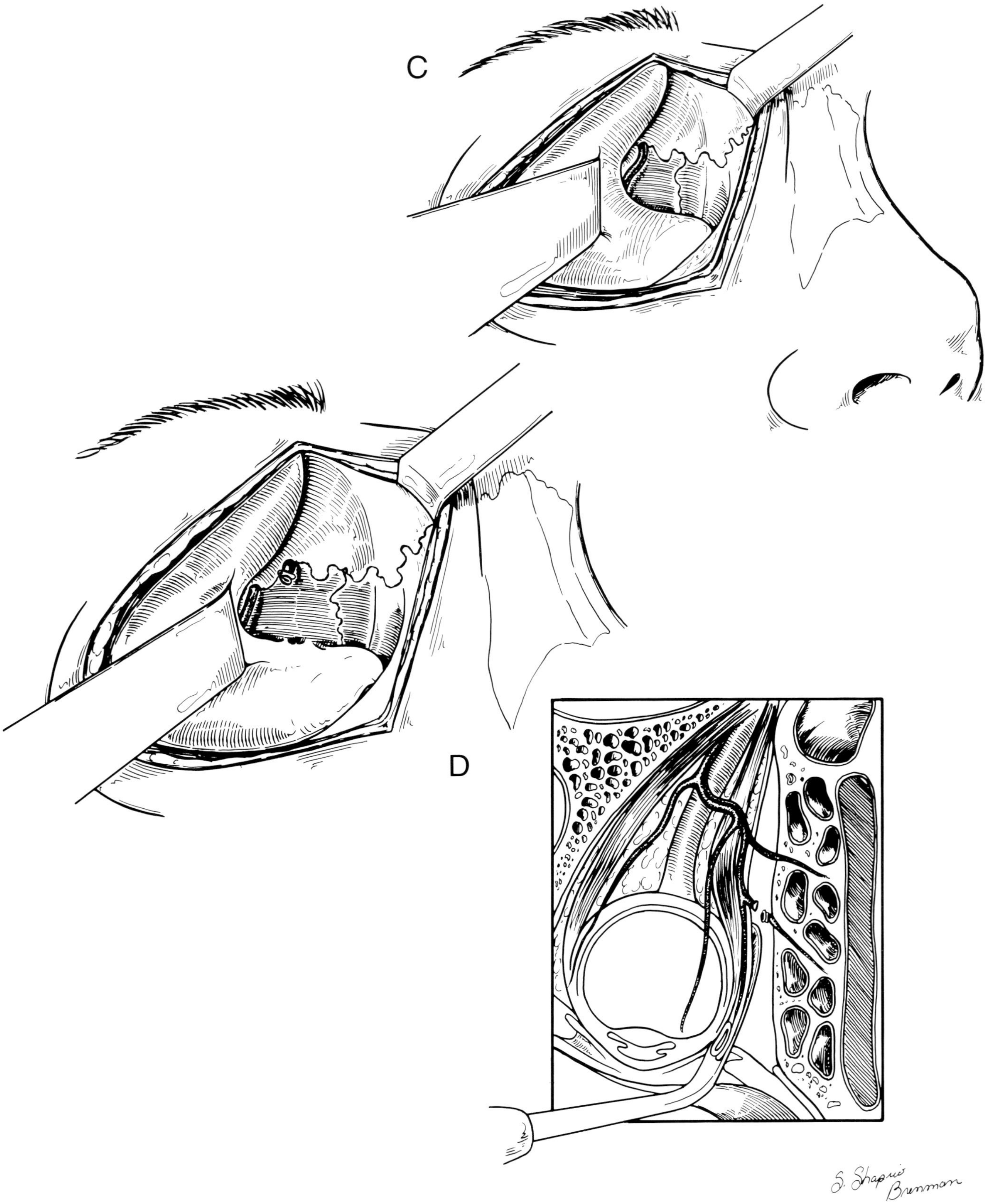


▶ **FIGURE 11-6**

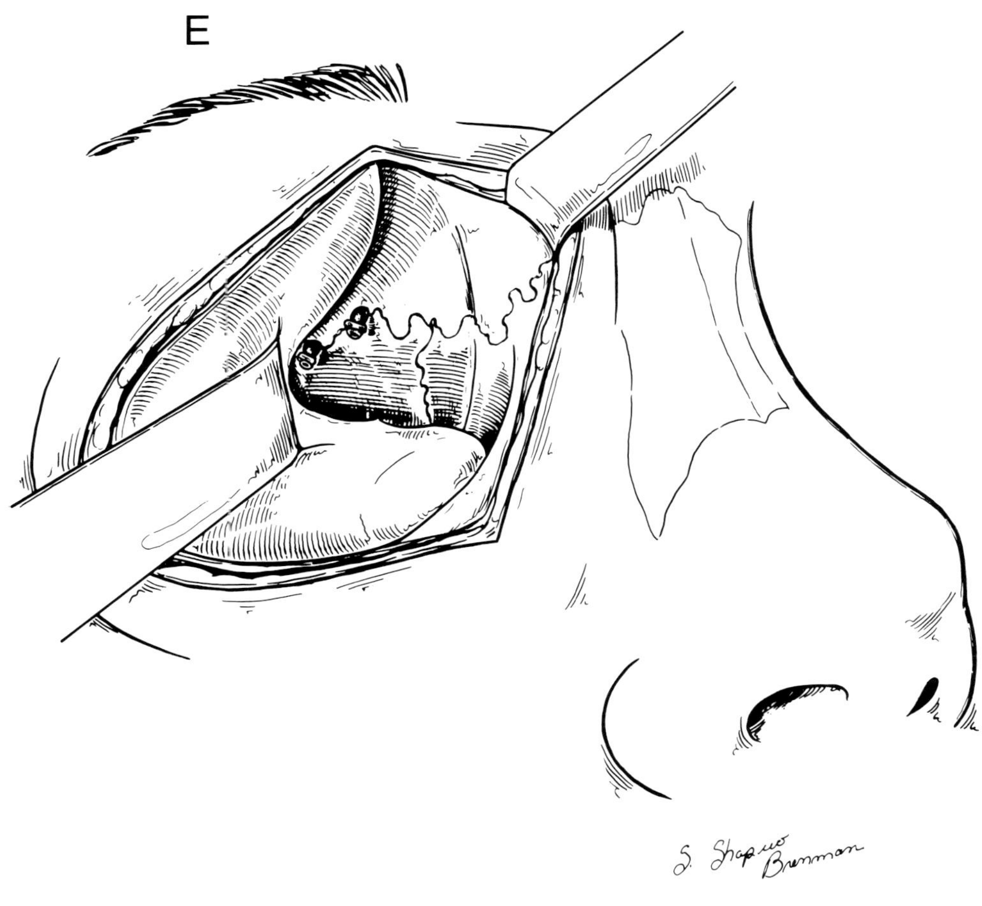


▶ **FIGURE 11-6**

## ▶ 11-7 SEPTAL GRAFT FOR TELANGIECTASIA

Hereditary telangiectasia with a single or multiple hemangiomas of the nasal septum can be a cause of recurrent and debilitating epistaxis.

### Indications

Removal of septal mucosa with skin grafting is indicated in the case of recurrent epistaxis secondary to hereditary telangiectasia that has not responded to packing or cautery.

### Preoperative Evaluation

Preoperative evaluation includes a complete endoscopic examination of the nasal cavities. Angiography may be performed to localize the hemangiomas and also to evaluate the suitability for embolization of the malformation.

### Operative Technique

1. Septal grafting is best performed utilizing general anesthesia and topical vasoconstriction with 4% cocaine (alternately, any combination of a topical vasoconstrictor and local anesthetic may be used).
2. One percent lidocaine with 1:100,000 epinephrine is injected in the subcutaneous tissue of the alar rim and the anterior septum. The septum is exposed by an alar incision in the nasolabial crease from its attachment at the septum to the inferior edge of the nasal bone. This exposes the anterior septum (Fig. 11–7**A**).
3. Additional exposure can be obtained by extending the incision along the lateral border of the nose (Fig. 11–7**B**).
4. The septal mucosa is incised down to, but not through, the nasal septal perichondrium surrounding the area to be removed (Fig. 11–7**C**).
5. The mucosa is elevated and removed with a sharp elevator taking care to keep the perichondrium intact over the septum (Fig. 11–7**D**).
6. A split-thickness skin graft 0.012 to 0.015/in is taken from a relatively hairless area of the body (e.g., lateral hip above the bathing suit line) and secured in place with 5-0 Vicryl suture (Fig. 11–7**E**).
7. The alar incision is closed with interrupted chromic subcutaneous sutures and 5-0 interrupted subcuticular absorbable sutures in the skin (Fig. 11–7**F**).
8. The nose is then packed with Gelfoam moistened with an antibiotic-containing otic suspension. The Gelfoam usually becomes soggy and falls out in a few days.
9. Antibiotic ointment should be applied twice daily to the nostril for 2 weeks following removal of the pack.
10. Antibiotics are administered for 7 to 10 days.

### Complications

1. Partial necrosis of graft
2. Continued epistaxis

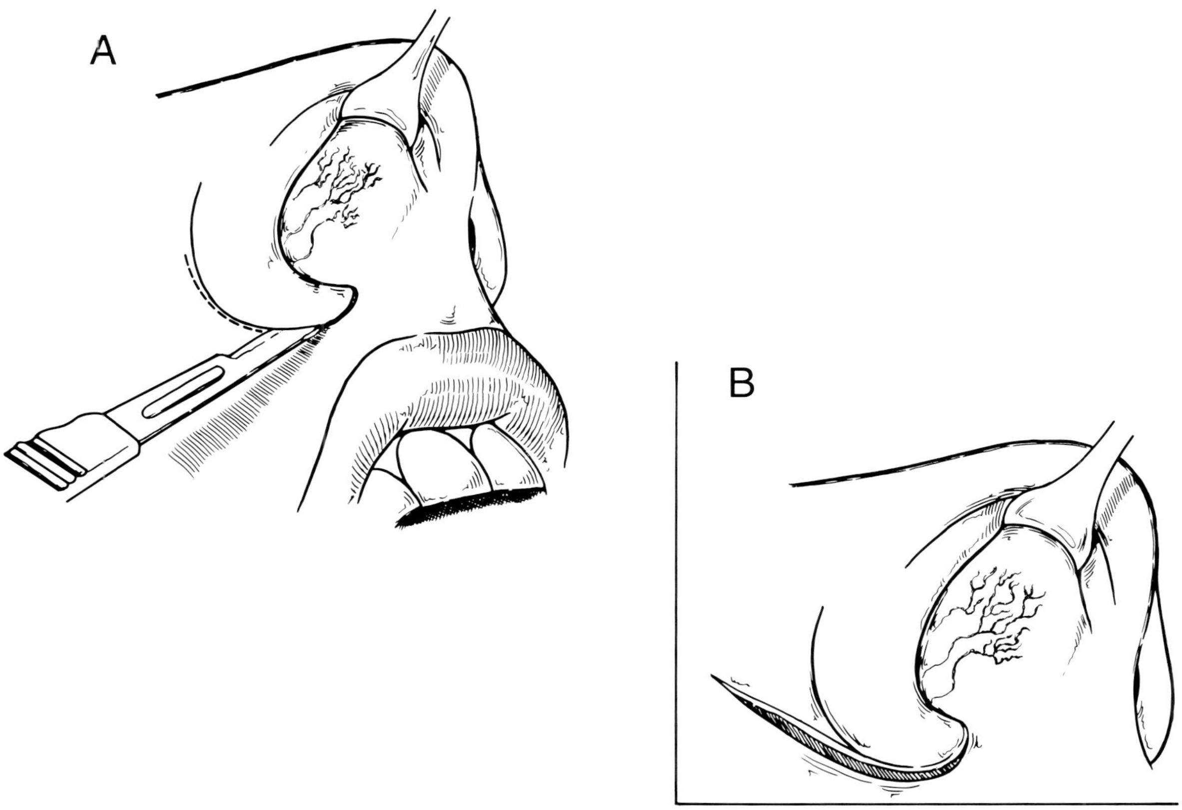


▶ **FIGURE 11-7**

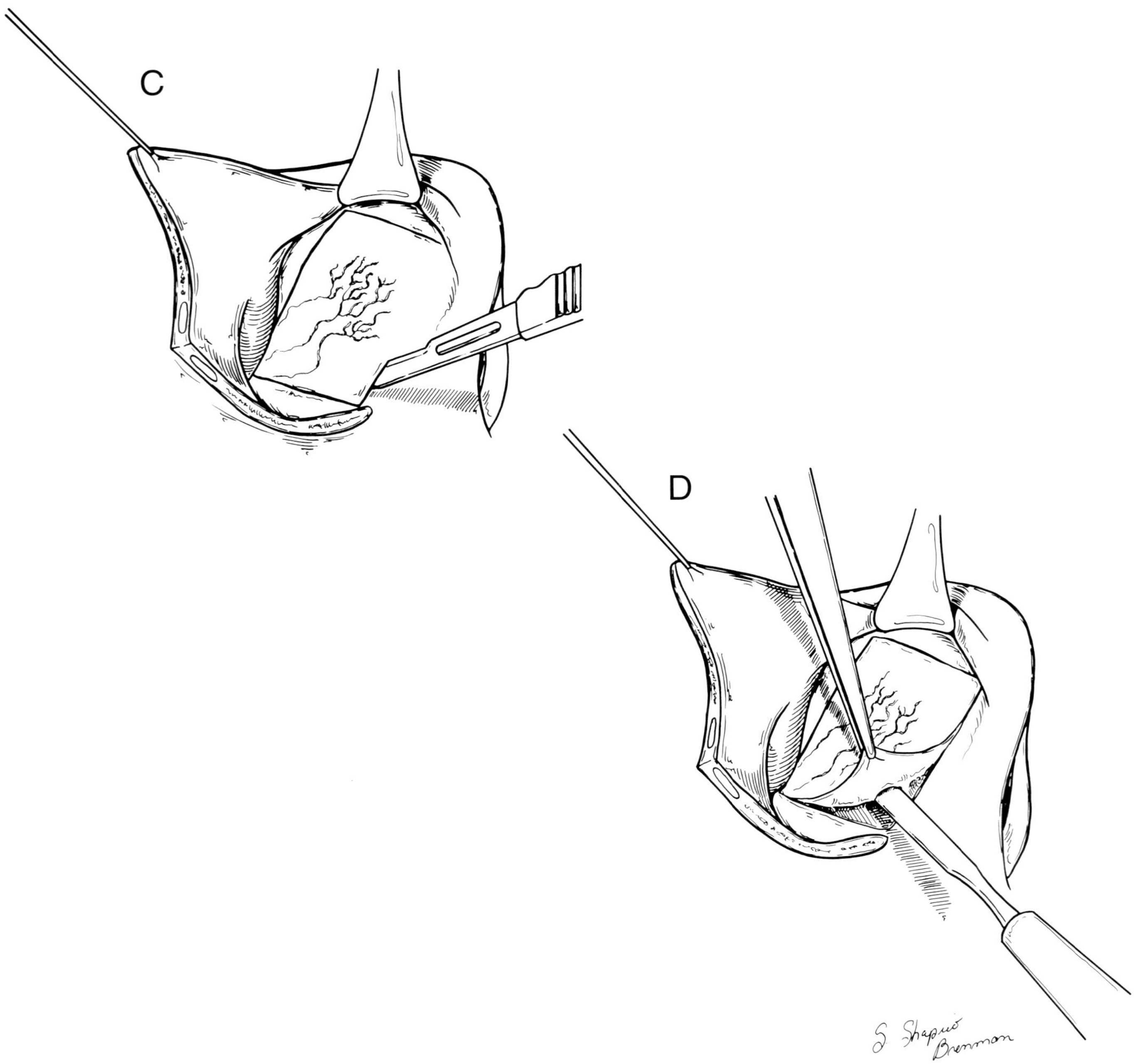


▶ **FIGURE 11-7**

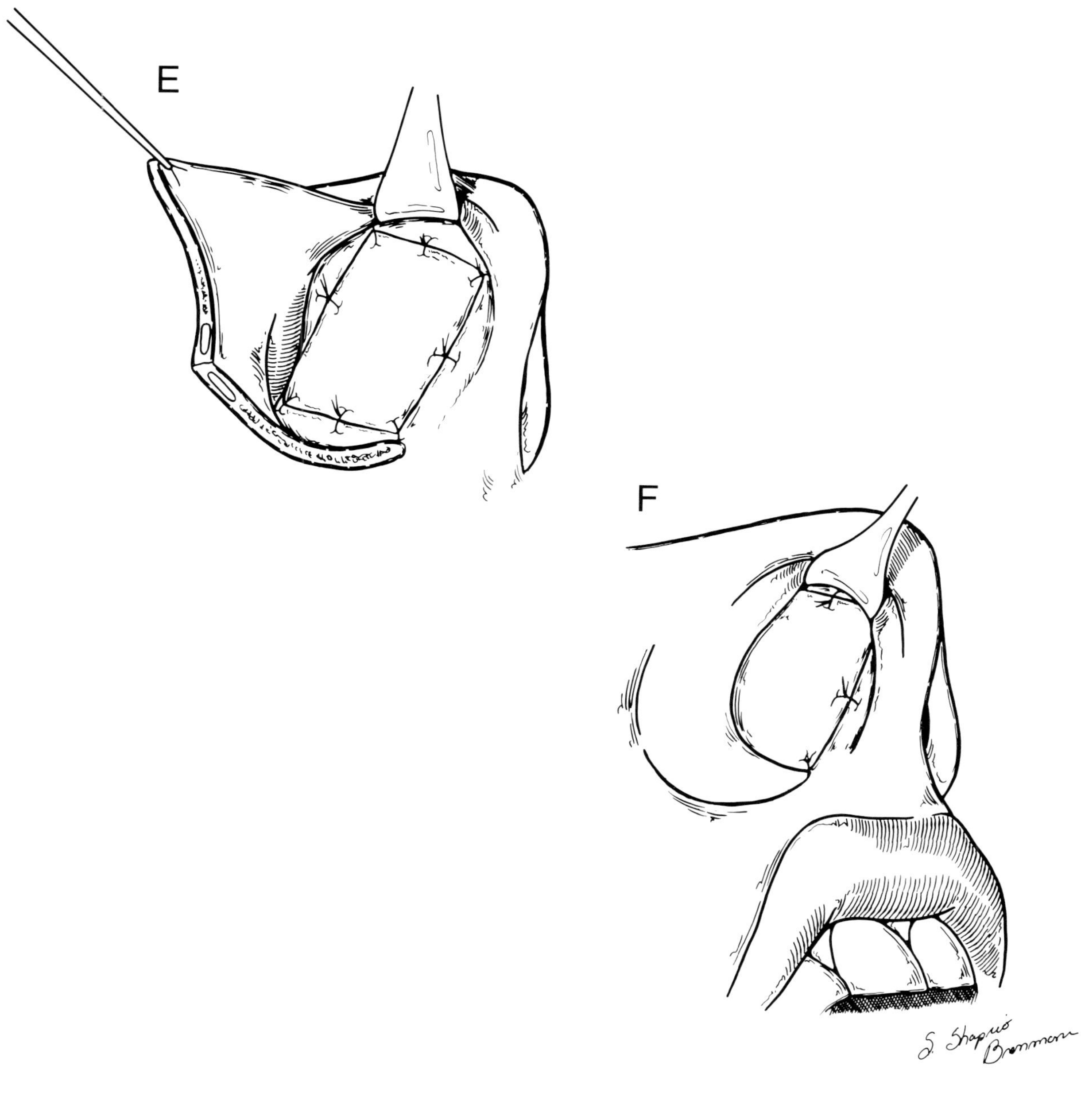


▶ **FIGURE 11-7**

## ▶ 11-8 NASAL VESTIBULOPLASTY

Vestibuloplasty is a procedure designed to surgically close the nostril.

### Indications

On very rare occasions when nasal bleeding has been resistant to all measures and vascular lesions and neoplasms have been ruled out, vestibuloplasty may be helpful. This procedure may be reversed after a sufficient symptom-free interval (e.g., 1 year).

### Preoperative Evaluation

Preoperative evaluation includes computed tomography (CT) and, possibly, angiography to rule out other treatable causes of the epistaxis.

### Operative Technique

1. Vestibuloplasty is best undertaken utilizing general anesthesia.
2. The circumference of the nasal vestibule is injected with 1% lidocaine containing 1:100,000 epinephrine for hemostasis (Fig. 11–8**A**).
3. A circumferential incision is made through the skin 1 cm from the edge of the vestibule, along the septum, lower lateral cartilage (taking care *not* to include the cartilage in the flap), and the floor of the nose (Fig. 11–8**B**).
4. The skin flap is elevated retrograde around the vestibule to within 2 mm of the vestibular edge using a skin hook and sharp curved scissors (Fig. 11–8**C**). This provides sufficient elevation to suture the flap closed without tension.
5. The top and bottom of the skin flap are lifted with a skin hook, and the vestibule is closed with a 5-0 interrupted chromic mattress suture (Fig. 11–8**D**, **E**).
6. A small antibiotic-impregnated piece of gauze is placed gently in the remnant of the vestibule and the tip of the nose is splinted with adhesive tape to relieve tension and reduce motion (Fig. 11–8**F**).
7. The tape and packing are removed in 3 days.
8. Antibiotics are administered for 7 to 10 days.

### Complications

1. Incomplete closure of the nostril
2. Alar collapse

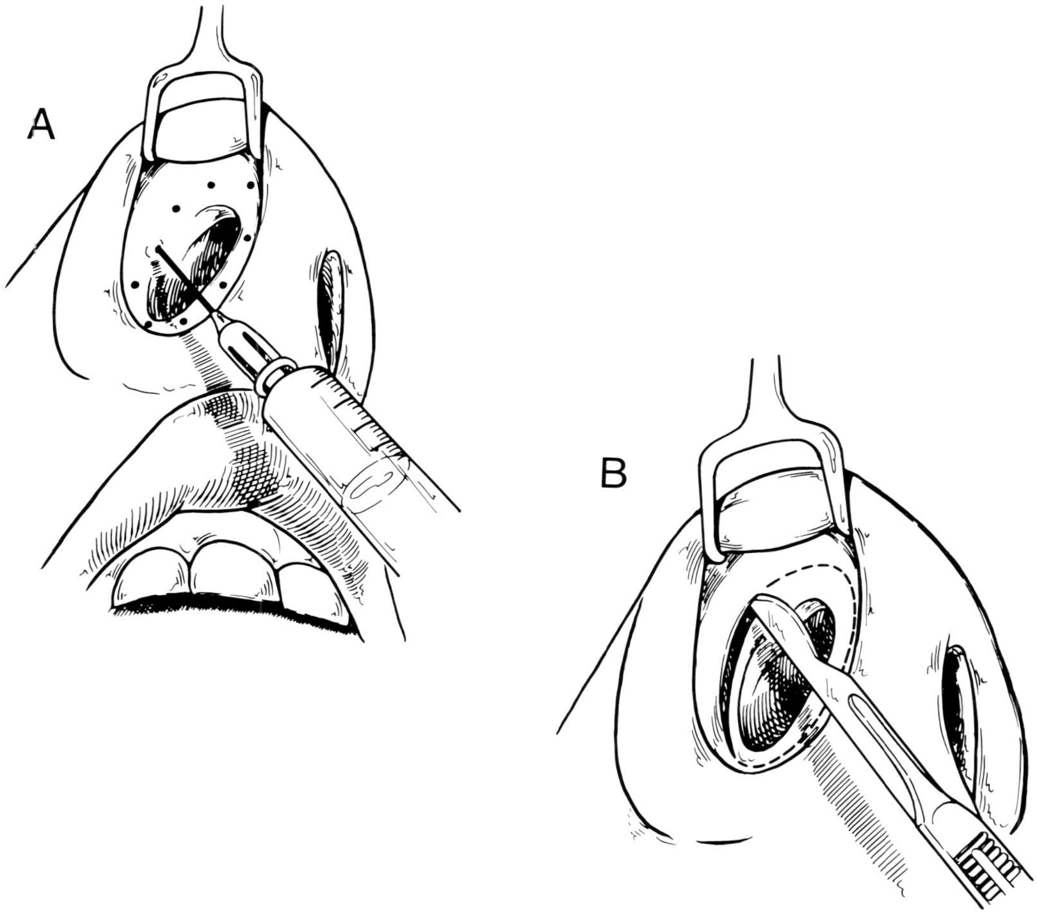


▶ **FIGURE 11-8**

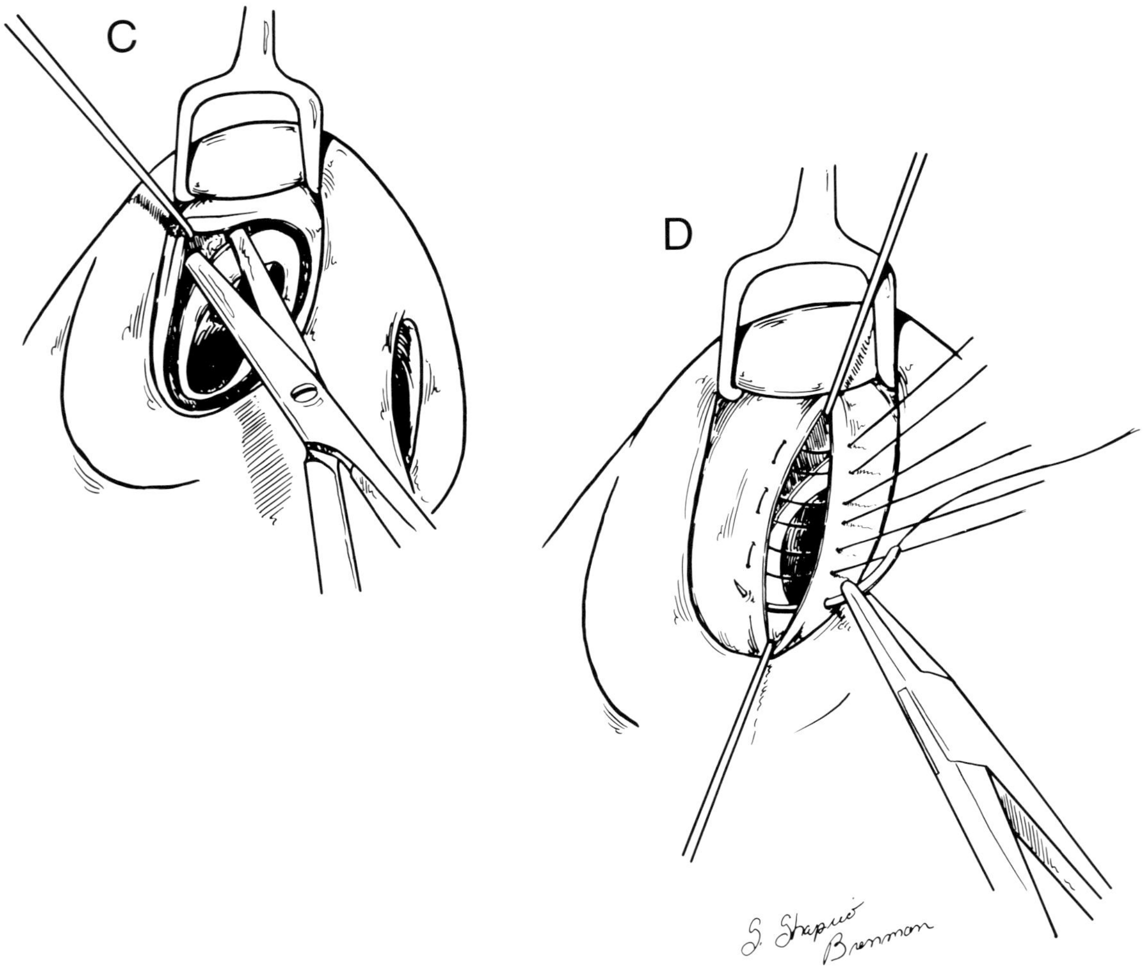


▶ **FIGURE 11-8**

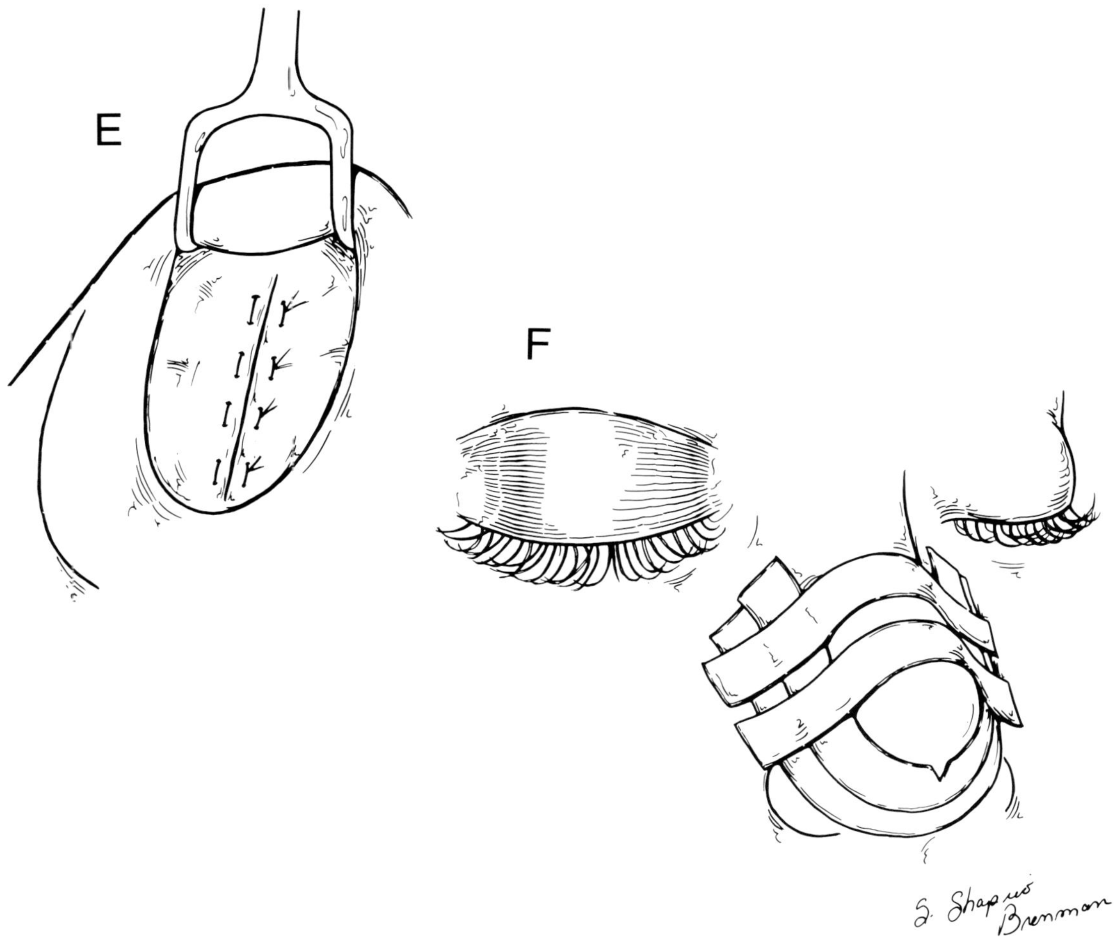


▶ **FIGURE 11-8**

# 12 ▶ Nasal Foreign Bodies

Children frequently put foreign bodies into their noses. Paper, vegetables (beans), and stones are common examples. A nasal foreign body should be suspected in any child with a foul-smelling unilateral nasal discharge.

## ▶ 12-1 REMOVAL OF NASAL FOREIGN BODIES

### Indications

Nasal foreign bodies should be removed expeditiously to avoid nasal and sinus infections.

### Preoperative Evaluation

The foreign body is usually seen on anterior rhinoscopy. Endoscopic examination may be helpful in locating a nasal foreign body. This is most easily done if the nasal cavity is suctioned and decongested with 4% cocaine (alternately, any combination of a topical vasoconstrictor and local anesthesia may be used). If a foreign body is not seen but is highly suspected, the examination should be performed under general anesthesia. Most nasal foreign bodies are radiolucent, so radiographs are rarely helpful.

### Operative Technique

1. Removal of nasal foreign bodies in small children usually requires immobilization with a Papoose Board. Older children may cooperate for removal of the foreign body utilizing topical anesthesia. Occasionally general anesthesia may be required.
2. The nasal mucosa is decongested with 4% cocaine dropped or sprayed into the nose (alternately, any combination of a topical vasoconstrictor and local anesthesia may be used).
3. After the nasal cavity is suctioned clear of mucus, the foreign body is removed under direct vision or endoscopically.
4. Rounded foreign bodies should be rolled to the anterior nare with a blunt hook (Fig. 12–1**A**).
5. Foreign bodies that can be grasped with a forceps can be removed in this fashion (Fig. 12–1**B**). Often, otologic forceps are useful in the removal of nasal foreign bodies.
6. Foreign bodies in the posterior nasal cavity or partially in the nasopharynx are always removed under general anesthesia to prevent aspiration. They can be grasped with forceps while placing a finger in the nasopharynx to prevent posterior displacement (Fig. 12–1**C**).

### Complications

1. Mucosal abrasion

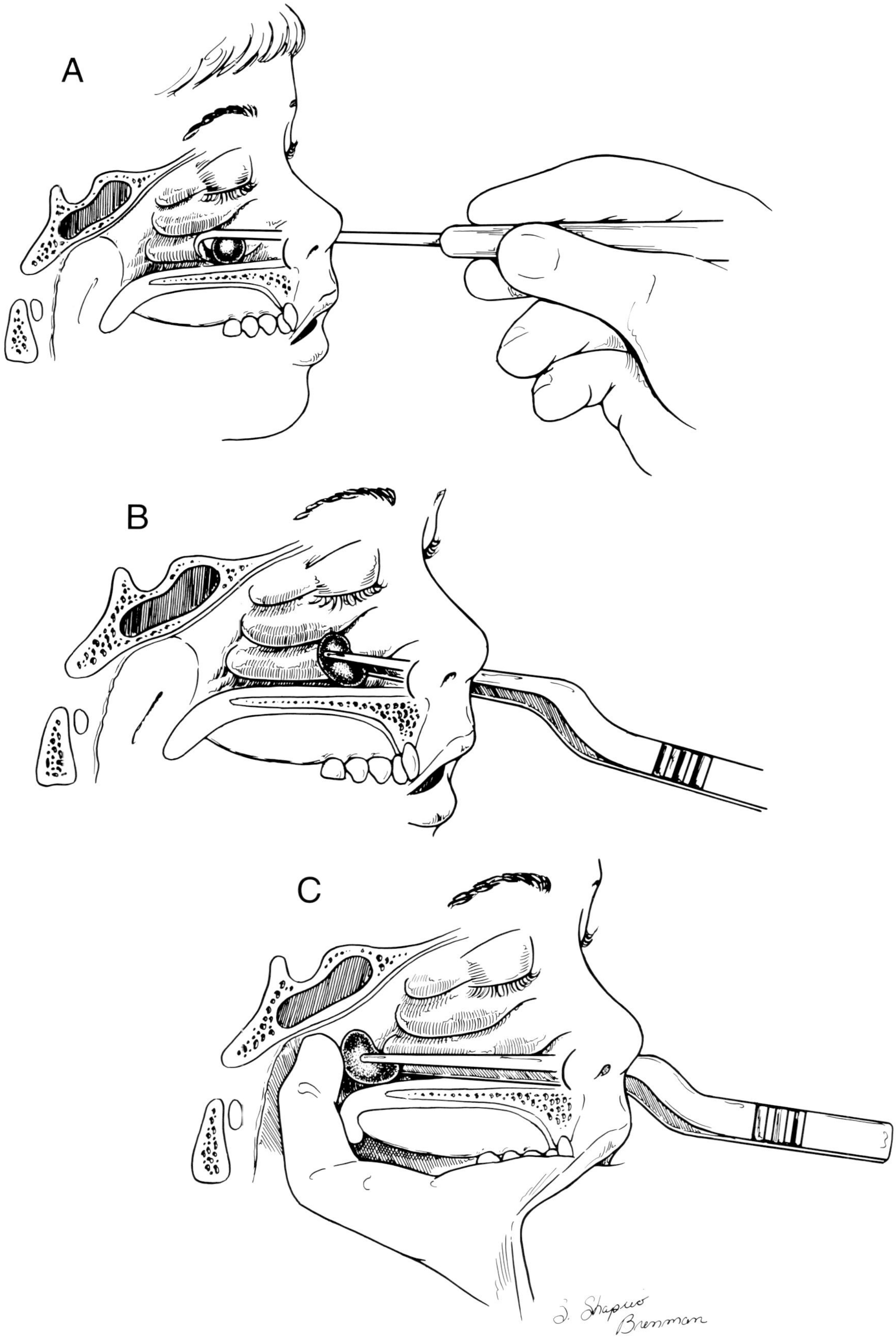


▶ **FIGURE 12-1**

# 13 ▶ Nasal Deformity

## ▶ 13-1 SEPTOPLASTY

Conservative septoplasty in children should be directed to the goal of improving breathing by reducing the deviation of the septum rather than achieving a "perfectly straight" septum. Septoplasty is usually not performed until the child is 4 to 5 years of age. However, septoplasty need not be withheld until the child is in his late teens as advocated in the past. With this in mind, an adequate improvement can be obtained utilizing minimal resection of cartilage without loss of nasal support or jeopardizing nasal growth.

### Indications

Septoplasty is indicated where there is sufficient septal deviation to cause nasal obstruction and/or recurrent epistaxis.

### Preoperative Evaluation

Visual examination or endoscopy after the nasal mucosa is vasoconstricted with 4% cocaine is adequate (alternately, any combination of a topical vasoconstrictor and local anesthetic may be used). Radiographic examination is not helpful.

### Operative Technique

1. Septoplasty in children and teenagers is best performed using general anesthesia. The nasal mucosa is injected bilaterally with 1% lidocaine with 1:100,000 epinephrine along the mucoperichondrial plane (Fig. 13–1**A**). Intranasal vasoconstriction is accomplished with 4% cocaine applied with neurosurgical cottonoids (alternately, any combination of a topical vasoconstrictor and local anesthetic may be used).
2. An incision is then made on one side of the nasal septum through the mucosa and perichondrium, but not through the septal cartilage (5 mm cephalad to the caudal edge) (Fig. 13–1**B**).
3. The mucoperichondrial flap is elevated with a sharp, flat elevator (e.g., Cottle elevator) (Fig. 13–1**C**, **D**).
4. If needed, the mucoperichondrial flap is elevated on the opposite side by dissecting the caudal end of the septum around to the opposite side (Fig. 13–1E) or by making an incision through the cartilage, but not through the contralateral mucosa (Fig. 13–1**F**) and elevating the mucoperichondrium.
5. Small strips of cartilage are removed or cut to permit repositioning of the cartilage. Care should be taken to preserve the dorsal and the caudal portions of the quadrangular cartilage to avoid loss of support (Fig. 13–1**G**, **H**). Resection of cartilage is kept to a minimum to prevent disturbance of subsequent nasal growth.
6. Thick areas and reduplications of bone or cartilage may be shaved with a knife or sharp chisel to reduce bulk (Fig. 13–1**I**).

7. Through-and-through sutures of 5-0 chromic are placed to secure the position of the cartilage and to reapproximate elevated mucoperichondrial flaps and to reduce the dead space (Fig. 13–1J).
8. The caudal incision is closed with 5-0 chromic sutures (Fig. 13–1J).
9. A Telfa strip or Merocel pack with a silk suture attached is placed on each side of the nose to apply gentle pressure to the septum (Fig. 13–1K).
10. The packing can be removed by pulling the silk sutures in 12 to 24 hours.
11. Antistaphylococcal antibiotics are administered for 7 days.

## Complications

1. Septal perforation
2. Saddle nose deformity
3. Persistent septal deviation
4. Synechiae

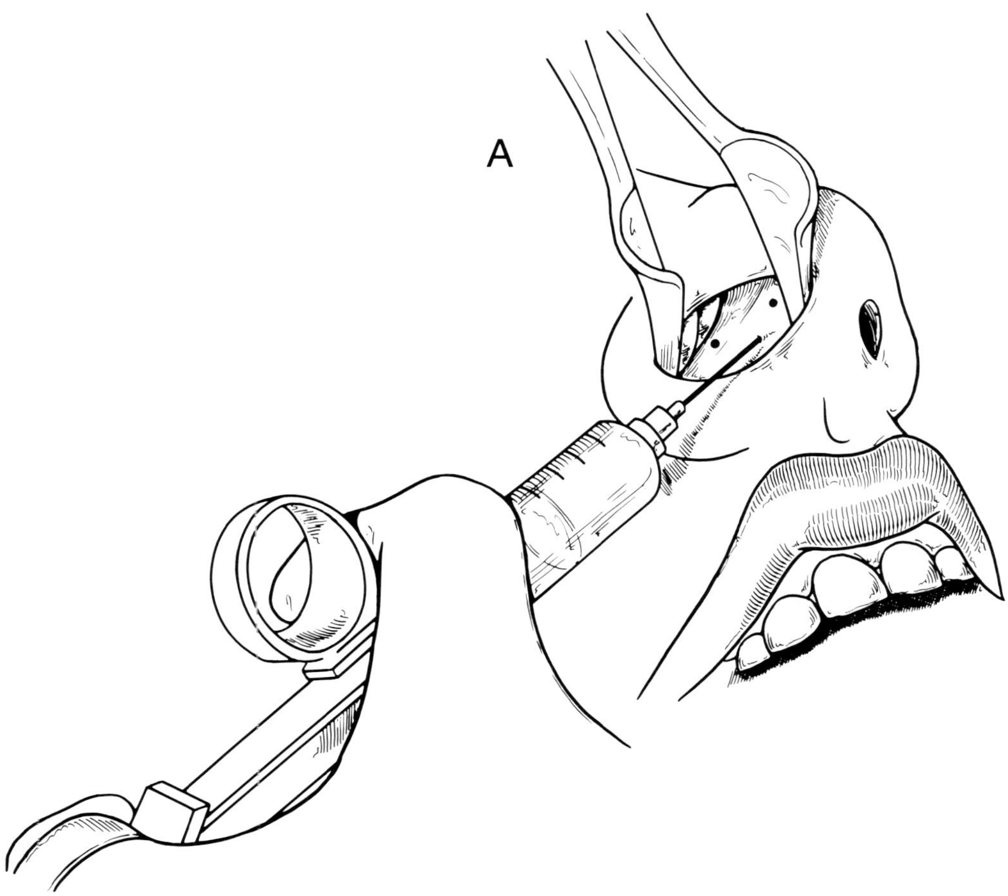


▶ **FIGURE 13-1**

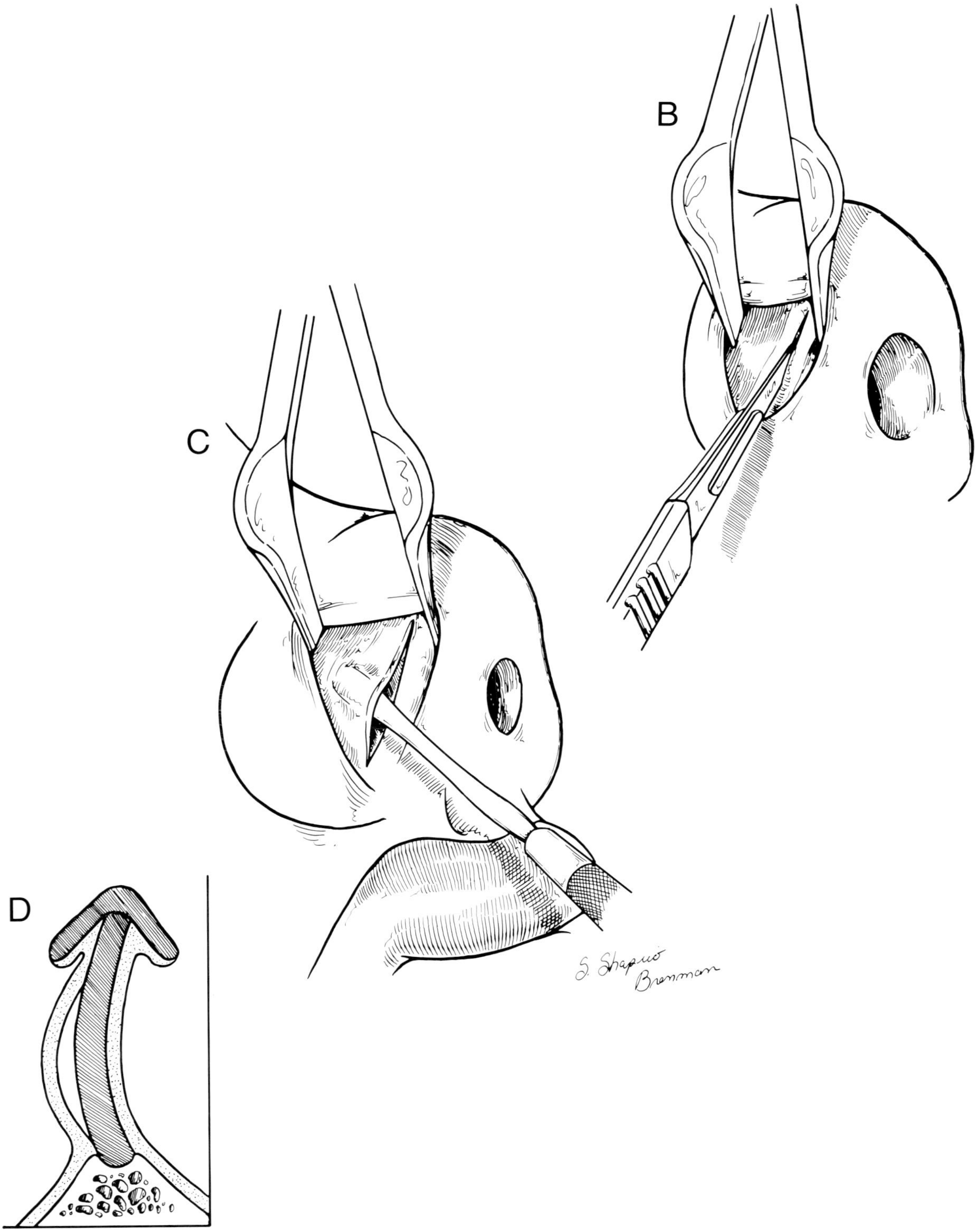


▶ **FIGURE 13-1**

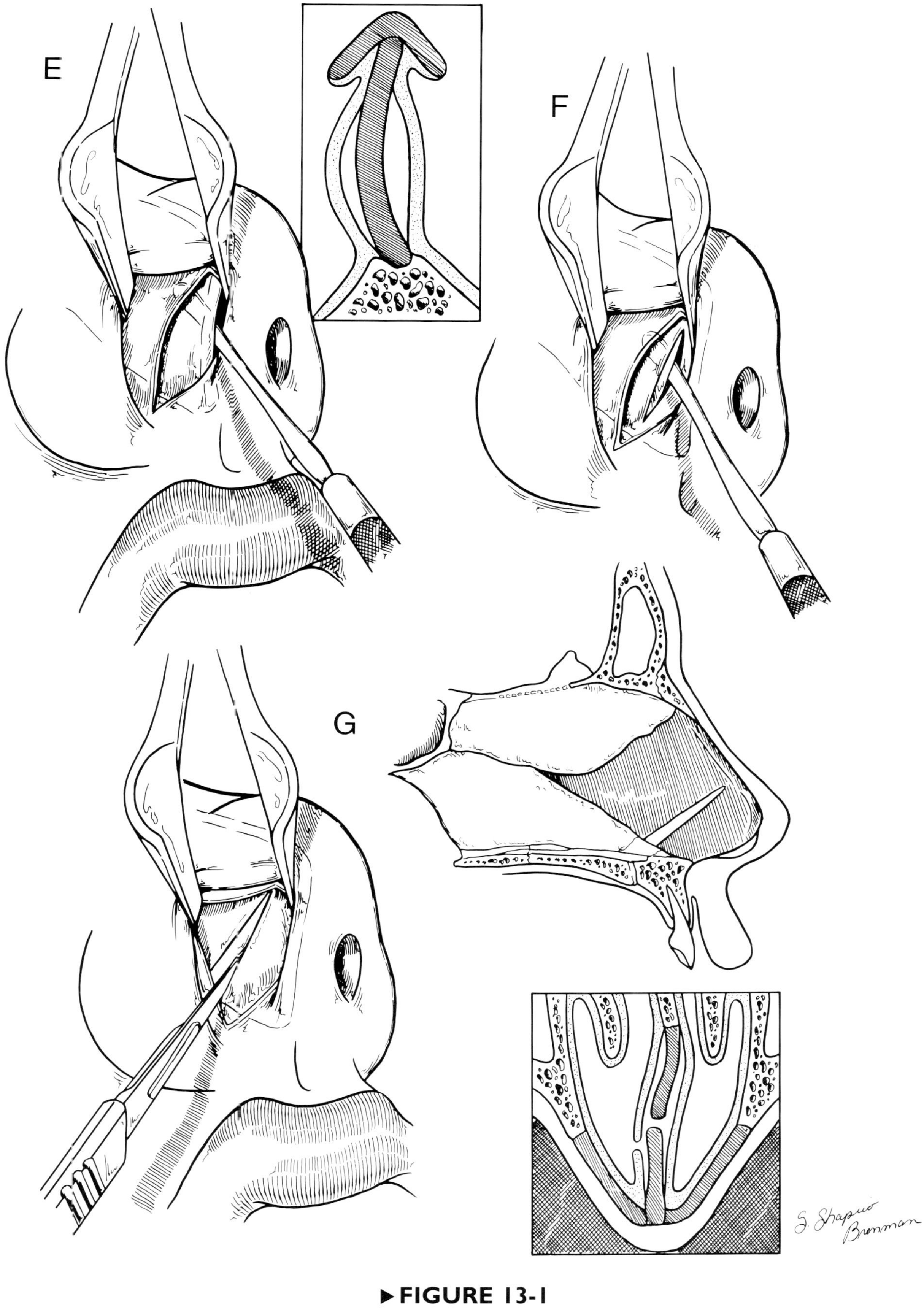


▶**FIGURE 13-1**

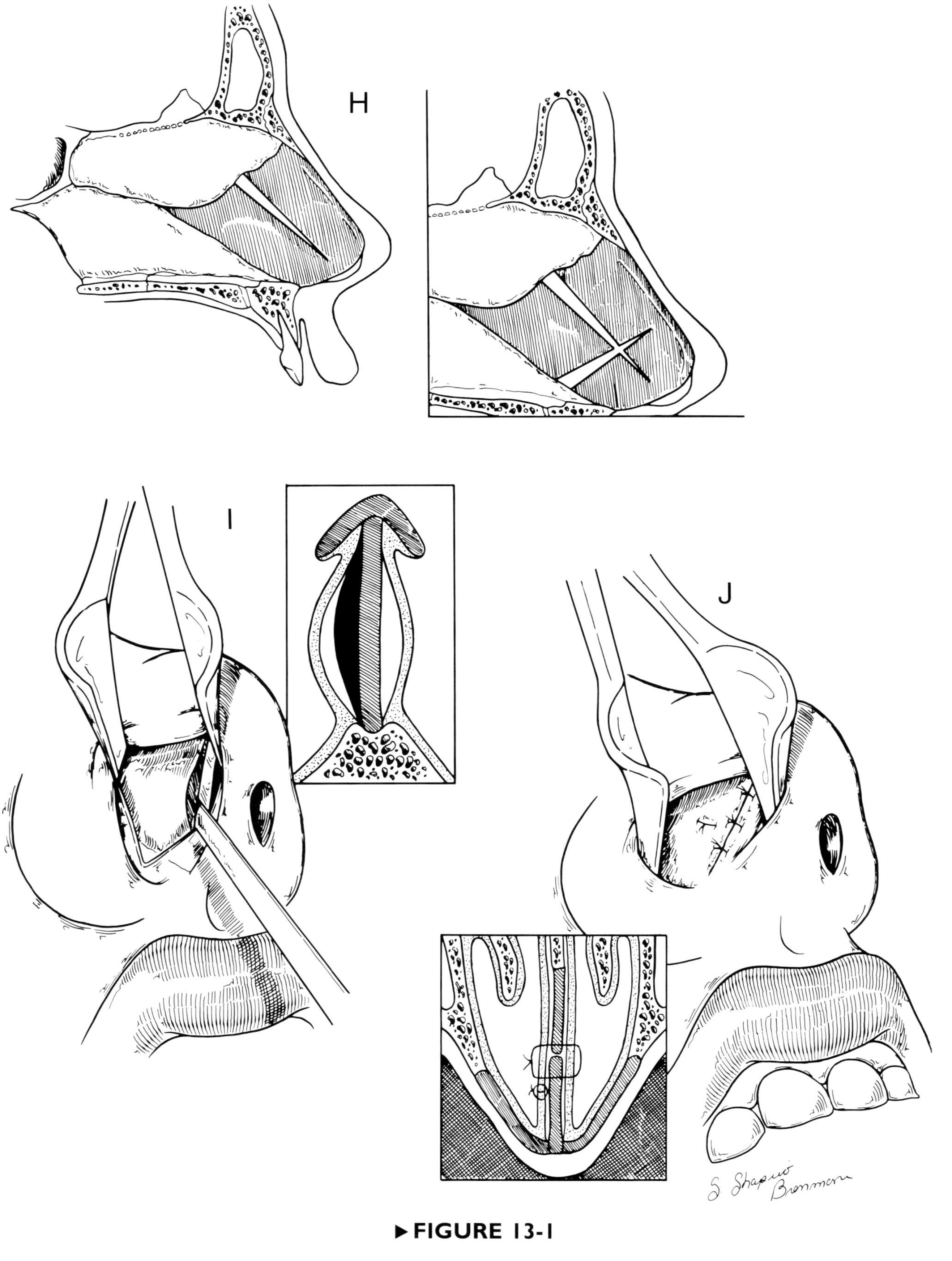


▶**FIGURE 13-1**

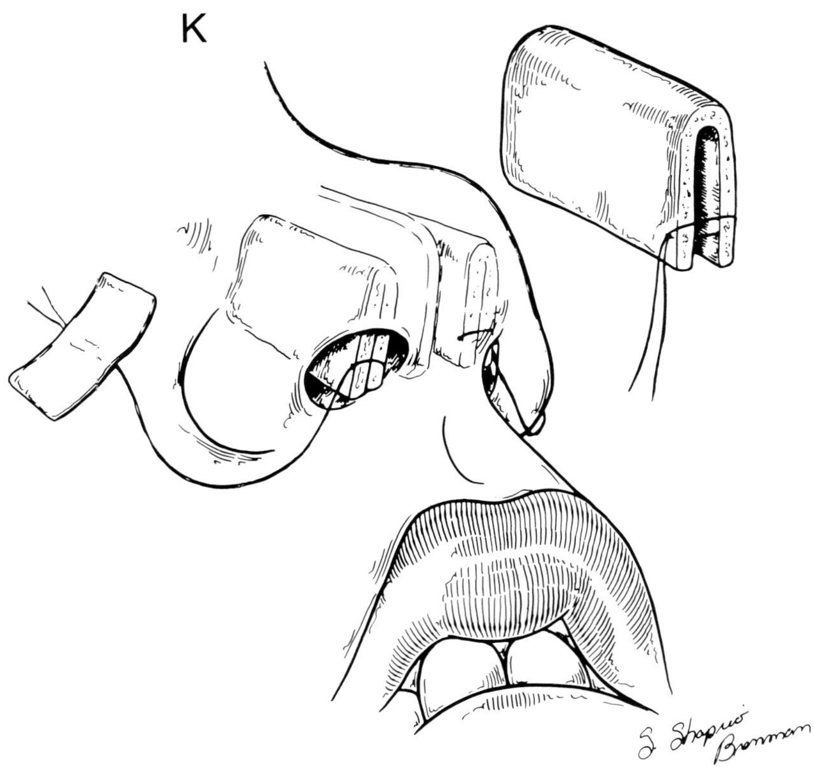


▶ **FIGURE 13-1**

## 13-2 CONSERVATIVE RHINOPLASTY

Conservative rhinoplasty is a procedure to straighten a congenitally or traumatically deviated nose and septum. Rhinoplasty in children is best deferred until the middle teenage years when resection of bone or cartilage is unlikely to alter growth of the nose.

Correction of the deviated nose in a child should be performed cautiously and conservatively taking into account the anatomy, severity of the deformity, and psychosocial circumstances.

### Indications

Rhinoplasty is indicated to straighten a congenitally or traumatically deformed nose.

### Preoperative Evaluation

Visual inspection of the nasal pyramid and nasal septum is essential because the external nasal deformity is often accompanied by a septal deviation. Both deformities must be corrected to obtain an adequate result. Radiographs are rarely helpful in this evaluation.

### Operative Technique

1. Rhinoplasty in children is best done utilizing general anesthesia and local injection of the nasal tissues with 1% lidocaine with 1:100,000 epinephrine. Intranasal vasoconstriction is accomplished with 4% cocaine applied with neurosurgical cottonoids (alternately, any combination of a topical vasoconstrictor and local anesthetic may be used).
2. The nasal septum is injected as described for septoplasty (see section 13–1).
3. A line of local anesthesia is placed on each side of the nose by injection 1% lidocaine with 1:100,000 epinephrine in the subcutaneous tissues halfway between the nasal dorsum and the lateral border of the nose (Fig. 13–2**A**).
4. The mucosa at the lower edge of the upper lateral cartilage is injected at multiple sites with just enough solution to blanch the tissues, but not enough to deform the nose (Fig. 13–2**B**).
5. The septum is corrected as described in septoplasty (see section 13–1).
6. An intercartilaginous incision is made at the lower edge of the upper lateral cartilage (Fig. 13–2**C**).
7. The skin over the dorsum of the nose is elevated by sharp dissection with a blunt scissors (Fig. 13–2**D**, **E**).
8. If the nasal septal deviation is high and the septum is adherent to the upper lateral cartilages, it is released by cutting the attachments with a knife or septal scissors while protecting the overlying skin of the nasal dorsum (Fig. 13–2**F**, **G**). Otherwise, the upper lateral cartilages are left attached to the septum.
9. The medial osteotomy is performed by placing a small osteotome at the caudal edge of the nasal bones along the septum. The osteotome is directed posterior-superiorly along the septum with gentle taps from a small mallet. The osteotomy is curved laterally to meet the point of return fracture expected from the lateral osteotomy (Fig. 13–2**H**).

10. For the lateral osteotomy, a small transverse incision is made with a knife down to the edge of the pyriform aperture just above the attachment of the inferior turbinate. Scissors are used to clean off remaining soft tissue attachments from the bony edge (Fig. 13–2**I**).
11. A small osteotome is placed in the incision. A lateral osteotomy is carried out with gentle taps from a small mallet as the osteotome advances along the lateral base of the nose (Fig. 13–2**J**).
12. The nasal pyramid is then mobilized manually and positioned in the midline (Fig. 13–2**K**).
13. A 2 × 4 cm piece of Telfa is folded and placed in each side of the nose to help reapproximate mucosal flaps and to stabilize the nasal structures (alternately, Merocel packing may be used). A long 3-0 silk suture is placed at the anterior edge of the packing to facilitate its removal in 12 to 24 hours (Fig. 13–2**L**).
14. A splint made of plaster or a prefabricated material is placed on the nose to protect the nasal pyramid. This can be removed in 7 days.
15. Antibiotics are administered for 7–10 days.

### In the Neonate

1. The neonate may have a severely deviated nose secondary to birth trauma. The nose should be replaced by firm digital pressure.
2. If the deviation has been present for more than a week, it may not be amenable to manual reduction.
3. Long-standing deviation (>2 weeks) should be left alone, as the deformity may usually correct itself in 1 to 3 months. The resulting position may not be perfect, but is usually quite acceptable.
4. If the nose remains severely deviated, it may be corrected after 4 years of age. Correction of lesser deformities should be delayed until the teenage years.

## Complications

1. Poor cosmetic/functional result
2. Septal perforation
3. Orbital hemorrhage

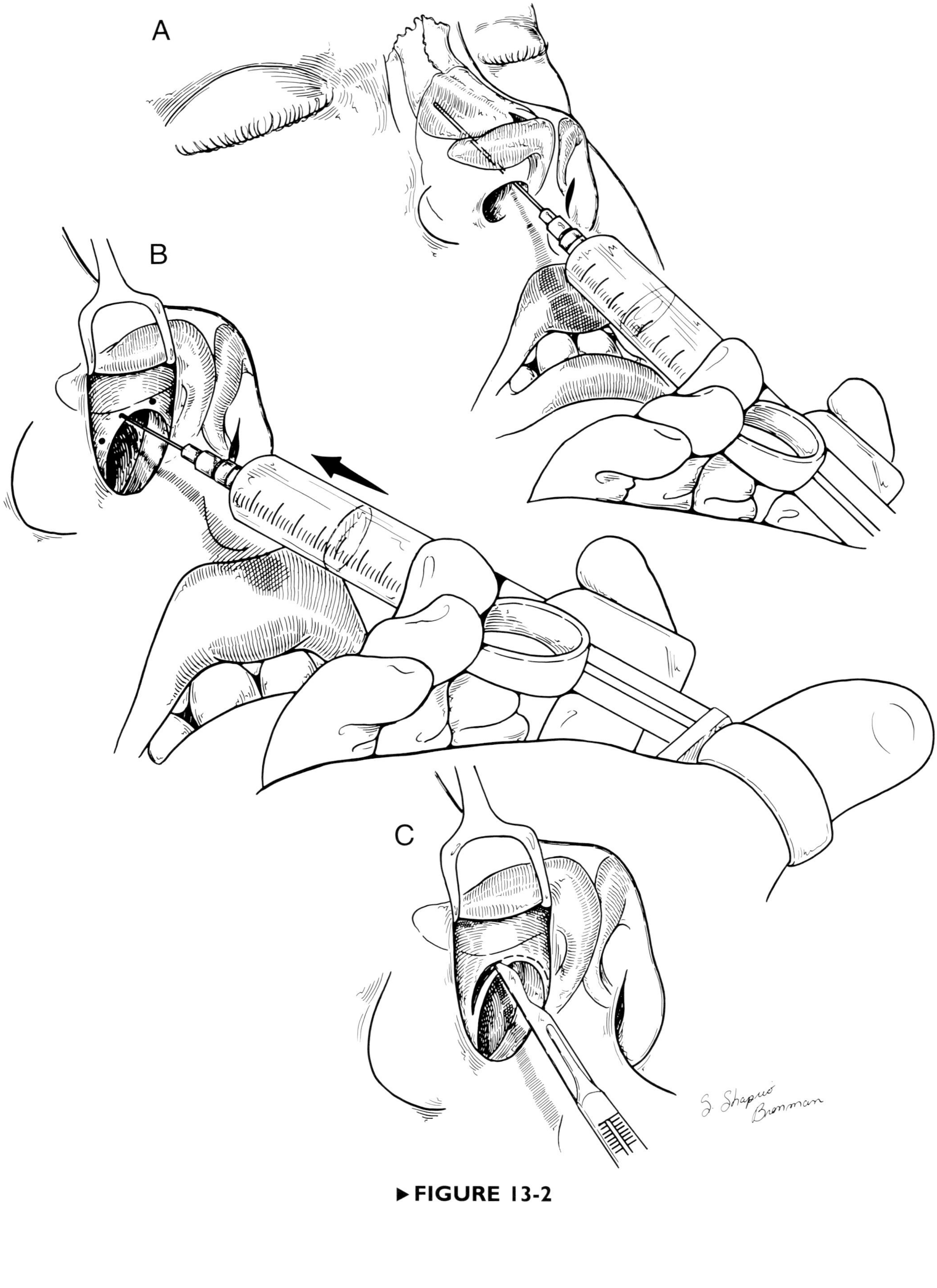


▶ **FIGURE 13-2**

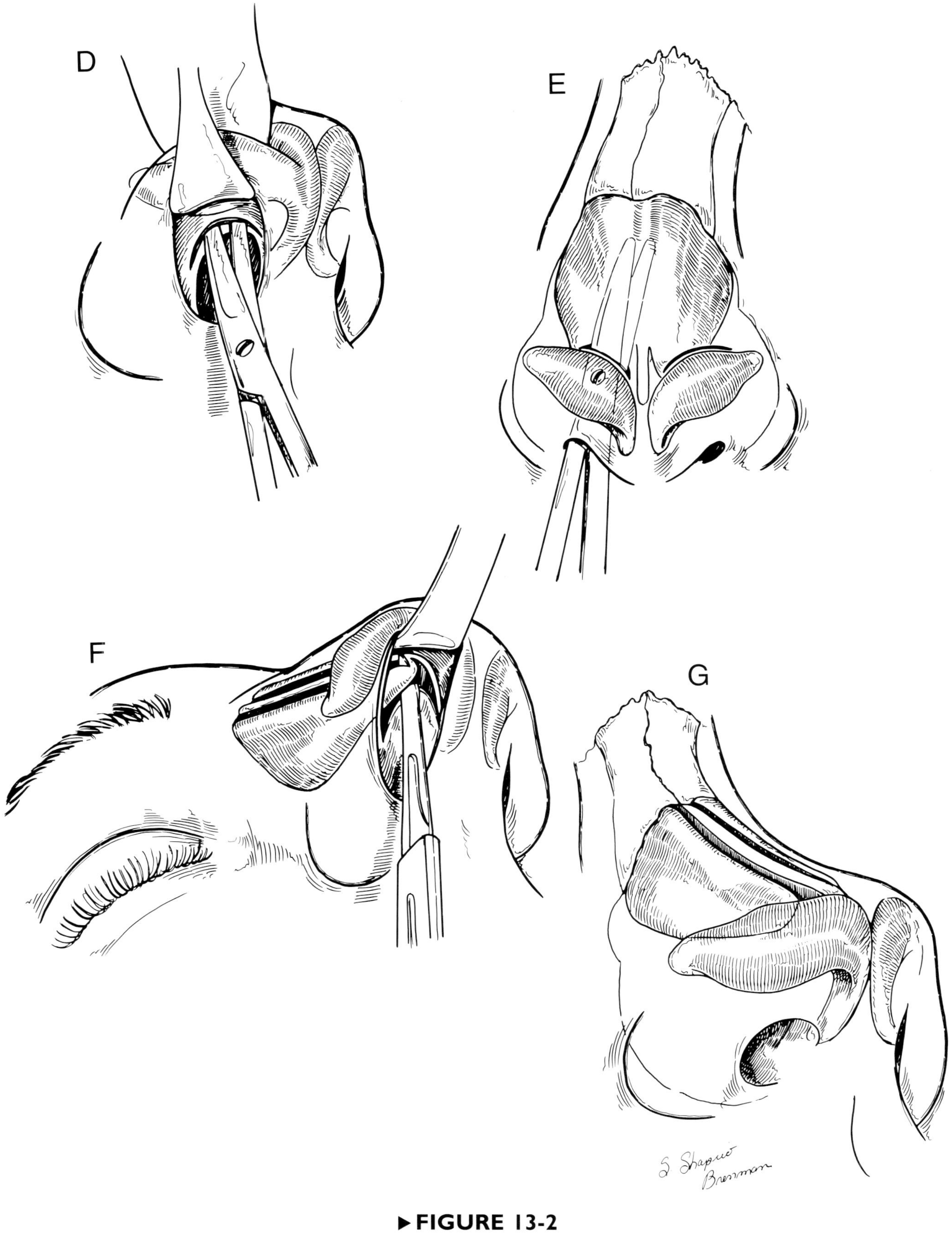


▸**FIGURE 13-2**

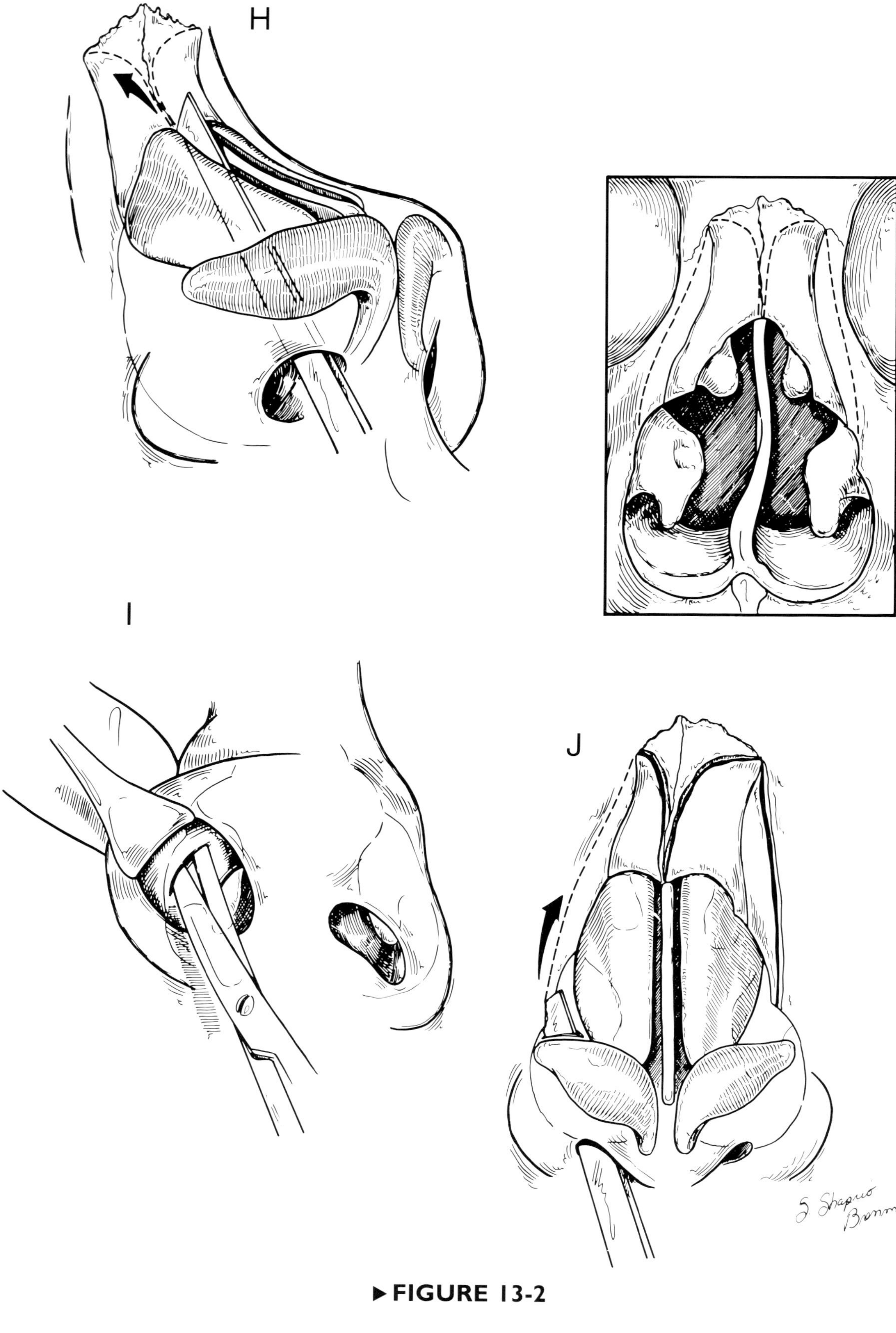


▶**FIGURE 13-2**

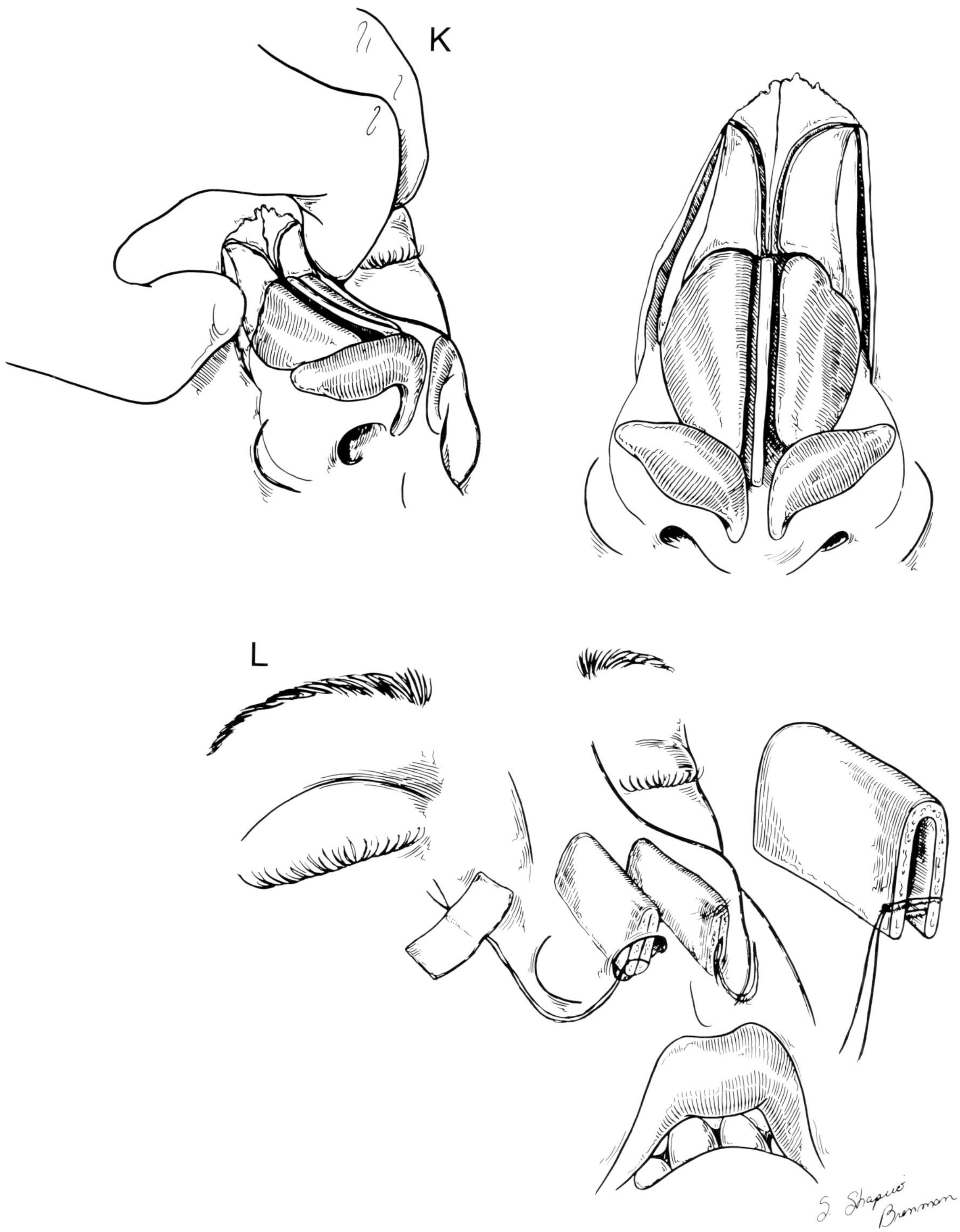


▶ **FIGURE 13-2**

# 14 ▶ Nasal Tumors

## ▶ 14-1 LATERAL RHINOTOMY

Lateral rhinotomy is a technique to provide increased exposure of the nasal cavity. Small anterior intranasal tumors often can be exposed utilizing the alar approach described for skin grafting of the septum (see section 11–7, Septal Graft for Telangiectasia). Nasal septal or lateral nasal wall tumors are best approached through a lateral rhinotomy.

### Indications

The presence of a mass in the lateral wall or septum requires a lateral rhinotomy for adequate exposure.

### Preoperative Evaluation

Preoperative evaluation of intranasal tumors includes anterior and posterior rhinoscopy. Computed tomography (CT) is necessary to determine the size and extent of the tumor.

### Operative Technique

1. Removal of the intranasal tumors should be carried out under general anesthesia.
2. One percent lidocaine with 1:100,000 epinephrine is injected in the line of the proposed incision to aid in hemostasis.
3. The ala is released with a 15 knife blade to the anterior edge of the pyriform aperture (Fig. 14–1**A, B**).
4. For additional exposure, the incision is continued along the lateral border of the nose or to the lower edge of the bony rim of the orbit. The incision can be further extended, if needed, along the inferior eyelid to provide additional lateral exposure through the anterior wall of the maxillary sinus. Extension of the incision superiorly along a line one-half the distance between the medial canthus and the dorsum of the nose permits access to the ethmoid area to provide lateral exposure of a high and/or deep tumor (Fig. 14–1**C**).
5. The nasal bone is cut along its lateral border with the maxilla using a small osteotome (Fig. 14–1**D**). The bony cut is then angled medially to complete the fracture at the junction of the nasal bone and the bony nasal septum (Fig. 14–1**E**).
6. Lateral and posterior exposure is obtained by opening the maxillary and/or ethmoid sinuses (Fig. 14–1**F**). Bone is removed with a bone rongeur and forceps.
7. The tumor is then removed by sharp dissection with a scissors or knife (Fig. 14–1**G**).
8. The nasal bone is returned to its normal position.
9. The incision is closed with 3-0 chromic sutures in the subcutaneous tissues.

**10.** The skin is closed with 4-0 interrupted subcuticular chromic sutures (Fig. 14–1H).

## Complications

1. Infraorbital nerve injury
2. Orbital hemorrhage
3. Cerebrospinal fluid leak
4. Nasal deformity

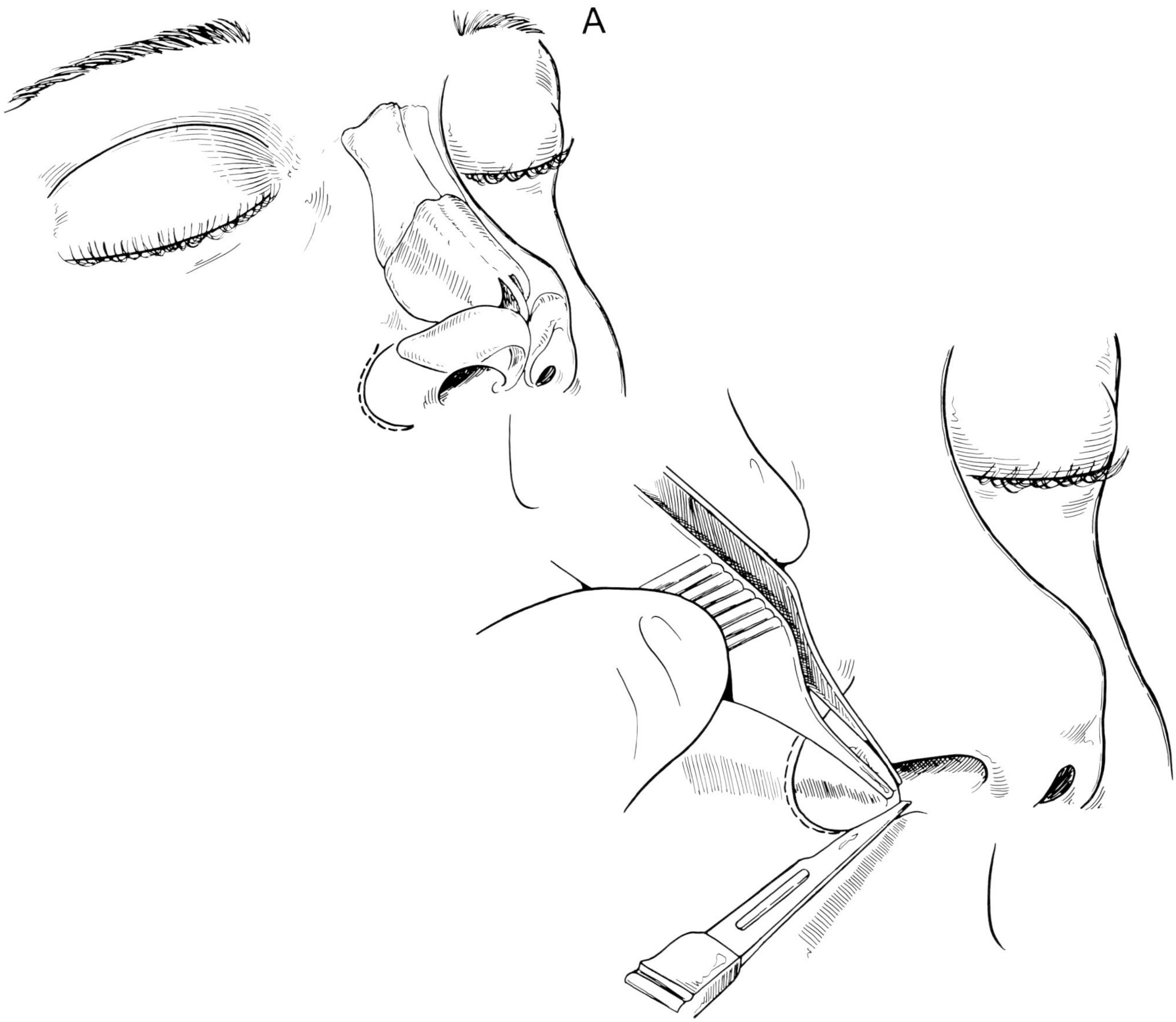


▶ **FIGURE 14-1**

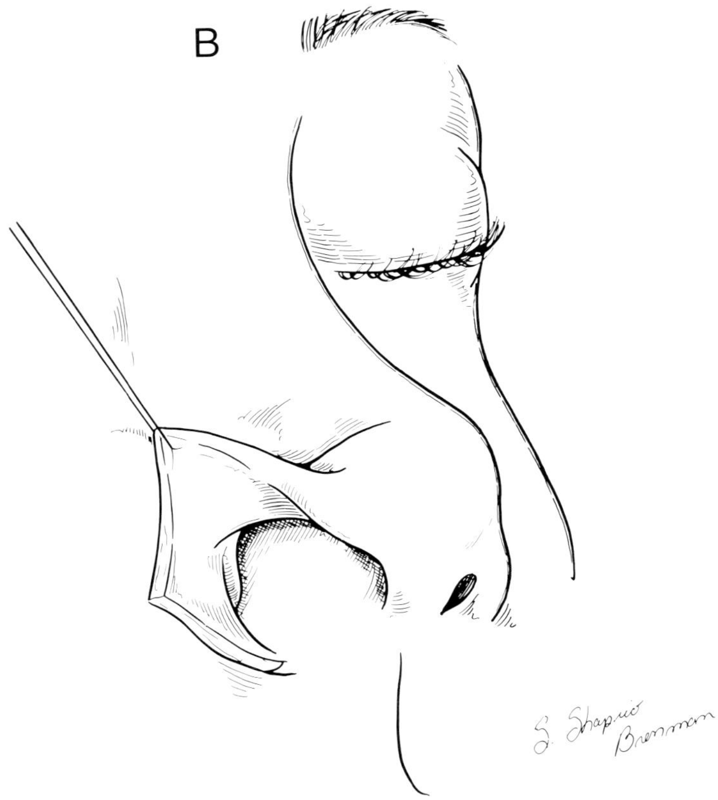


▶ **FIGURE 14-1**

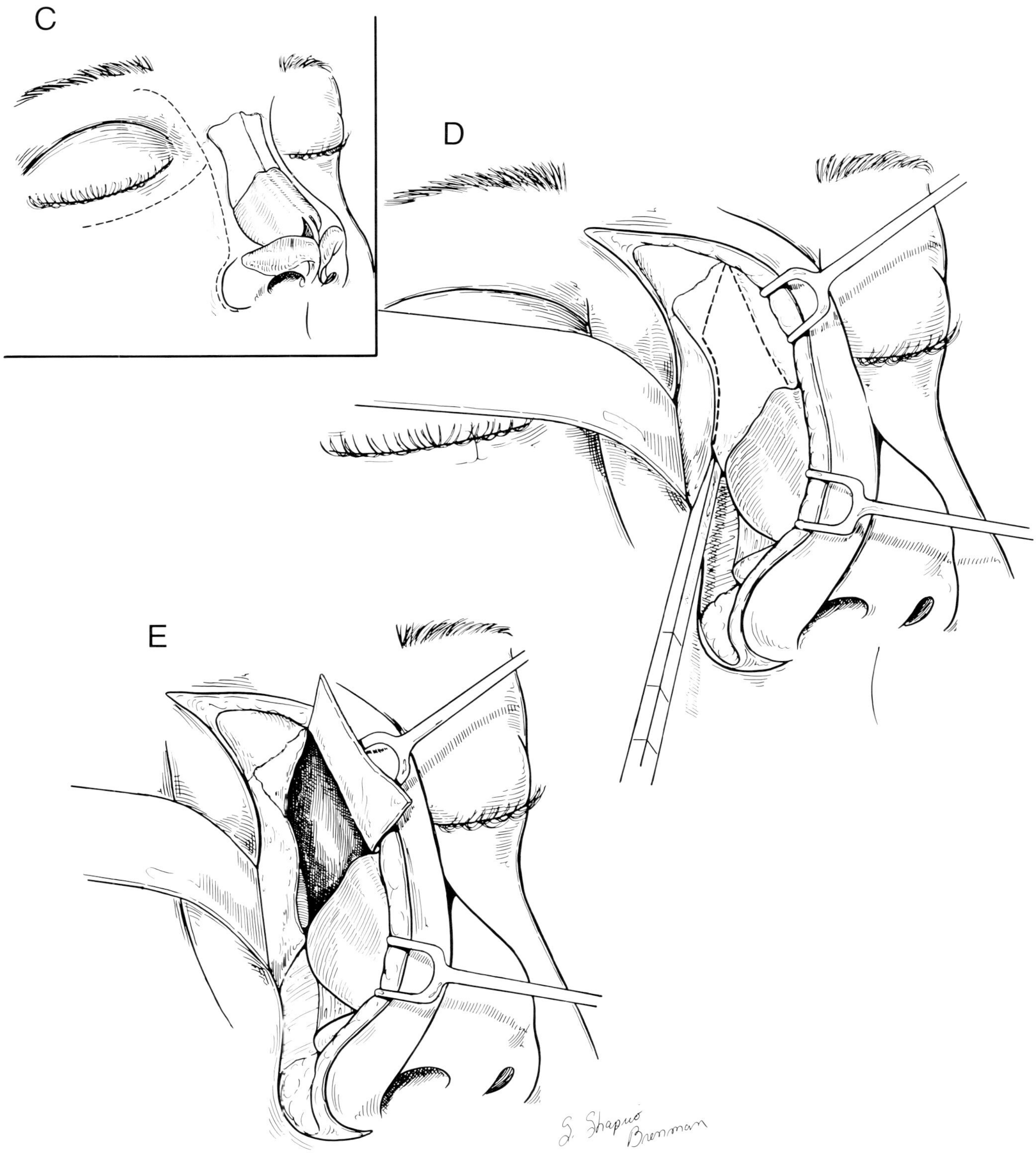


▶ **FIGURE 14-1**

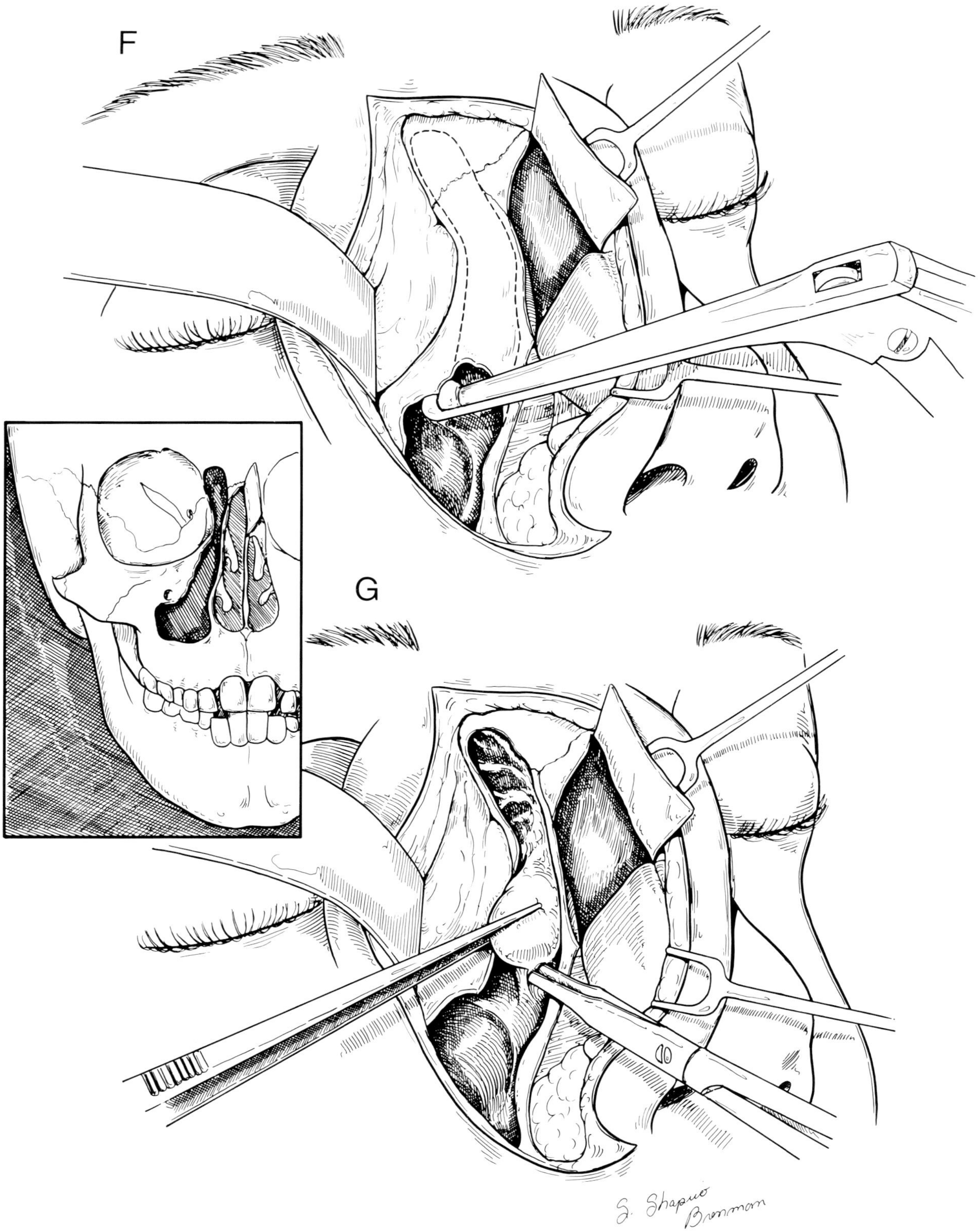


▶**FIGURE 14-1**

H

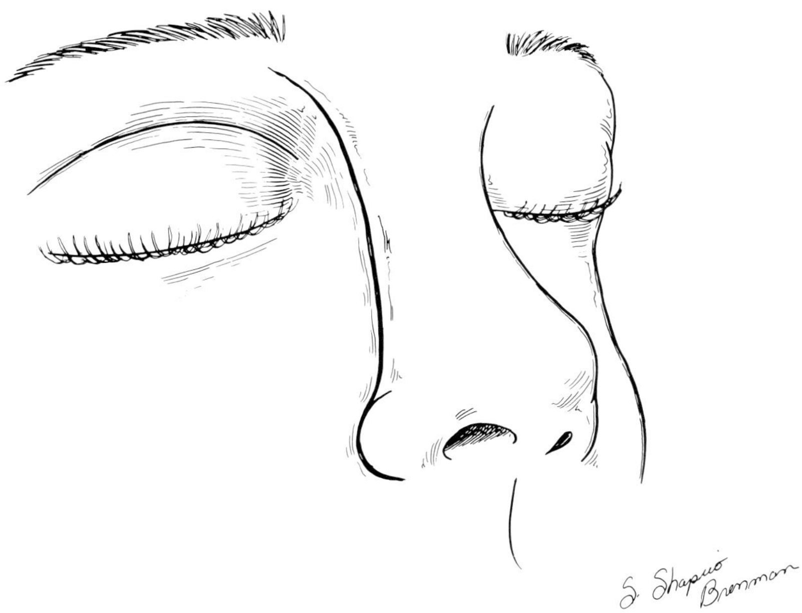


▶ **FIGURE 14-1**

## ▶ 14-2 NASAL POLYPECTOMY

Nasal polyps are uncommon in children and adolescents. They may occur unilaterally or bilaterally. The etiologies of nasal polyps in children include chronic infection, allergy, and cystic fibrosis.

### Indications

The indication for nasal polypectomy is chronic nasal obstruction and/or infection that has not resolved with medical therapy.

### Preoperative Evaluation

Nasal endoscopy is extremely important prior to operative intervention. Computed tomography (CT) is helpful to assess the condition of the nose and sinuses prior to nasal polypectomy. Unilateral sinus disease suggests an infectious etiology. Resection of unilateral polyps is likely to provide drainage and is usually not associated with recurrence. Diffuse bilateral sinus disease, however, suggests an allergic etiology or cystic fibrosis. Simple polypectomy is seldom curative. Sinus surgery is almost always required to provide long-term relief of symptoms.

### Operative Technique

1. Nasal polypectomy in children and adolescents is best carried out under general anesthesia.
2. Topical 4% cocaine (alternately, any combination of a topical vasoconstrictor and local anesthetic may be used) is placed in the nasal cavity on cotton pledgets to decongest the mucosa and provide improved visibility.
3. Polyps are usually pedunculated and should be removed as close to their base as possible.
4. A nasal snare or forceps is advanced into the nasal cavity and manipulated around the base of the polyp (Fig. 14–2**A**). The wire is tightened around the stalk and the polyp is avulsed.
5. Smaller nasal polyps and residual tags are removed with a biting forceps (Fig. 14–2**B**).
6. Antral choanal polyps can be removed by grasping the base of the polyp with a forceps while pushing the polyp forward from the nasopharynx with the index finger of the opposite hand (Fig. 14–2**C**). On rare occasions, the polyp is too large to remove through the anterior nare and must be delivered into the nasopharynx.
7. If the origin of the polyp is the maxillary sinus and the dumbbell component of the polyp is not removed with the forceps, a Caldwell Luc or functional endoscopic sinus surgery should be performed to remove the residual tissue from the sinus to prevent recurrence.

### Complications

1. Recurrence of polyps
2. Nasal synechiae

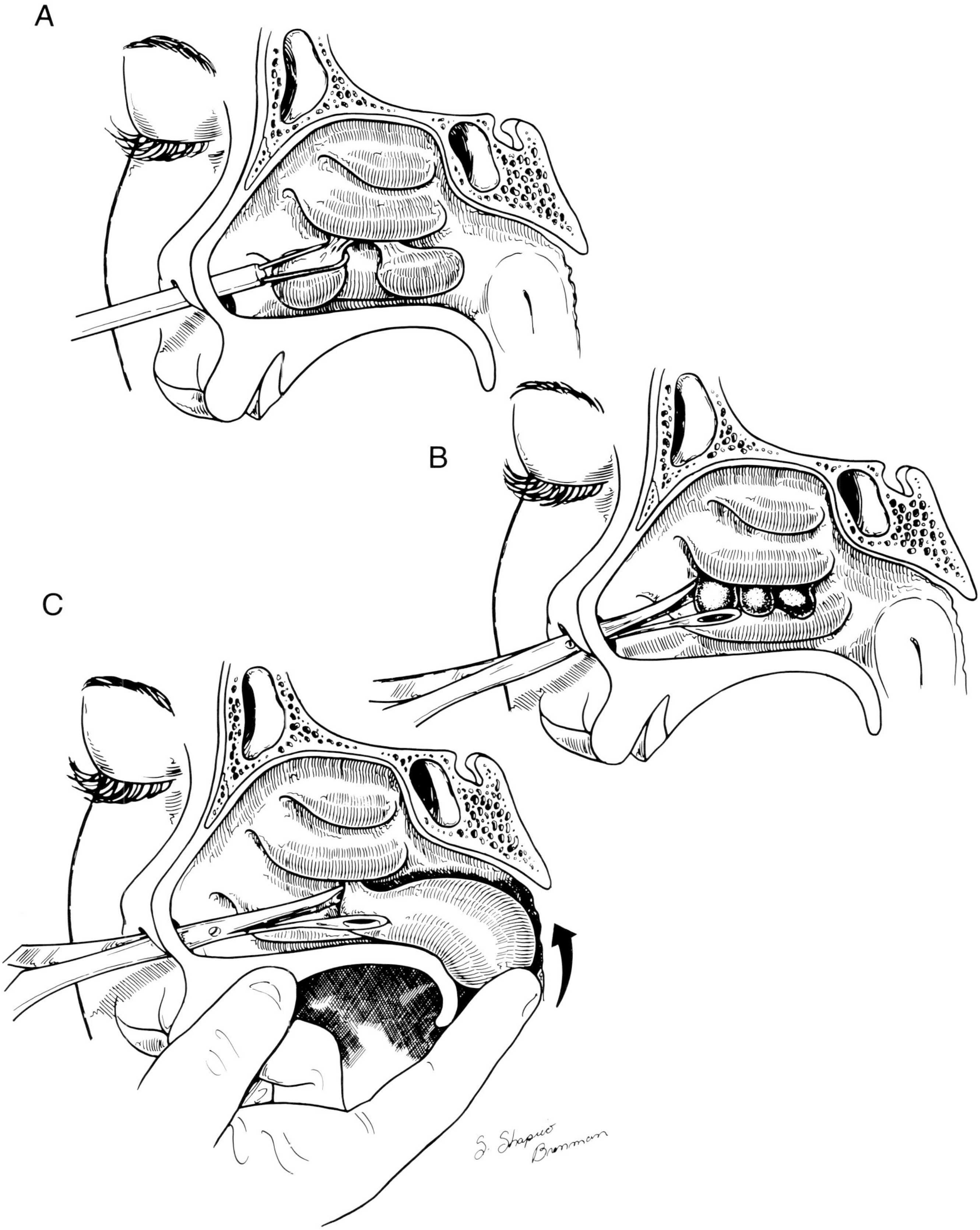


▶ **FIGURE 14-2**

## ▶ 14-3 EXCISION OF NASAL DERMOID CYST

A dermoid cyst is a congenital lesion that appears as a subcutaneous mass on the dorsum of the nose. Often, there is a single opening on the skin that has hairs protruding from it.

### Indications

Surgery is indicated for all dermoid cysts because they enlarge and may become infected. Surgery is best carried out before infection occurs.

### Preoperative Evaluation

Preoperative evaluation with CT defines the extent and location of the cyst. The CT will be necessary to rule out an encephalocele or the very rare cyst that involves the frontal sinus.

### Operative Technique

1. General anesthesia is utilized in the removal of nasal dermoids.
2. One percent lidocaine with 1:100,000 epinephrine is injected in the line of the proposed incision.
3. A vertical incision with an ellipse around the pit or pits is made on the dorsum of the nose (Fig. 14–3**A**).
4. The skin flaps are elevated and retracted laterally. The sinus and underlying cyst are dissected from their surrounding attachments with a sharp scissors (Fig. 14–3**B**).
5. Any tract is followed to its end and removed. The tract usually lies in a trough in the septal cartilage at the attachment of the upper lateral cartilages.
6. If the tract enters the nose under the nasal bones, a medial osteotomy is performed with a chisel (without removing or elevating periosteum) (Fig. 14–3C).
7. A small clamp is used to lift up the nasal bones to expose the remainder of the cyst (Fig. 14–3**D, E**).
8. The tract and cyst are then dissected free from their attachments to the underlying nasal structures.
9. The nasal bones are replaced and the periosteum is sutured with 4-0 chromic sutures (Fig. 14–3**F**).
10. The incision is closed with 4-0 interrupted subcuticular chromic sutures and a thin rubber band drain is left in the wound. Steri-strips are applied to the nasal dorsum (Fig. 14–3**G**).
11. The rubber band drain is removed in 24 hours.
12. If the dermoid cyst was infected at the time of operation, antibiotics are administered for 7 to 10 days.

### Complications

1. Recurrence secondary to incomplete removal of the cyst

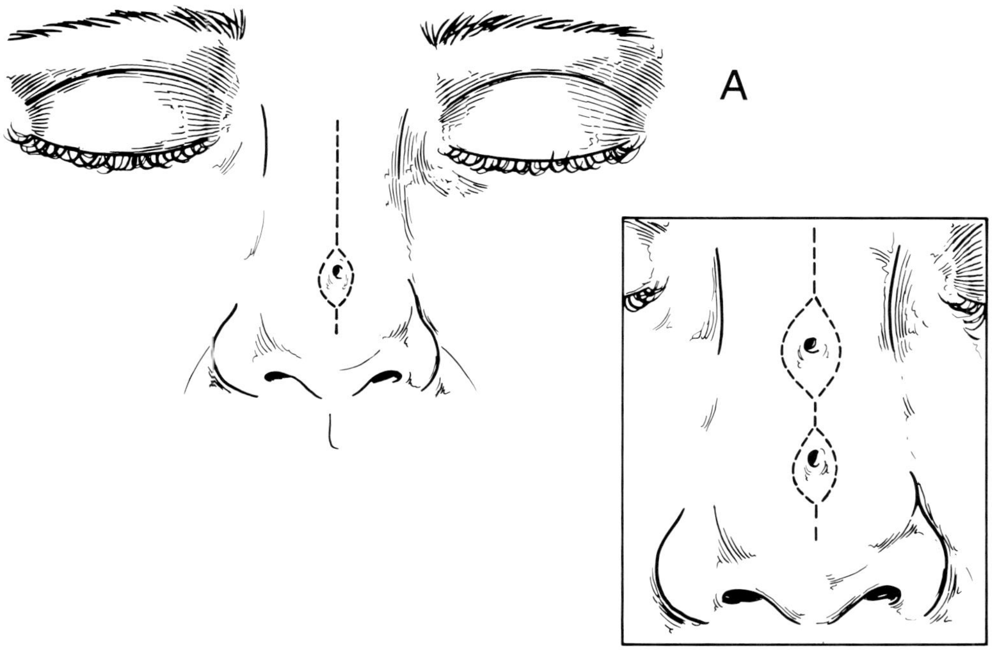


▶ **FIGURE 14-3**

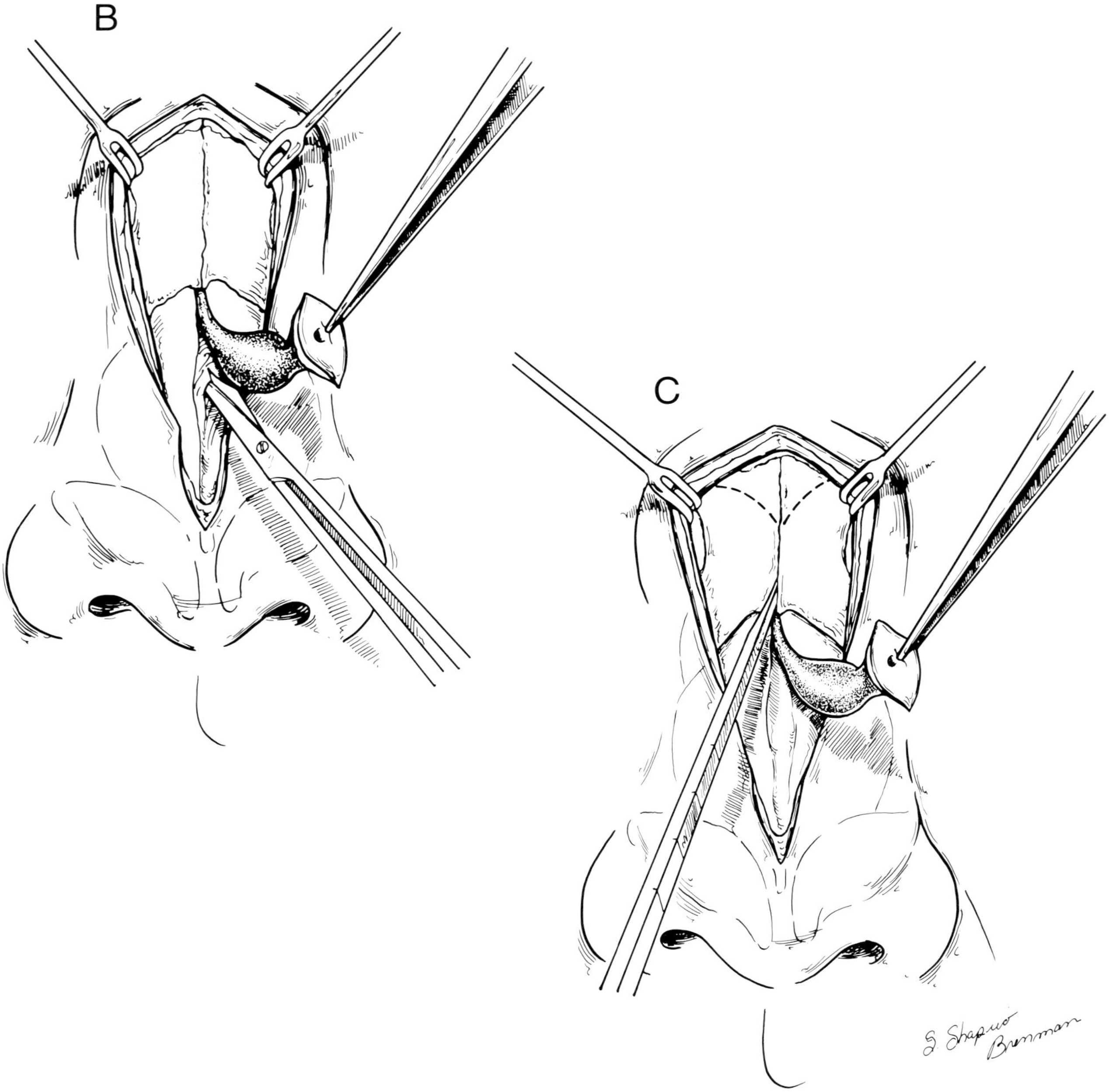


▶ **FIGURE 14-3**

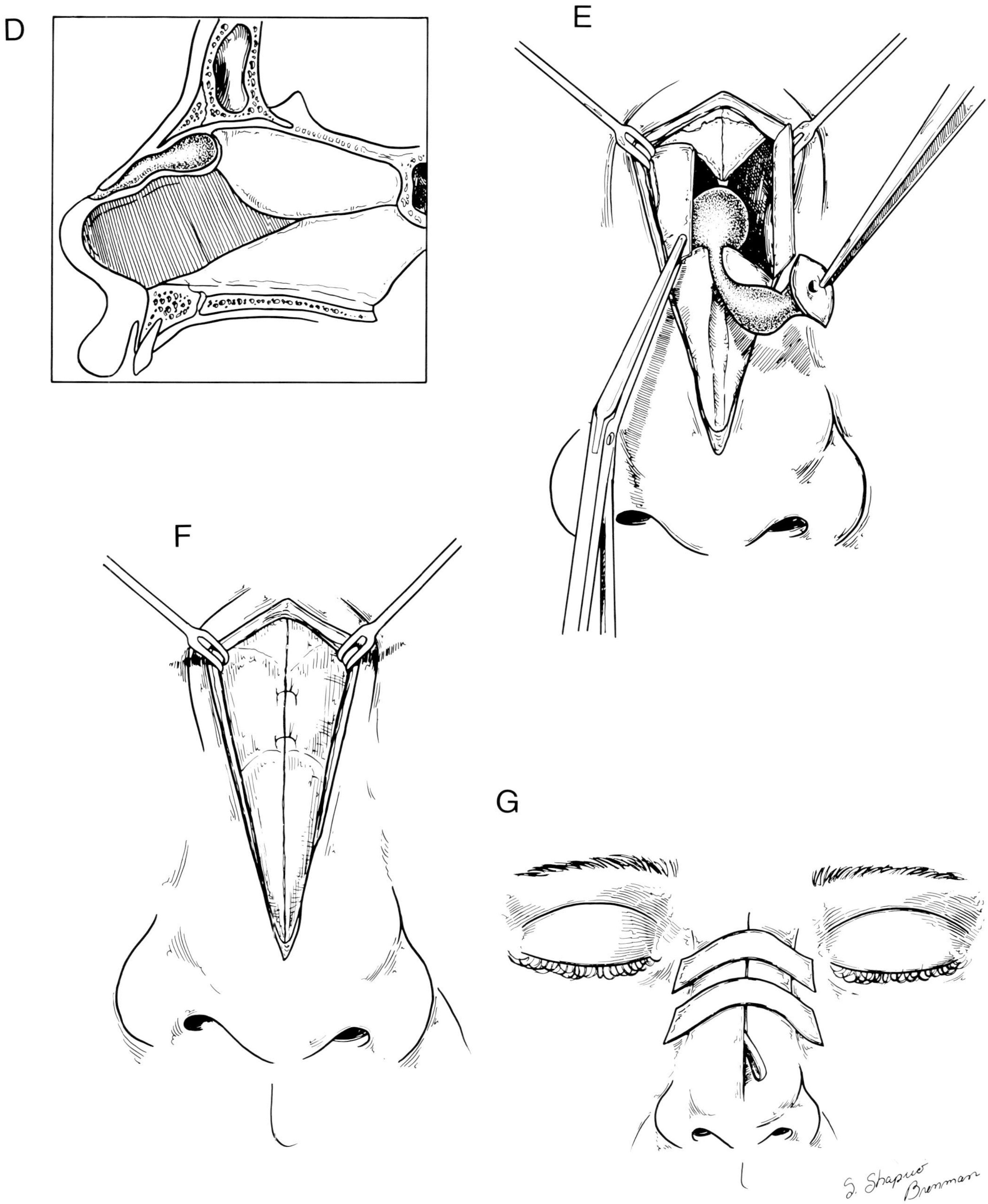


▶ **FIGURE 14-3**

## ▶ 14-4 RESECTION OF LYMPHANGIOMA OF THE NASAL TIP

Congenital lymphangiomas of the nasal tip are uncommon but can present a significant cosmetic problem in a young child. Small lymphangiomas causing minimal deformity are best left alone.

### Indications

Large disfiguring lymphangiomas should be excised or debulked when the child is 4 to 5 years of age.

### Preoperative Evaluation

A complete and careful nasal examination is essential and preoperative pictures are helpful to evaluate postoperative results. A CT or magnetic resonance imaging (MRI) scan may be helpful to rule out deep extension of the lesion.

### Operative Technique

1. Excision of a nasal lymphangioma is performed utilizing a general anesthetic supplemented by 1% lidocaine with 1:100,000 epinephrine for hemostasis.
2. An incision is made down to but not through the perichondrium in the nasal vestibule bilaterally and across the base of the columella (Fig. 14–4**A**).
3. If better dorsal nasal exposure is needed, the incisions can be extended into the nasolabial groove (Fig. 14–4**A**).
4. The skin of the nasal tip is elevated by blunt and sharp dissection with a scissors taking care not to perforate the overlying skin (Fig. 14–4**B**).
5. After the skin is reflected, the lymphangioma can be debulked and shaped with a scissors or surgical laser. Both the $CO_2$ and KPT laser are well suited for sculpting lymphangioma (Fig. 14–4**C**).
6. No attempt should be made to excise all of the lymphangioma.
7. The skin is draped over the nasal tip, distributing the excess evenly. No skin is resected. The incision is closed with 5-0 mild chromic sutures that do not require removal, or 5-0 subcuticular Vicryl sutures (Fig. 14–4**D**).
8. A nasal dressing with Steri-strips is applied to help shape the nose (Fig. 14–4**E**).
9. The Steri-strips are removed in 7 to 10 days. The excess skin shrinks to accommodate the debulked nasal tip in a few weeks.
10. Antibiotics are administered for 7 to 10 days.

### Complications

1. Poor cosmetic result

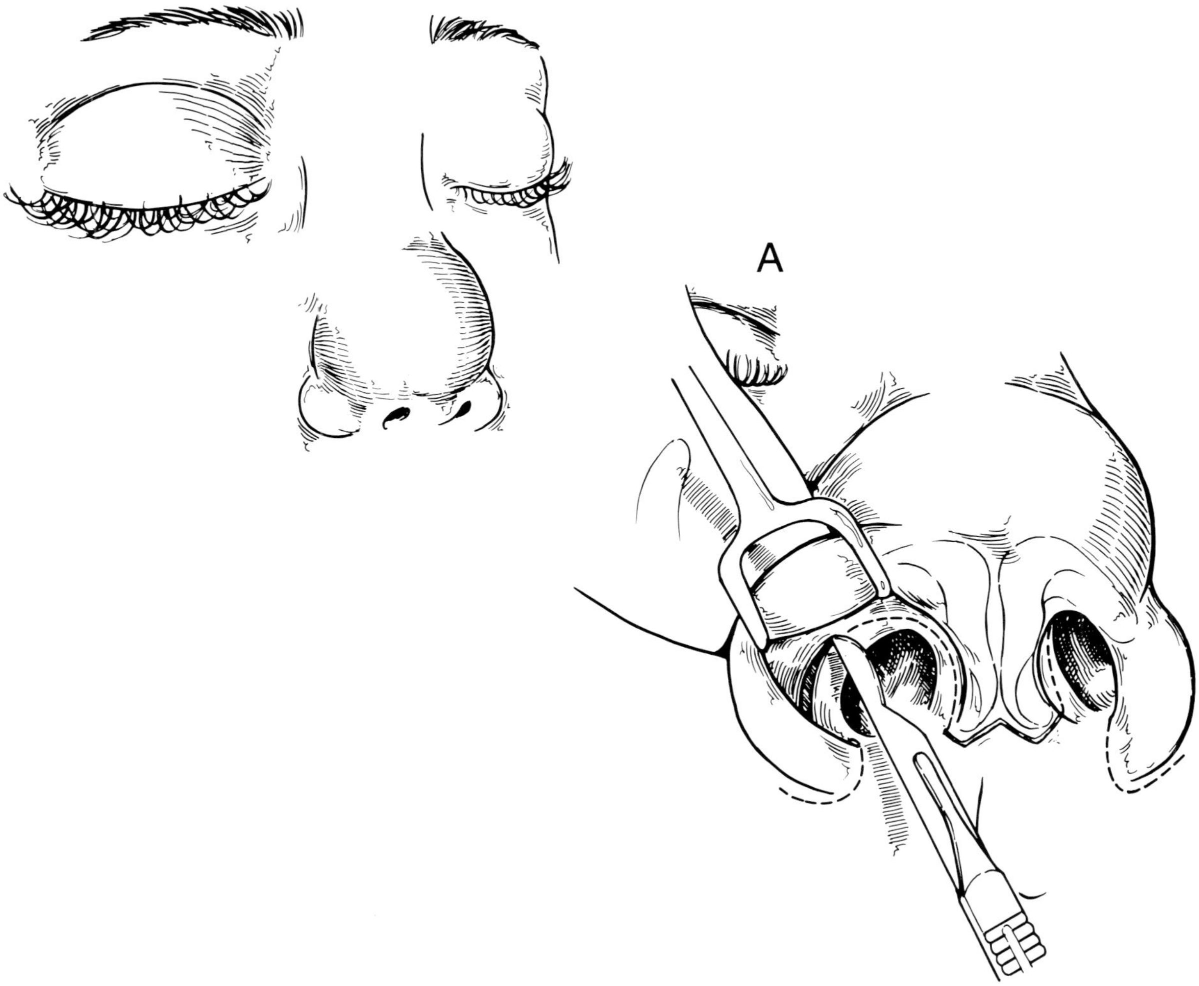


▶ **FIGURE 14-4**

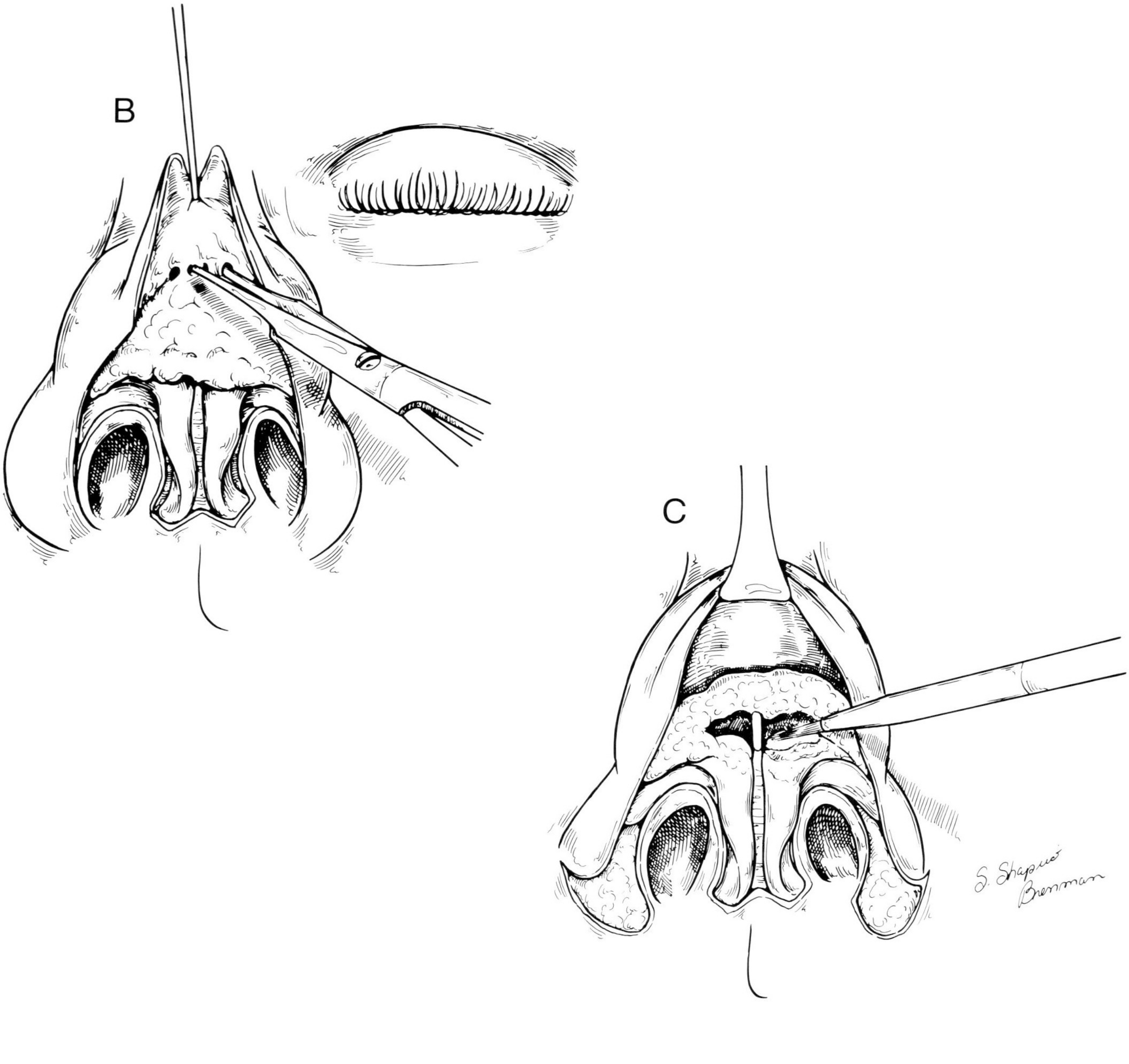


▶ **FIGURE 14-4**

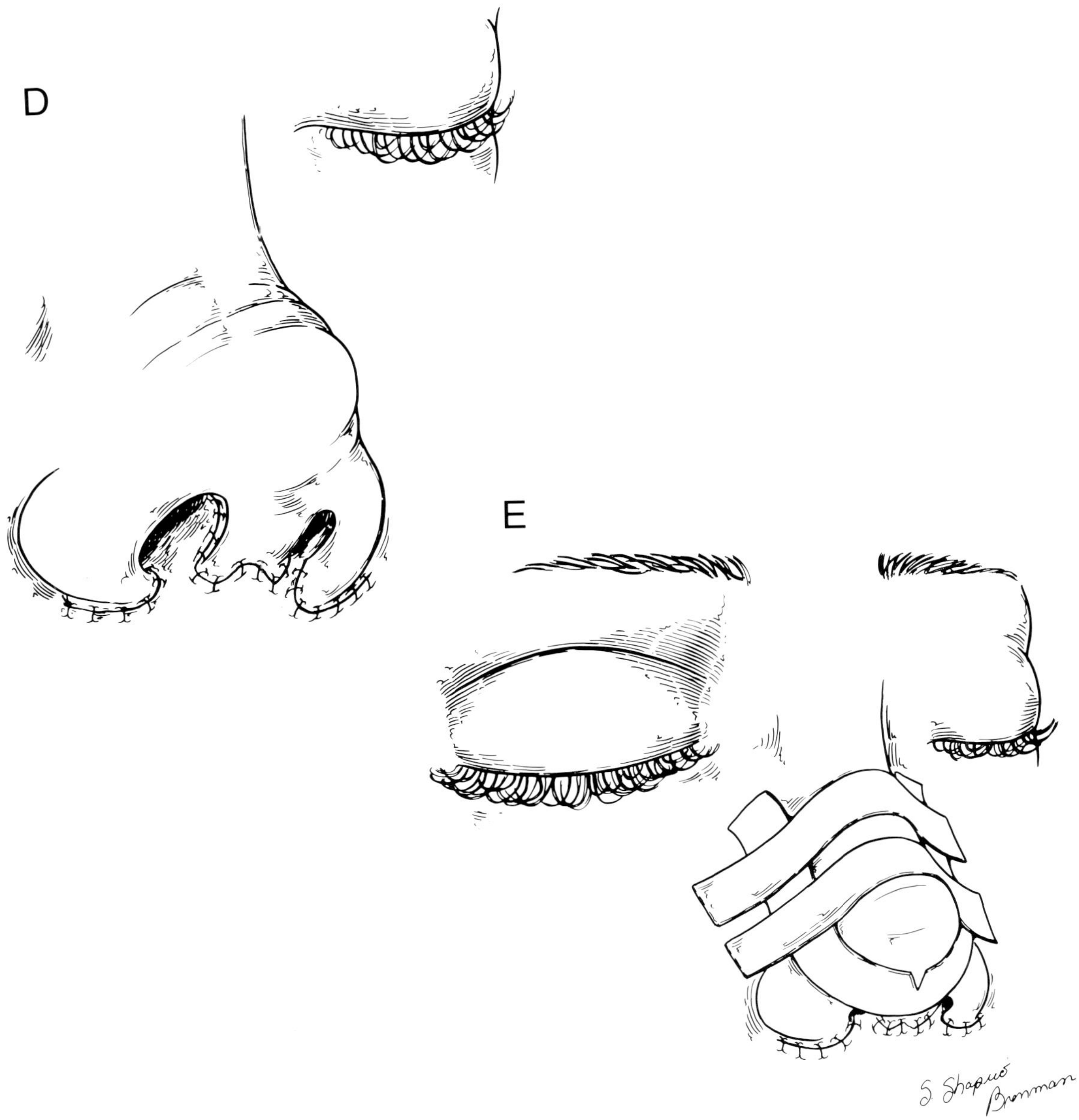


▸ **FIGURE 14-4**

# 15 ▸ Choanal Atresia

Choanal atresia is an incomplete opening between the posterior nasal cavity and the nasopharynx. The condition may be unilateral (Fig. 15–1**A**) or bilateral (see section 15–2, Fig. 15–2**A**). Unilateral choanal atresia usually presents with chronic unilateral rhinorrhea but causes little or no respiratory distress.

Because neonates are obligate nasal breathers, bilateral atresia causes severe respiratory distress. When the neonate cries, he opens his mouth to breathe and the distress subsides. The initial distress can be managed with a McGovern nipple (large nipple with cross-cuts in the end) to open the mouth and displace the tongue inferiorly to permit oral breathing. An oral-gastric tube may also provide a path for the infant to breathe. However, the child may have difficulty feeding and maintaining weight.

## ▸ 15-1 TRANSNASAL REPAIR OF CHOANAL ATRESIA

### Indications

Repair of choanal atresia is necessary when conservative management is ineffective in sustaining adequate respiration and nutrition. The transnasal approach is generally tried first.

### Preoperative Evaluation

A computed tomography (CT) scan is essential to define the shape of the nasal chambers and determine whether the atresia is membranous or bony.

### Operative Technique

1. Choanal atresia repair is performed using general anesthesia. Oral tracheal intubation with an oral RAE tube facilitates access to the nasopharynx (Fig. 15–1**B**).
2. Four percent cocaine on cotton or neurosurgical pledgets is placed in the nose for vasoconstriction (alternately, any combination of a topical vasoconstrictor and local anesthetic may be used).
3. A McIver tonsil gag is used to expose the oropharynx and the nasopharynx (Fig. 15–1**B**). The choanae can be visualized with a mirror or a nasopharyngoscope.
4. The atresia plate is perforated by gentle pressure with a Frazier suction tip or urethral sound that is directed along the floor of the nose (Fig. 15–1**C**). Its passage into the nasopharynx is visualized with a mirror or confirmed by palpation of the surgeon's finger in the nasopharynx. The atresia plate may also be perforated with a drill (Fig. 15–1**D**). Care must be taken to avoid traversing the nasopharynx and causing injury to the base of the skull.
5. The opening is then enlarged in all directions with either a cutting drill or rongeurs (Fig. 15–1**E**). This may be facilitated by endoscopic visualization.
6. When the choanae are open, $\frac{1}{4}$ to $\frac{1}{2}$ cm of posterior nasal septum is removed with a reverse rongeur, back-biting forceps, or a drill. This is an important step in avoiding stenosis of the newly opened choanae (Fig. 15–1**F**).

7. A section of endotracheal tube is then placed in each nostril, extending into the nasopharynx to stent the choana (Fig. 15–1G).
8. The anterior ends of the stents should be placed inside the vestibule to avoid necrosis of the ala or columella. They are sutured in place by a nonabsorbable suture through both tubes and the septum (Fig. 15–1H). The stents should extend to just inside the nasal vestibule (Fig. 15–1I) so that there is no pressure on the columella or alar rim. The stents are left in place for 4 to 6 weeks. They are usually removed utilizing a brief general anesthetic. This permits a close inspection of the opened choanae and removal of any granulation tissue.
9. If the choanae begin to stenose after the stents are removed, dilatation with a urethral sound at intervals of 4 to 6 weeks may be necessary until the choanae stays open. The sounds should be passed along the floor of the nose on each side and the tip directed down into the nasopharynx (Fig. 15–1J). This may be done without a general anesthetic in very young children.
10. Antibiotics are administered as long as the stents are in place.

## Complications

1. Choanal stenosis
2. Trauma to brainstem

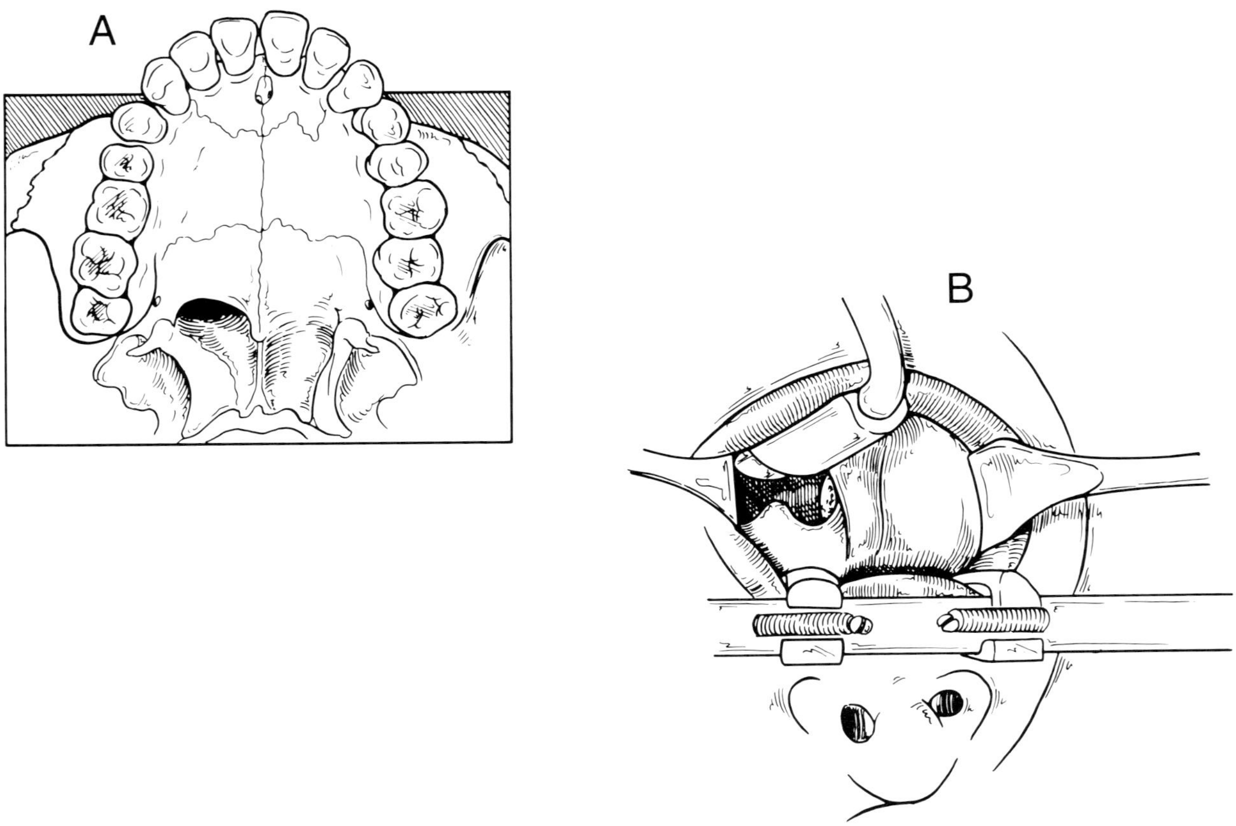


▶ **FIGURE 15-1**

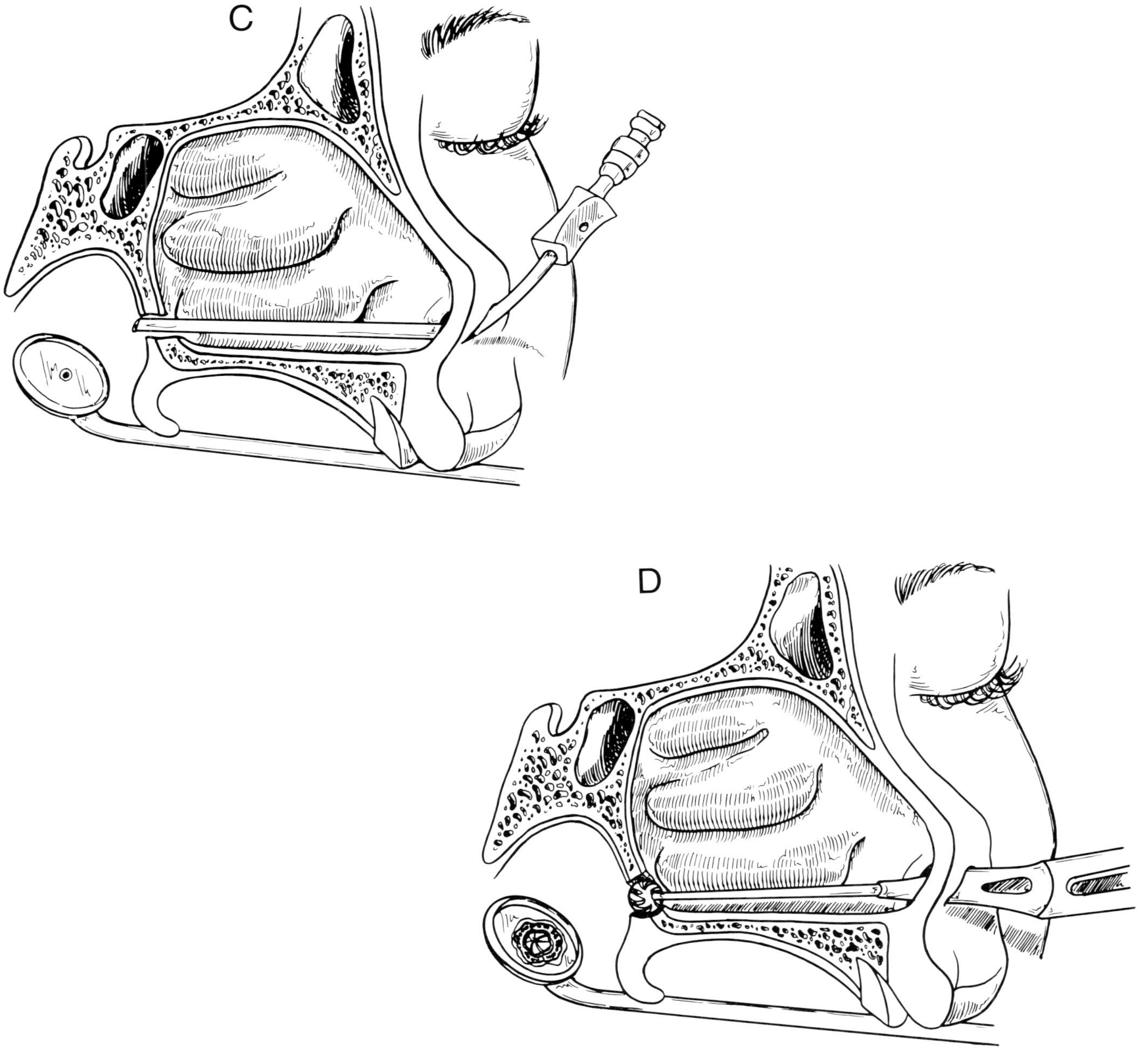


▶**FIGURE 15-1**

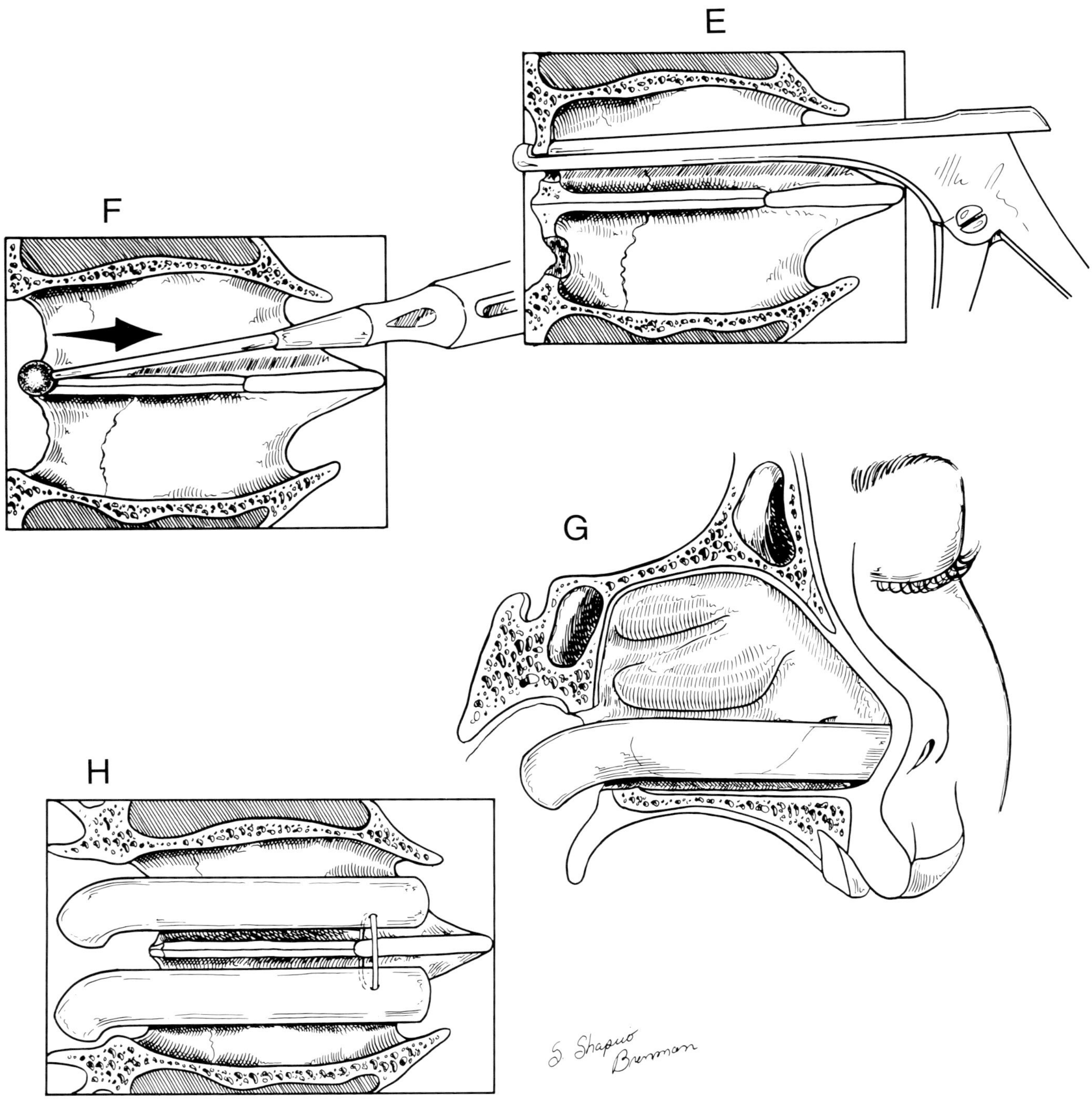


▶ **FIGURE 15-1**

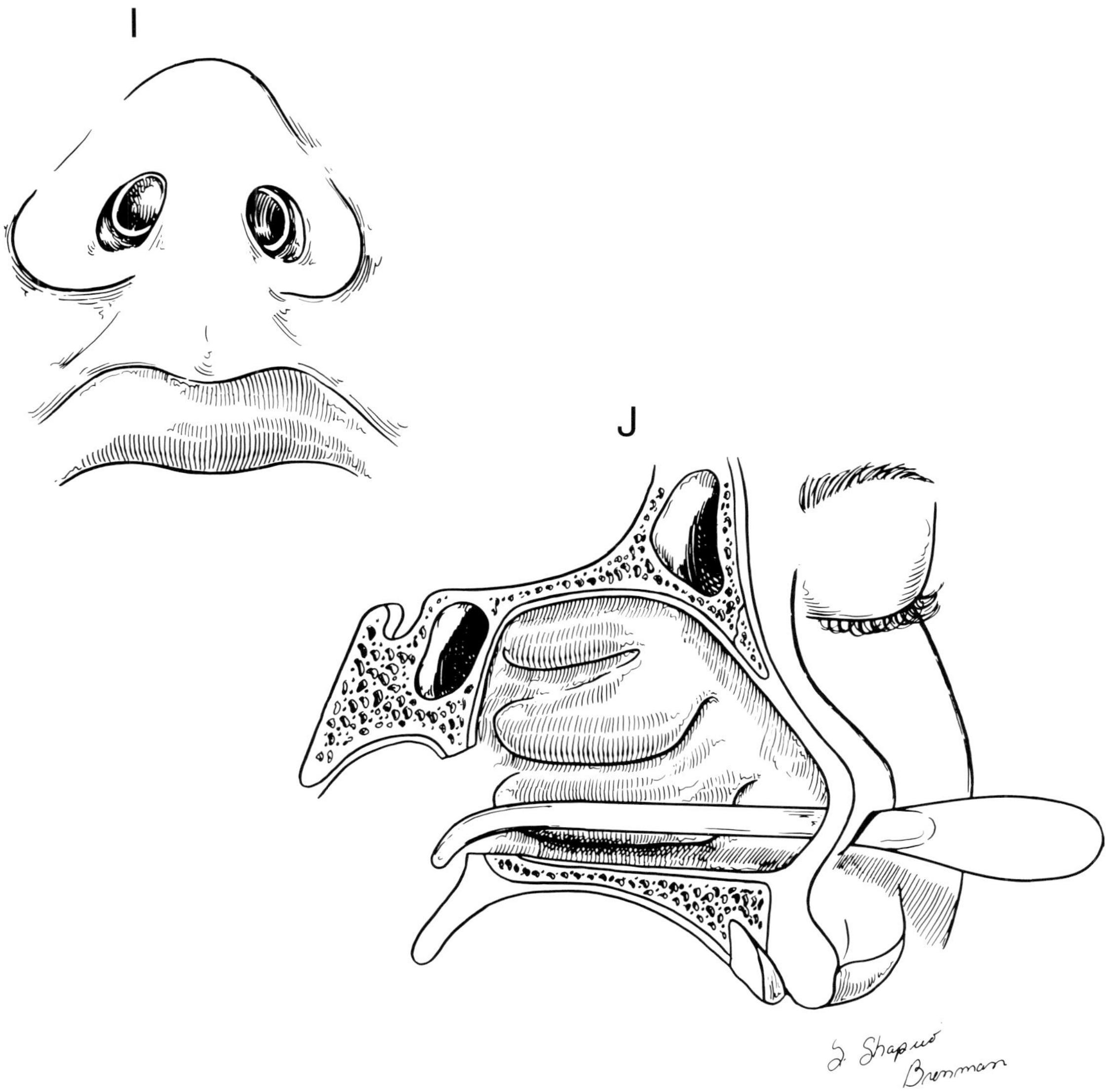


▶ **FIGURE 15-1**

## ▶ 15-2 TRANSPALATAL REPAIR OF CHOANAL ATRESIA

### Indications

The transpalatal approach may be used for primary repair of choanal atresia or for revision of failed transnasal repairs.

### Operative Technique

1. The transpalatal repair is done using general anesthesia administered through an oral RAE tube. A tonsil McIver gag is placed for exposure (Fig. 15–2**A**).
2. The midportion and edge of the hard palate are injected with 1% lidocaine with 1:100,000 epinephrine for hemostasis (Fig. 15–2**A**).
3. A longitudinal midline incision is made through the mucosa, submucosa, and periosteum of the palate to just beyond the edge of the hard palate (Fig. 15–2**B**).
4. The palatal soft tissues are elevated from the bone of the hard palate and retracted laterally. The muscular attachments of the soft palate are cut transversely from the posterior edge of the hard palate to expose the posterior choana in the nasopharynx (Fig. 15-2**C**).
5. The bone of the hard palate and choanal atresia is removed with a drill or bone rongeurs (Fig. 15-2**D**).
6. A portion of the posterior bony nasal septum is similarly removed (Fig. 15-2**E**).
7. Endotracheal tube stents are placed from the nose into the nasopharynx to stent the area (Fig. 15-2**F**) as described in the transnasal repair (see section 15–1).
8. The incision is then closed by suturing the periosteum and muscle with 3-0 chromic sutures. The mucosa is closed with interrupted 3-0 chromic sutures (Fig. 15-2**G**).
9. If the choanae begin to stenose after the stents are removed, dilatation with a urethral sound at intervals or 4 to 6 weeks may be necessary until the choanae stays open. The sounds should be passed along the floor of the nose on each side and the tip directed down into the nasopharynx (see section 15–1). This may be done without a general anesthetic in very young children.

### Complications

1. Choanal stenosis
2. Palatal fistula

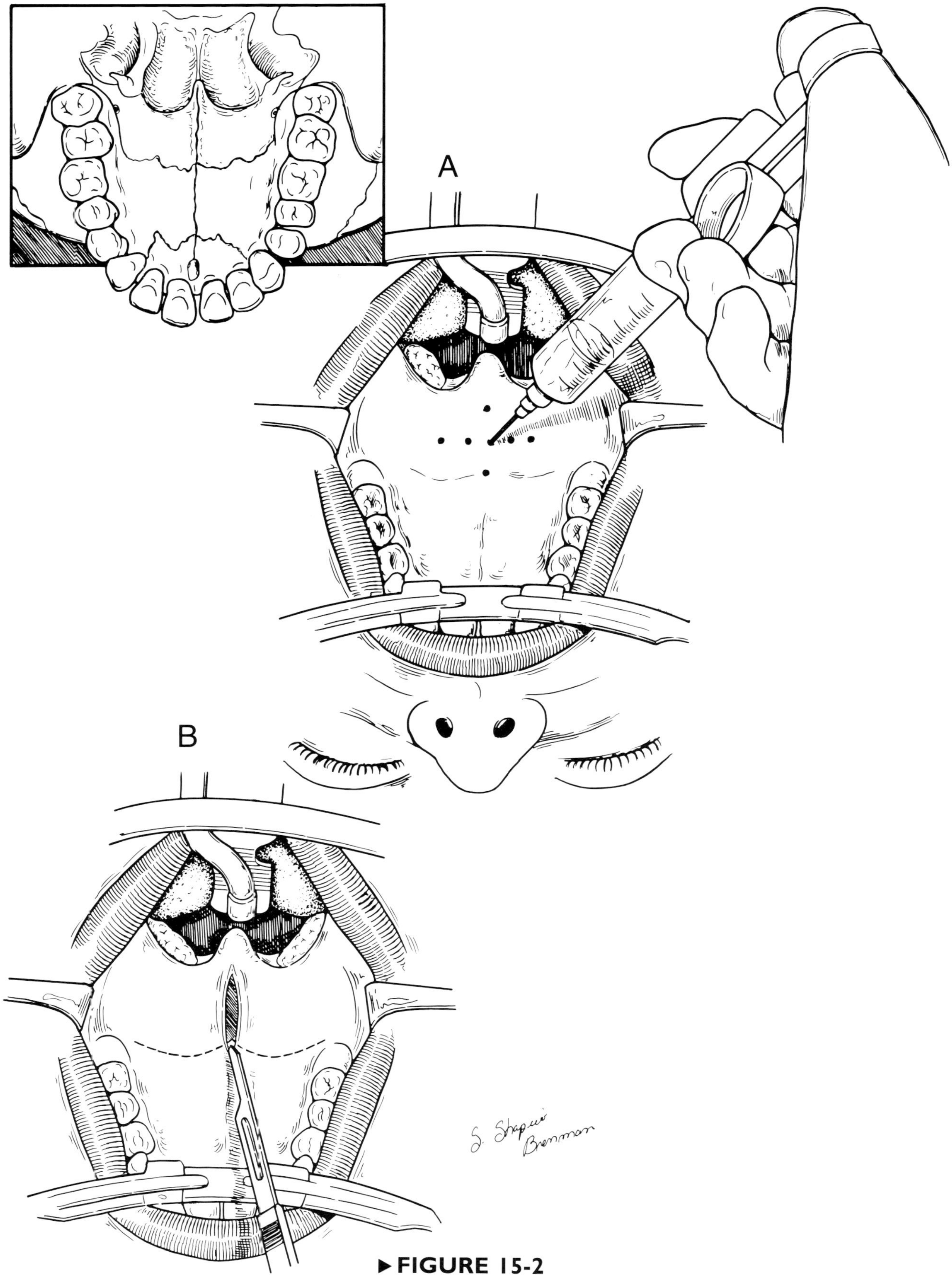


▶ **FIGURE 15-2**

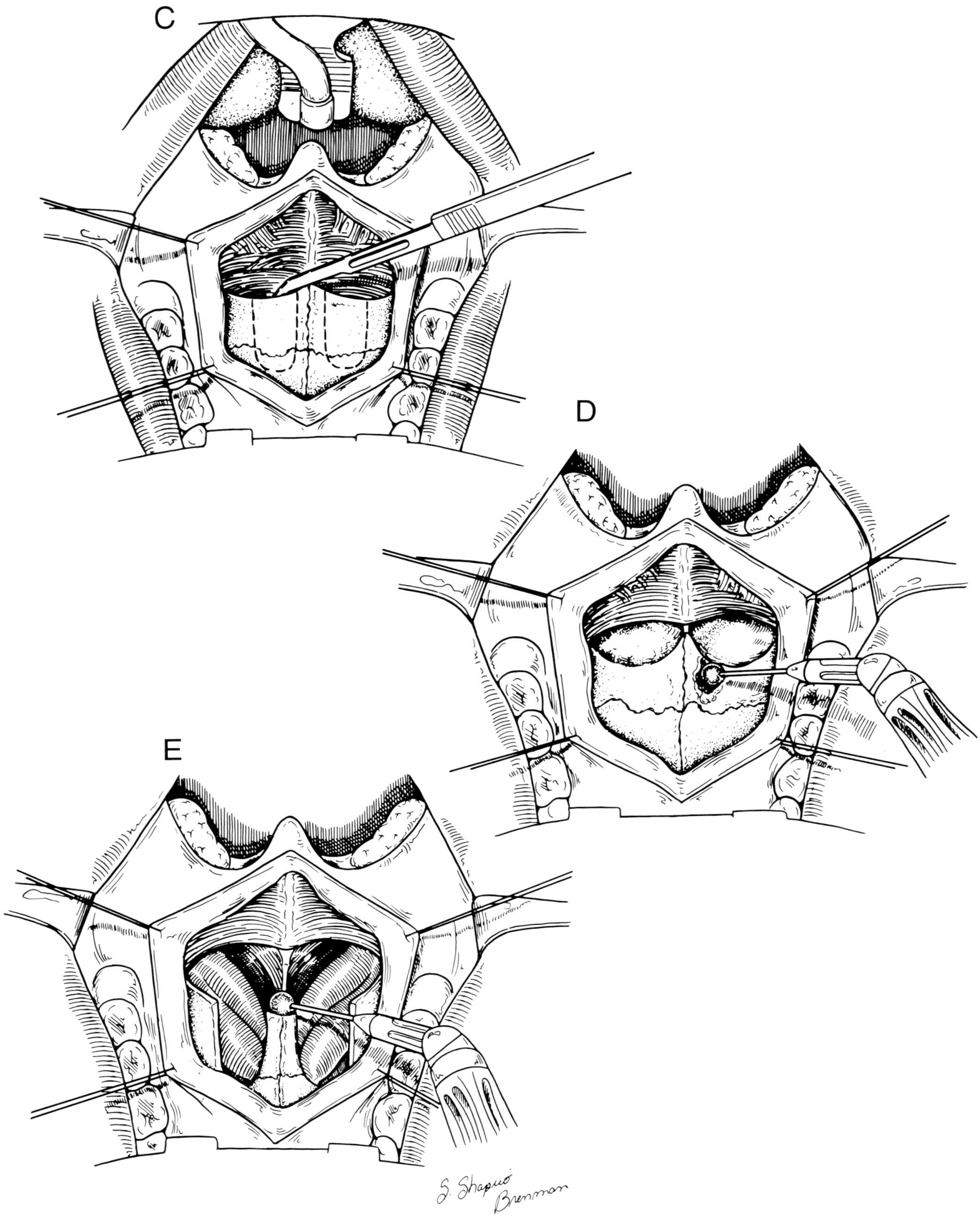


▶ **FIGURE 15-2**

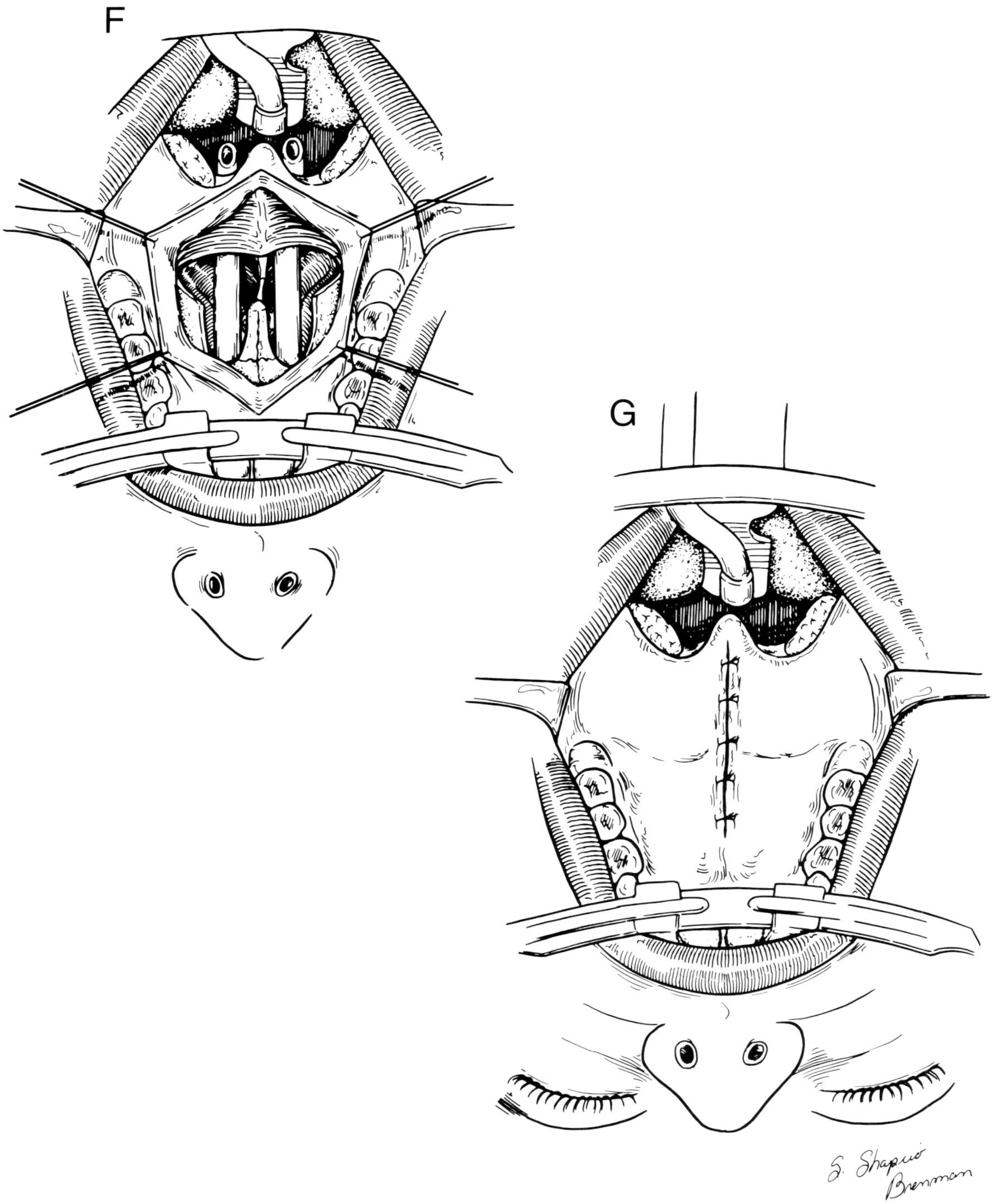


▶ **FIGURE 15-2**

PART III

# NASOPHARYNX, ORAL CAVITY AND OROPHARYNX

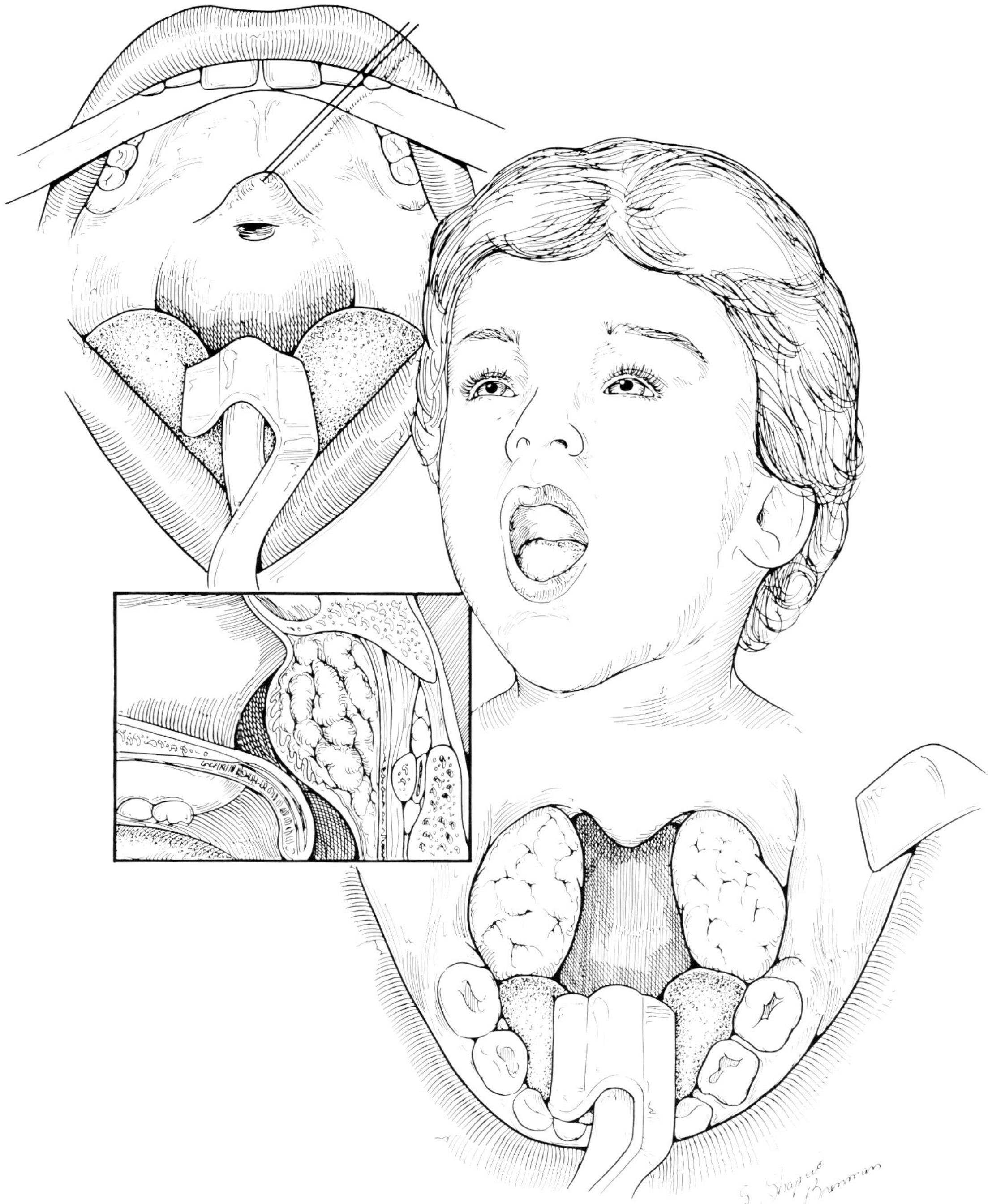

# 16 ▸ Nasopharyngeal Stenosis

Nasopharyngeal stenosis usually occurs when there is extensive scarring following an adenoidectomy or adenotonsillectomy.

## ▸ 16-1 REPAIR OF NASOPHARYNGEAL STENOSIS

### Indications

Repair of nasopharyngeal stenosis is required to treat nasal obstruction and to improve mucus drainage posteriorly.

### Preoperative Evaluation

Flexible nasopharyngoscopy or indirect mirror nasopharyngoscopy is required prior to repair of the stenosis. Radiographs are of little help.

### Operative Technique

1. Repair of nasopharyngeal stenosis is done under general endotracheal anesthesia through an oral RAE tube with a mouth gag in place to expose the pharynx (Fig. 16–1**A**).
2. The nasopharyngeal lumen is examined utilizing a nasopharyngeal mirror (Fig. 16–1**A**).
3. An incision is made from the lateral edge of the nasopharyngeal lumen across the posterior pharyngeal wall to the lateral wall of the pharynx (line 1, Fig. 16–1**B**).
4. The incision is continued across the lower edge of the lumen and then inferiorly on the opposite side of the pharynx (line 2, Fig. 16–1**B**).
5. The flap is completed by making a back cut sloping superiorly on the posterior inferior wall of the oropharynx (line 3, Fig. 16–1**B**).
6. The uvula is elevated and retracted with 4-0 prolene suture, and a mucosal muscle flap is then elevated with a scissors in the plane of the fascia of the posterior pharyngeal wall (Fig. 16–1**C, D**).
7. The flap is rotated superiorly opening the nasopharynx and sutured in place with 4-0 interrupted Vicryl suture (Fig. 16–1**E**).
8. The hypopharyngeal incision does not require complete closure.
9. A nasopharyngeal airway is left in place overnight.
10. The patient is kept on intravenous antibiotics for 10 days.
11. One laterally based flap is usually sufficient to open the nasopharyngeal airway. However, if the postoperative airway is not sufficient, the procedure can be repeated with a flap based on the other side in 3 to 4 months.

### Complications

1. Restenosis of nasopharynx

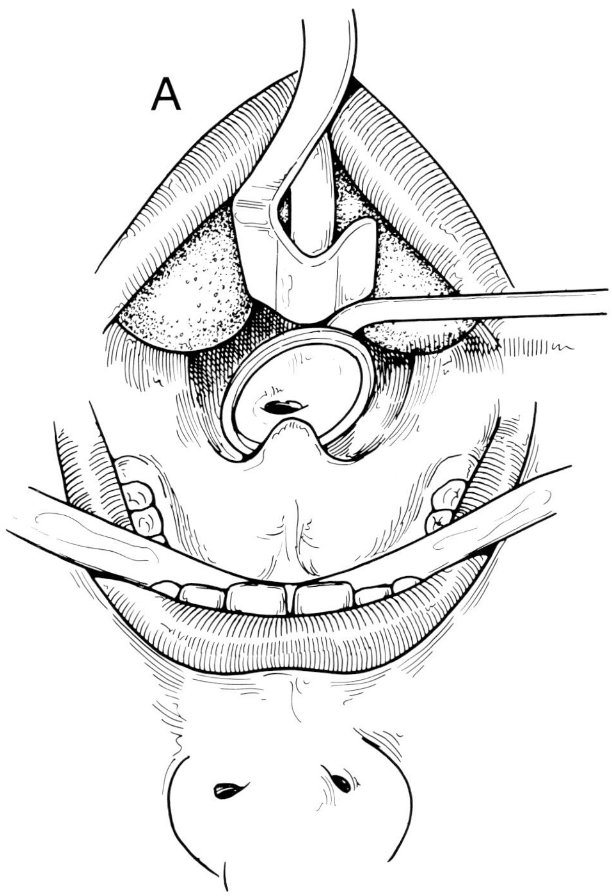


▶ **FIGURE 16-1**

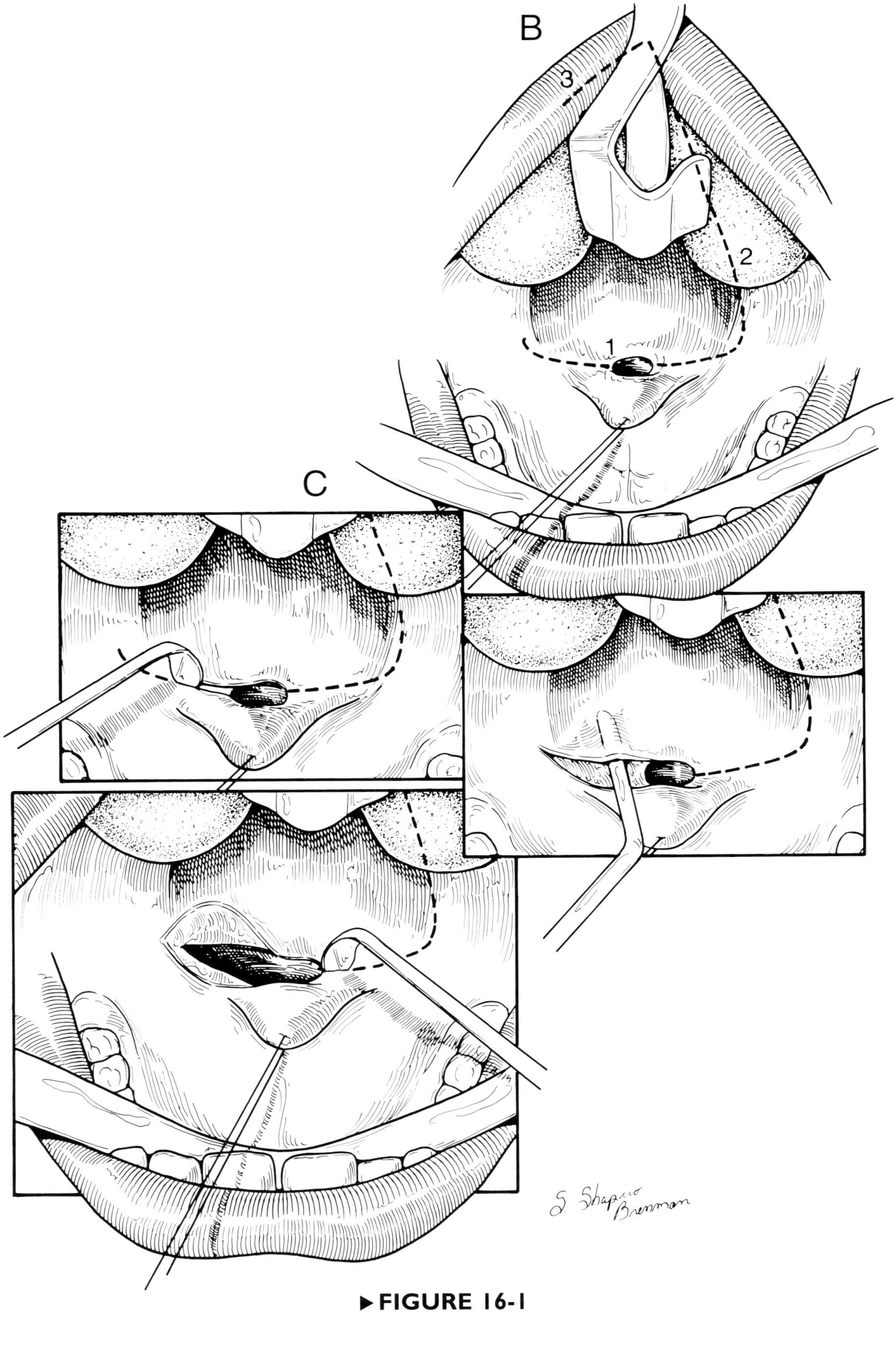


▶**FIGURE 16-1**

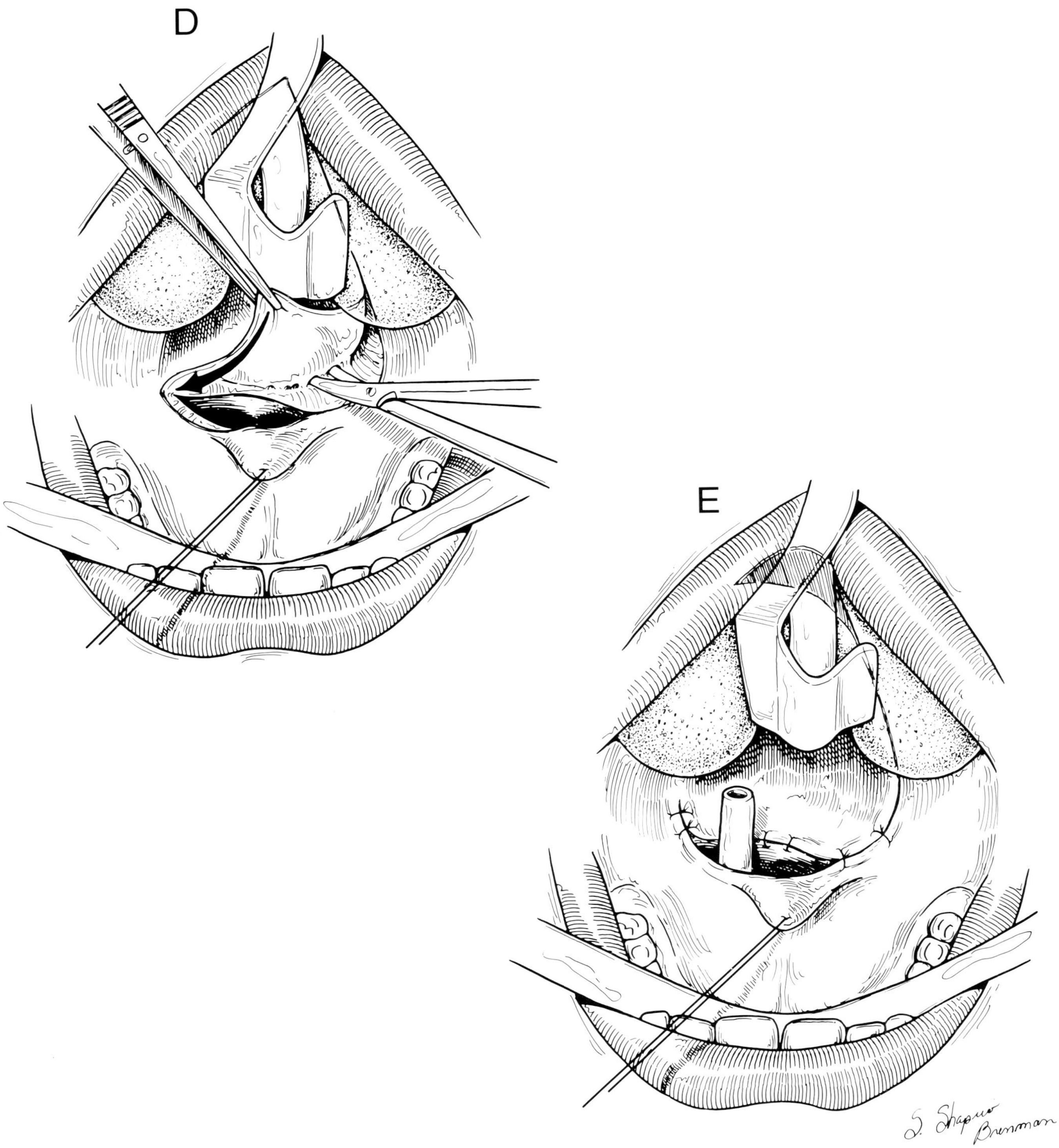


▶**FIGURE 16-1**

# 17 ▸ Nasopharyngeal Angiofibroma

## ▸ 17-1 EXCISION OF NASOPHARYNGEAL ANGIOFIBROMA

Nasopharyngeal angiofibromas are found almost exclusively in teenage boys and present with recurrent severe epistaxis and nasal obstruction.

### Indications

Nasopharyngeal angiofibromas are excised to prevent recurrent epistaxis, nasopharyngeal obstruction, and intracranial extension.

### Preoperative Evaluation

The preoperative evaluation of a nasopharyngeal angiofibroma includes computed tomography (CT) scan, magnetic resonance imaging (MRI) with MR angiogram, and arteriography with arterial embolization. Embolization is usually performed 24 to 72 hours prior to resection to reduce intraoperative blood loss.

### Operative Technique

1. Transpalatal excision of an angiofibroma is performed utilizing general anesthesia administered through an oral RAE tube. A Dingman mouth gag is placed for exposure of the palate (Fig. 17–1**A**).
2. The midline of the palate is injected with 1% lidocaine with 1:100,000 epinephrine for hemostasis (Fig. 17–1**A**).
3. A midline palatal splitting incision is made with a knife through the soft palate and through the soft tissue overlying the hard palate (Fig. 17–1**B**).
4. The muscular attachments and soft tissue flaps are reflected laterally exposing the hard palate (Fig. 17–1**C**).
5. The bone of the hard palate is removed with a drill or bone rongeurs exposing the angiofibroma. A portion of the posterior nasal septum may also be removed (Fig. 17–1**D**).
6. The angiofibroma is excised by dissection with a knife or scissors from its surrounding attachments (Fig. 17–1**E**, **F**).
7. Hemostasis is obtained by suction cautery.
8. The palate incision is closed in two layers. The mucosa on the nasal side is closed with 4-0 interrupted chromic suture. The oral mucosa and muscle are closed with deep 3-0 interrupted Vicryl suture (Fig. 17–1**G**).
9. Additional exposure for very large extracranial lesions may be obtained through a lateral rhinotomy incision (see section 14–1, Lateral Rhinotomy).

### Complications

1. Palatal fistula
2. Laceration of internal maxillary artery
3. Cerebral spinal fluid leak

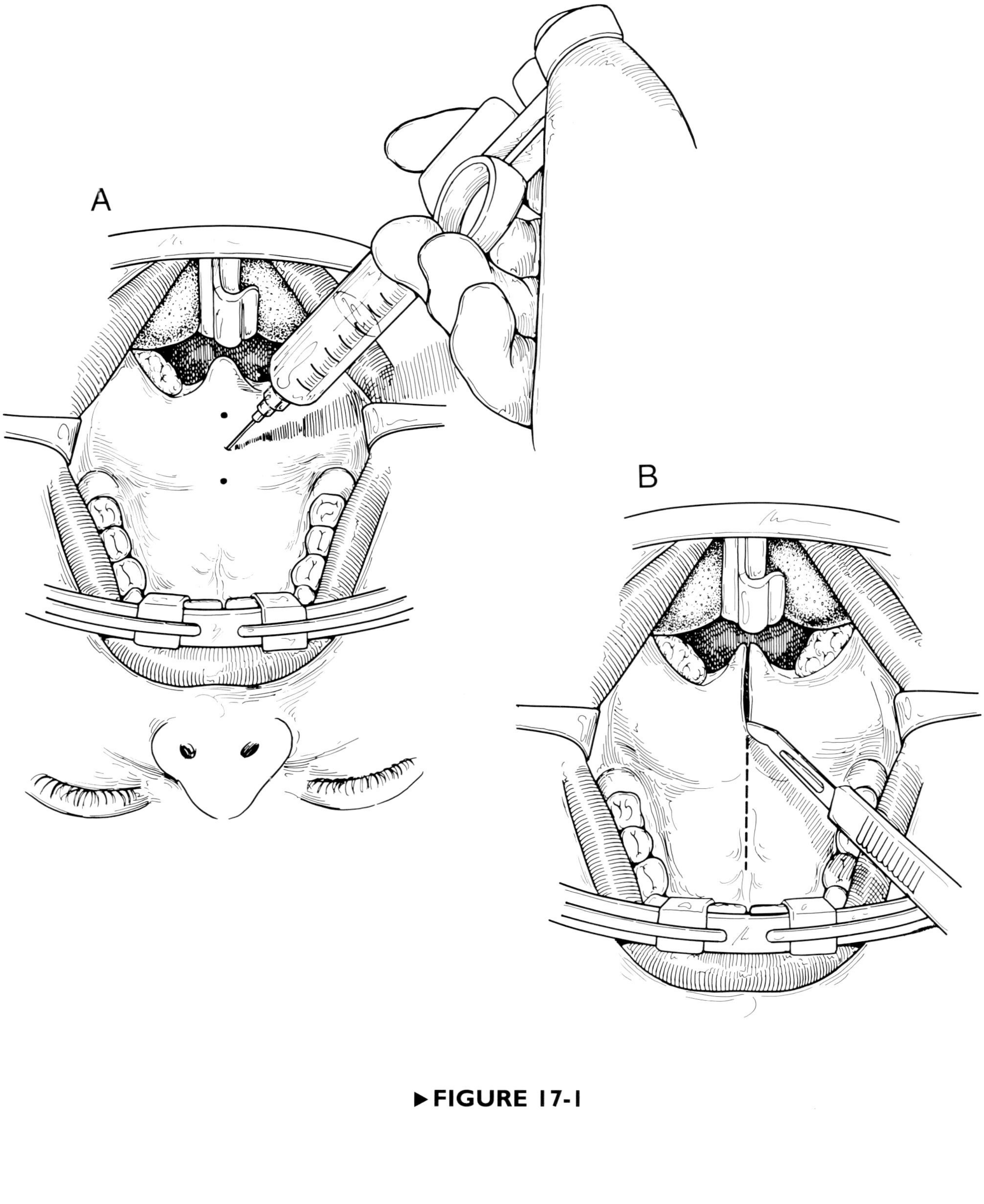


▶**FIGURE 17-1**

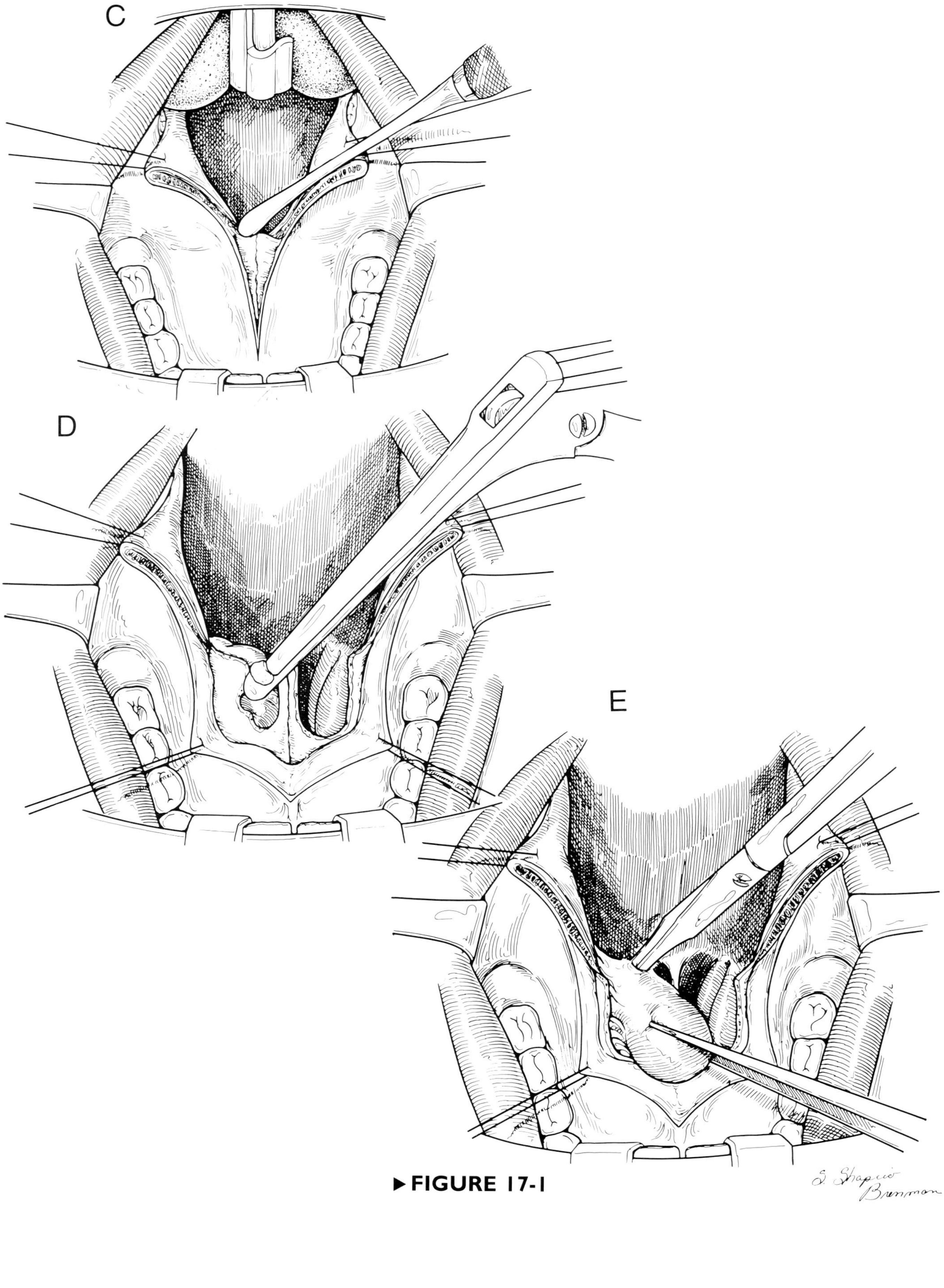


▶**FIGURE 17-1**

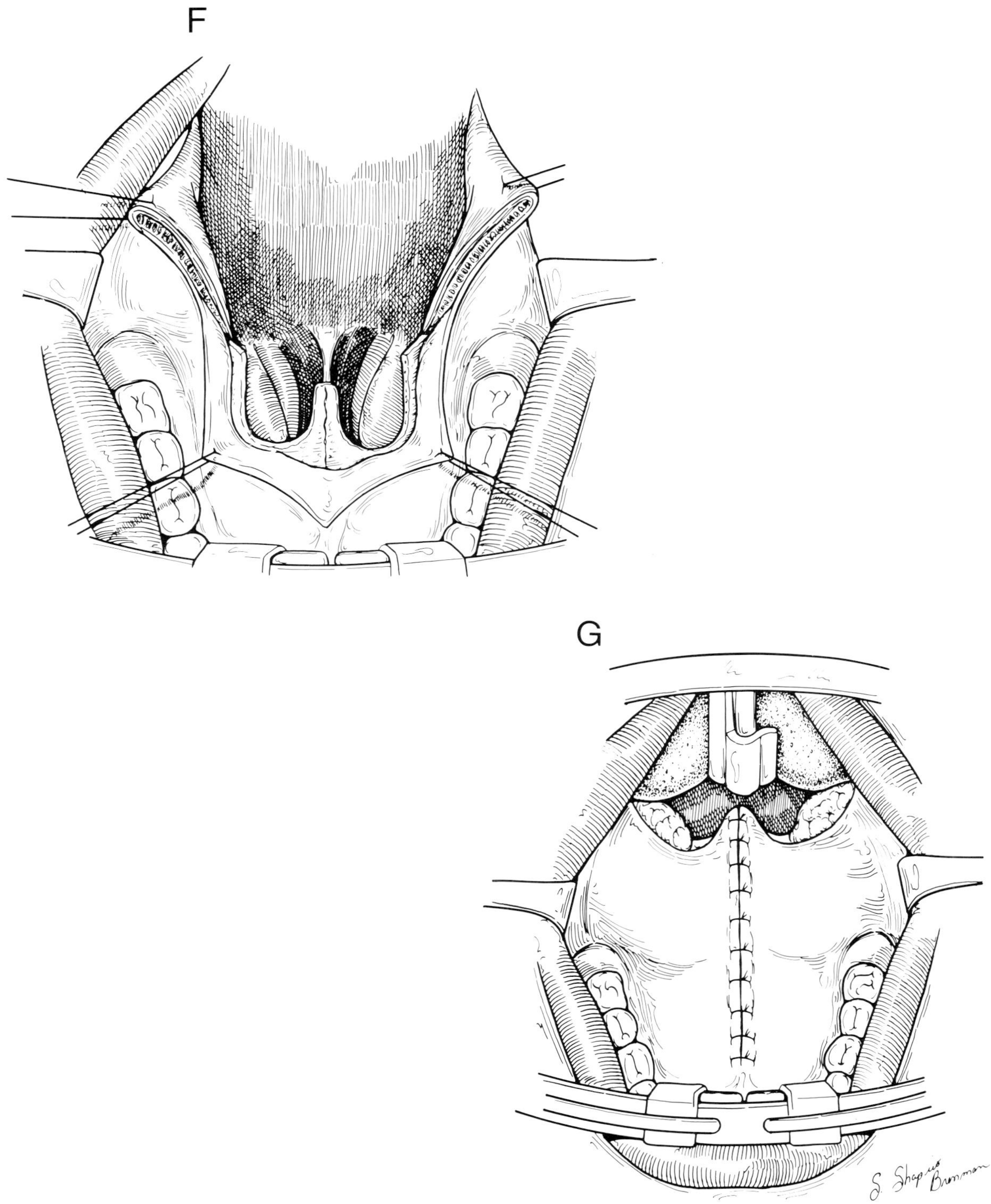


▶ **FIGURE 17-1**

# 18 ▸ Velopharyngeal Insufficiency (VPI)

Velopharyngeal insufficiency (VPI) may be caused by congenital neuromuscular dysfunction or an anatomic abnormality that prevents adequate pharyngeal closure. VPI may also occur after pharyngeal surgery.

## ▸ 18-1 PALATOPHARYNGOPLASTY (PHARYNGEAL FLAP)

Palatopharyngoplasty is an operation designed to correct velopharyngeal incompetence (VPI).

### Indications

Palatopharyngoplasty is indicated when VPI is severe enough to cause a speech or voice disorder that has not improved with speech therapy or the possible use of a palatal lift prosthesis.

### Preoperative Evaluation

Preoperative evaluation includes flexible nasopharyngoscopy and video fluoroscopy of the palate and pharynx during speech.

### Operative Technique

1. Palatopharyngoplasty is performed under general endotracheal anesthesia through an oral RAE tube with a mouth gag in place and the patient positioned on a shoulder roll with the head extended (see section 21–1, Tonsillectomy, Fig. 21–1**A**).
2. The lower border of the palate and the posterior pharyngeal wall are injected with 1% lidocaine with 1:100,000 epinephrine (Fig. 18–1**A**).
3. A 4-0 prolene suture is placed through the uvula, and the palate is everted (Fig. 18–1**B**).
4. An incision is made with a knife into the mucosa and muscle on the nasopharyngeal surface of the palate (Fig. 18–1**B**).
5. Pharyngeal incisions are then made laterally (Fig. 18–1**C**) and the flap elevated with a clamp or scissors (Fig. 18–1**D**) to create a pointed superiorly based flap (Fig. 18–1**E**).
6. The mucosal-muscle flap is released with a clamp and scissors (Fig. 18–1**D**, **E**, **F**). Endotracheal tube stents are placed to create lateral ports (Fig. 18–1**F**).
7. The anterior portion of the pharyngeal flap is sutured to the posterior edge of the palate incision with 4-0 Vicryl suture (Fig. 18–1**G**). Tube stents are placed to create lateral ports.
8. Tension-releasing sutures of 4-0 Vicryl are passed through the flap and tied on the anterior surface of the palate (Fig. 18–1**H**).

9. The inferior edge of the palate incision is then sutured to the deep surface of the posterior pharyngeal flap (Fig. 18–1**I**).
10. As much of the posterior pharyngeal wall as possible is closed with interrupted 4-0 Vicryl sutures (Fig. 18–1**J**).
11. If the palate is short and stiff, a midline palatal splitting incision is made after the palate and pharyngeal wall have been injected (Fig. 18–1**K**).
12. The palatal flaps are retracted laterally with 4-0 prolene suture (Fig. 18–1**L**).
13. Mucosal flaps are elevated from the nasal side of the palate (Fig. 18–1**M**).
14. The elevated pharyngeal flap from the posterior pharyngeal wall is sutured to the nasal mucosal edge of the split palate after tubes are placed for lateral ports. One through-and-through suture of 3-0 Vicryl is placed to reduce tension (Fig. 18–1**N, O**).
15. Endotracheal tube stents are placed to create lateral ports (Fig. 18–1**N**).
16. The palatal mucosal flaps are rotated back to the surface of the pharyngeal flap (Fig. 18–1**P**).
17. The palate incision is closed with 4-0 interrupted Vicryl sutures and the posterior pharyngeal defect is closed as much as possible (Fig. 18–1**Q**).
18. The nasal stents are removed in 24 to 36 hours.
19. The child is maintained on antibiotics for 7 days.

## Complications

1. Flap breakdown
2. Persistent velopharyngeal incompetence
3. Inadequate nasal airway

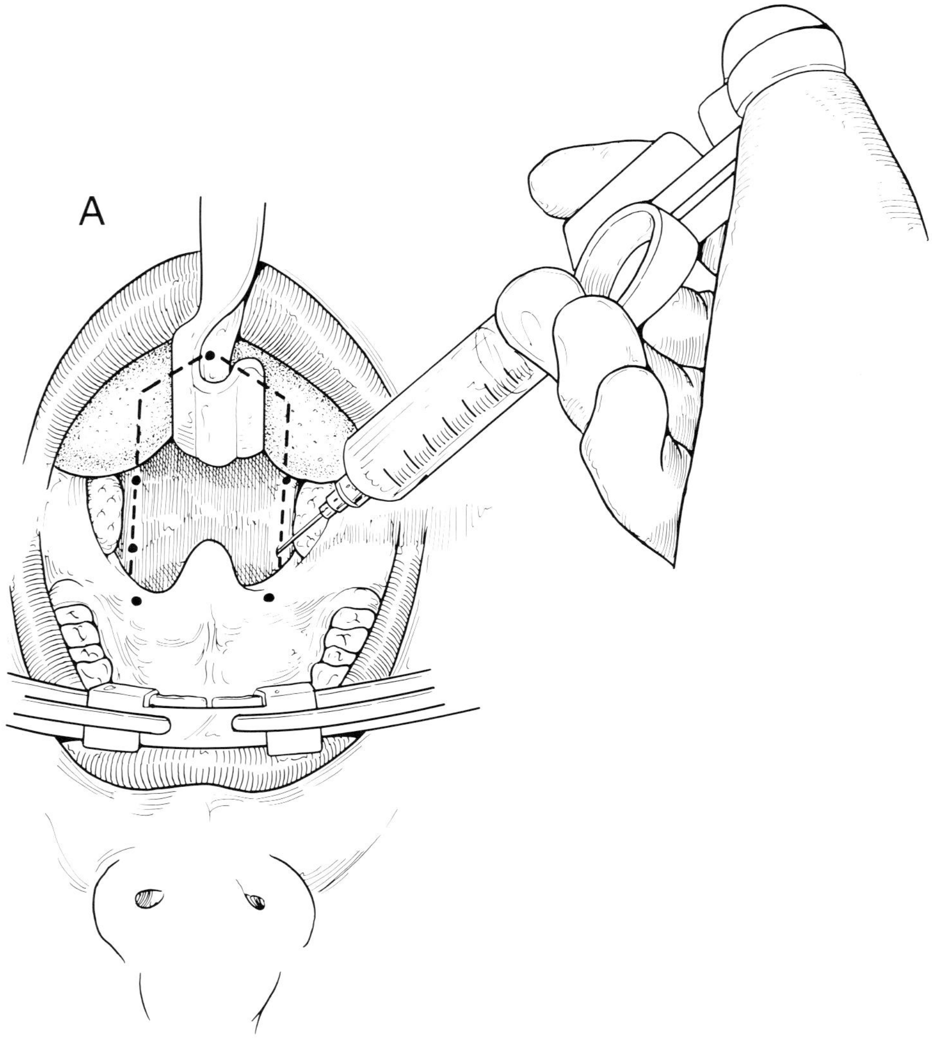


▶ **FIGURE 18-1**

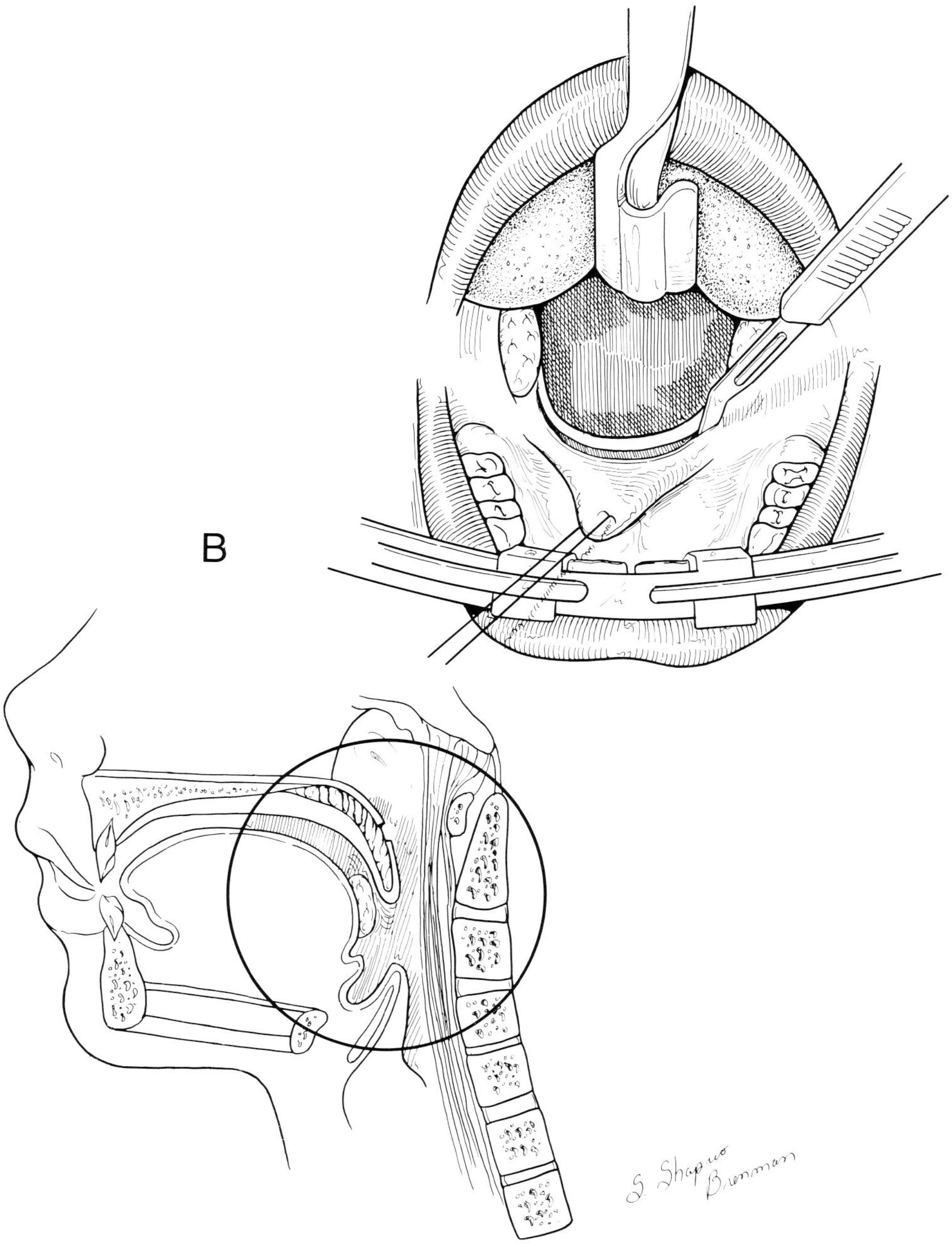


▶ **FIGURE 18-1**

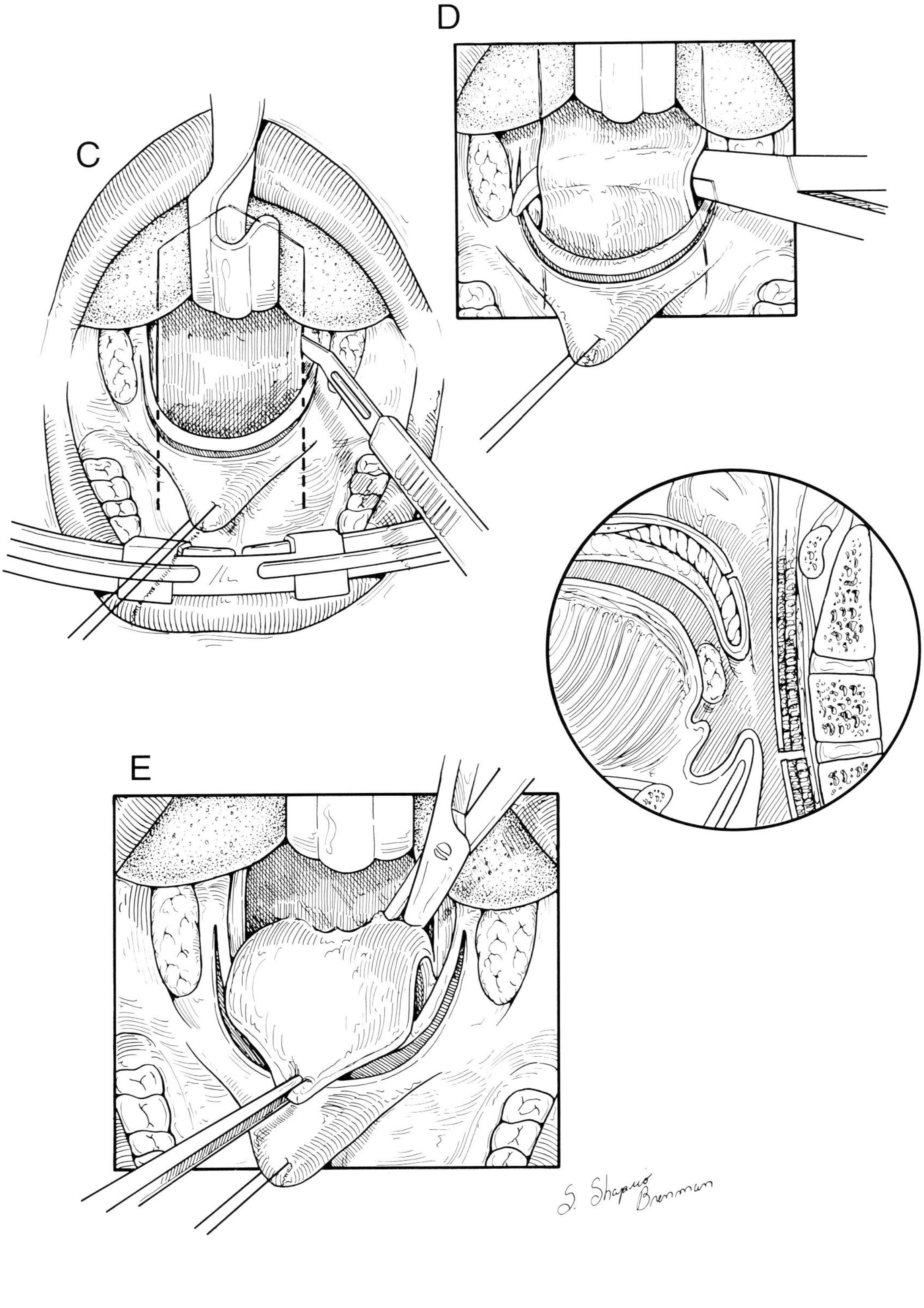


▶ **FIGURE 18-1**

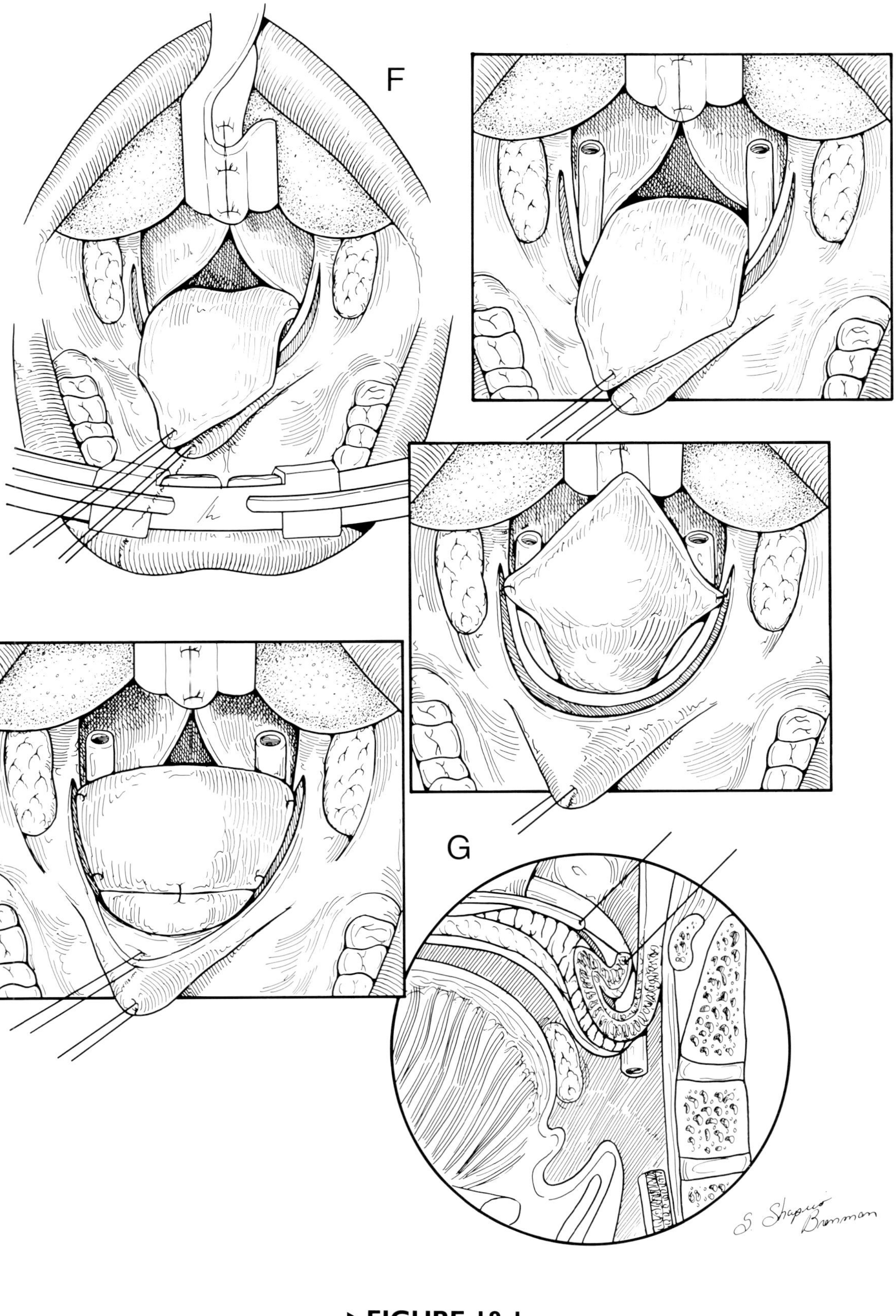


▶ **FIGURE 18-1**

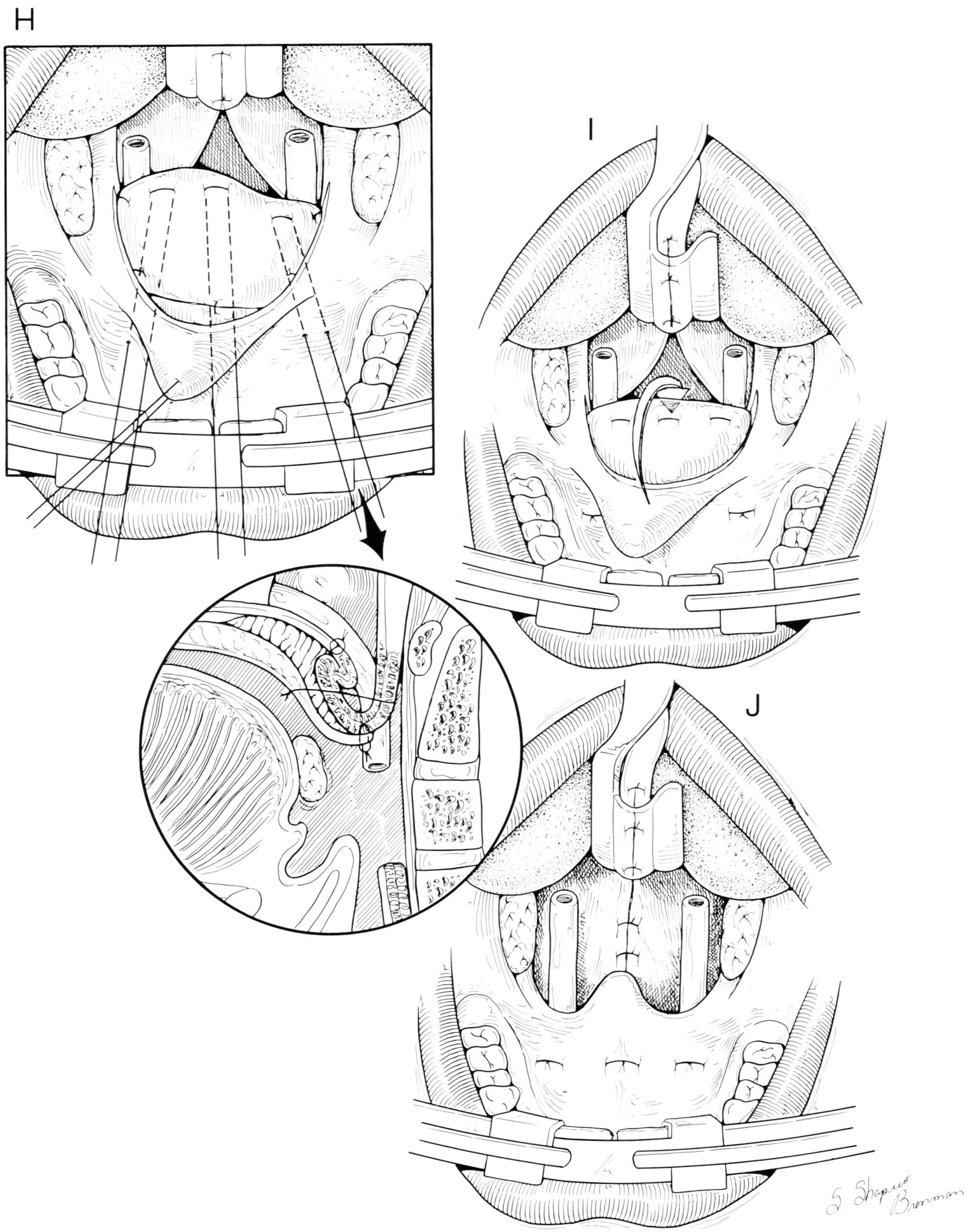


▶ **FIGURE 18-1**

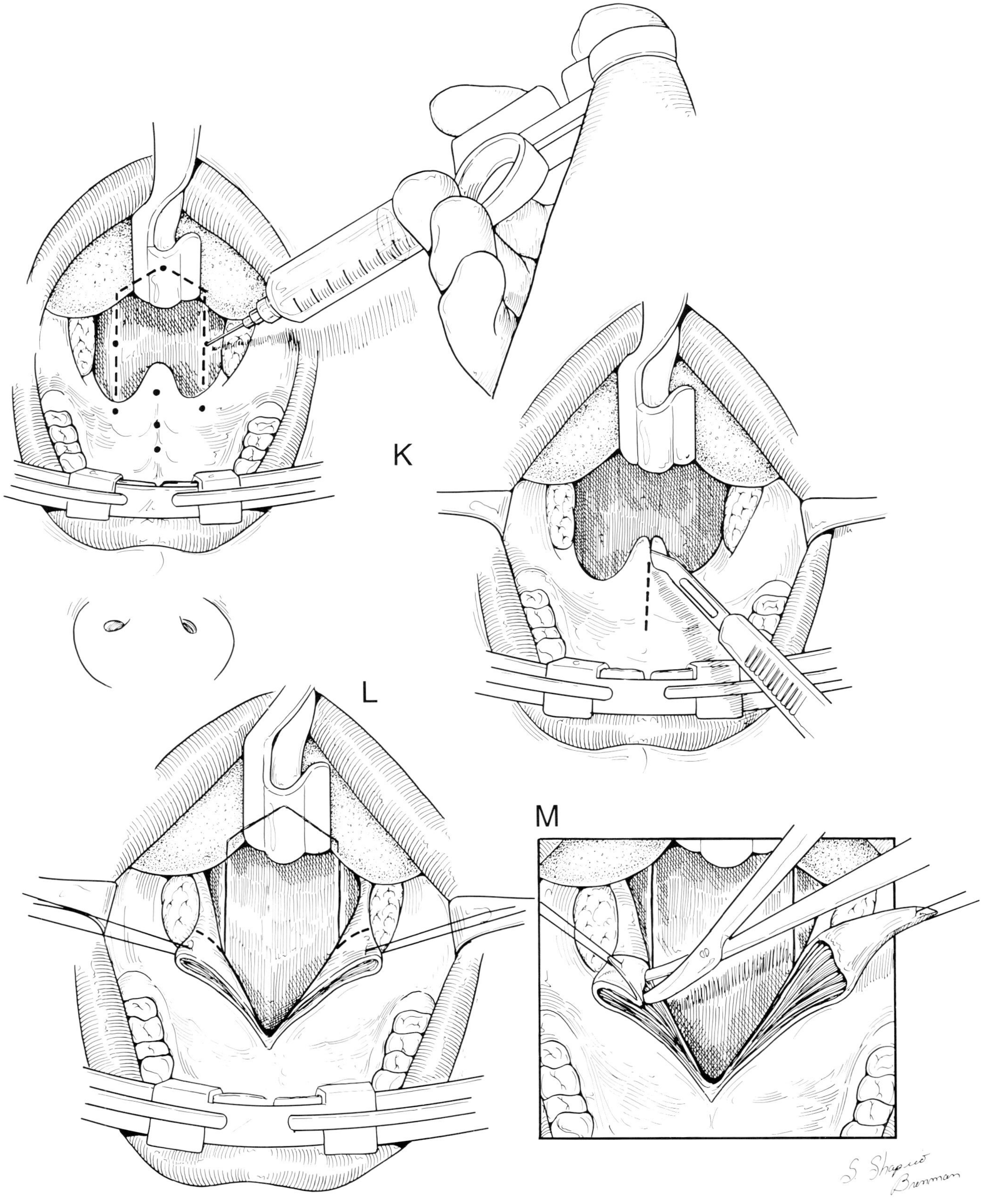


▶ **FIGURE 18-1**

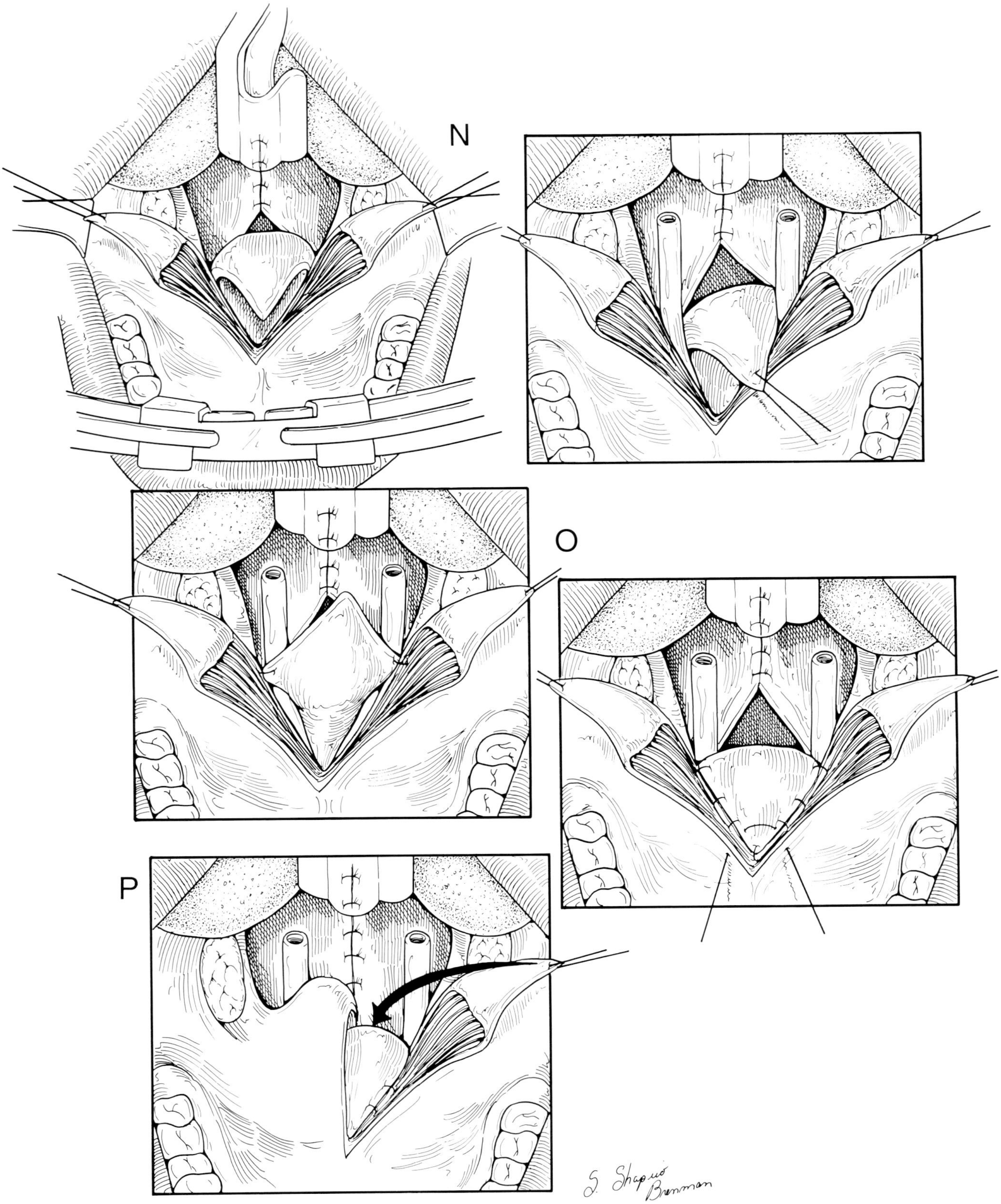


▶ **FIGURE 18-1**

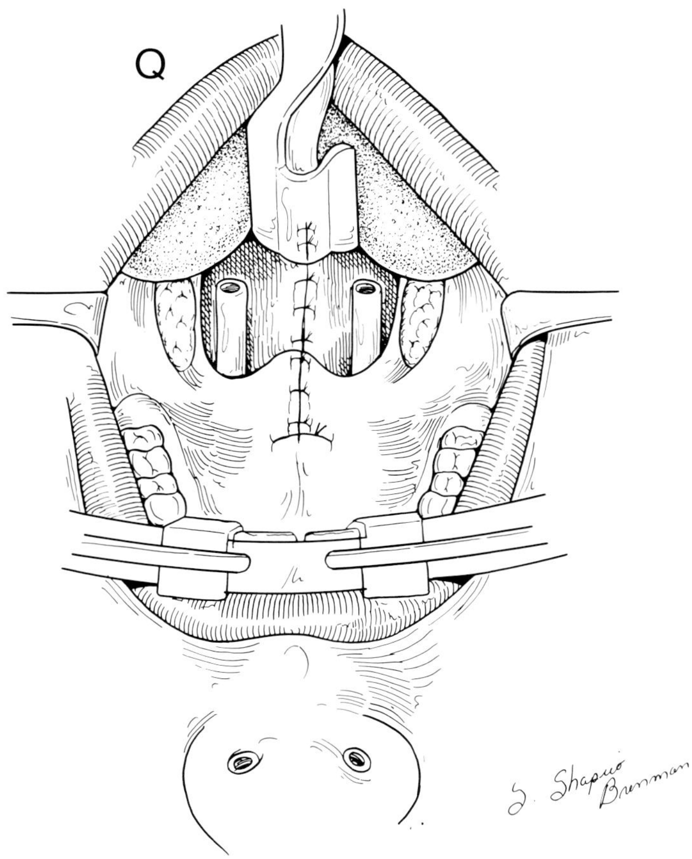


▶ **FIGURE 18-1**

## ▶ 18-2 PALATOPLASTY (PALATAL PUSH BACK)

### Indications

A palatoplasty is indicated in a patient with a submucous cleft palate and persistent velopharyngeal insufficiency (VPI) that has not responded to speech therapy.

### Preoperative Evaluation

The preoperative evaluation of VPI should include nasopharyngoscopy and fluoroscopy of the palate with phonation.

### Operative Technique

1. Under general orotracheal anesthesia administered through an oral RAE tube, a Dingman mouth gag is placed, and 1% lidocaine with 1:100,000 epinephrine is injected into the palate around the greater palatine artery, taking care not to inject directly into the artery (Fig. 18–2**A**).
2. A "W" incision is made with a knife down to the bone of the hard palate (Fig. 18–2**A**).
3. A palatal flap is elevated posteriorly with a periosteal elevator, preserving the palatine arteries (Fig. 18–2**B**).
4. The abnormal insertion of the levator palatini muscle is identified at the posterior border of the hard palate, and the muscle is detached from the bone (Fig. 18–2**C**).
5. The muscles are sutured together in the midline to create the levator sling using 4-0 Vicryl sutures (Fig. 18–2**D**).
6. The anterior palate is closed with 4-0 interrupted Vicryl sutures leaving the bare surface of the hard palate to heal by secondary intention (Fig. 18–2**E**).
7. The mucosa of the cleft of the uvula is excised and the lateral segments are sutured together with 4-0 interrupted Vicryl sutures (Fig. 18–2**F**).
8. The child is given a 7-day course of antibiotics.

### Complications

1. Persistent VPI
2. Palatal fistula

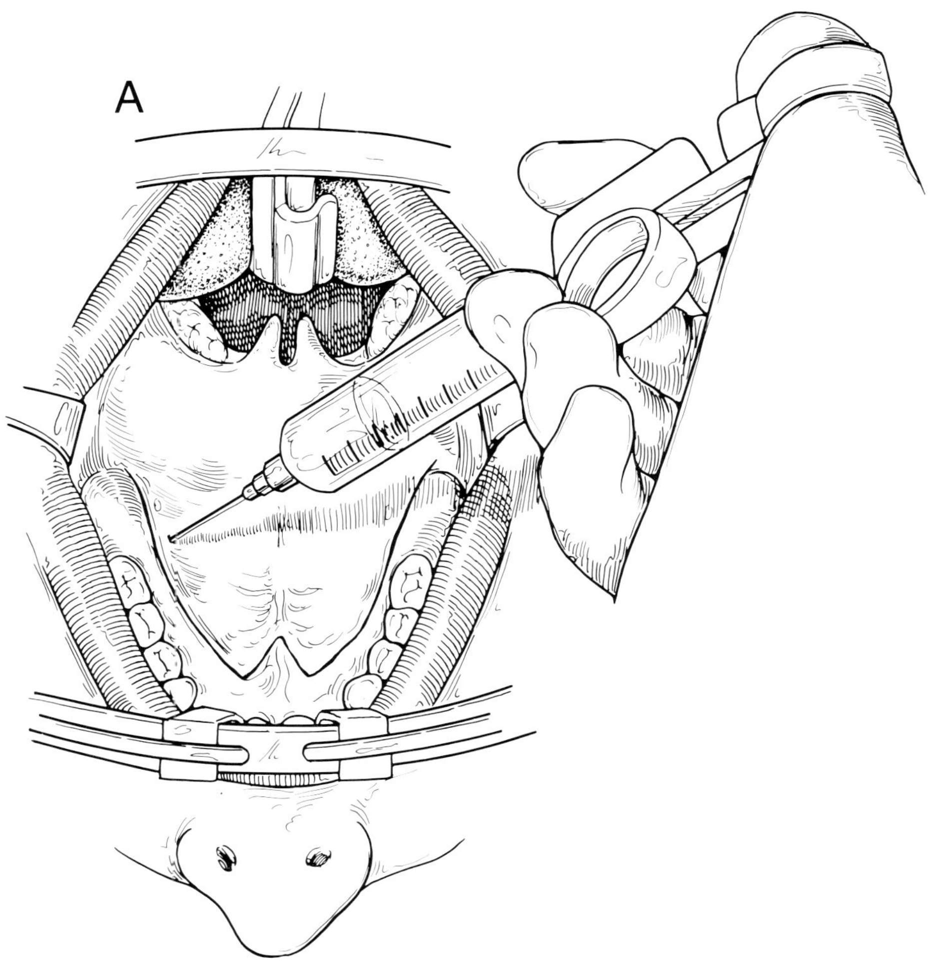


▶ **FIGURE 18-2**

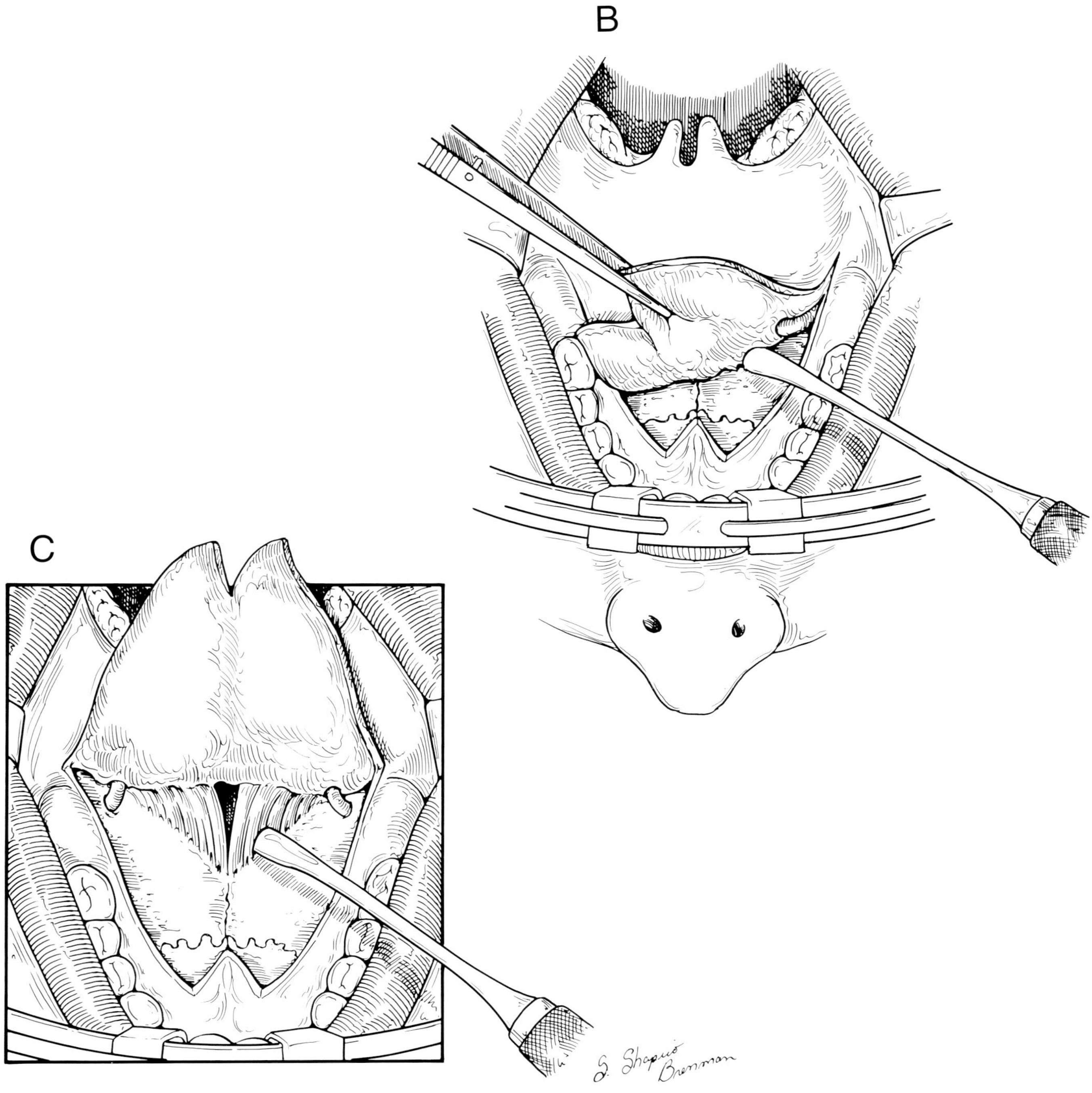


▶ **FIGURE 18-2**

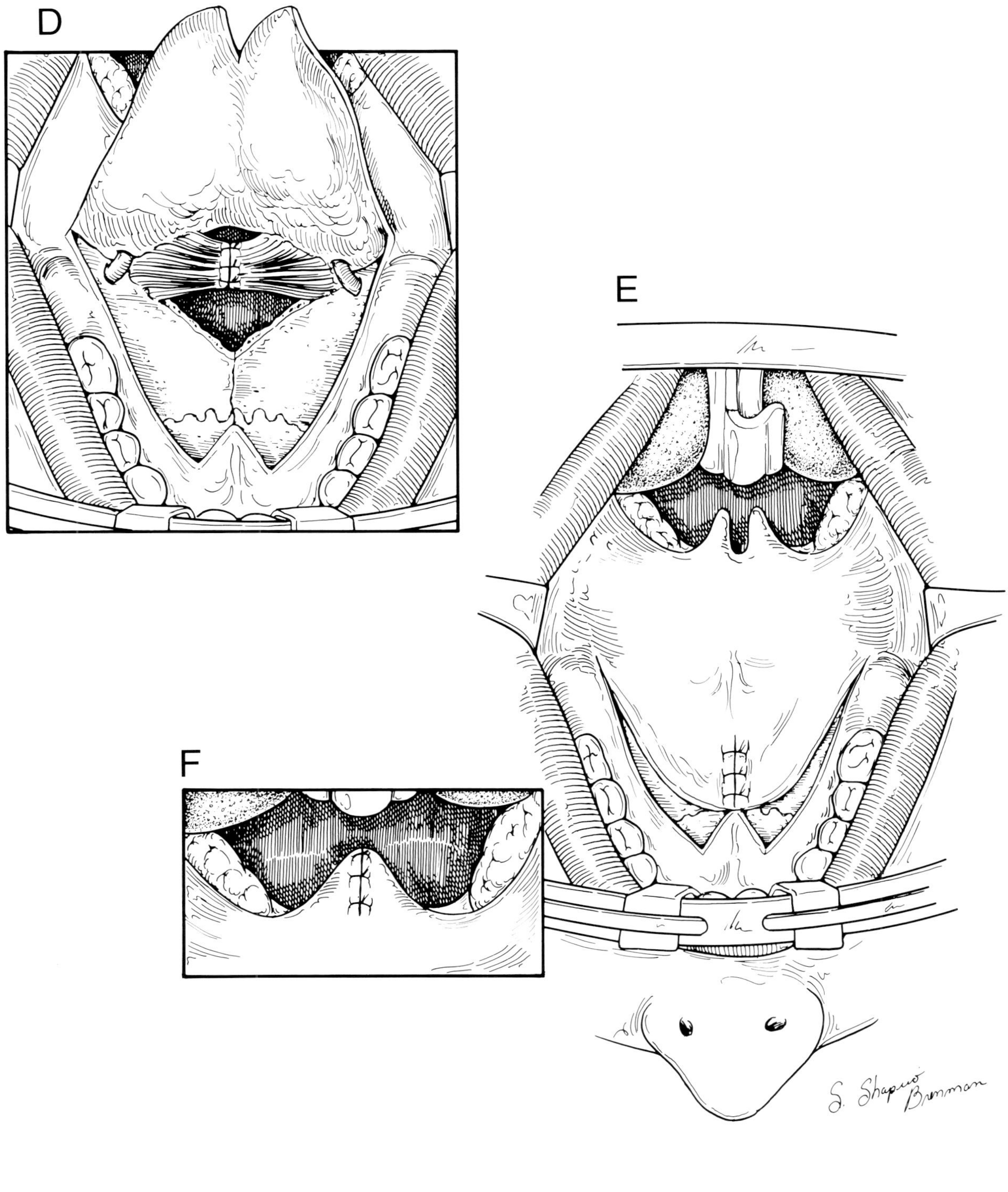


▶ **FIGURE 18-2**

# 19 ▶ Palatal Fistula

## ▶ 19-1 CLOSURE OF PALATAL FISTULA

A palatal fistula may occur following transpalatal surgery (e.g., choanal atresia and nasopharyngeal angiofibroma).

### Indications

A palatal fistula requires closure if it is associated with a leak of fluid or food into the nose.

### Preoperative Evaluation

The preoperative evaluation involves inspection of the palate. Video fluoroscopic examination of the palate may be useful to document leak of air or food into the nose.

### Operative Procedure

1. Closure of a palatal fistula is performed under general anesthesia administered through an oral RAE tube.
2. After a Dingman mouth gag is placed, the edges of the fistula are injected with 1% lidocaine and 1:100,000 epinephrine (Fig. 19–1**A**).
3. The fistula tract is excised with a knife making an ellipse through the oral mucosa of the palate and extending into the nasal or nasopharyngeal cavity (Fig. 19–1**B**).
4. Relaxing incisions are made on each side of the palate, and the palatal tissue is elevated with a periosteal elevator (Fig. 19–1**C**).
5. Elevated soft tissue is slid medially (Fig. 19–1**D**), and the midline incision is closed in two layers. The nasal mucosa is closed with 4-0 interrupted Vicryl, and the muscle with oral mucosa is closed with 3-0 interrupted Vicryl suture (Fig. 19–1**E**, **F**).
6. The lateral incisions are allowed to close by secondary intention.

### Complications

1. Recurrence of the palatal fistula

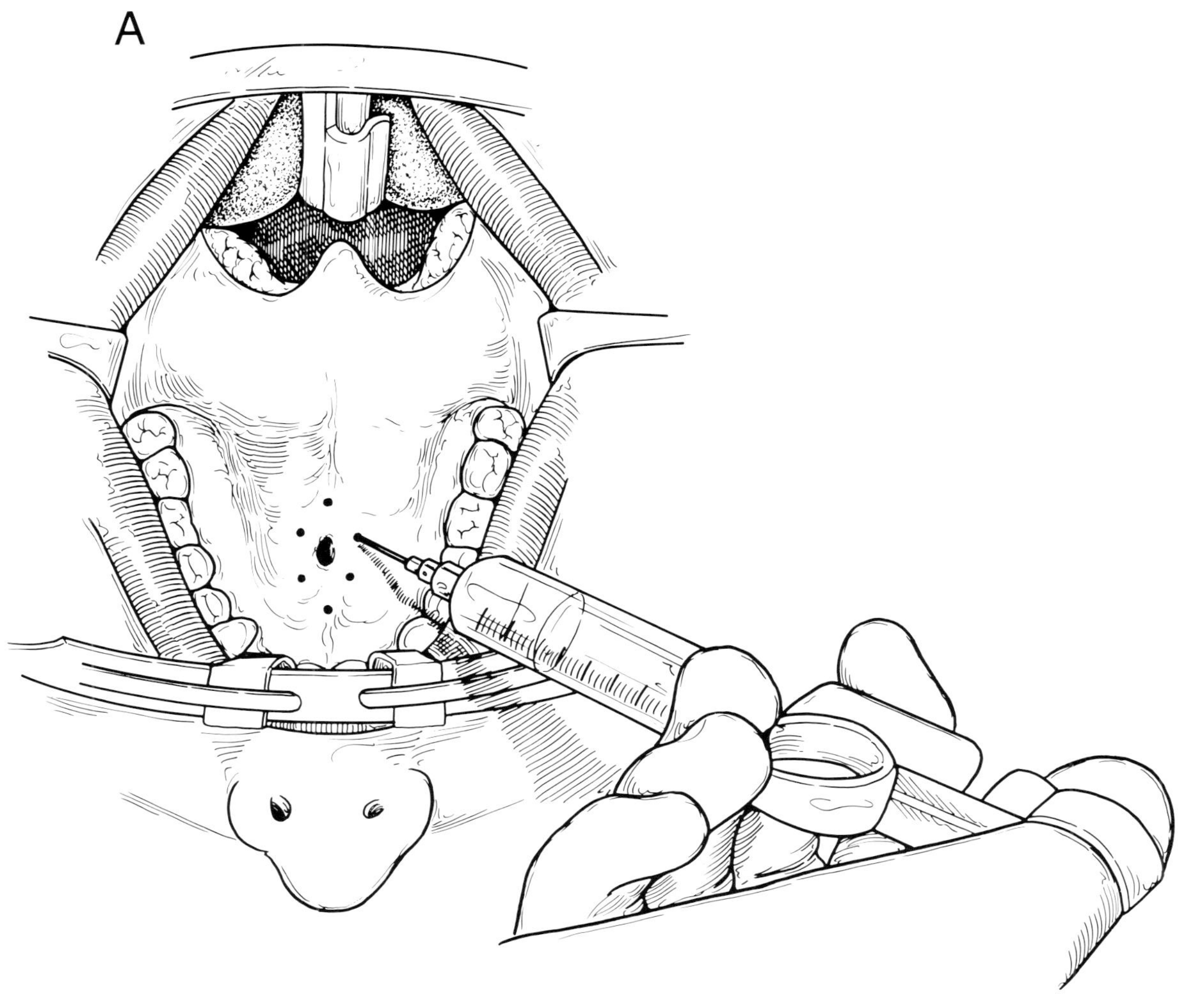


▶ **FIGURE 19-1**

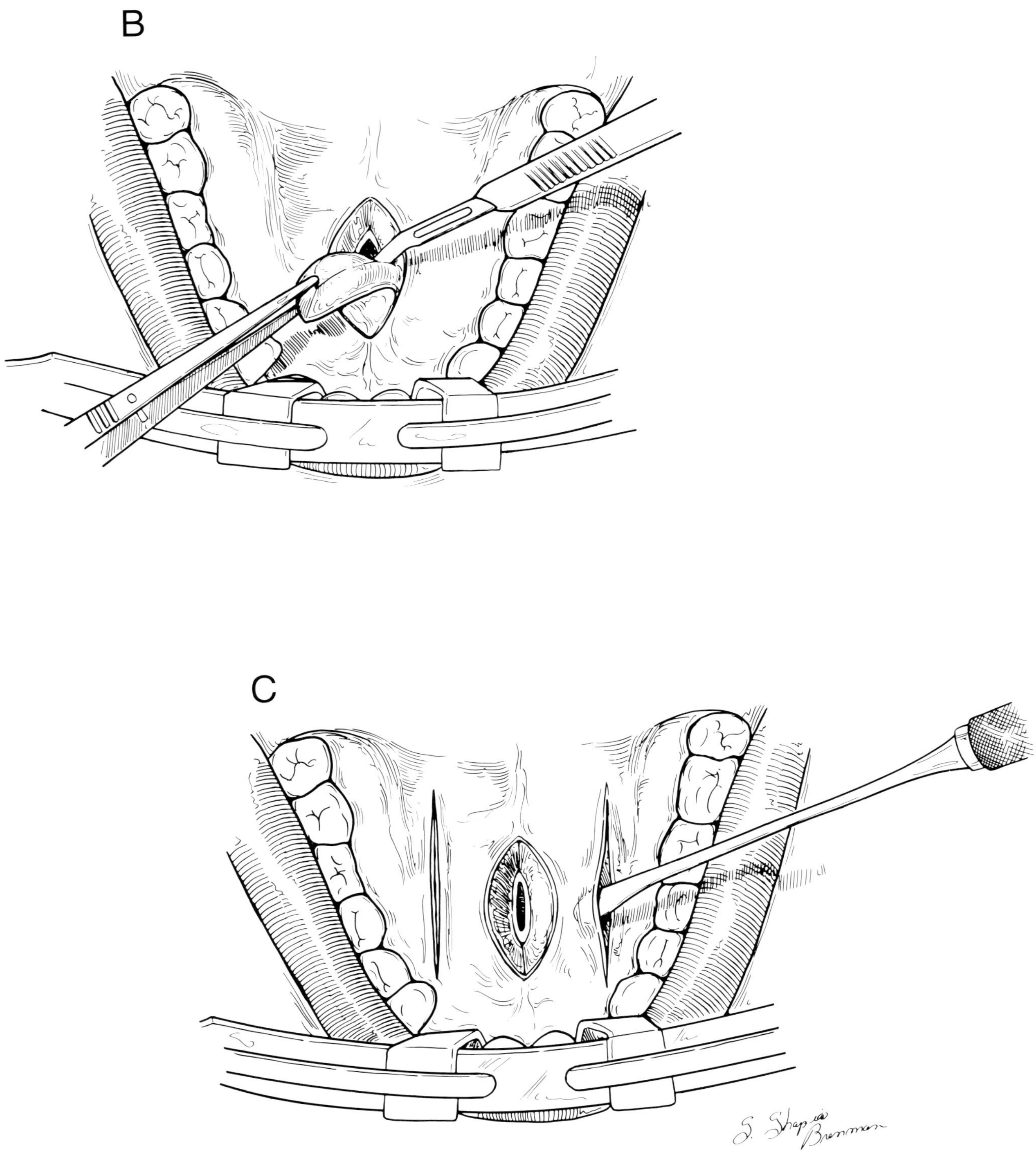


▶ **FIGURE 19-1**

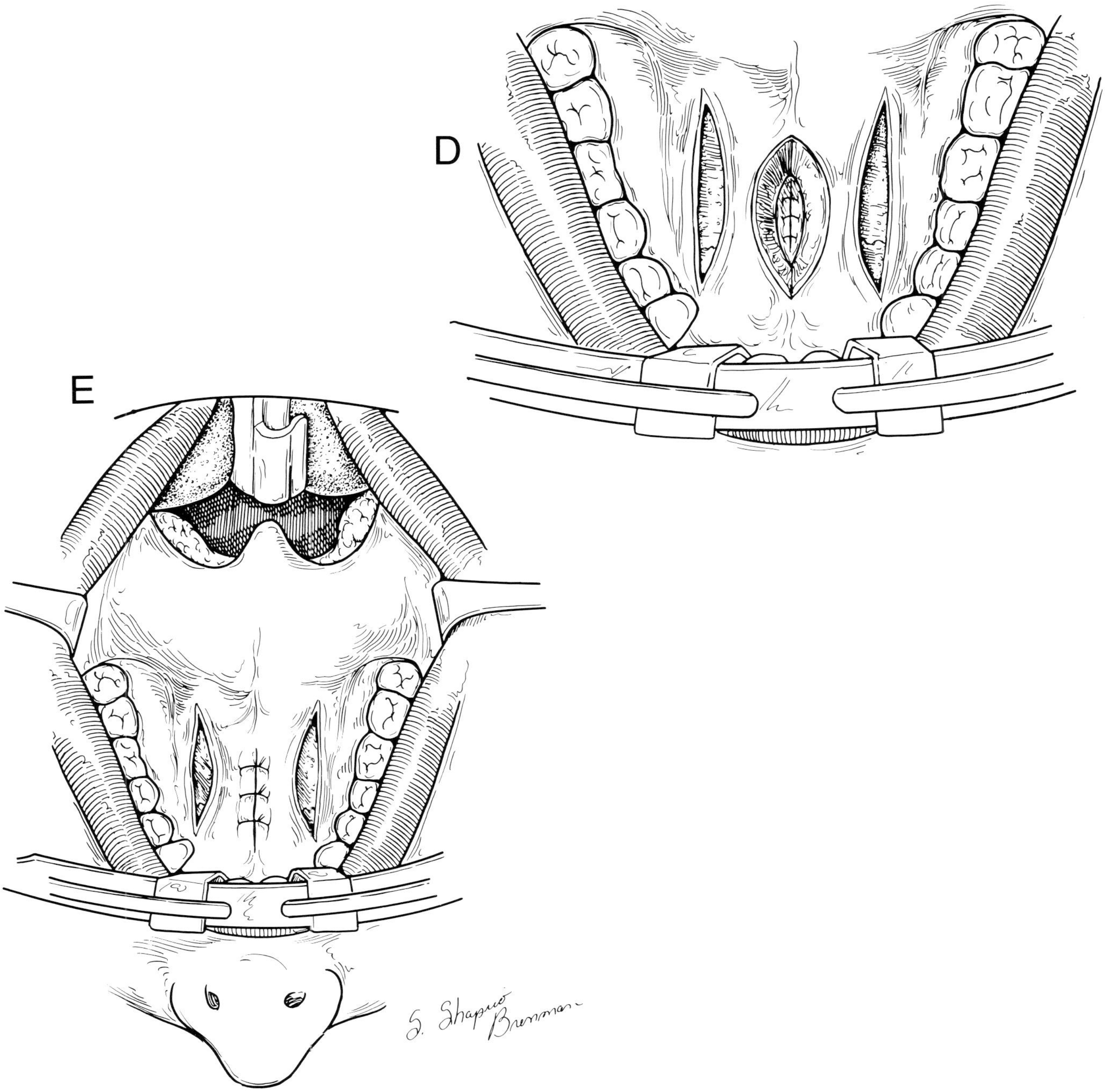


▶ **FIGURE 19-1**

# 20 ▶ Adenoid

Adenoid tissue may enlarge (hyperplasia) and/or become infected during bouts of pharyngitis.

## ▶ 20 - 1 ADENOIDECTOMY

### Indications

Adenoidectomy is indicated for the relief of nasal obstruction, sleep apnea, recurrence of chronic infection, and as part of the surgical therapy of chronic ear disease.

### Preoperative Evaluation

A lateral x-ray of the neck and nasoendoscopy are two reliable methods of assessing adenoid size. Careful evaluation of the palate to detect a submucous cleft palate and occult submucous cleft palate is necessary to minimize the incidence of velopharyngeal insufficiency after adenoidectomy. The classic triad of a submucous cleft palate is seen with careful inspection of the palate: the abnormal insertion of levator palatini muscle, the zona pellucida, and palpation of the posterior border of the hard palate for a notch in place of the posterior nasal spine. The occult (or hidden) submucous cleft palate can only be determined by nasoendoscopy. Nasoendoscopy is not required in all cases planned for adenoidectomy.

### Operative Technique

1. Adenoidectomy is performed under general anesthesia administered through an oral RAE tube. The patient is placed in the Rose position as for a tonsillectomy (see section 21–1, Figure 21–1**A**). Care is taken not to overextend the neck in patients suspected of having cervical spine abnormality.
2. The hard palate is carefully palpated to exclude the presence of a submucous cleft palate (Fig. 20–1**A**).
3. Red rubber catheters are placed through the nose to retract the palate (Fig. 20–1**B**).
4. Alternatively, a fine suture may be placed in the base of the uvula on the nasal surface to act as a retractor (Fig. 20–1**C**).
5. A mirror is used to inspect the nasopharynx (Fig. 20–1**D**). It is important to visually inspect and palpate the posterior wall of the nasopharynx for any signs of abnormal arterial pulsation. A variety of arterial malformations, including severe tortuousity of the internal carotid artery can occur in the nasopharynx.
6. Using the mirror for visualization, a sharp curette of suitable width is placed at the base of the vomer under direct vision (Fig. 20–1**E**).
7. The mirror is removed, and, using the thumb as a fulcrum (Fig. 20–1**F**), the adenoid tissue is carefully removed in one slow, gentle sweep of the curette. Any residual adenoid tissue in the posterior choanae is removed using a small

angled curette, again placed under direct vision (Fig. 20–1G). Alternatively, the entire adenoid can be removed with a suction cautery.

8. If curette is used, the nasopharynx is packed for a minimum of 2 minutes before suction cautery is used to coagulate any persistent bleeding vessels and to remove any residual adenoid tissue (Fig. 20–1H).

9. It is important to remove as much of the adenoid tissue as possible (Fig. 20–1I). Residual adenoid tissue often makes it difficult to obtain adequate hemostasis and may lead to regrowth of the adenoid and recurrence of nasopharyngeal obstruction. Care should be taken, however, not to be too aggressive in removing all the adenoid tissue surrounding the eustachian tube for fear of causing scarring at the end of the tube, or nasopharyngeal stenosis.

## Complications

1. Velopharyngeal insufficiency
2. Nasopharyngeal stenosis
3. Recurrent granuloma formation

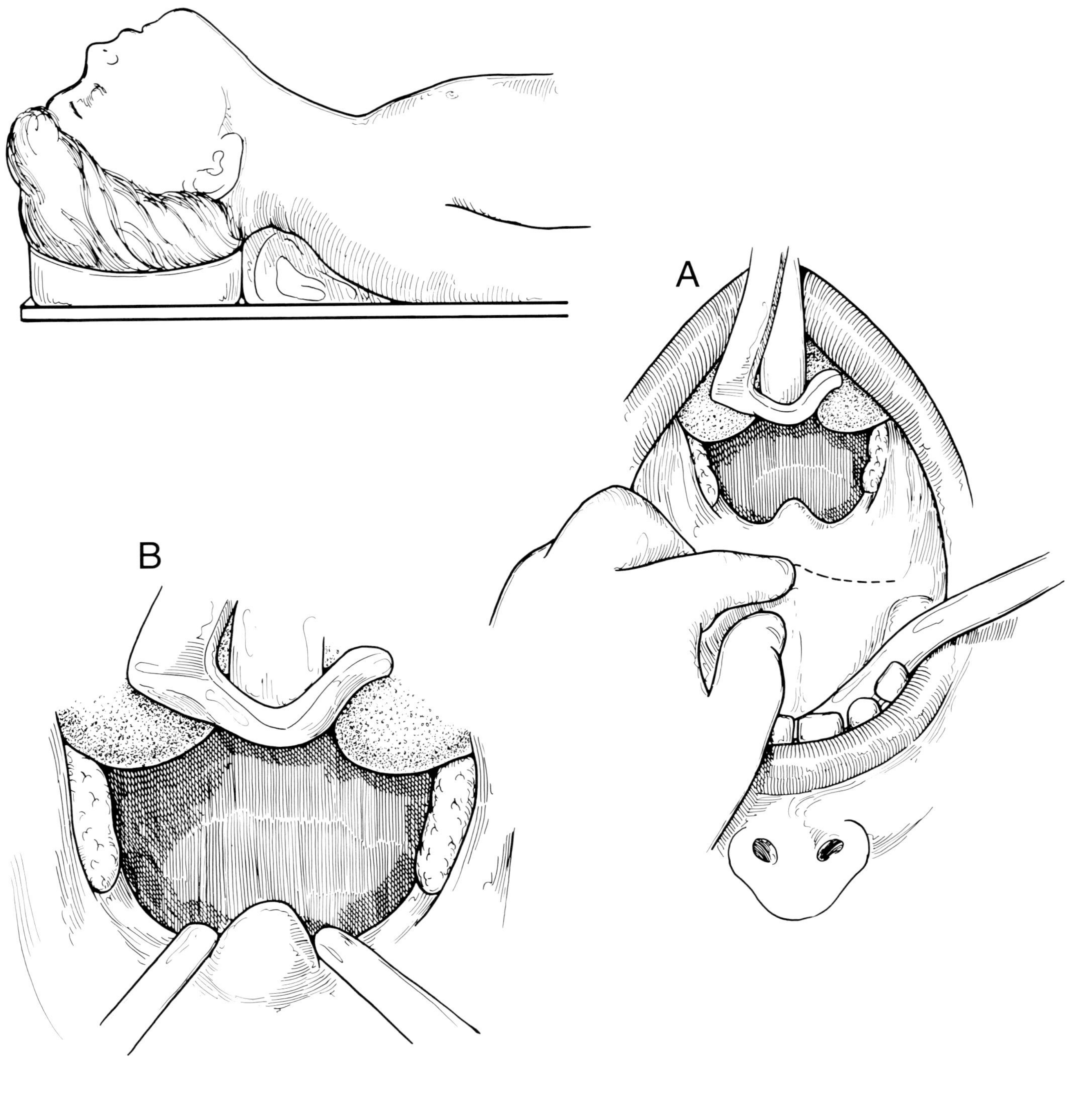


▶ **FIGURE 20-1**

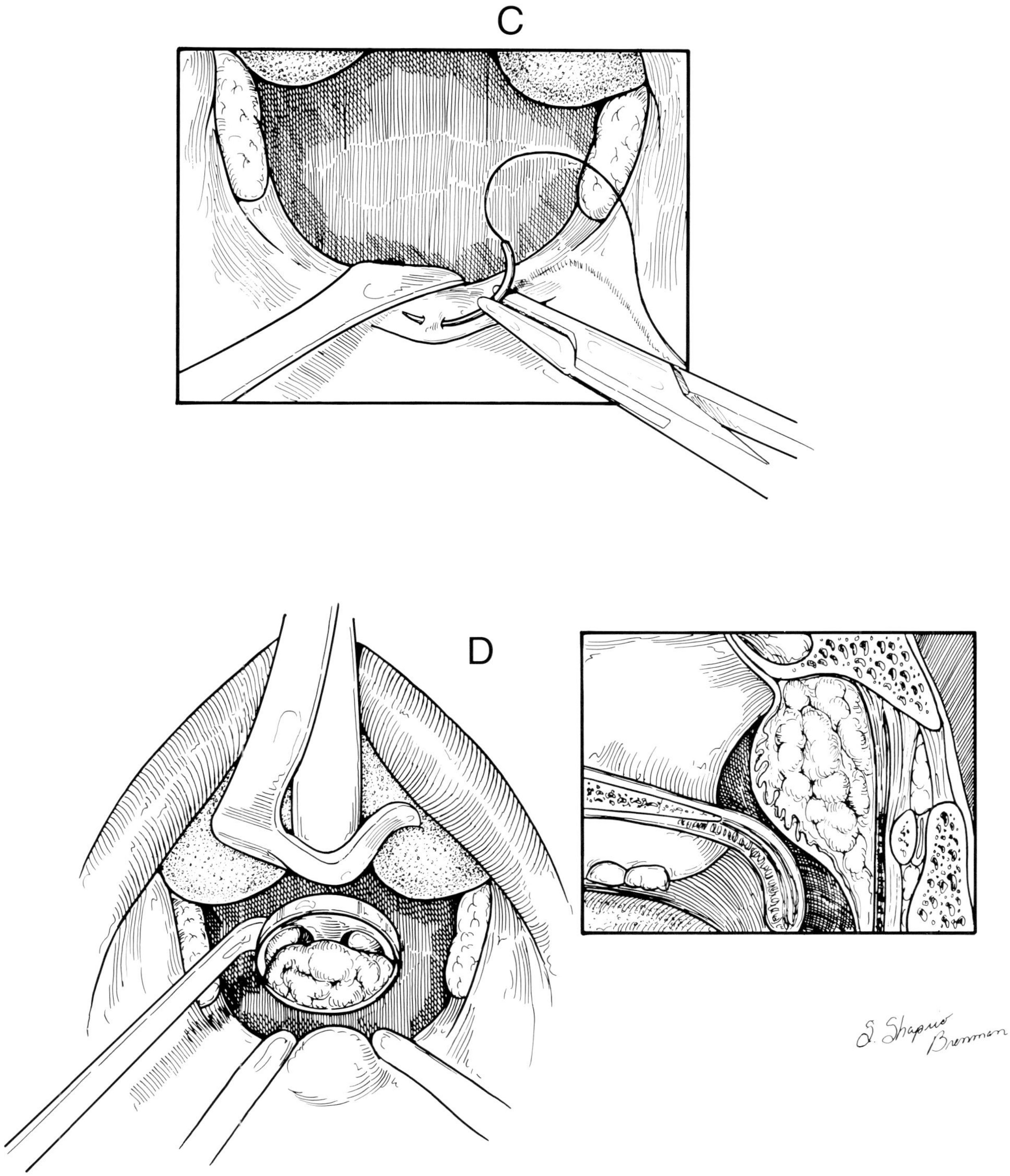


▶ **FIGURE 20-1**

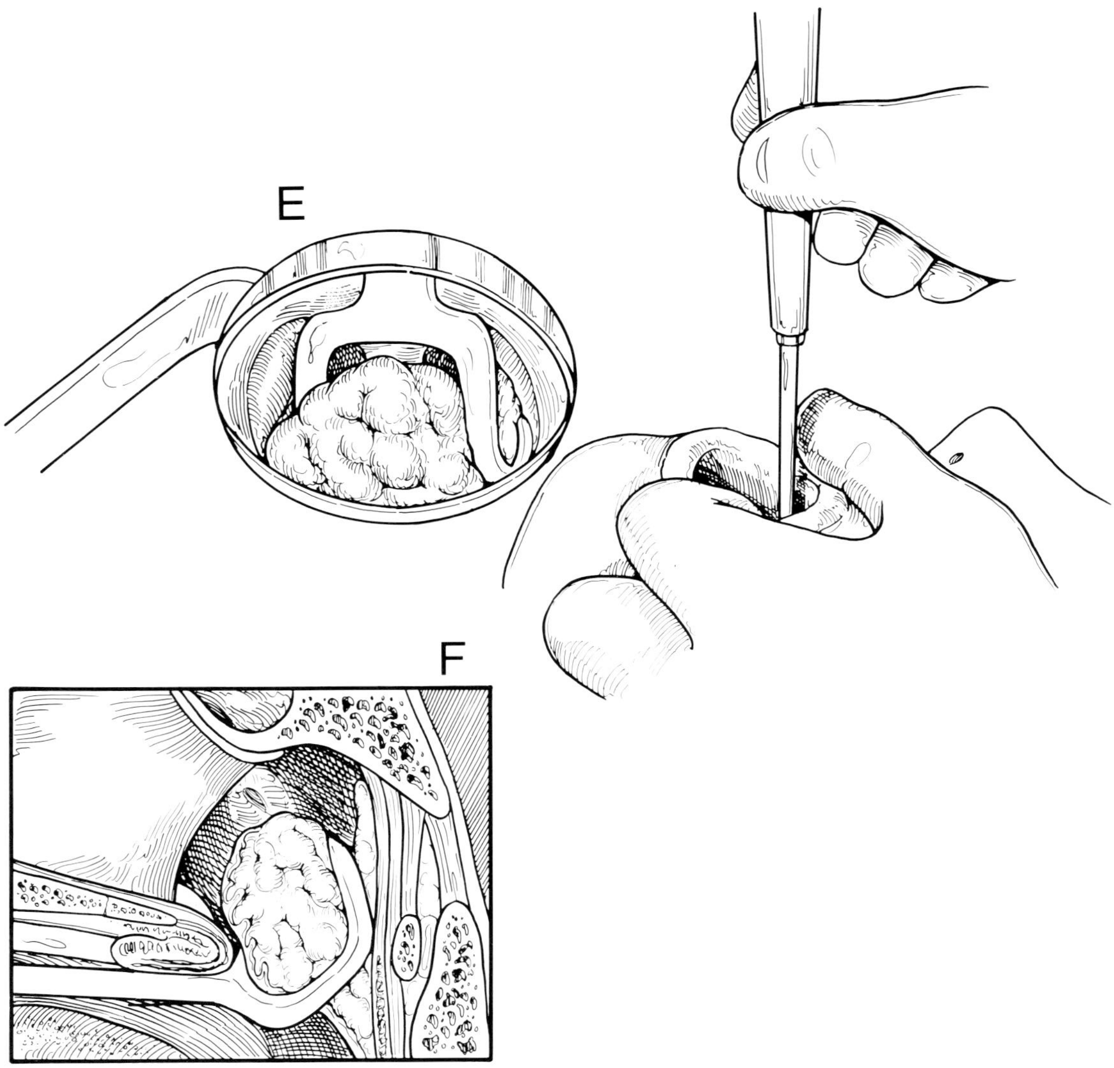


▶ **FIGURE 20-1**

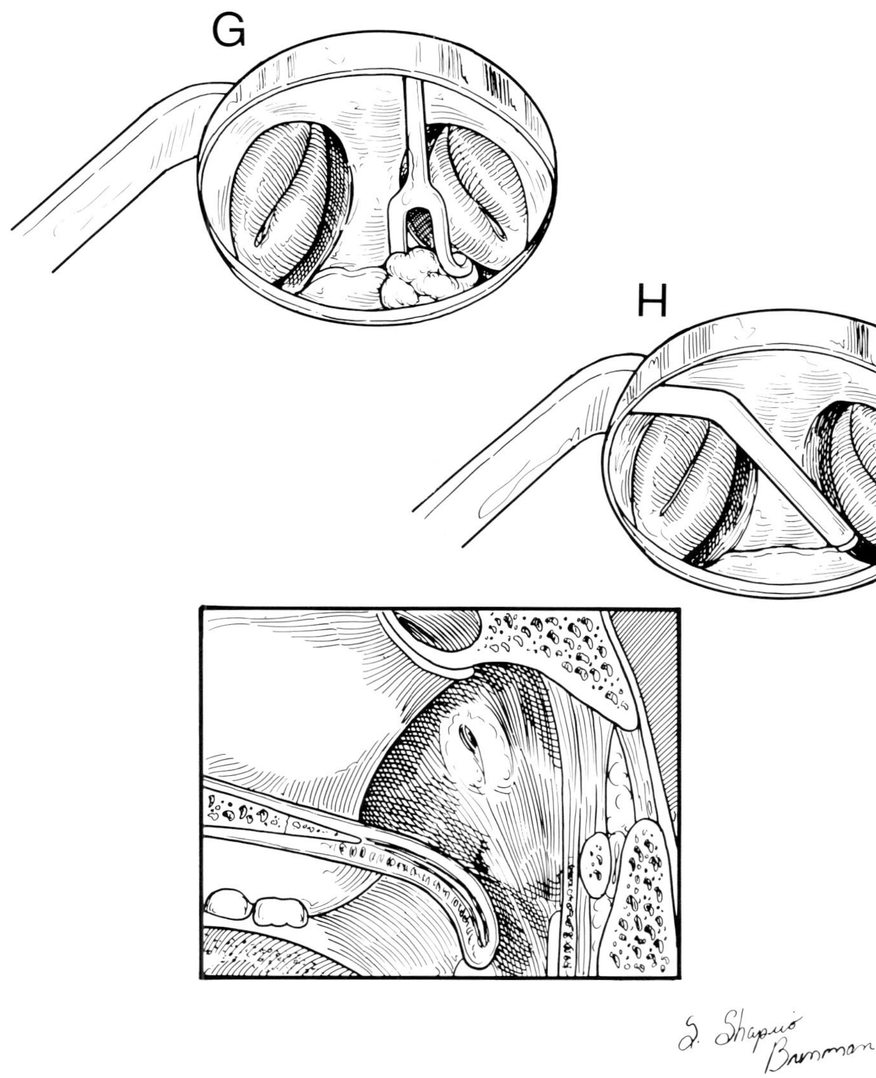


▶ **FIGURE 20-1**

# 21 ▶ Tonsils

Tonsillar hyperplasia and recurrent pharyngotonsillitis are common conditions in children. Tonsillar hyperplasia may cause sleep disorders and apnea. Recurrent infection, often debilitating, may be associated with complications of streptococcal infection.

## ▶ 21 - 1 TONSILLECTOMY

### Indications

Removal of the pharyngeal tonsils is indicated to relieve pharyngeal obstruction and to reduce the frequency and severity of pharyngeal infection.

### Preoperative Evaluation

The history and physical examination are usually sufficient to determine the need for tonsillectomy. Radiographs are not helpful in the evaluation of tonsillar disease.

### Operative Technique

1. Tonsillectomy is usually performed under general anesthesia through an oral RAE tube. The procedure may be performed under local anesthesia in cooperative adolescents. The patient is placed in the Rose position at the end of the operating table. A shoulder roll is placed under the shoulders and the head rests in a doughnut (Fig. 21–1**A**).
2. A tonsil gag is introduced and opened, keeping the tongue in the midline.
3. The posterior and lateral walls of the pharynx are carefully inspected and palpated to detect abnormally positioned vessels (Fig. 21–1**B**).
4. The hard palate is palpated to detect a submucous cleft palate (Fig. 21–1**C**).
5. The superior pole of the right tonsil is grasped with an Allis clamp, and the mucosal cuts on the anterior and posterior tonsillar pillars are outlined with a protected cautery, preserving as much mucosa as possible (Fig. 21–1**D**). The guarded cautery blade prevents inadvertent burns.
6. Using careful dissection, the plane of the tonsillar capsule is located (Fig. 21–1**E**).
7. The tonsil is removed by dissection with the cautery as the tonsil is retracted medially with the Allis clamp (Fig. 21–1**H**). Larger vessels, when encountered, may need additional cauterization.
8. The attachment of the inferior portion of the pharyngeal tonsil to the lingual tonsil is transected with the cautery (Fig. 21–1**F**).
9. Residual bleeding vessels are cauterized with a suction cautery while the tonsil fossa is exposed using a hemostat or Hurd dissector for retraction (Fig. 21–1**G**).

**10.** The recessed superior pole of the tonsillar fossa is best visualized using a mirror (Fig. 21–1H).

**11.** This procedure is repeated on the opposite side.

**12.** When the tonsillectomy is completed, the mouth gag is released for a brief period and then reopened to inspect the oral cavity to make sure that there is no further bleeding from vessels that might have been compressed by the mouth gag. The gag is then carefully removed from the oral cavity to avoid accidental extubation of the patient.

## Complications

1. Incomplete tonsil removal
2. Velopharyngeal insufficiency
3. Pharyngeal stenosis

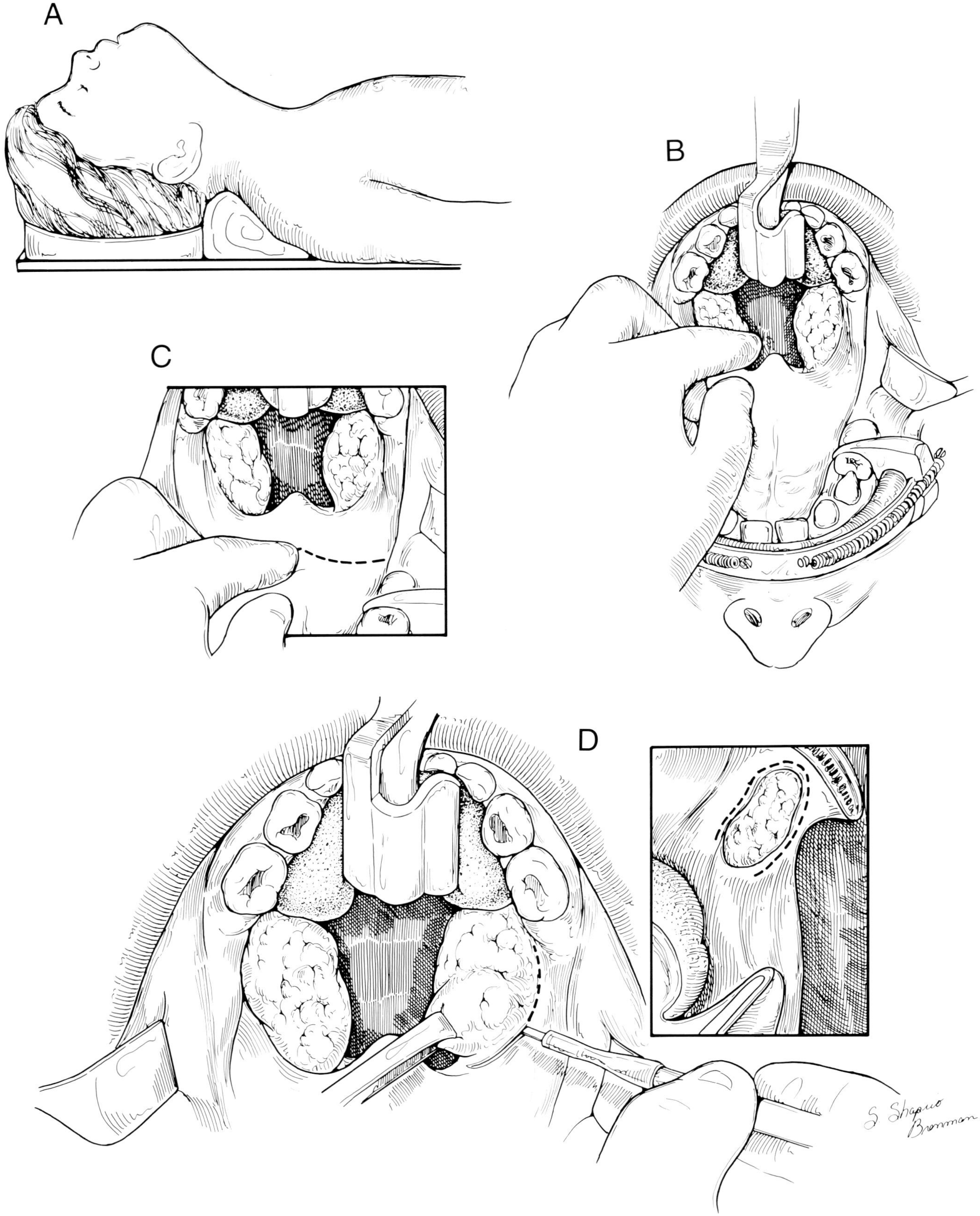


▶ **FIGURE 21-1**

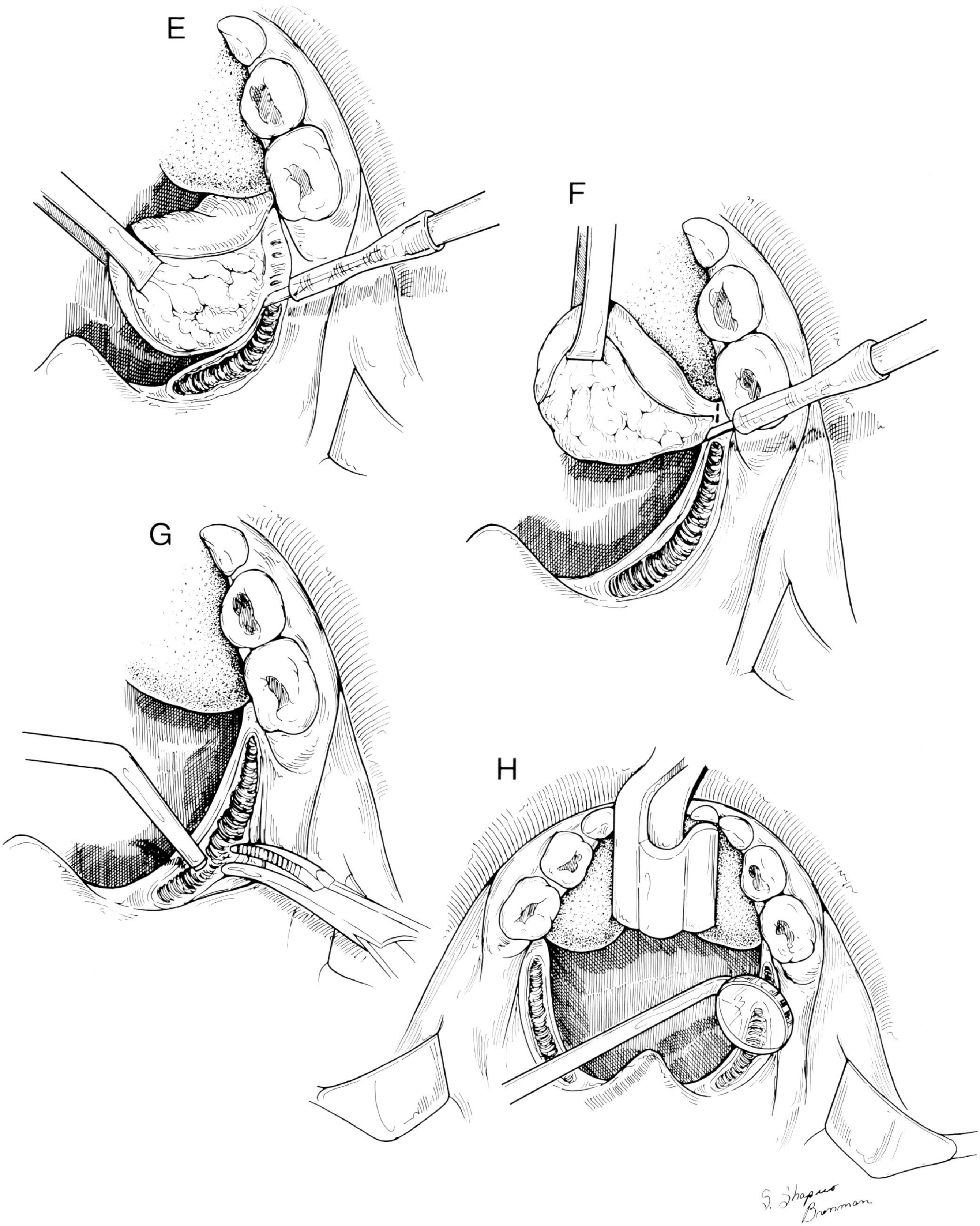


▸ **FIGURE 21-1**

# 22 ▸ Tongue

## ▸ 22-1 FRENULOPLASTY

Ankyloglossia is an uncommon cause of speech or feeding problems. Severe, thick ankyloglossia may cause pressure against the teeth or trauma to the lingual frenulum itself by rubbing against the lower teeth. Thin webs may be divided with a scissors in the outpatient setting.

### Indications

Frenuloplasty is indicated for symptomatic severe ankyloglossia.

### Preoperative Evaluation

Inspection of the floor of the mouth or frenulum is sufficient. No additional evaluation is required.

### Operative Technique

1. Frenuloplasty in children is performed using general anesthesia by nasotracheal intubation, or with an oral tracheal tube taped to one side of the mouth.
2. The tongue is grasped with a toothed forceps and the frenulum is stretched (Fig. 22–1**A**).
3. The frenulum is crushed with a straight clamp above the submandibular ducts, taking care to avoid injury to the orifices (Fig. 22–1**B**).
4. The crushed frenulum is cut with a scissors to the base of the sublingual area, releasing the frenulum (Fig. 22–1**C**).
5. This releases the tongue and leaves a mucosal defect on the tongue, extending to the floor of the mouth (Fig. 22–1**D**).
6. Three or four 4-0 interrupted chromic sutures are placed to close the incision on the ventral surface of the tongue (Fig. 22–1**E**). No sutures are placed in the floor of the mouth because of potential injury to the submandibular ducts (Fig. 22–1**E**).

### Complications

1. Submandibular duct injury
2. Recurrence of ankyloglossia
3. Submandibular gland swelling

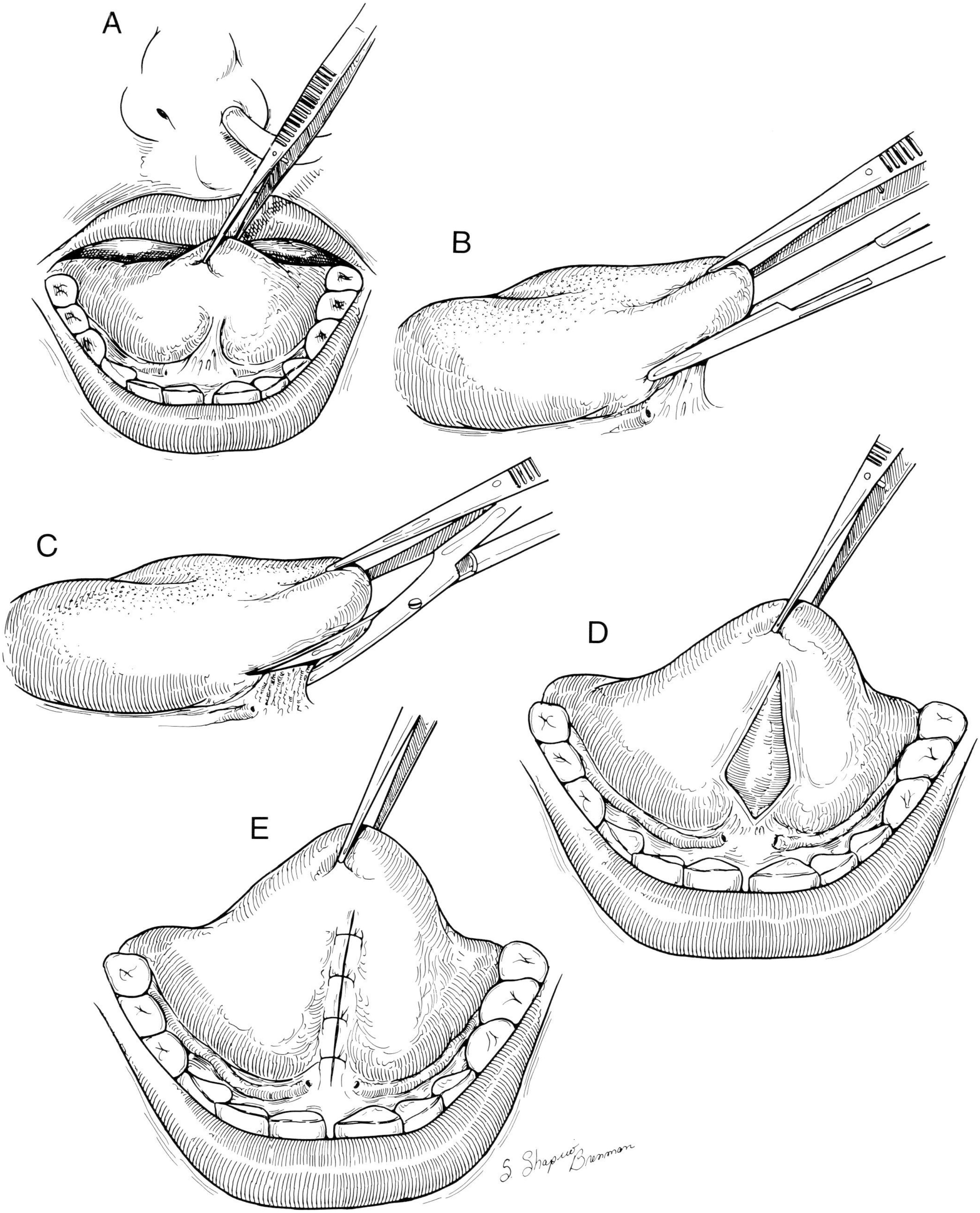


▶ **FIGURE 22-1**

## ▶ 22-2 EXCISION OF DISCRETE LESIONS OF THE TONGUE

Discrete lesions of the tongue such as papillomas, granulomas and fibromas may present in children.

### Indications

Suspicious lesions on the anterior third of the tongue require excisional biopsy.

### Preoperative Evaluation

Inspection of the lesion is all that is required. No further evaluation is needed.

### Operative Technique

1. Discrete lesions of the tongue are excised using general anesthesia administered through nasotracheal intubation to facilitate intraoral exposure.
2. A 3-0 silk suture is passed through the anterior portion of the tongue and used for traction (Fig. 22–2**A**).
3. One percent lidocaine with 1:100,000 epinephrine is injected subcutaneously at the site of the incision to aid in hemostasis.
4. The lesion is excised with an elliptical incision through mucosa and into the underlying muscle (Fig. 22–2**B**, **C**).
5. The incision is closed with a single layer of 3-0 interrupted chromic suture (Fig. 22–2**D**).

### Complications

1. Wound dehiscence

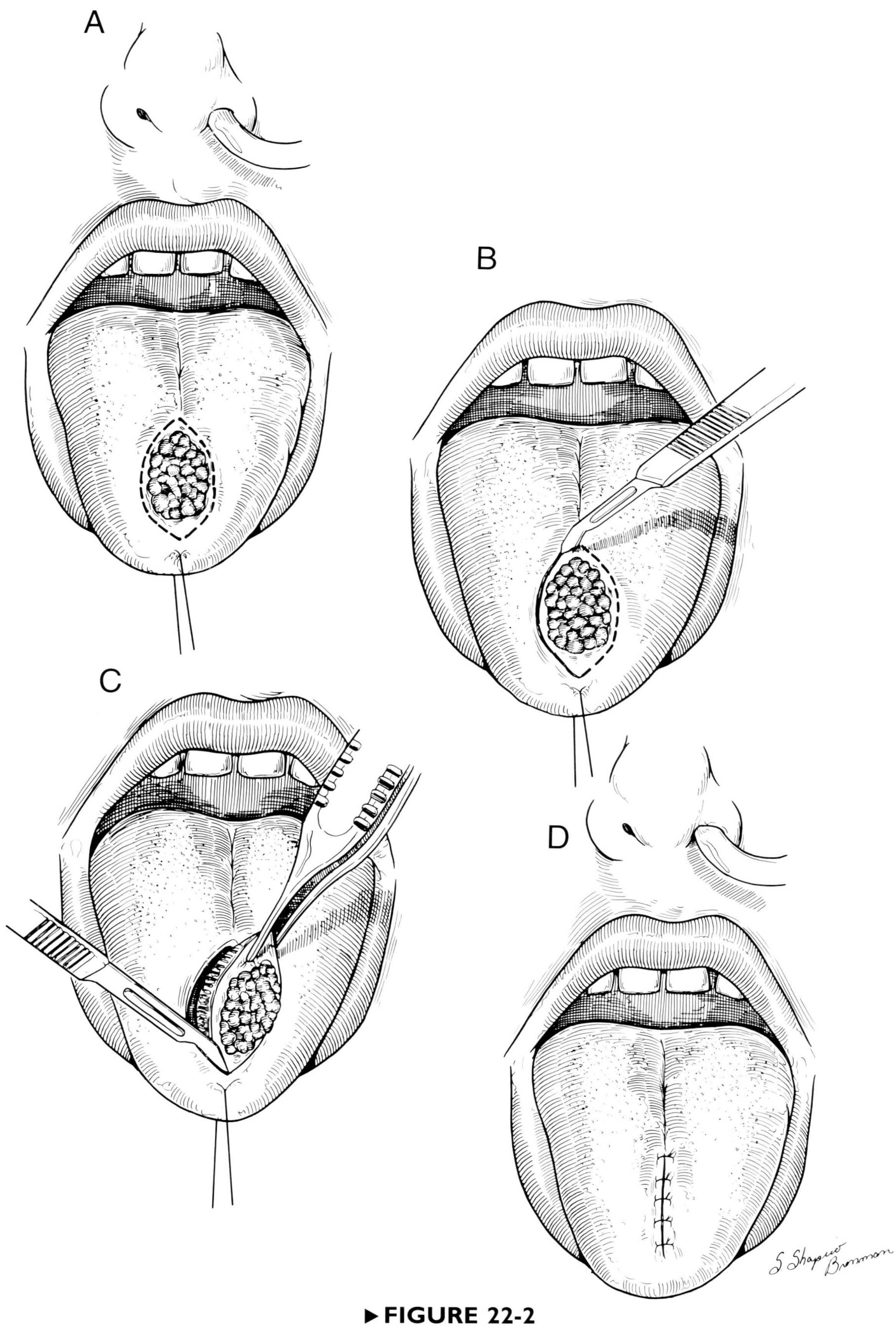


▶ **FIGURE 22-2**

## ▶ 22-3 EXCISION OF DIFFUSE LESIONS OF THE TONGUE

Diffuse lesions of the tongue are usually hemangiomas or lymphangiomas.

### Indications

Surgical treatment of lymphangiomas or hemangiomas of the tongue is required when there is recurrent bleeding, tissue necrosis, infection, or airway obstruction. A large lesion may cause disfigurement, dysphagia, or an articulation disorder.

### Preoperative Evaluation

Inspection of the lesion is usually the only evaluation required. A computed tomography (CT) scan or magnetic resonance angiogram (MRA) scan may be helpful to define the extent of involvement of the floor of mouth. Preoperative embolization is recommended for large vascular lesions.

### Operative Technique

1. Surgery for diffuse lesions of the tongue is performed utilizing general anesthesia by nasotracheal intubation.
2. A 3-0 silk suture in the tip of the tongue is used for traction (Fig. 22–3**A**).
3. A $CO_2$ or KTP laser is used to vaporize and "sculpt" the lesion until it is flush with the surface of tongue muscle (Fig. 22–3**B, C**).
4. Deep or large defects may require closure using multiple figure-of-eight knots of 3-0 or 4-0 chromic suture.

### Complications

1. Recurrence of the lesion
2. Tongue swelling with airway obstruction

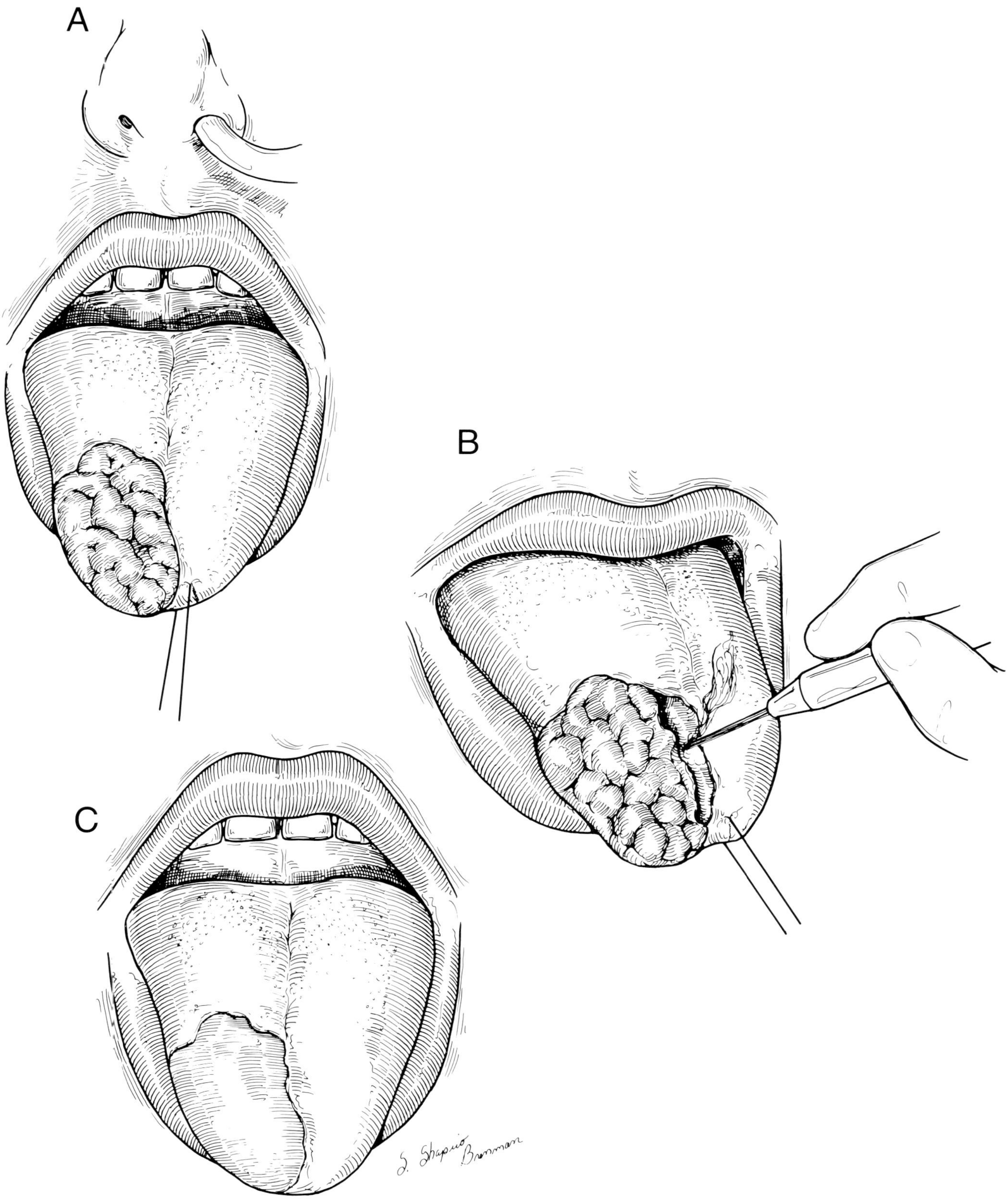


▶ **FIGURE 22-3**

## ▶ 22-4 TONGUE REDUCTION

Macroglossia often causes feeding and breathing difficulties. Tongue reduction by excision provides reliable results and limited postoperative morbidity. Two of the most commonly used techniques involve excision of the lateral and anterior borders of the tongue or removal of a central wedge of tongue tissue. These two procedures, used separately or together, are usually sufficient to accomplish tongue reduction.

### Indications

Tongue reduction is performed when the protuberant tongue causes oral dysfunction such as problems with oral hygiene, airway compromise, deglutition, articulation, and orthognathic complications. The child's appearance may be psychologically distressing to both the parents and the child.

### Preoperative Evaluation

Inspection of the tongue and evaluation of the complications of macroglossia is sufficient. A preoperative speech evaluation should be obtained if appropriate for the child's age.

### Operative Technique

1. Tongue reduction is best performed using a general anesthesia through a nasotracheal tube.
2. The lines of excision are drawn on the tongue with a marking pencil (Fig. 22–4**A, D**); 3-0 silk sutures are used for traction.
3. One percent lidocaine with 1:100,000 epinephrine is injected subcutaneously at the site of the incision to aid in hemostasis.
4. Smooth intestinal clamps or nonabsorbable hemostatic sutures are placed at the posterior portion of the tongue to compress the lingual arteries and their branches.
5. The appropriate portion of tongue tissue is removed with a knife or cutting cautery to achieve the desired result (Fig. 22–4**B, E**).
6. The wound is closed with deep and mucosal 3-0 Vicryl suture after hemostasis is obtained (Fig. 22–4**C, F**).
7. Dexamethasone is given intraoperatively and tapered over 3 days postoperatively.
8. The patient is usually kept intubated for 12 to 24 hours and broad-spectrum antibiotics are given for 10 to 14 days.

### Complications

1. Tongue swelling and airway obstruction
2. Wound dehiscence

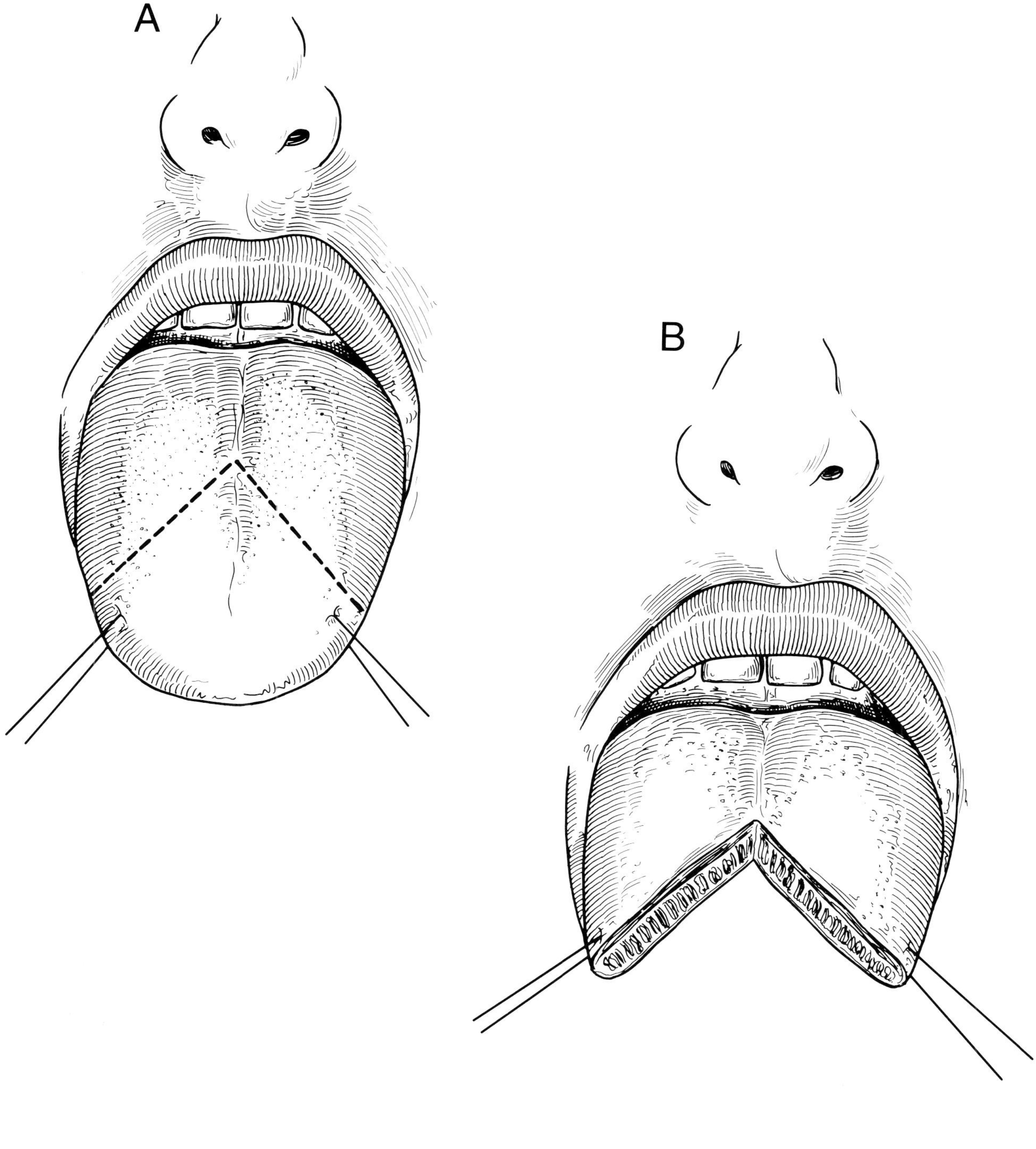


▶ **FIGURE 22-4**

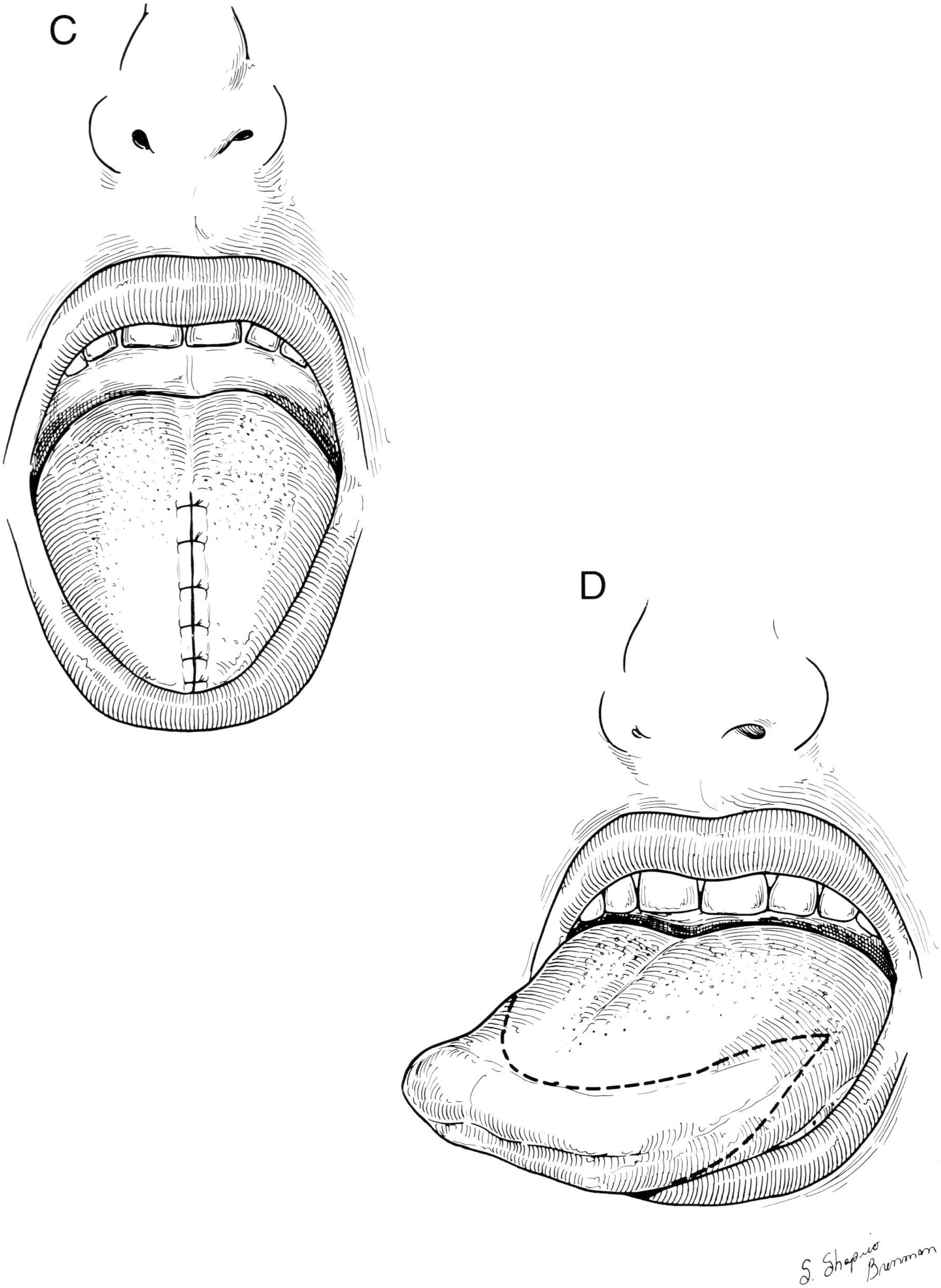


▶ **FIGURE 22-4**

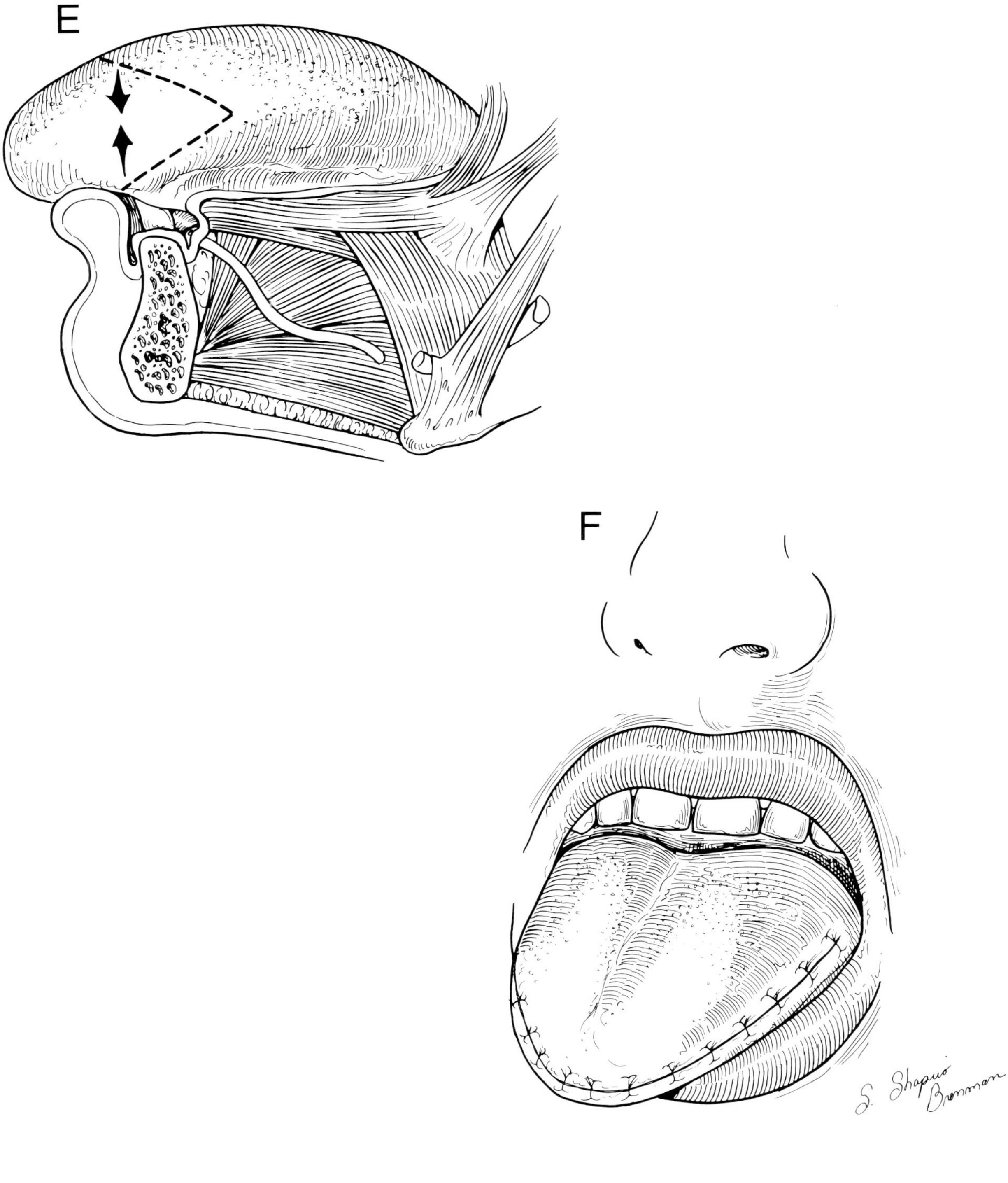


▶ **FIGURE 22-4**

# 23 ▸ Tumors of the Oral Cavity and Jaw

## ▸ 23-1 EXCISION OF FIBROUS DYSPLASIA

Fibrous dysplasia is a benign locally invasive fibro-osseous disorder. In its most common monostotic form, it involves the maxilla more often than the mandible. The lesion usually presents with an obvious deformity of the involved bony structure (Fig. 23–1**A**).

### Indications

Surgery is indicated both to confirm the diagnosis and to sculpt the lesion to restore normal anatomy and function. Radical excision of this lesion is never indicated. Repeat procedures may be required to treat this slow-growing lesion.

### Preoperative Evaluation

Computed tomography (CT) scan of the affected bony area is mandatory before surgical intervention.

### Operative Procedure

1. General anesthesia is administered through a nasal endotracheal tube placed in the uninvolved side. If the lesion involved the maxilla, the usual approach to this area is the gingival-buccal approach as in the Caldwell-Luc procedure (see section 24–3, Fig. 24–3**A**).
2. One percent lidocaine with 1:100,000 epinephrine is injected into the gingivobuccal sulcus (Fig. 23–1**B**).
3. An incision in the gingival-buccal sulcus 5 mm above the gum line is made with a #15 blade. The incision is carried down to the periosteum of the maxilla with the cutting cautery (Fig. 23–1**C**).
4. A periosteal elevator is used to elevate the soft tissues of the cheek off of the face of the maxilla until the infraorbital nerve is identified (Fig. 23–1**D**).
5. If there is a thin layer of normal bony cortex, this is cracked and removed with a small curved clamp or elevator (Fig. 23–1**E**).
6. The tumor is debulked with a knife or large cup forceps (Takahashi) or curette, depending upon its gritty nature. When the desired contour has been obtained, the operation is terminated (Fig. 23–1**F**).
7. If there is a patent maxillary sinus cavity, an inferior antrostomy (see section 24–3) should be performed.
8. The mucosa of the cheek is sutured loosely with interrupted 4-0 chromic sutures. These sutures are left in place until they dissolve on their own (Fig. 23–1**G**).

**Complications**

1. Recurrence from incomplete excision
2. Ocular injury
3. Infraorbital nerve injury

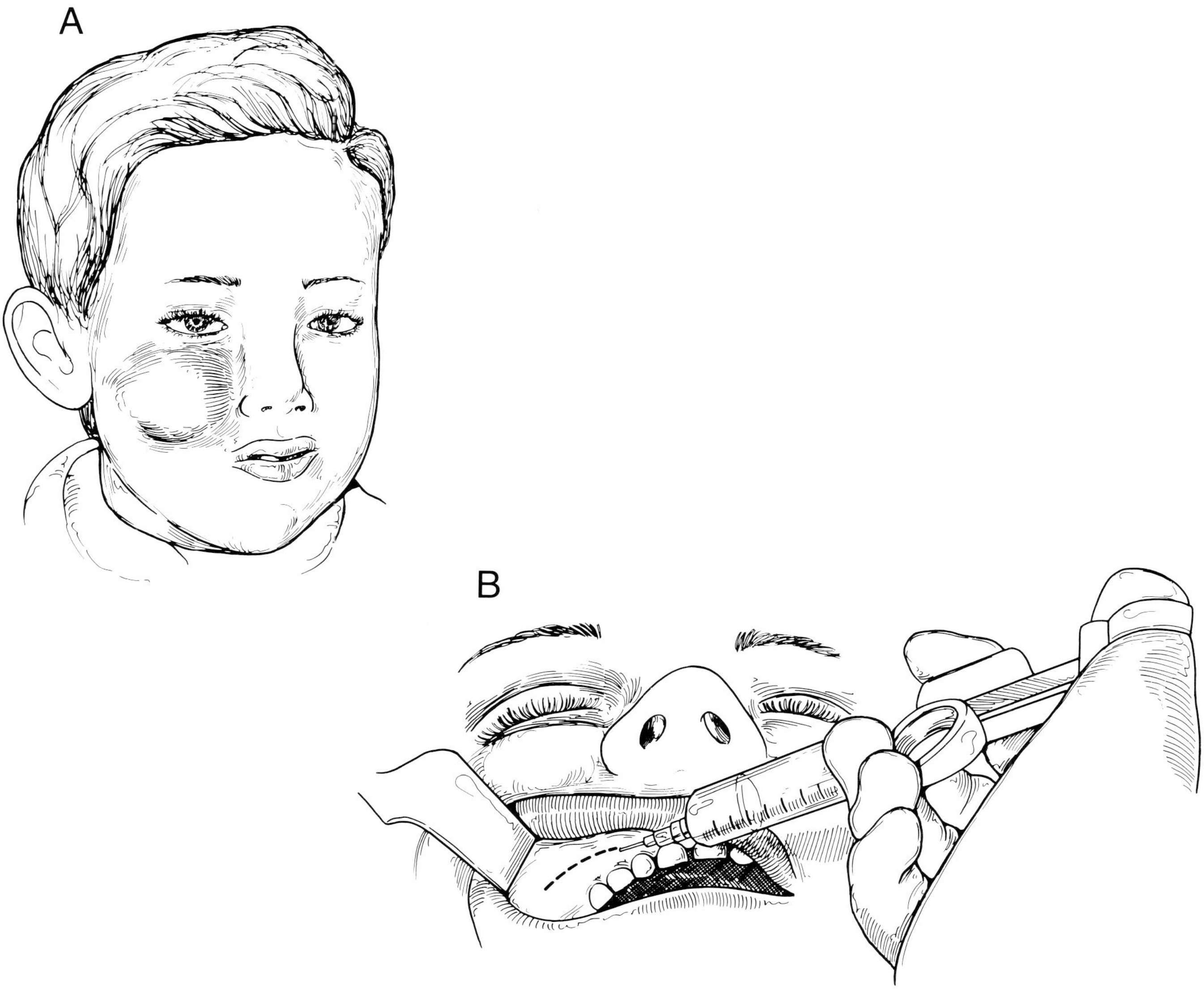


▶ **FIGURE 23-1**

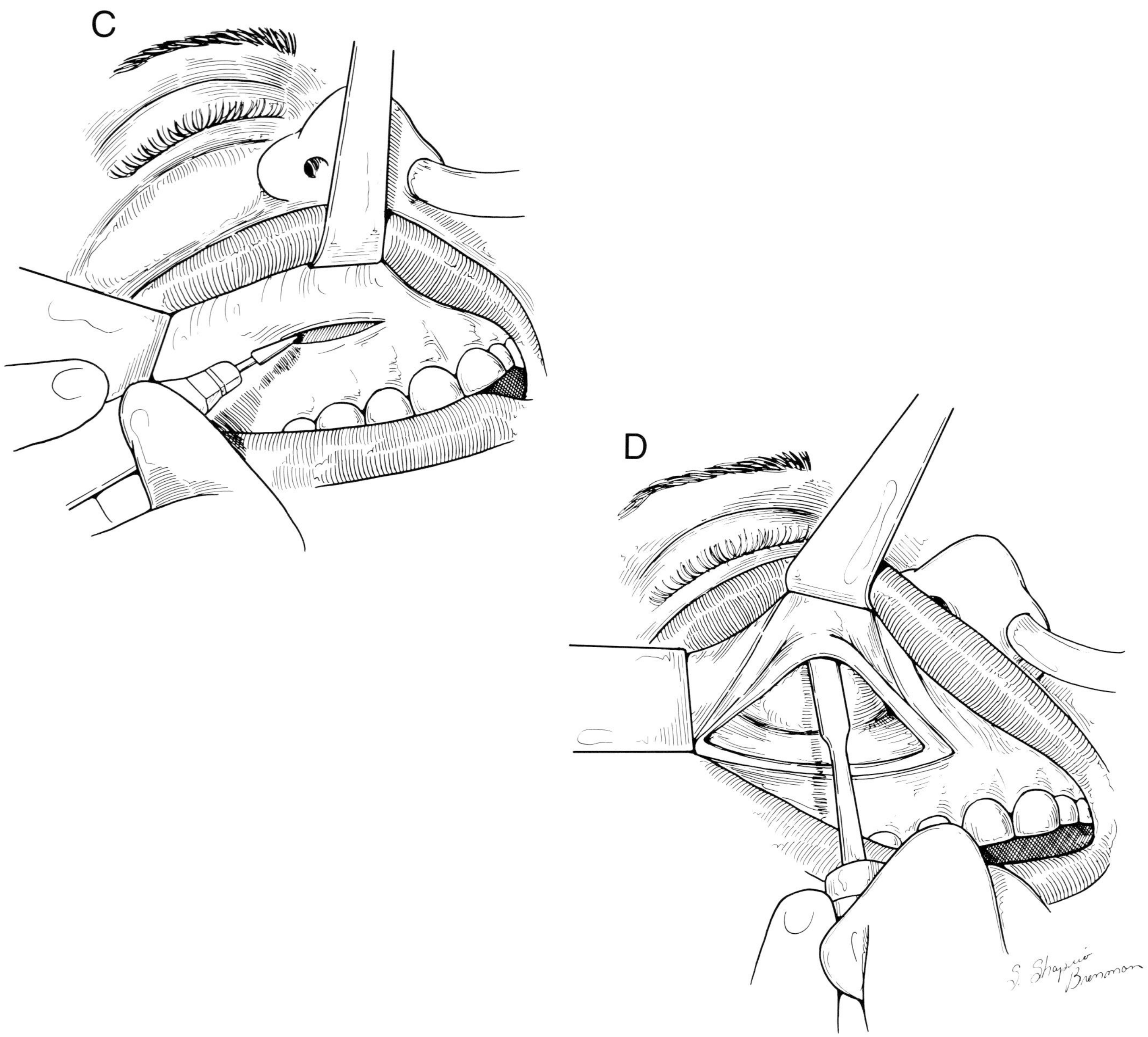


▶ **FIGURE 23-1**

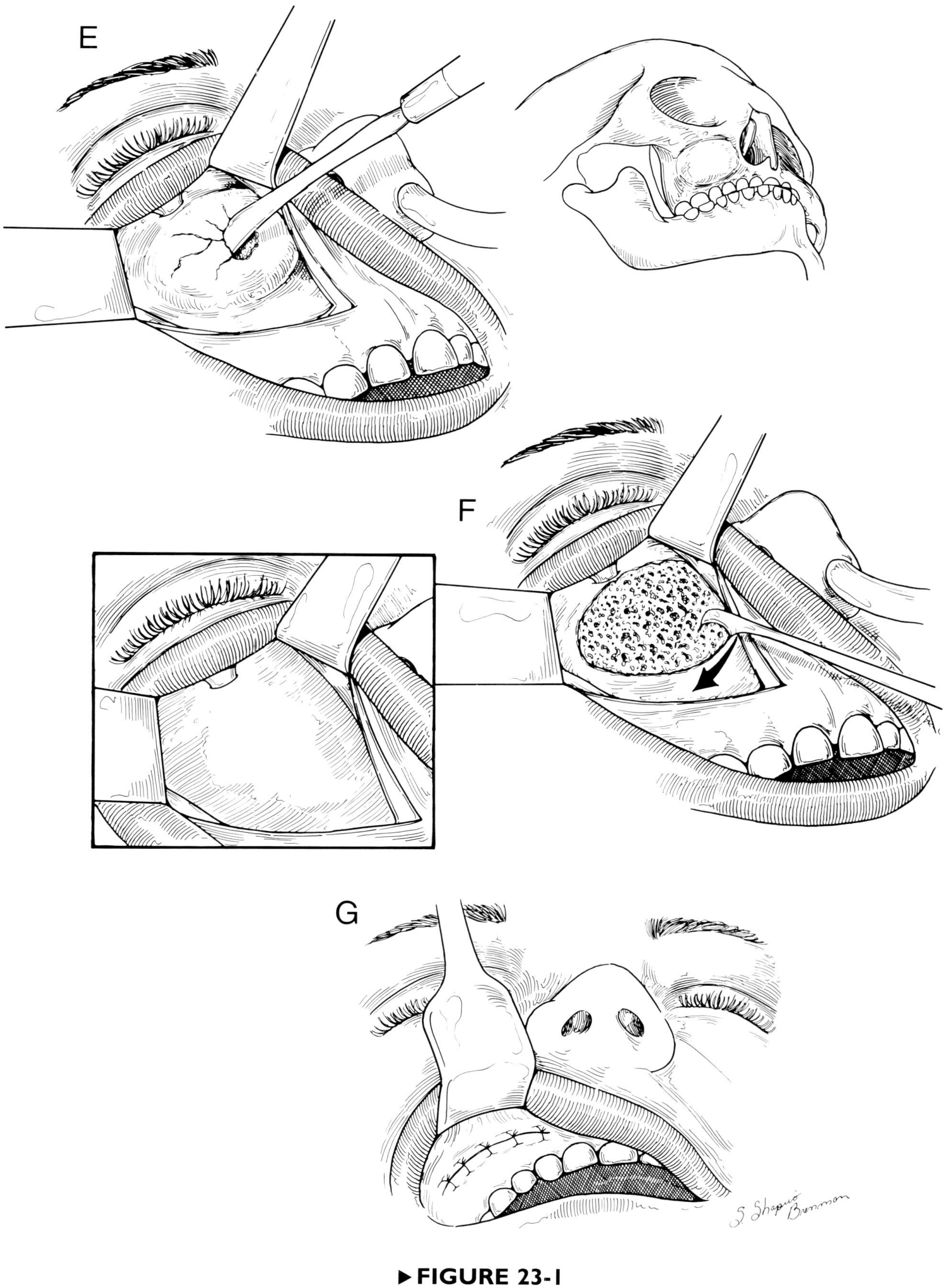


▶ **FIGURE 23-1**

## ▶ 23-2 EXCISION OF BENIGN FIBRO-OSSEOUS TUMORS

Benign fibro-osseous tumors include a variety of slow-growing lesions, such as ossifying fibroma, aneurysmal bone cyst, and osteomas that create a pseudocapsule of compressed normal tissue. These often occur in the area of the ethmoid or maxillary sinus.

### Indications

The presence of the bony lesion is the indication for removal (Fig. 23–2**A**). Complete removal of the lesion is required to prevent recurrence.

### Preoperative Evaluation

Computed tomography (CT) scan of the area is mandatory before surgical treatment.

### Operative Procedure

1. General anesthesia is administered through a nasal endotracheal tube placed in the uninvolved side. One percent lidocaine with 1:100,000 epinephrine is injected in the proposed incision site. For maxillary sinus lesions, a gingivobuccal sulcus incision is utilized (see section 24–3). If the lesion is in the ethmoid area, a Lynch incision that extends along the side of the nose is utilized (see section 25–3).
2. An incision is made with a #15 blade down to the periosteum overlying the involved bone (Fig. 23–2**B**).
3. If there is normal bone overlying the lesion, the bone is cracked and removed using osteotomes and small bone-biting rongeurs (Fig. 23–2**C**).
4. The lesion is removed piecemeal with cup forceps, curettes, and periosteal elevators (such as the Freer). It is important to remove all of the tumor to prevent recurrence (Fig. 23–2**D**).
5. The resulting cavity is loosely packed with antibiotic-impregnated gauze, which can be brought out into the nose through the middle meatus or inferior meatus for ethmoid or maxillary lesions, respectively. The packing is removed in 24 to 36 hours (Fig. 23–2**E**).
6. The incision is closed with interrupted 4-0 chromic sutures in the gingivobuccal sulcus or subcuticular sutures in the ethmoid area (Fig. 23–2**F**).
7. Antibiotics are prescribed for 7 to 10 days to prevent infection in the cavity that is usually connected to a paranasal sinus.

### Complications

1. Recurrence from incomplete excision
2. Ocular injury
3. Infraorbital nerve injury

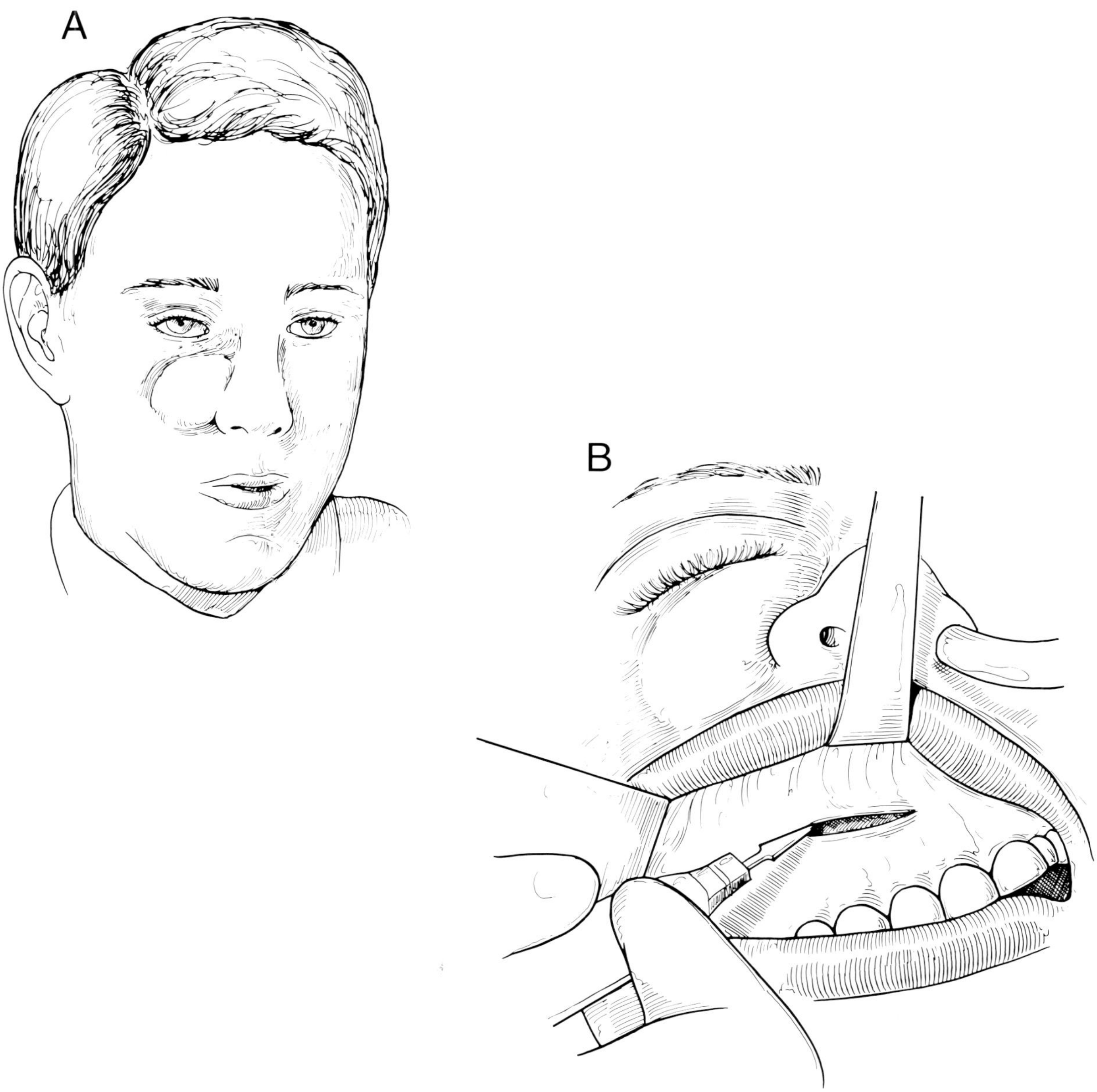


▶ **FIGURE 23-2**

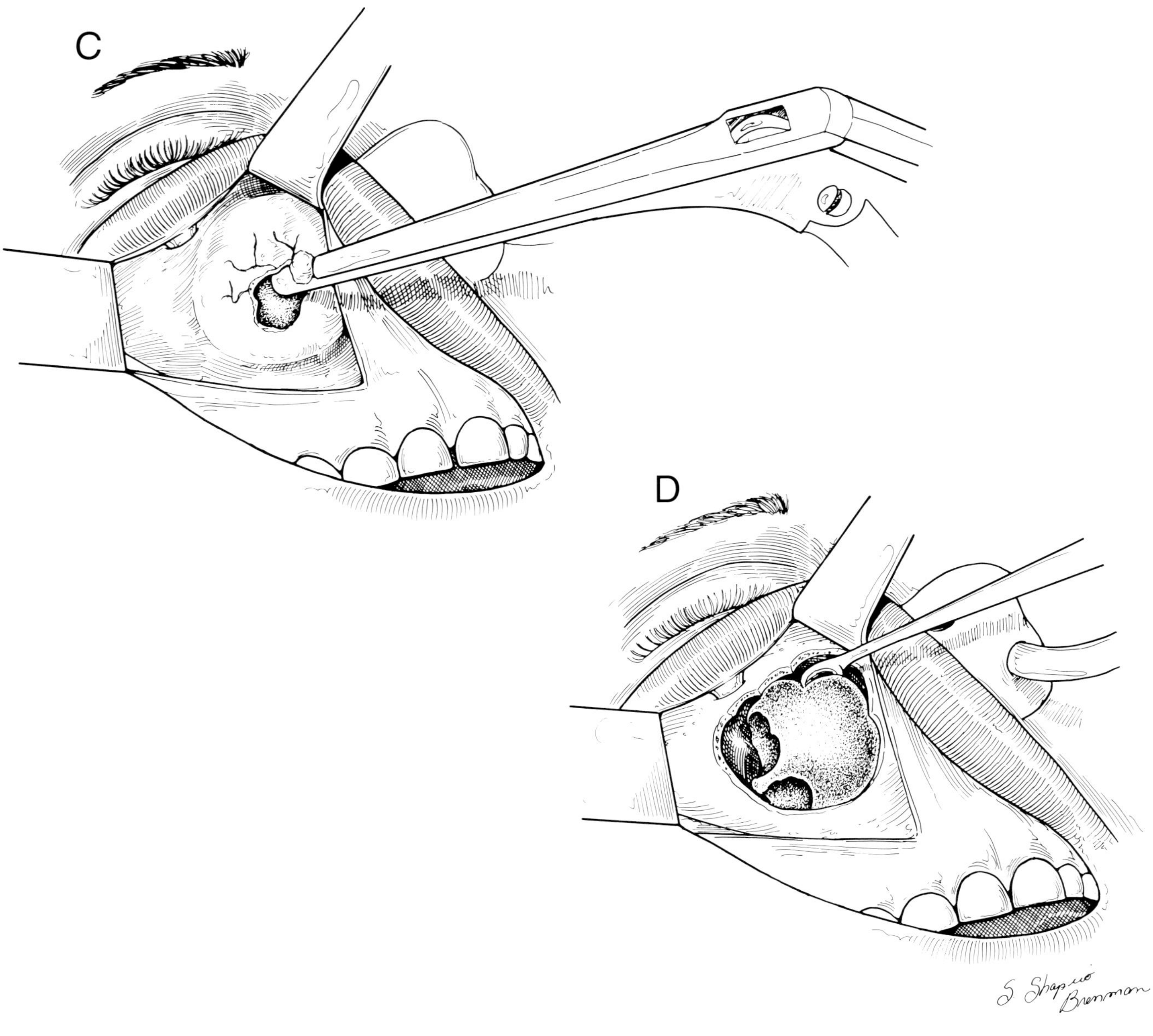


▶ **FIGURE 23-2**

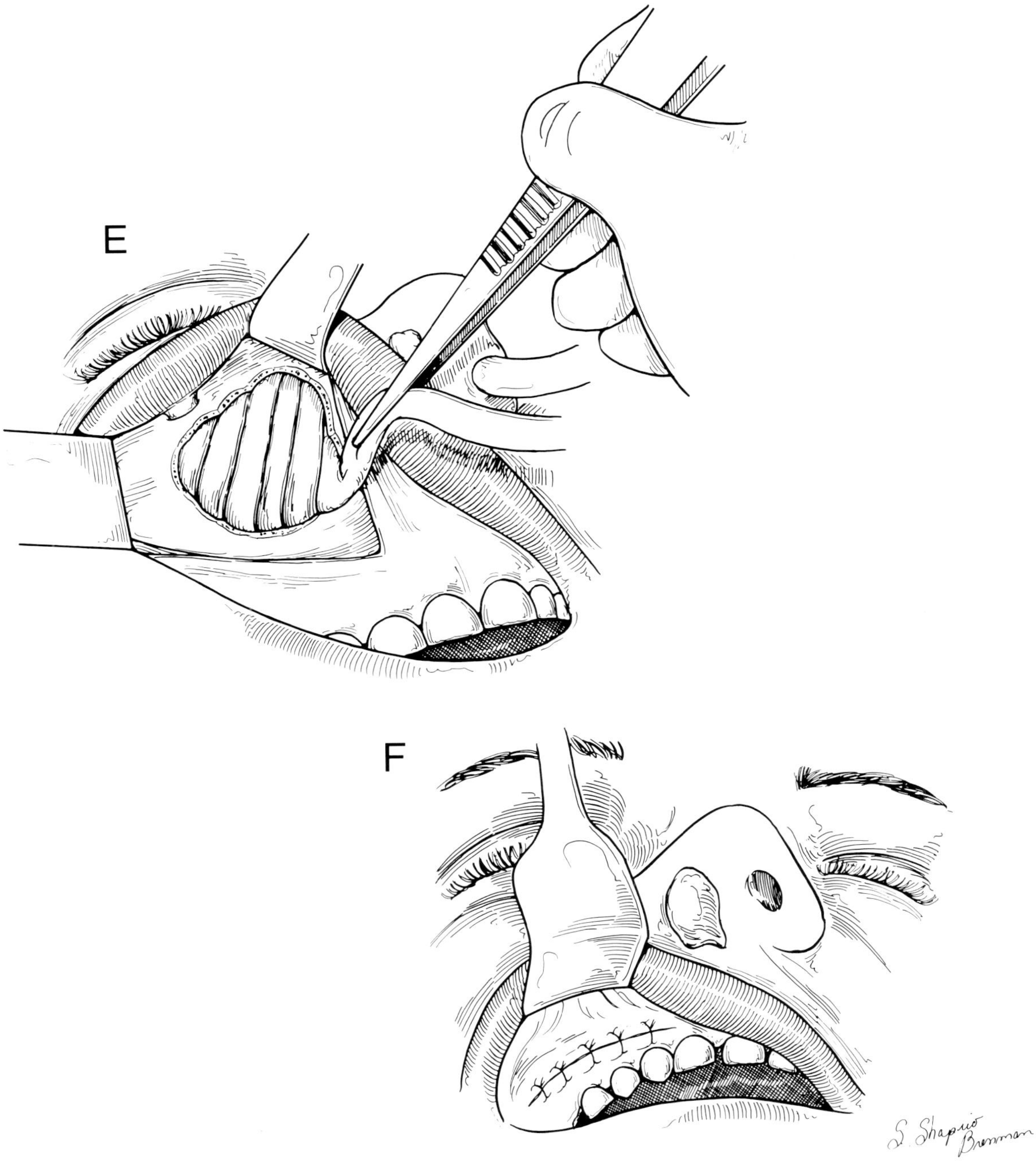


▶ **FIGURE 23-2**

## ▶ 23-3 EXCISION OF PALATAL TUMORS

Palatal tumors may involve the hard and/or soft palate.

### Indications

The presence of a lesion of the hard and/or soft palate is the indication for surgical excision of the lesion.

### Preoperative Evaluation

Computed tomography (CT) scans are not required in the preoperative evaluation of these lesions unless they extend into the nasopharynx or nasal cavity. Attention must be directed to preserving normal palatal function. This is especially important in lesions of the soft palate where velopharyngeal insufficiency can result from excess tissue removal.

### Operative Procedure

1. The patient is placed on a shoulder roll and in a position similar to that used when performing a tonsillectomy. General anesthesia is administered through an oral RAE tube. A Dingman mouth gag is used to provide adequate exposure.
2. One percent lidocaine with 1:100,000 epinephrine is injected submucosally around the lesion (Fig. 23–3**A**).
3. An elliptical incision is utilized to encompass the lesion (Fig. 23–3**B**).
4. Sharp dissection with a knife or scissors is performed to excise the lesion.
5. If a large defect is created in the soft palate, and there is the possibility of postoperative velopharyngeal insufficiency, a rotation flap is created and moved in from the adjacent hard palate (Fig. 23–3**C, D**). Care is taken not to cut or compromise the blood supply to the palate via the laterally placed palatal vessels.
6. The flap is rotated into the defect and sutured into place with interrupted 4-0 chromic sutures (Fig. 23–3**E**).
7. The defect in the mucosa overlying the hard palate is allowed to heal by secondary intention.
8. Superficial lesions of the mucosa of the hard palate are excised with an elliptical incision (Fig. 23–3**F**) and the mucosal defect is left to heal by secondary intention (Fig. 23–3**G**).
9. If the lesion involves the underlying bone of the soft palate, the bone is removed with rongeurs or osteotomes (Fig. 23–3**H**).
10. Lateral relaxing incisions can be created to permit undermining and medial movement of the mucosa to allow closure of the incision and to prevent an oronasal fistula (Fig. 23–3**I**). (If necessary, a rotation flap from an adjacent portion of the hard palate can be created, as described above.) Small defects in the mucosa overlying intact portions of the bony maxilla are allowed to heal by secondary intention.

### Complications

1. Velopharyngeal insufficiency
2. Oronasal fistula

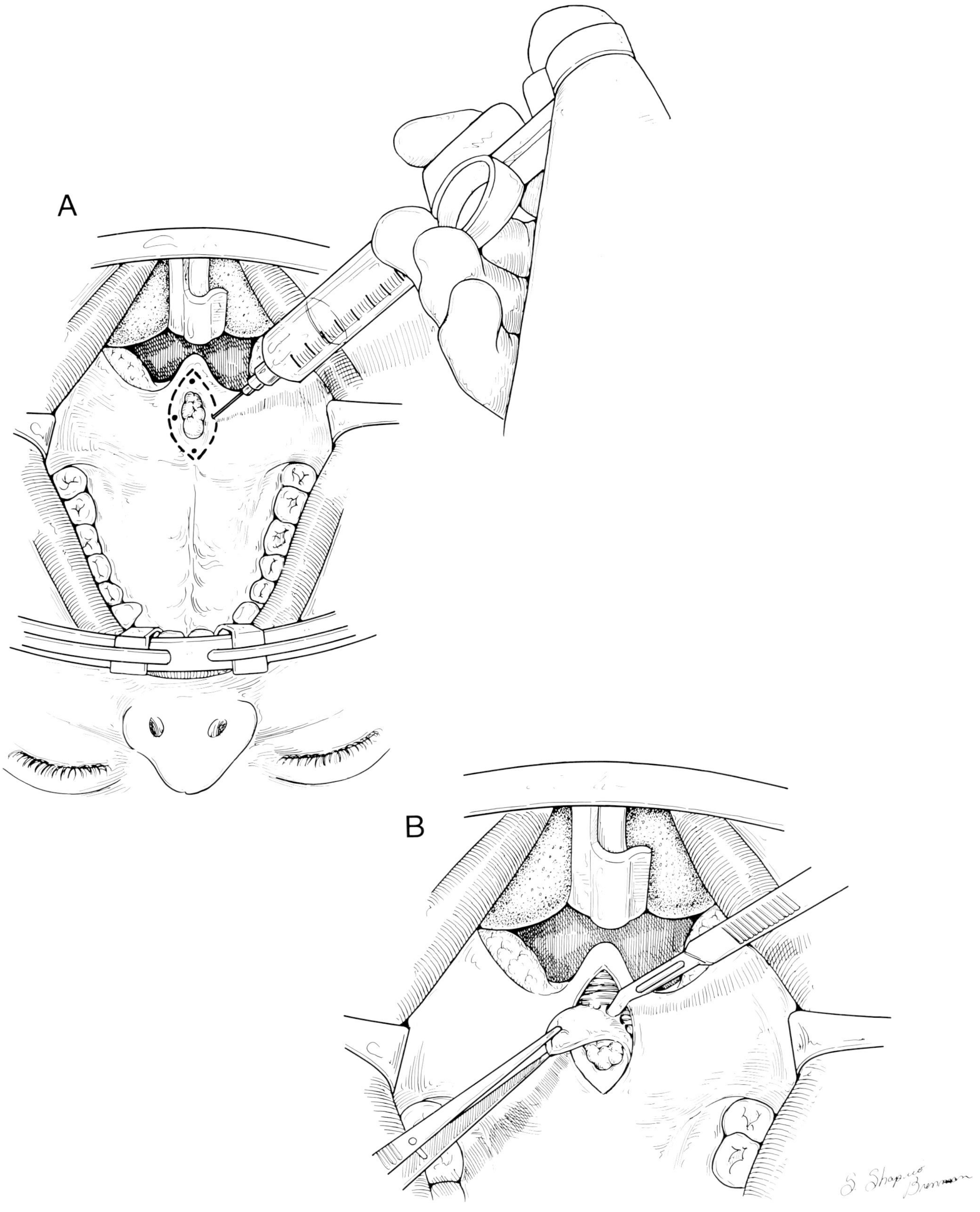


▶ **FIGURE 23-3**

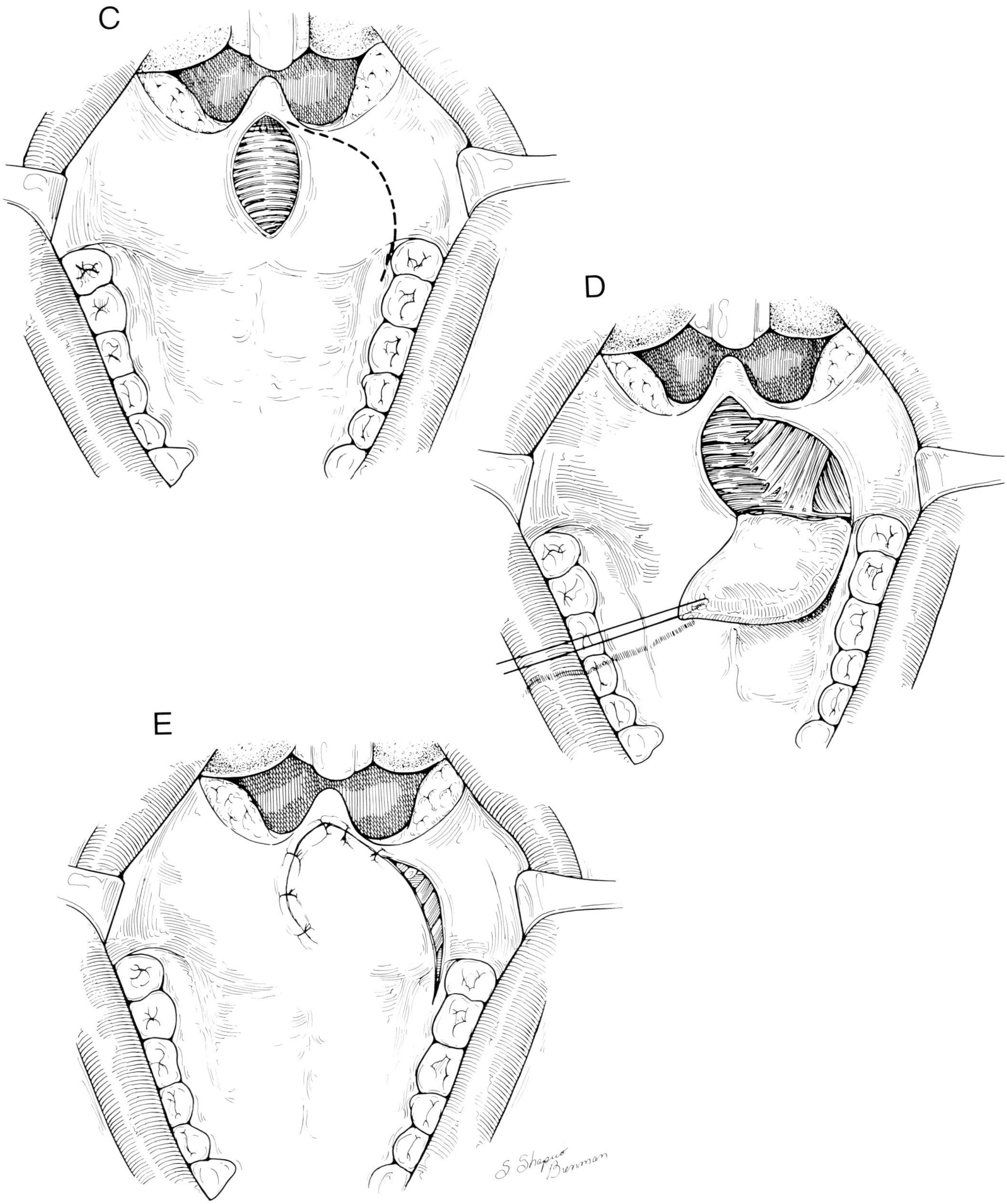


▶ **FIGURE 23-3**

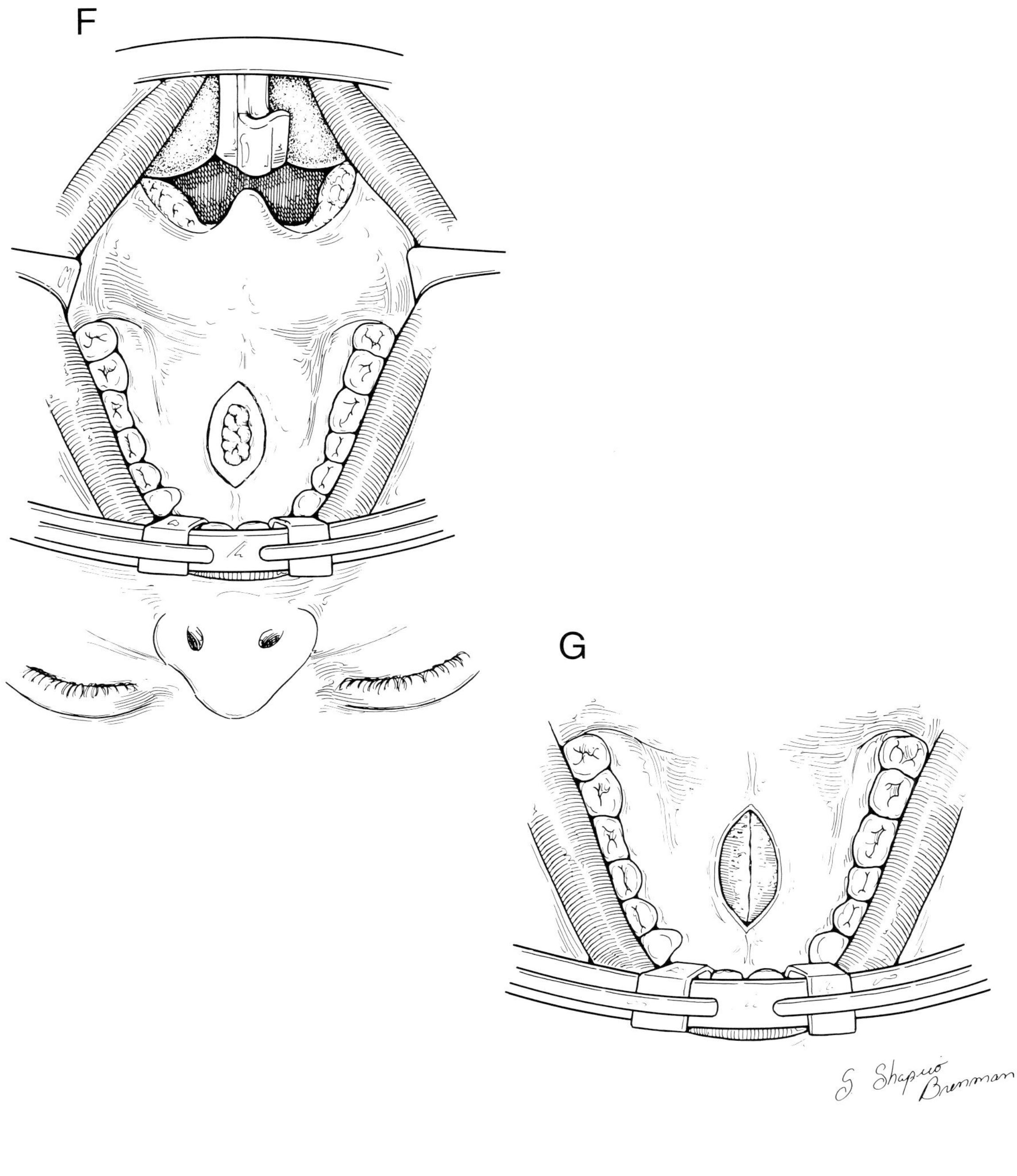


▸ **FIGURE 23-3**

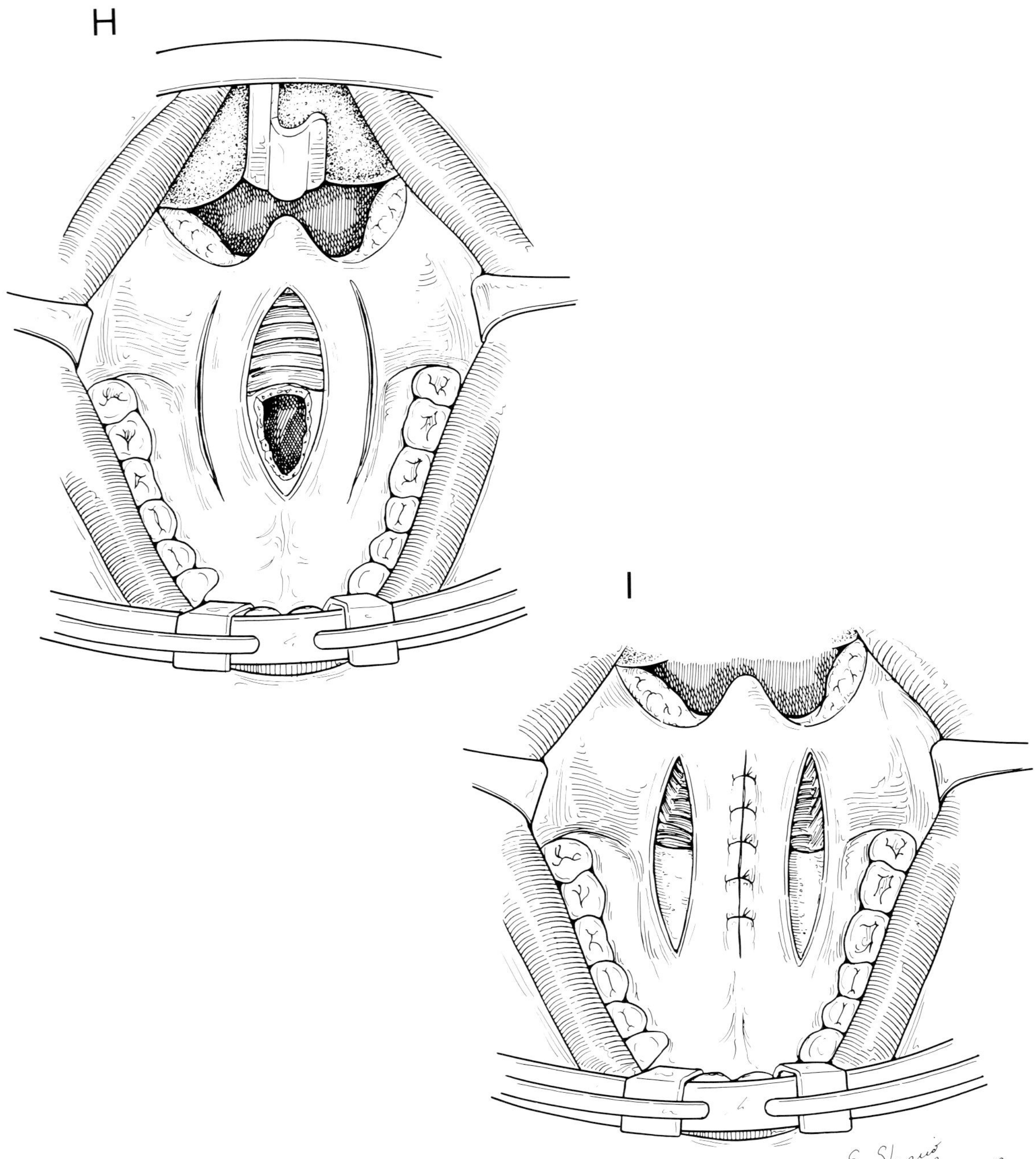


▶ **FIGURE 23-3**

PART IV

# Sinus Surgery

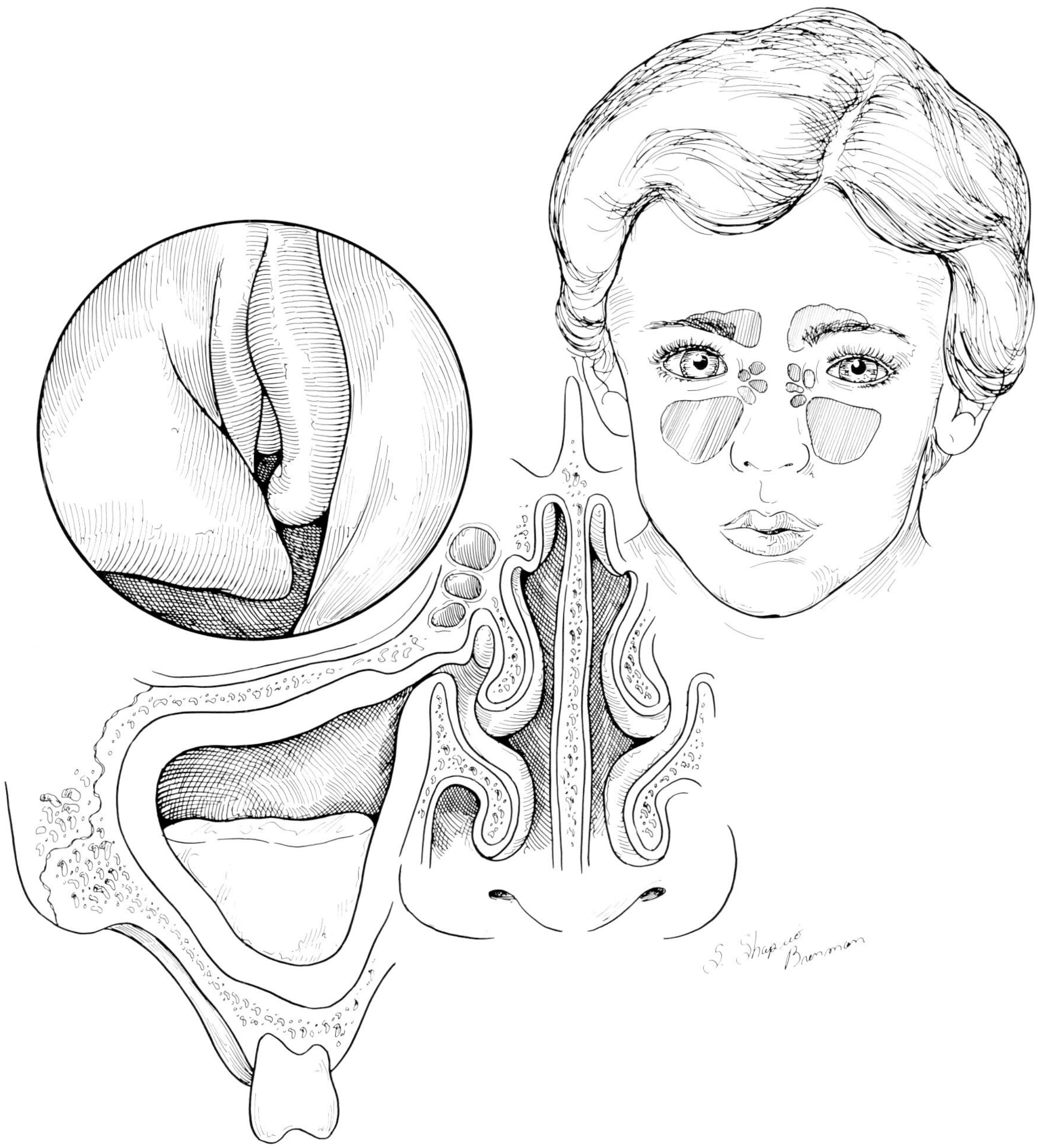

# 24 ▸ Maxillary Sinus

Maxillary sinusitis commonly occurs with upper respiratory infections. These infections usually clear with antibiotic therapy and rarely require surgical intervention.

## ▸ 24 - 1 ANTRAL LAVAGE

### Indications

Maxillary sinus lavage is indicated in the management of both acute and chronic maxillary sinusitis to aspirate secretions to determine the causative organisms of the sinusitis. The secondary benefit of the procedure is to allow for irrigation of the sinus to hasten resolution of the sinusitis.

### Preoperative Evaluation

Preoperative evaluation includes a complete examination of the nose, pharynx, and paranasal sinus area. While plain sinus radiographs may be helpful in directing attention to specific sinuses, a computed tomography (CT) scan gives much better detail of the bony and mucosal structure.

### Operative Technique

1. General anesthesia via endotracheal tube is utilized in most cases.
2. The nasal cavity is examined using the nasal speculum and secretions are removed (Fig. 24–1A). Four percent cocaine (alternately, any combination of a topical vasoconstrictor and local anesthetic may be used) on a cotton pledget is placed in the inferior meatus to aid in hemostasis and to shrink the nasal mucosa for better visibility (Fig. 24–1B).
3. The curved nasal antral cannula is placed under direct vision in the inferior meatus making sure that its point is posterior to the anterior maxillary face and that it points slightly upward toward the superior lateral aspect of the sinus (Fig. 24–1C). Constant pressure is applied until the trocar enters the maxillary sinus. This is usually signaled by an audible crack and sudden ease of penetration.
4. The obturator portion of the cannula is withdrawn and an irrigating extension attached.
5. Aspiration of the sinus is performed. Placement of the cannula in the sinus cavity is confirmed by aspiration of air or secretions (Fig. 24–1D). If no air or secretions are aspirated, the cannula is gently manipulated until this occurs.
6. Once appropriate position in the sinus is confirmed, secretions are aspirated and sent for culture and sensitivity. Saline is then used to irrigate the maxillary sinus (Fig. 24–1E). Care is taken to make sure that no air is pushed into the soft tissues of the face.
7. Saline from the irrigation of the sinus will appear at the anterior nasal cavity or in the oropharynx.

**8.** The cannula is withdrawn and the nasal cavity is inspected. If there is significant bleeding, a cotton pledget soaked in cocaine can be placed once again in the inferior meatus. If a specific bleeding point can be identified, electrocautery can be utilized to control the bleeding.

## Complications

1. Epistaxis
2. Subcutaneous emphysema
3. Orbital hemorrhage

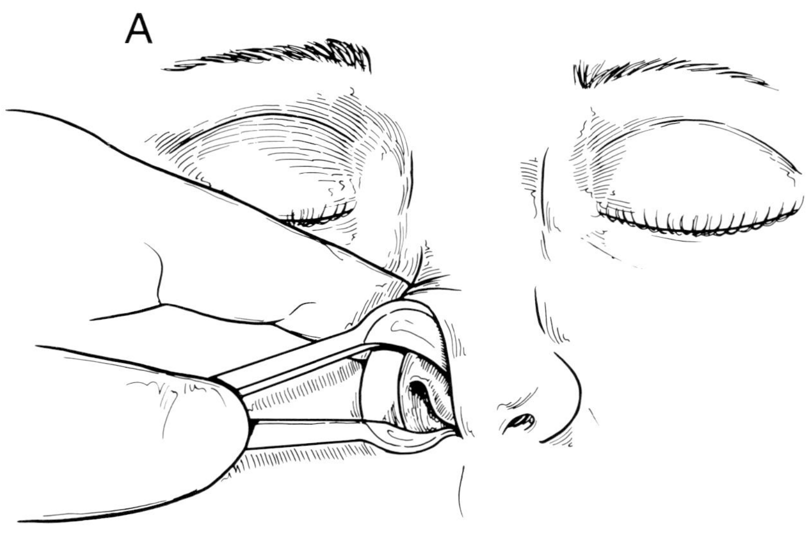


▶ **FIGURE 24-1**

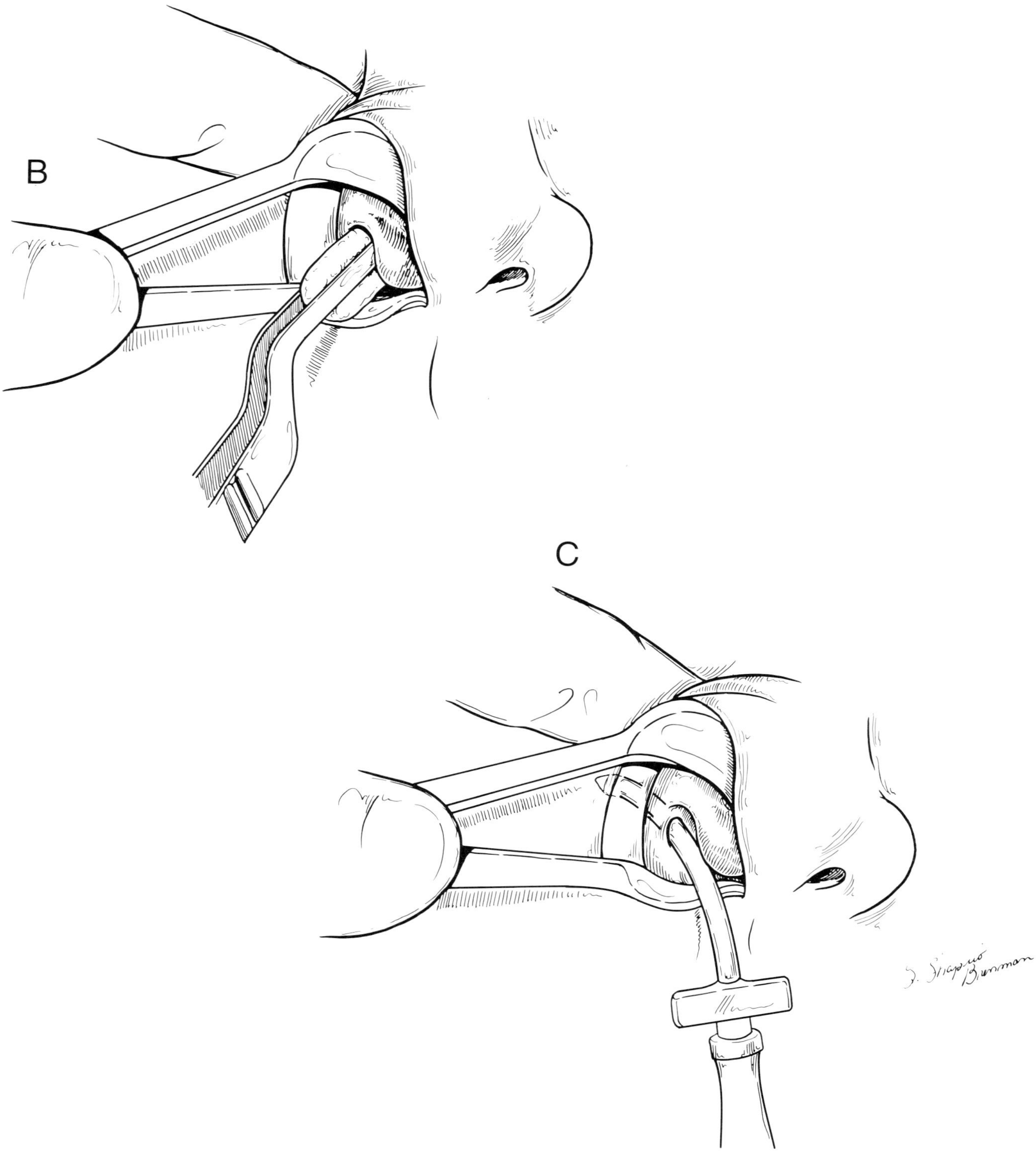


▶ **FIGURE 24-1**

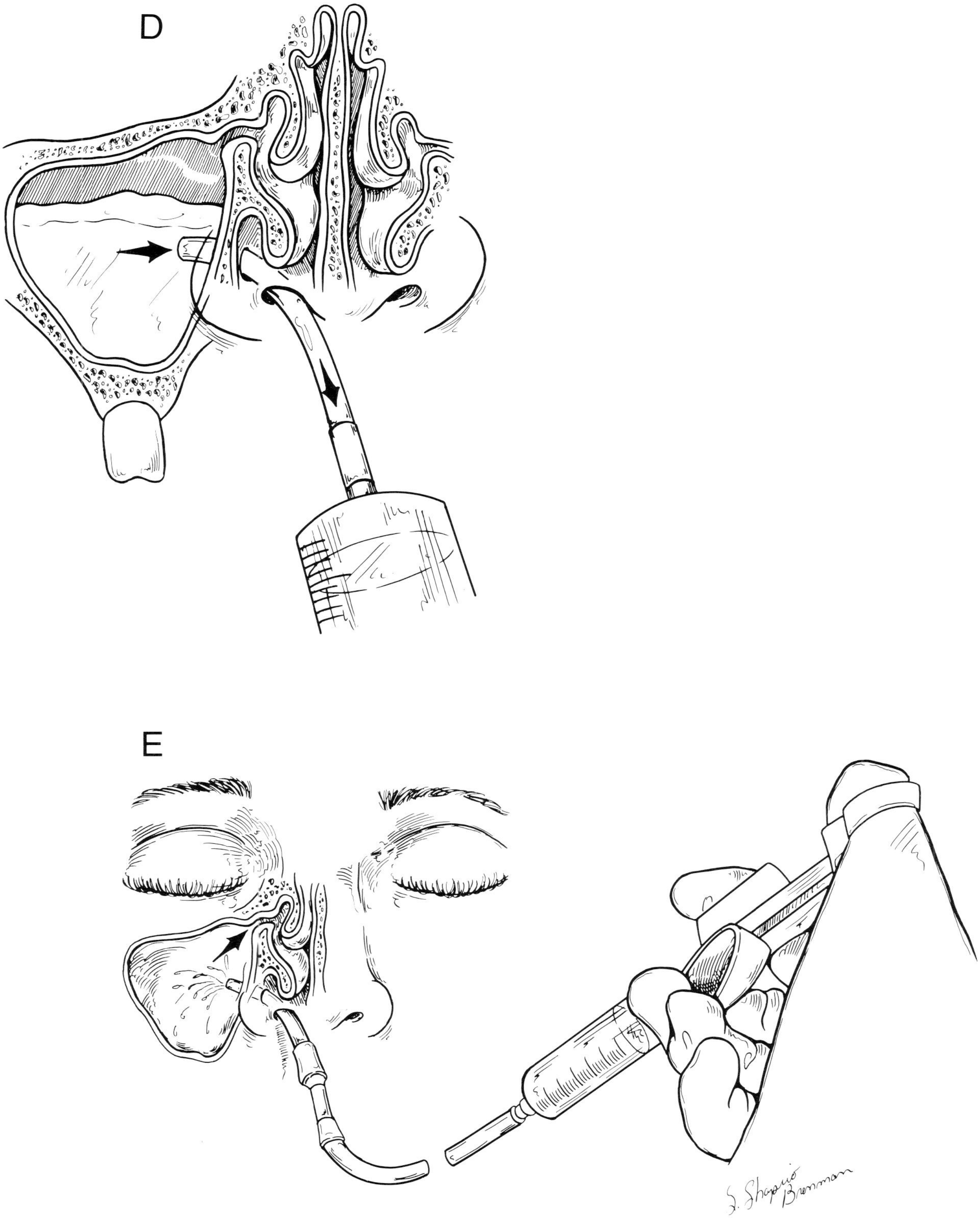


▶ **FIGURE 24-1**

## ▶ 24-2 INTRANASAL ANTROSTOMY

Intranasal antrostomy is a procedure to create a communication between the nose and maxillary sinus through the inferior meatus. The procedure allows for the creation of a long-term drainage site while also allowing for telescopic access to the maxillary sinus. In this way, thickened mucosa can be removed and suspicious tissue biopsied.

### Indications

The creation of an intranasal antrostomy is indicated in the treatment of chronic sinus disease that does not respond to conventional antibiotic treatment.

### Preoperative Evaluation

A complete nasal examination and sinus computed tomography (CT) scans are mandatory before maxillary sinus surgery.

### Operative Technique

1. General anesthesia is administered through an oral RAE endotracheal tube is the preferred method.
2. The nasal cavity is inspected using a nasal speculum and excess secretions are removed with a suction. A cotton pledget soaked in 4% cocaine is placed in the inferior meatus to aid in hemostasis and to shrink the nasal mucosa for better visualization (alternately, any combination of a topical vasoconstrictor and local anesthetic may be used) (Fig. 24–2**A**). One percent lidocaine with 1:100,000 epinephrine is injected into the lateral wall of the inferior meatus and the anterior and lateral aspects of the inferior turbinate to further aid in the process.
3. A Freer elevator is placed in the inferior meatus and the inferior turbinate is fractured upward and medially to further open the entrance into the inferior meatus (Fig. 24–2**B**).
4. A curved mosquito clamp is then used to punch a small hole in the medial wall of the maxillary sinus (Fig. 24–2**C**). Care is taken to avoid the posterior aspects of the medial maxillary wall, which contain the pterygomaxillary vessels, and to avoid the nasal lacrimal duct, which is anterior and superior in the inferior meatus (Fig. 24–2**D**).
5. The antrostomy is enlarged using rongeurs and cup forceps until an adequate lumen has been created (Fig. 24–2**E**). Redundant mucosa and polypoid tissue are gently removed from the maxillary sinus through this site (Fig. 24–2**F**).
6. A telescope can be used to inspect the maxillary sinus and to aid in biopsy of suspicious tissue (Fig. 24–2**G**). Irrigation of the sinus can be performed if indicated.
7. Excess bleeding is controlled with electrocautery or with a small piece of Gelfoam packing. It is usually not necessary to pack the nose with any more-substantial packing.
8. The inferior turbinate is left in its out-fractured position. It will assume its more normal position over time.
9. A broad-spectrum antibiotic is administered for 7 to 10 days.

## Complications

1. Nasloacrimal duct injury
2. Bleeding from sphenopalatine artery

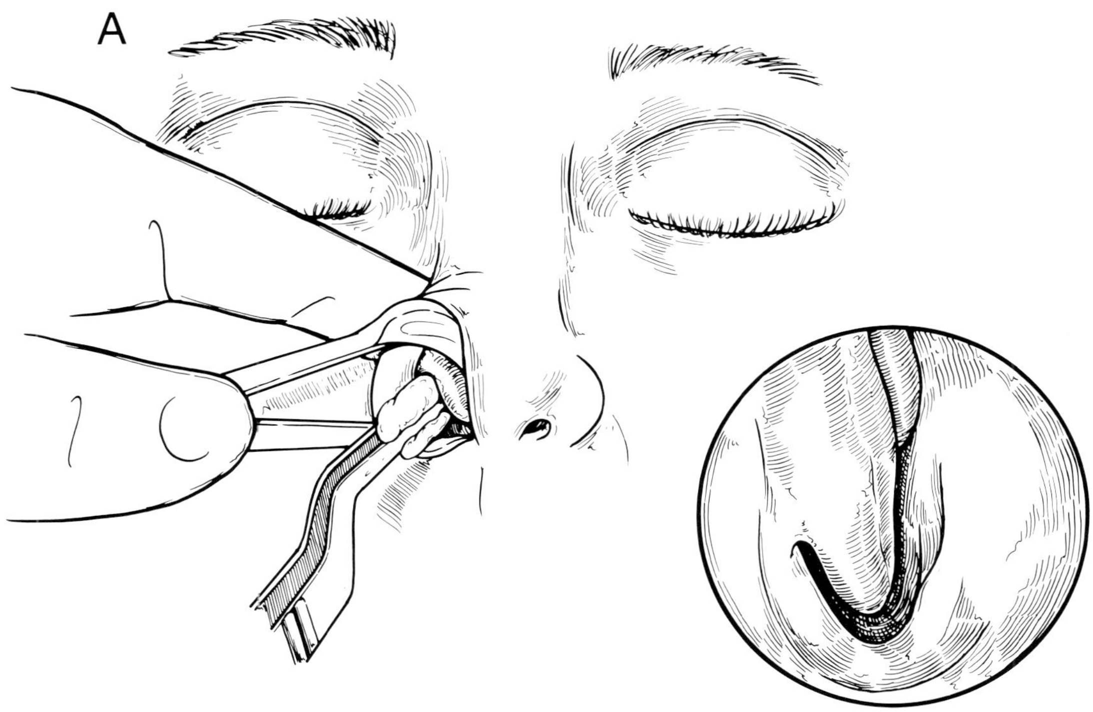


▶ **FIGURE 24-2**

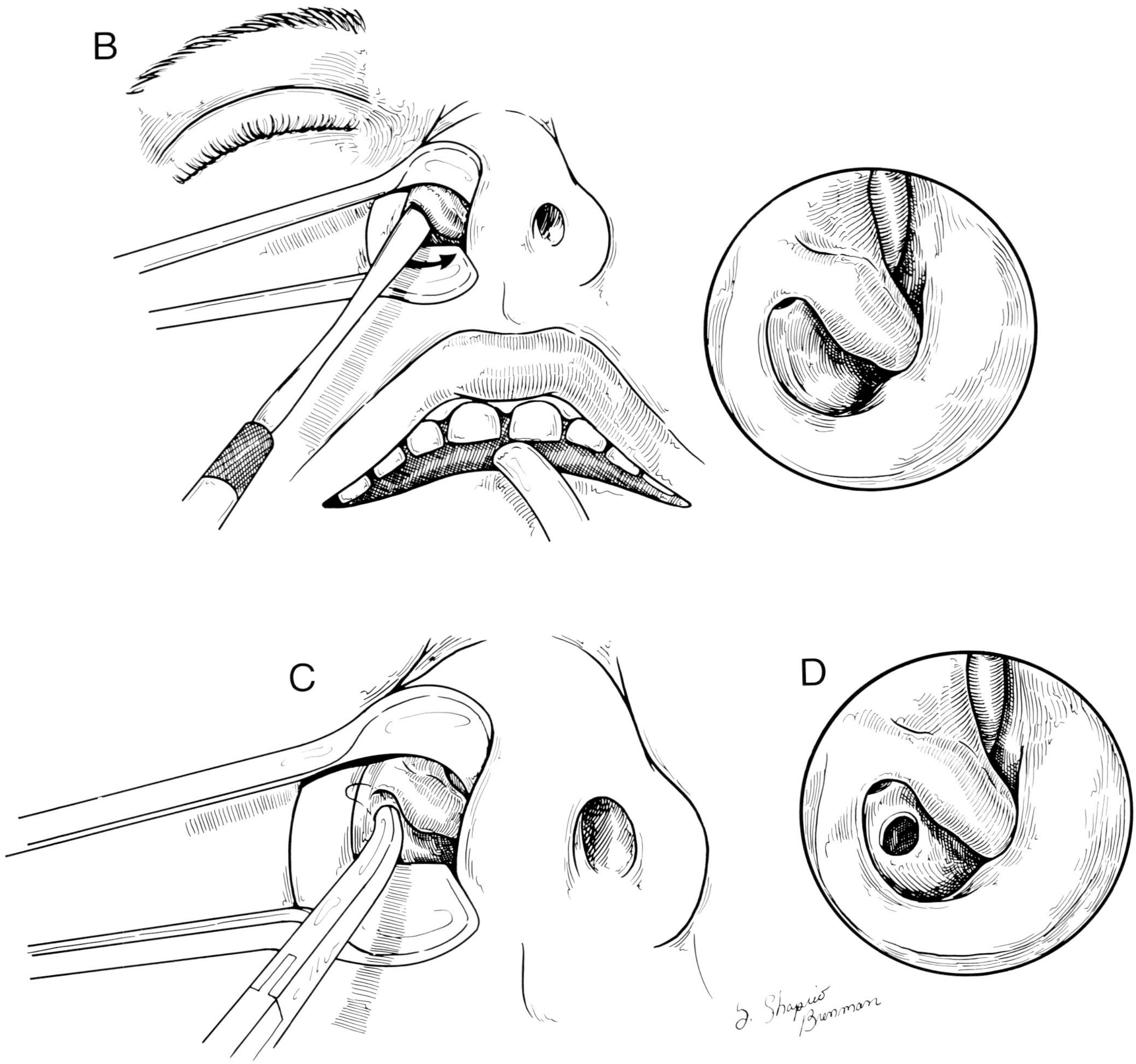


▶ **FIGURE 24-2**

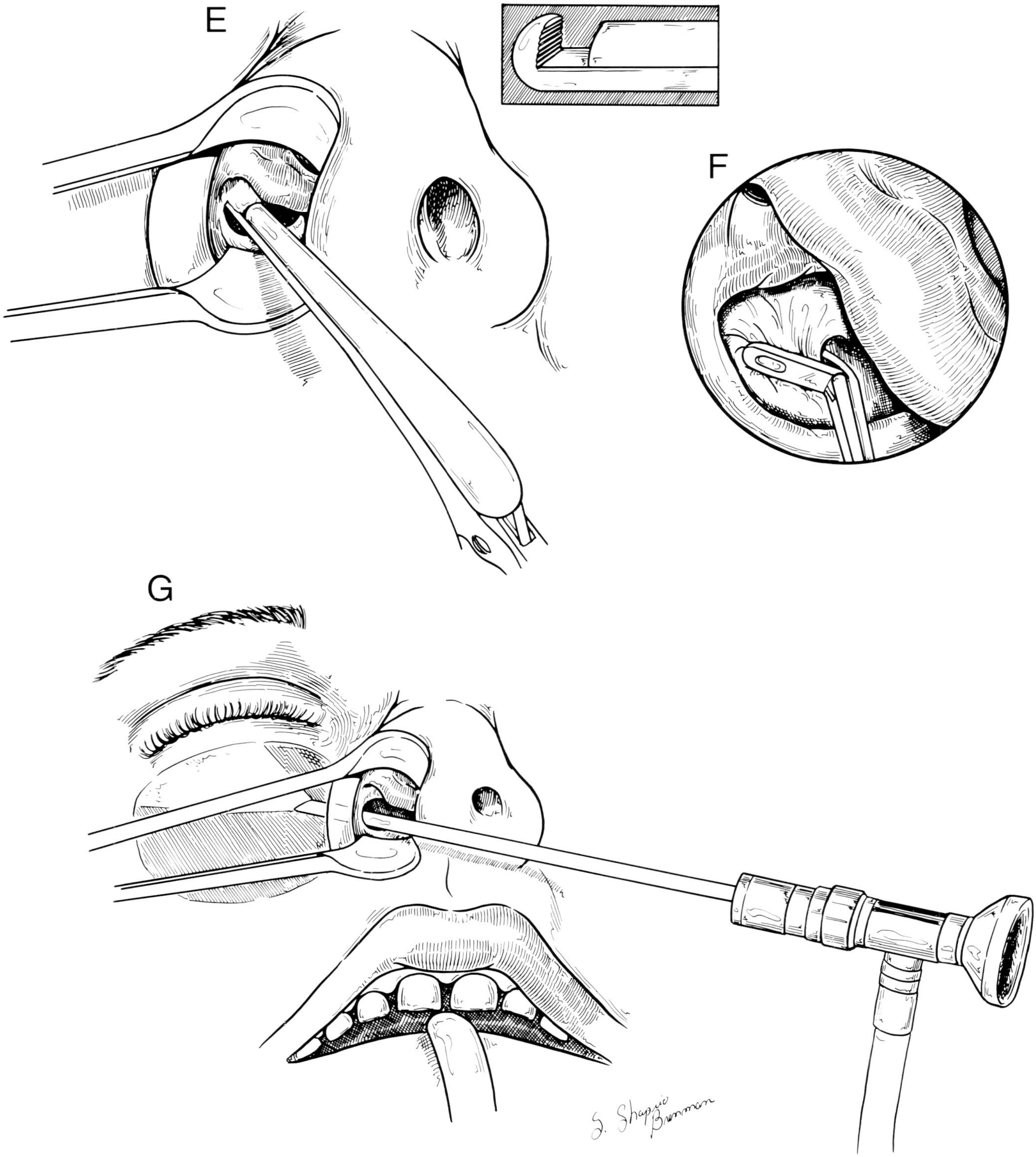


▶ **FIGURE 24-2**

## ▶ 24-3 CALDWELL-LUC

The Caldwell-Luc procedure is a useful operation in the treatment of conditions involving and surrounding the maxillary sinus. The operation, which creates an anterior opening into the maxillary sinus, allows inspection of the maxillary sinus cavity, removal of pathologically hypertrophied mucosa, and creation of a nasal antral window. In addition, the approach permits inspection of the orbital floor in treatment of orbital floor and maxillary fractures. Access to the pterygopalatine space and the ethmoid sinuses can be obtained through the maxillary sinus utilizing the Caldwell-Luc operation.

### Indications

Chronic maxillary sinusitis, unresponsive to medical management, orbital floor fractures, malar fractures, severe epistaxis requiring ligation of the internal maxillary artery, and neoplasms of the maxillary sinus are all indications for the Caldwell-Luc approach.

### Preoperative Evaluation

A complete nasal examination and sinus computed tomography (CT) scans are mandatory before maxillary sinus surgery.

### Operative Technique

1. General anesthesia is administered through a nasal RAE tube inserted in the side of the nose opposite to the sinus requiring operation. Alternatively, an oral RAE endotracheal tube may be used, taped in the midline or to the uninvolved side.
2. A cotton pledget soaked with 4% cocaine is placed in the inferior meatus to aid in hemostasis and to permit better visualization when the nasal antral window is created (alternately, any combination of a topical vasoconstrictor and local anesthetic may be used). One percent lidocaine with 1:100,000 epinephrine is injected in the gingival buccal sulcus (Fig. 24–3**A**).
3. A horizontal incision is made in the mucosa approximately 5 to 8 mm superior to the gumline. This allows for creation of an inferior flap of tissue so that the incision can be closed at the end of the procedure. The incision is extended from the area of the pyriform aperture to the first premolar and taken down to the face of the anterior maxillary wall (Fig. 24–3**B**).
4. The periosteum is incised with a blade or electrocautery. The soft tissues of the mucosa and periosteum are elevated superiorly with a periosteal elevator until the infraorbital nerve is identified (Fig. 24–3**C**).
5. A 4-mm osteotome is used to punch a square hole in the face of the maxillary sinus, taking care to avoid the infraorbital nerve superiorly and the tooth roots inferiorly (Fig. 24–3**D**).
6. The fragment of bone is elevated out with the osteotome or a small mosquito clamp. The mucosa of the maxillary sinus is identified and incised if not already entered. Secretions in the maxillary sinus can be cultured at this time.
7. The opening into the maxillary sinus is enlarged using Kerrison rongeurs, again making sure not to injure the infraorbital nerve or the developing tooth buds (Fig. 24–3**E**). Polypoid and hypertrophied tissue is removed from the sinus cavity utilizing a Freer elevator and cup forceps (Fig. 24–3**F**).

**8.** Care is taken to leave uninvolved mucosa intact. The orbital floor and entrance to the ethmoid sinuses can now be inspected by direct vision or by utilizing a telescope.

**9.** A nasal antral window is usually created after a Caldwell-Luc operation to allow for long-term drainage. A curved mosquito clamp is placed in the inferior meatus of the nose (Fig. 24–3**G**) and gently pushed laterally while the operating surgeon has the medial wall of the maxillary sinus under direct vision (Fig. 24–3**H**).

**10.** The clamp is spread and Kerrison rongeurs are used to further enlarge the window from the maxillary sinus side (Fig. 24–3**I**).

**11.** Packing the maxillary sinus is usually not necessary unless there is excessive bleeding or it is necessary to pack up the orbital floor in the treatment of a maxillary fracture. Antibiotic-impregnated gauze, if necessary, is introduced into the maxillary sinus through the nasal-antral window. The gauze is pulled back and forth to "file" down any rough edges on the nasal-antral window to ensure smooth postoperative removal of the packing (Fig. 24–3**J**). The packing is layered into the sinus (Fig. 24–3**K**) and the leading end is left in the anterior nasal cavity.

**12.** The gingival-buccal incision is closed loosely with interrupted 4-0 chromic sutures (Fig. 24–3**L**). This allows for drainage of blood and secretions should they accumulate in the maxillary sinus. The packing is removed in 24 to 36 hours.

**13.** A broad-spectrum antibiotic is administered for 7 to 10 days.

## Complications

1. Infraorbital nerve damage
2. Nasolacrimal duct damage
3. Oroantral fistula
4. Tooth root trauma

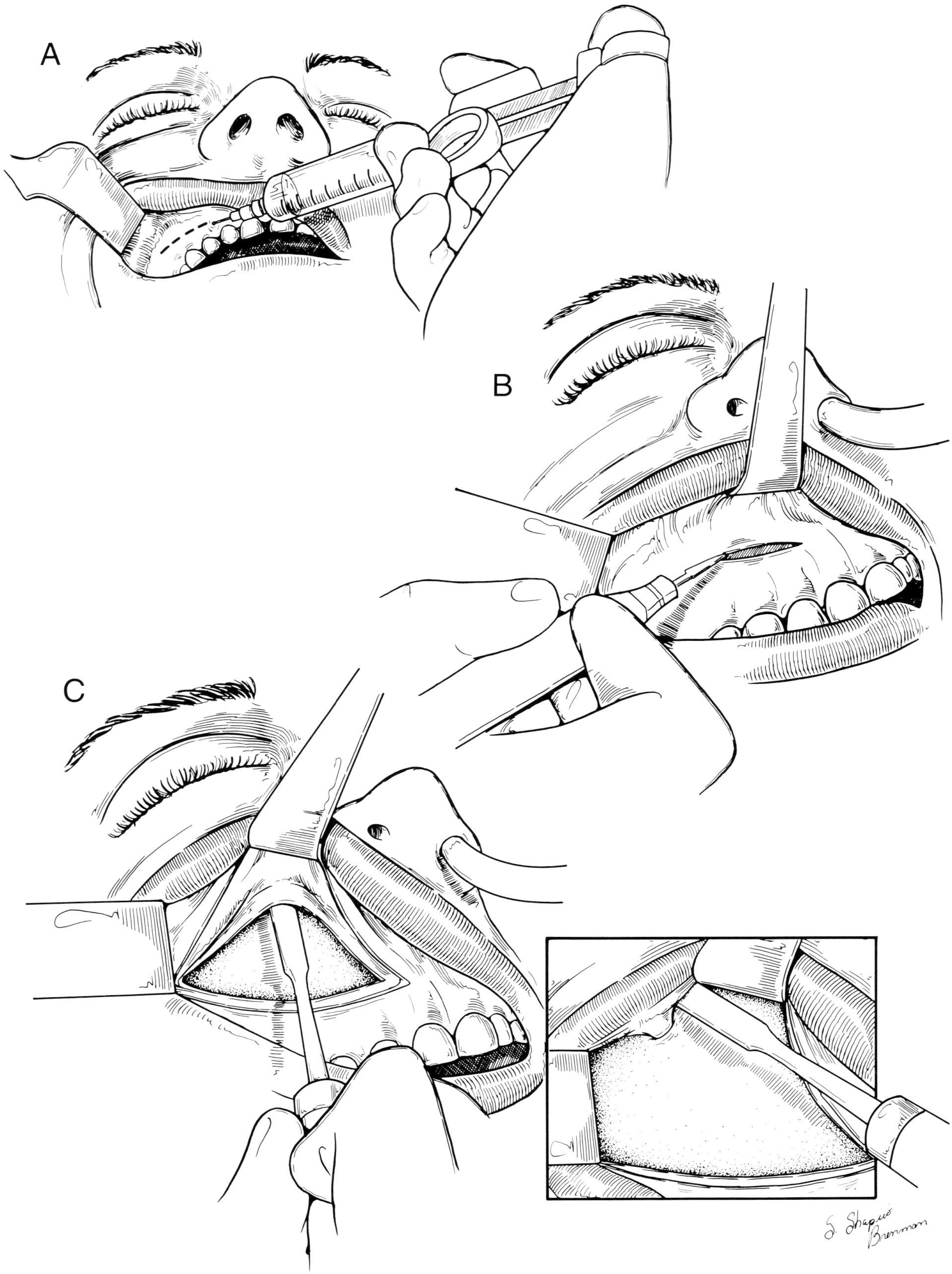


▶ **FIGURE 24-3**

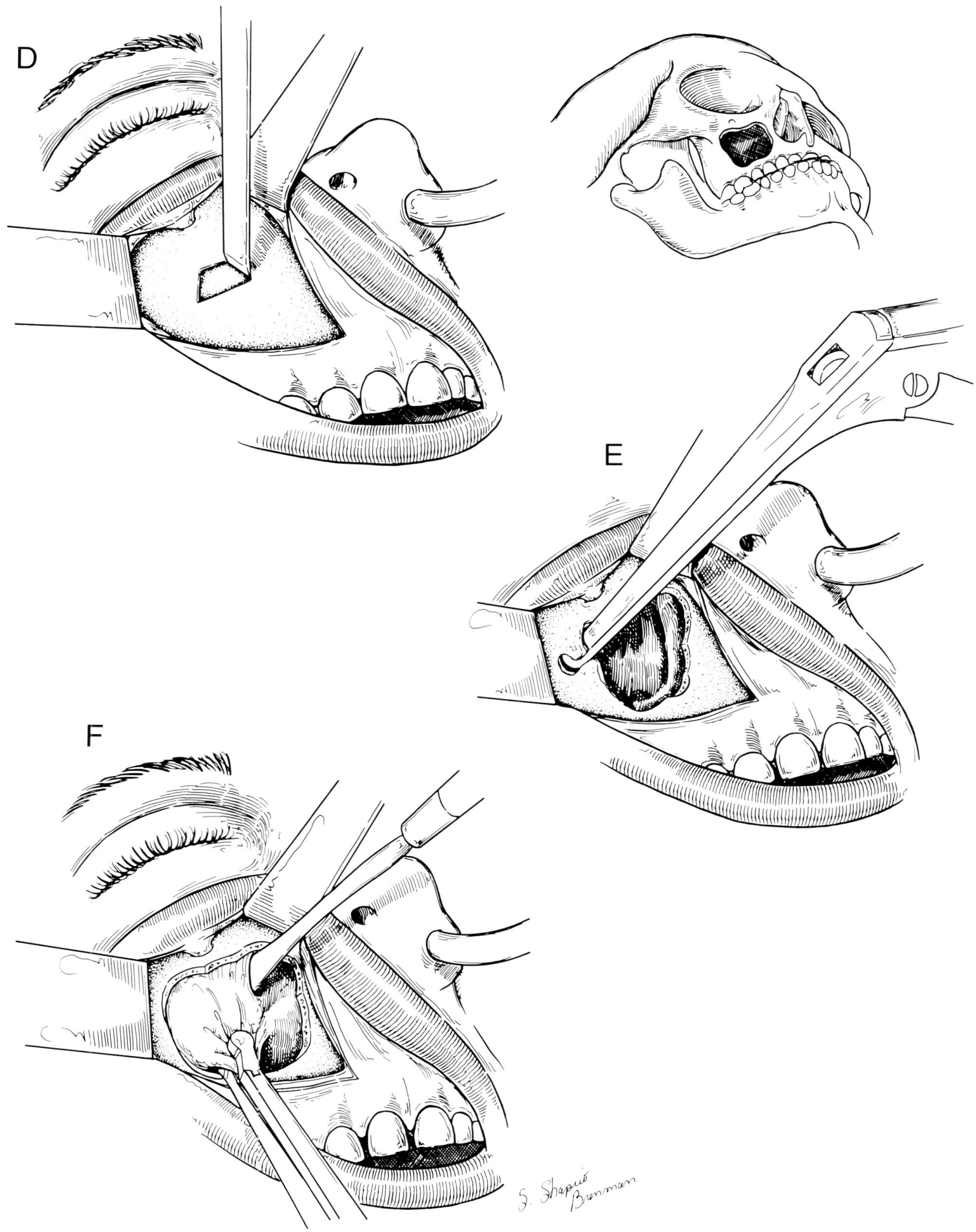


▶ **FIGURE 24-3**

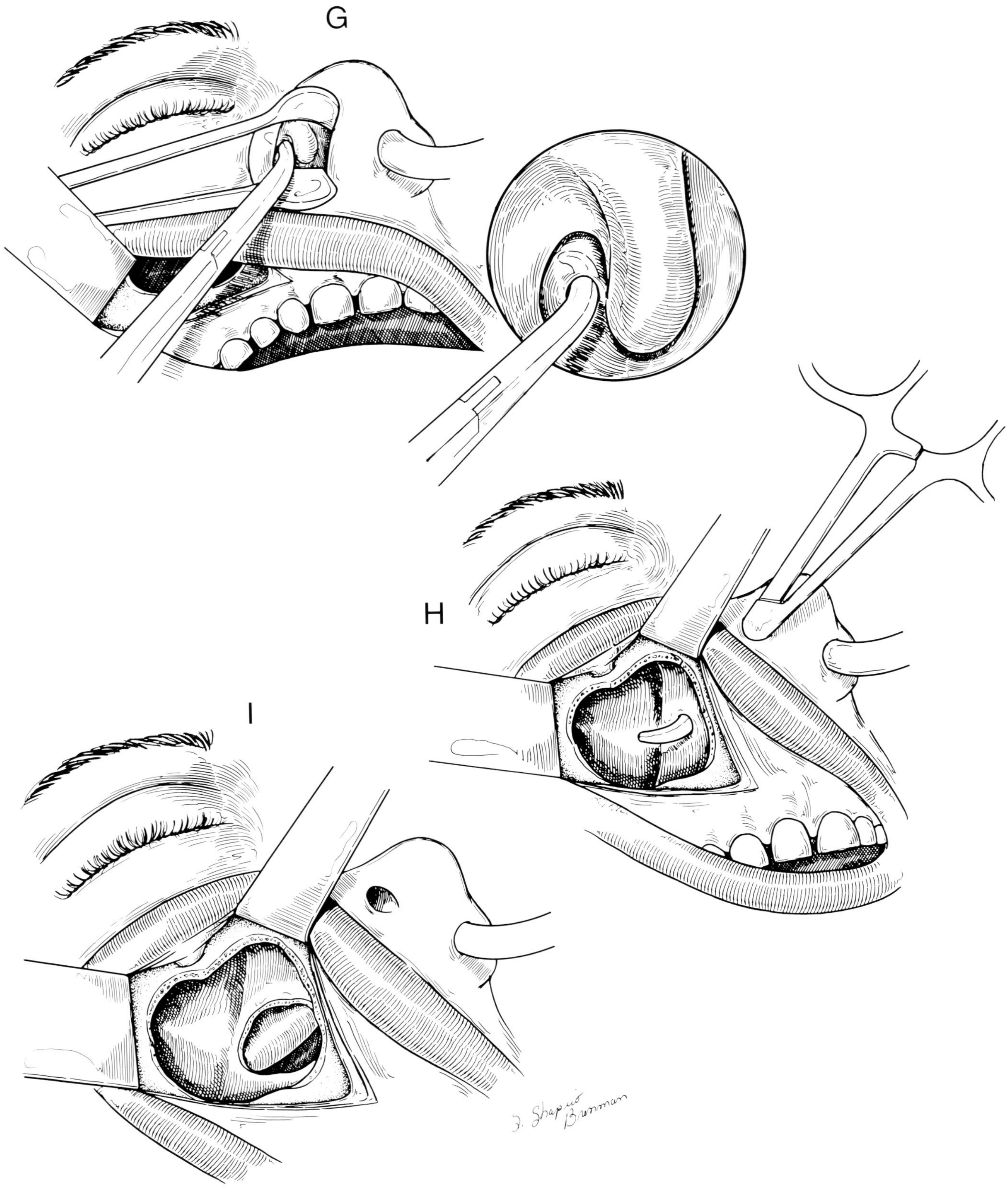


▶**FIGURE 24-3**

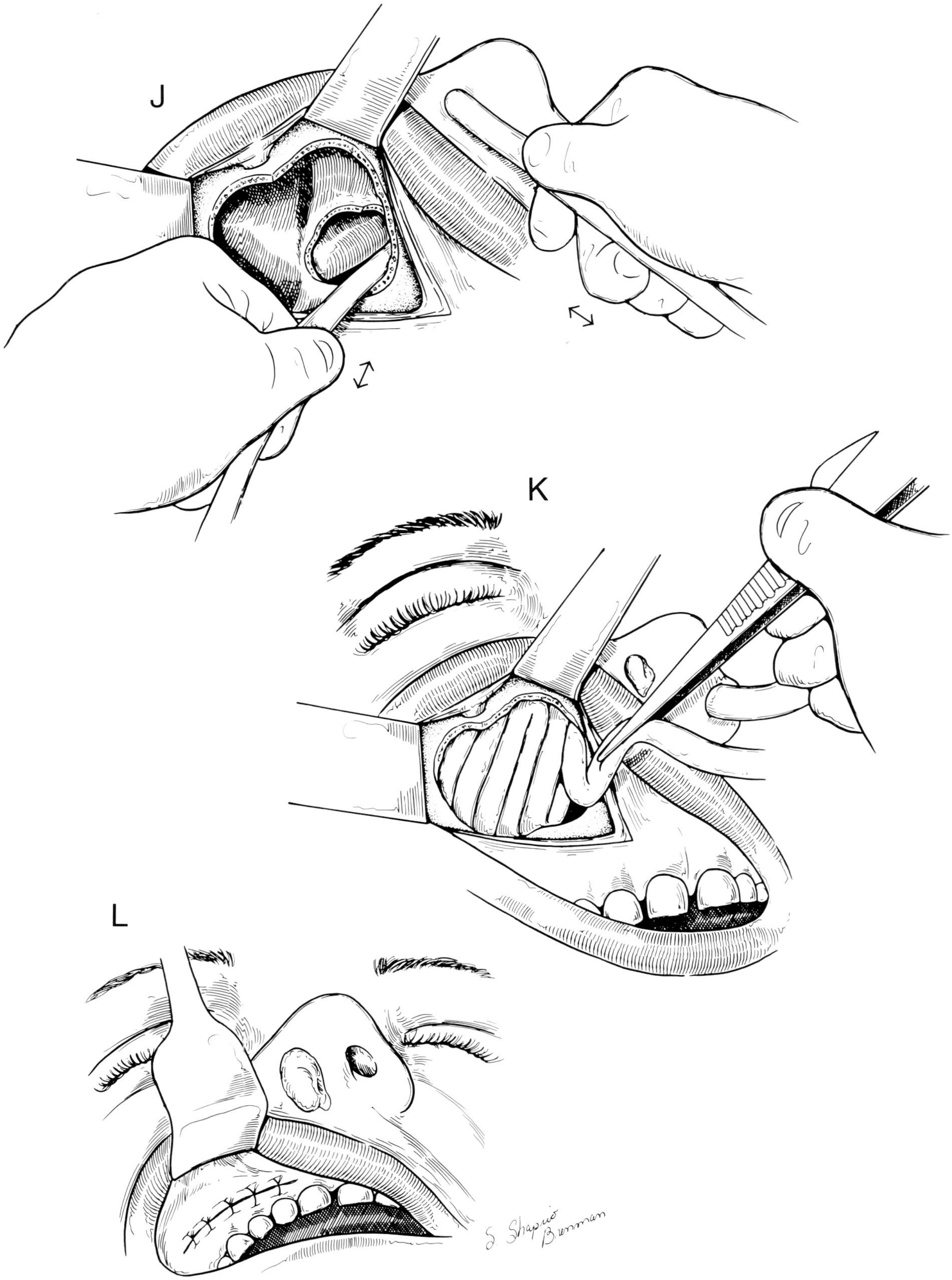


▶ **FIGURE 24-3**

# 25 ▶ Ethmoid Sinus

Ethmoid sinusitis commonly occurs with upper respiratory tract infections. These infections usually respond to antibiotics and rarely require surgical treatment. Ethmoidectomy is a procedure to open the ethmoid sinus system, and to provide drainage into the nose. Removal of the ethmoid air cells is indicated in the treatment of chronic ethmoid sinusitis and periorbital abscess secondary to ethmoiditis. Rarely, ethmoidectomy is required to biopsy or treat a neoplasm.

## ▶ 25 - 1 INTRANASAL ETHMOIDECTOMY

### Indications

Intranasal ethmoidectomy may be indicated in conjunction with nasal polypectomy in the treatment of chronic sinusitis.

### Preoperative Evaluation

A complete nasal examination and sinus computed tomography (CT) scans are mandatory before surgery on the ethmoid sinuses.

### Operative Technique

1. General anesthesia is administered through an endotracheal tube.
2. Cotton pledgets with 4% cocaine are placed in the inferior, middle, and superior meatus to aid in hemostasis and to shrink nasal mucosa to facilitate visualization (alternately, any combination of a topical vasoconstrictor and local anesthesia may be used) (Fig. 25–1**A**). One percent lidocaine with 1:100,000 epinephrine is injected in the inferior and middle turbinate and the adjacent areas of the nasal septum to further this process (Fig. 25–1**B**). The middle meatus is widely open after the vasoconstriction occurs (Fig. 25–1**C**).
3. Large nasal polyps are removed with a nasal snare or with cup forceps as described in the section on the nose (see section 14–2).
4. Under direct visualization, a ring curette is introduced into the middle meatus and gently brought anteriorly hugging the lateral edge of the middle turbinate (Fig. 25–1**D**). By remaining lateral to the middle turbinate, the cribriform plate area is avoided. Care must also be taken not to wander too far laterally because the lamina papyracea can be violated and the contents of the globe damaged.
5. Takahashi and other cup forceps are used to gently remove pieces of bone and mucosa that have been loosened by the ring curette (Fig. 25–1**E**).
6. If there is extensive pneumatization of the middle turbinate, it may be necessary to remove a portion of the turbinate to exenterate those cells. However, care should be taken not to avulse the complete turbinate because this removes a valuable landmark and will put the cribriform plate area at increased risk. The resultant cavity is seen in Figure 25–1**F**.

7. Antibiotic-impregnated gauze is then layered into the middle meatus for hemostasis. The pack is left in place 24 to 36 hours (Fig. 25–1G).
8. A broad-spectrum antibiotic is administered for 7 to 10 days.

## Complications

1. Orbital injury
2. CSF rhinorrhea
3. Olfactory nerve injury

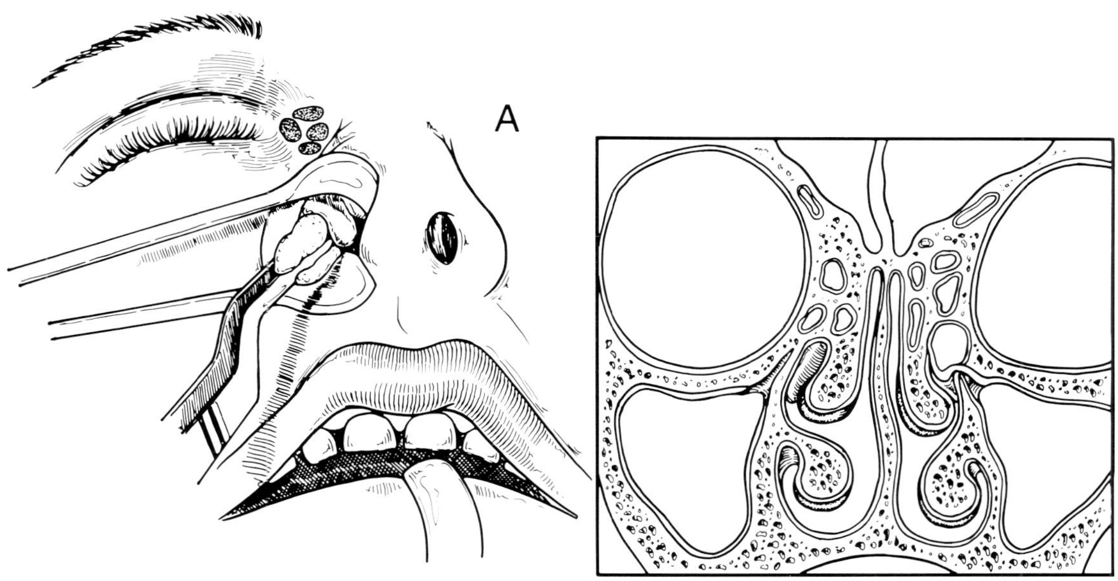


▶ **FIGURE 25-1**

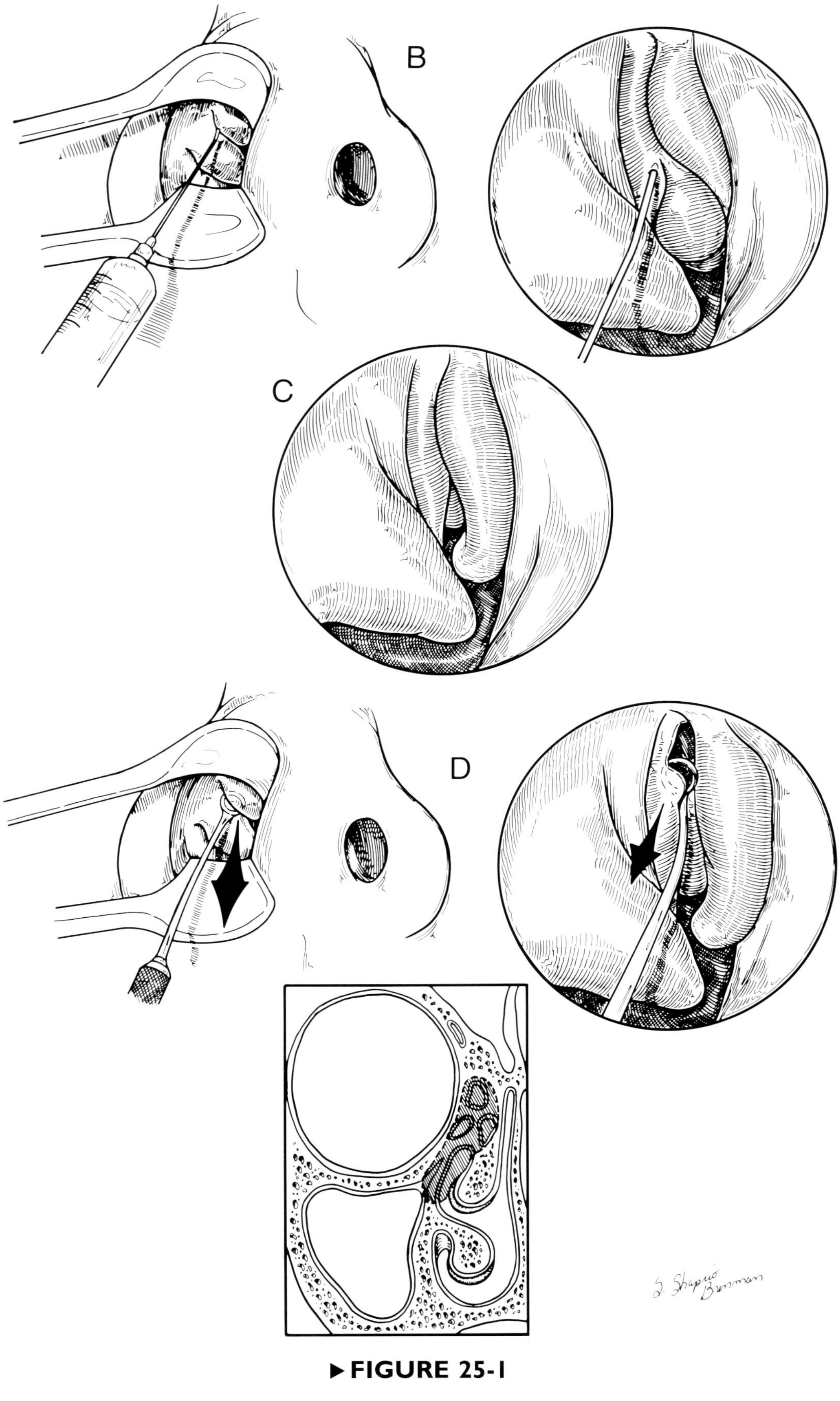


▶ **FIGURE 25-1**

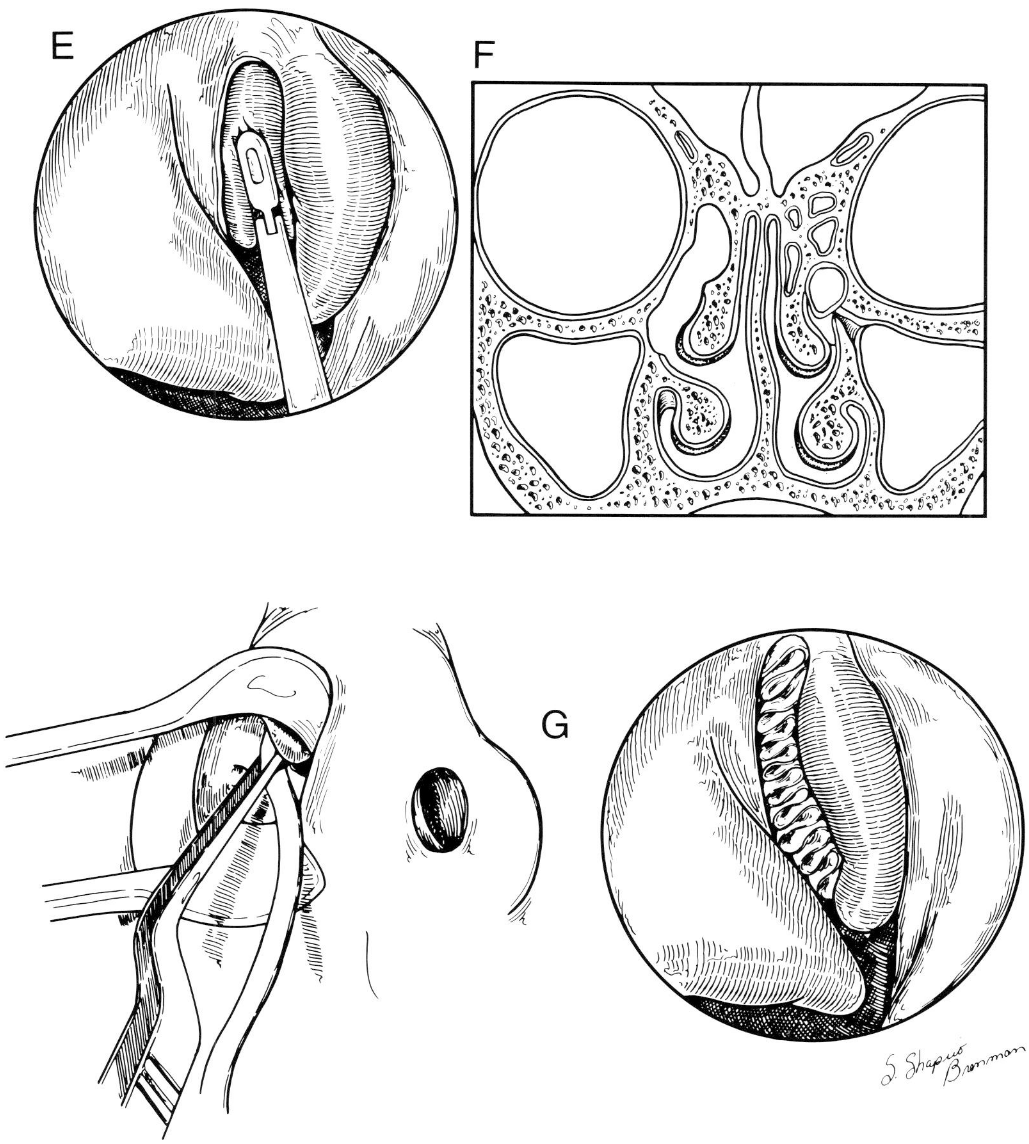


▶**FIGURE 25-1**

## ▶ 25-2 TRANSANTRAL ETHMOIDECTOMY

### Indications

If a Caldwell-Luc operation is being performed to treat chronic maxillary sinusitis, a transantral ethmoidectomy may be useful in exenterating ethmoid cells, particularly in conjunction with an intranasal approach.

### Preoperative Evaluation

Sinus computed tomography (CT) scan is required prior to surgery.

### Operative Technique

1. After a standard Caldwell-Luc operation, the orbital floor is identified. Dissection is begun in the superior medial corner of the maxillary sinus where it joins the ethmoid system. Dissection is accomplished with a ring curette gently opening the ethmoid labyrinth into the maxillary sinus (Fig. 25–2**A**). The same caution with regard to the cribriform plate and the lamina papyracea as discussed in the intranasal technique must be exercised during the transantral approach. The resultant cavity is seen in Figure 25–2**B**.
2. Packing with antibiotic-impregnated gauze is usually required. The packing may be brought out through the nose or through the antral window, which usually is part of the Caldwell-Luc operation. This packing is removed in 24 to 36 hours.
3. A broad-spectrum antibiotic is administered for 7 to 10 days.

### Complications

1. Infraorbital nerve damage
2. Nasolacrimal duct damage
3. Oroantral fistula
4. Orbital trauma
5. CSF rhinorrhea

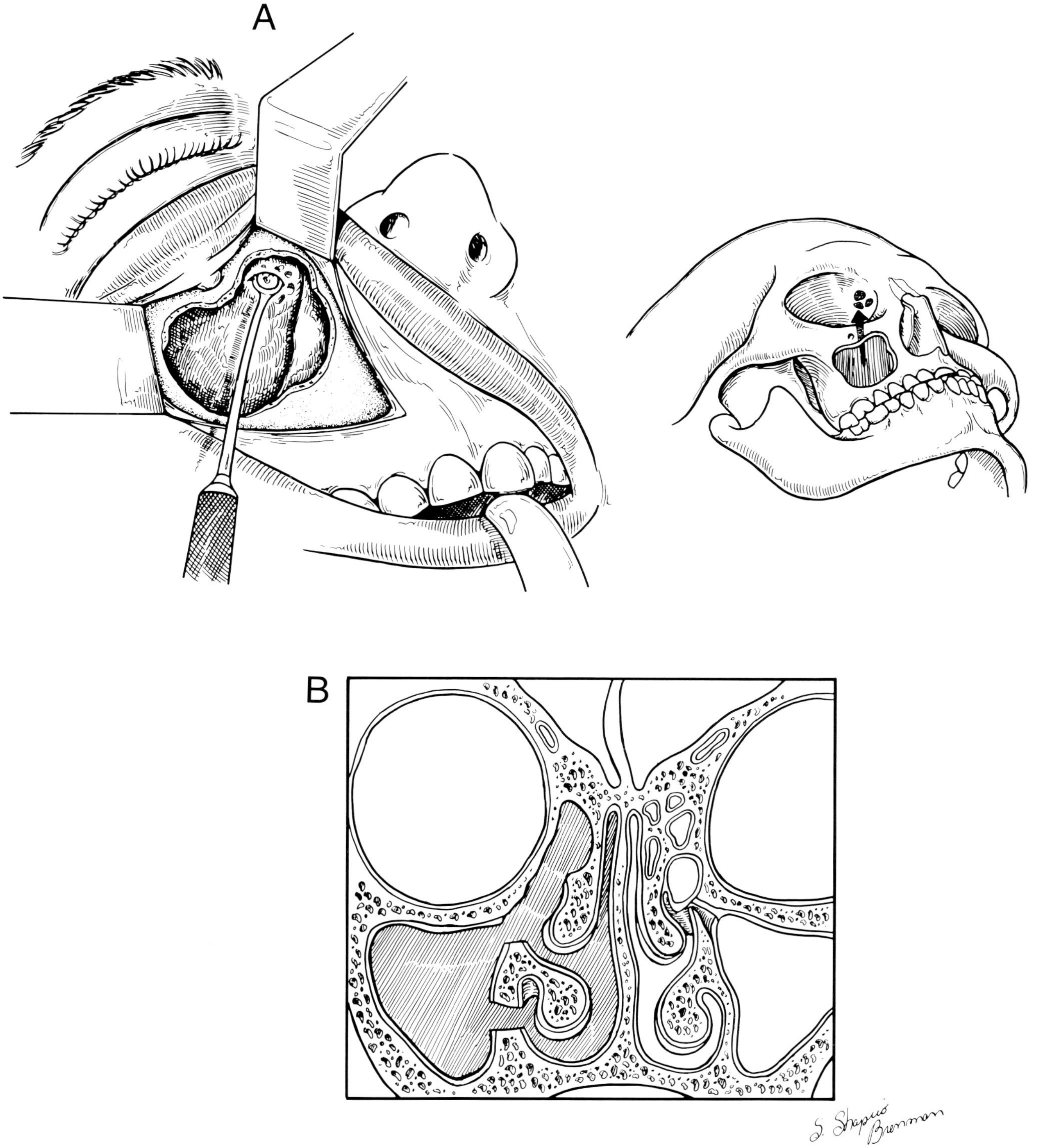


▶**FIGURE 25-2**

## ▶ 25 - 3 EXTERNAL ETHMOIDECTOMY

### Indications

External ethmoidectomy is indicated in the treatment of acute periorbital abscess secondary to ethmoiditis and to biopsy the ethmoid sinus for suspected neoplasm.

### Preoperative Evaluation

Sinus computed tomography (CT) scan is required prior to surgery.

### Operative Technique

1. General anesthesia is administered through an endotracheal tube.
2. A tarsorrhaphy suture of 6-0 nylon is used to keep the lids closed and the cornea protected during the procedure (Fig. 25–3**A**).
3. One percent lidocaine with 1:100,000 epinephrine is injected subcutaneously along the proposed incision plane and especially deep into the periosteum. A curvilinear incision is outlined starting slightly under the eyebrow coming down onto the nasal bone hallway between the medial canthus and the nasal dorsum (Fig. 25–3**A**). The incision is made with a #15 blade through the periosteum.
4. Bleeding vessels are identified, clamped, and tied, especially the angular vein.
5. The periosteum and soft tissues on the nasal side are gently elevated and retracted. Silk sutures through the subcutaneous tissue can be useful for retraction (Fig. 25–3**B**).
6. Malleable retractors are then used to gently retract orbital contents laterally as the Freer elevator is used to elevate periosteum and soft tissue off of the medial wall of the orbit (Fig. 25–3**B**).
7. The lacrimal sac is elevated inferiorly and laterally from its fossa (Fig. 25–3**C**).
8. The anterior ethmoid artery is identified, clipped, and divided (Fig. 25–3**C**, **D**). Dissection is taken only as far back as the posterior ethmoid artery. This is to ensure safety to the more posterior optic nerve.
9. If the lamina papyracea is intact, it is opened at a point below the level of the ethmoid arteries and posterior to the lacrimal fossa. This can usually be done with a very fine mosquito forceps or with a ring curette (Fig. 25–3**E**). Polypoid mucosa is gently removed using cupped forceps and a ring curette.
10. The opening in the lamina papyracea is gently enlarged superiorly to the level of the ethmoid arteries because this corresponds to the level of the cribriform plate (Fig. 25–3**F**). Care is taken not to injure the lacrimal apparatus inferiorly or the cribriform plate superiorly. Dissection can be taken anteriorly to the limits of the anterior ethmoid cells and posteriorly to the face of the sphenoid. The resultant cavity is seen in Figure 25–3**G**.
11. A curved clamp or a curette placed in the middle meatus through the nose should be apparent in the surgical field, thus demonstrating continuity between the enlarged ethmoid cavity and the nasal cavity (Fig. 25–3**H**). If a Caldwell-Luc has been performed, continuity can be ascertained through the transantral approach to the ethmoid cells.

**12.** The ethmoid cavity is packed lightly with antibiotic-impregnated gauze, which is brought out through the anterior naris. Care is taken not to place undue pressure on the orbital contents (Fig. 25–3**I**).

**13.** The orbital incision is closed in two layers. The deep layer of periosteum and subcutaneous tissue are closed with interrupted 4-0 chromic sutures. The skin is closed with interrupted or running 5-0 nylon sutures (Fig. 25–3**J**).

**14.** The packing is removed in 24 to 36 hours.

**15.** A broad-spectrum antibiotic is administered for 7 to 10 days.

## Complications

1. Orbital trauma
2. CSF rhinorrhea
3. Nasolacrimal damage

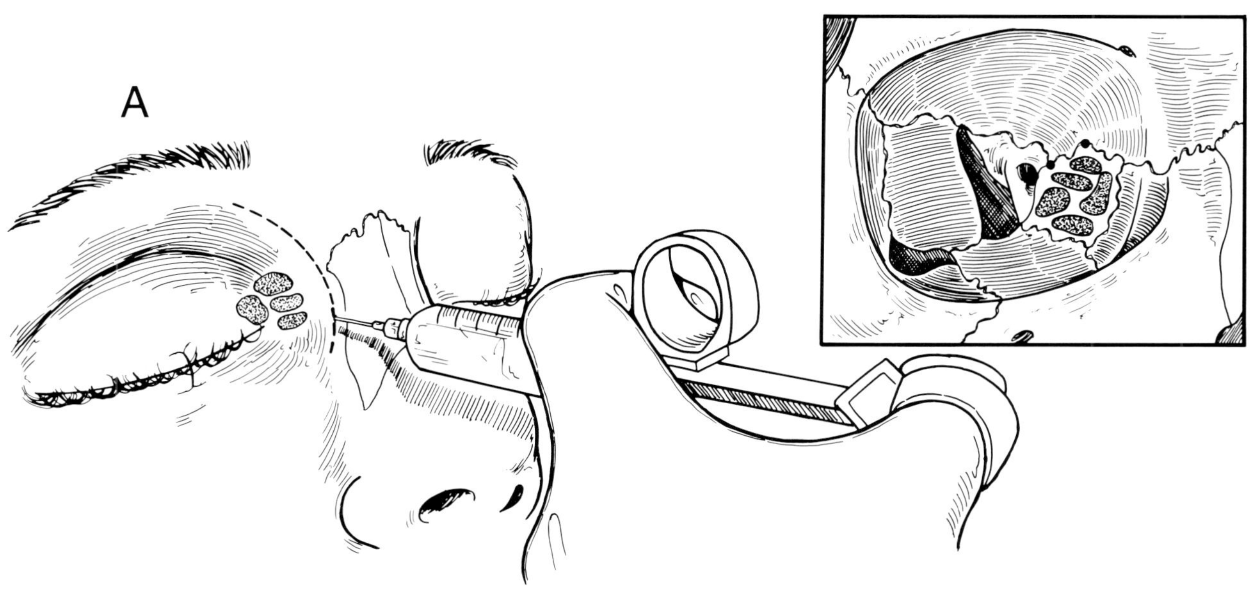


▶**FIGURE 25-3**

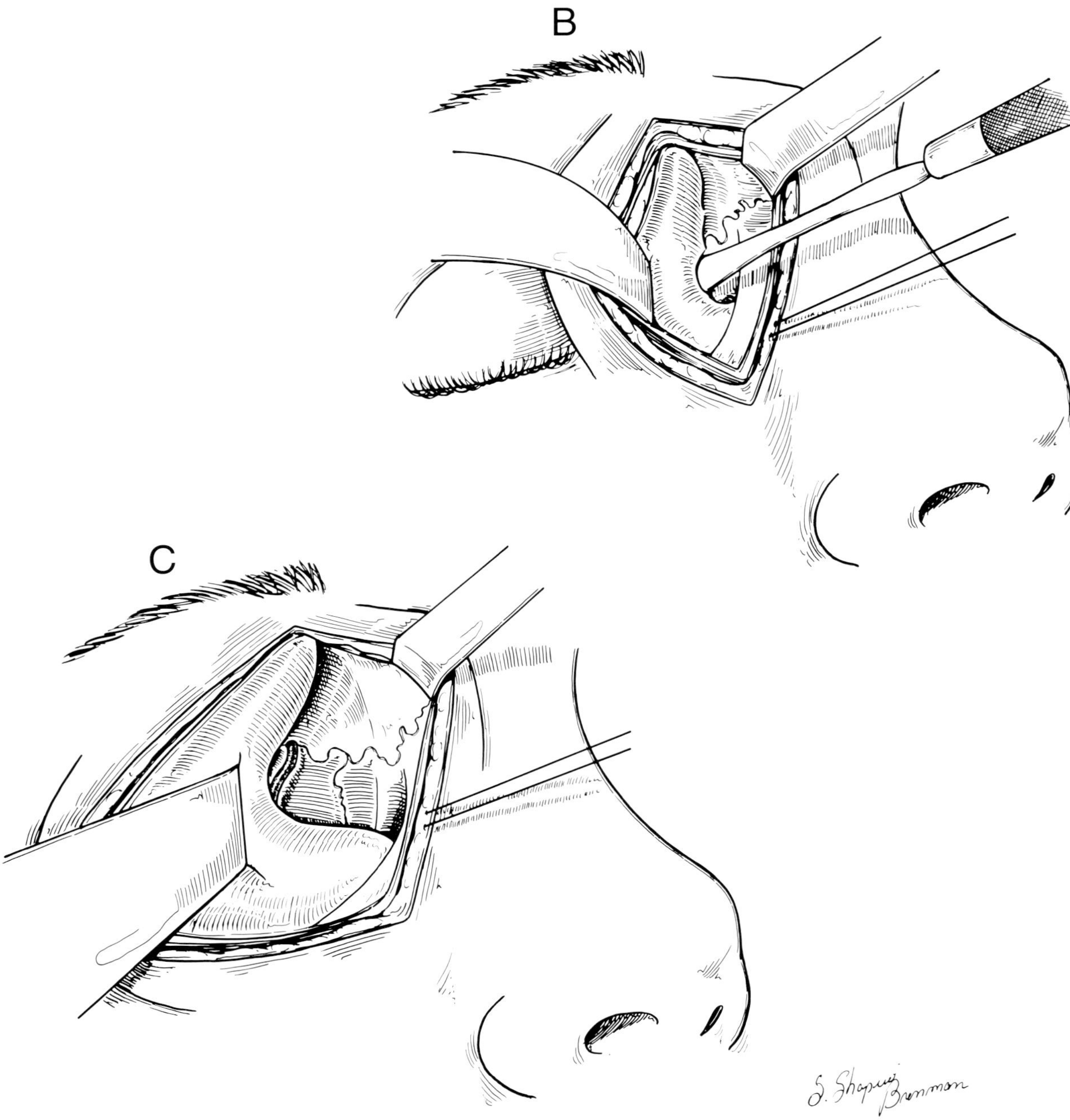


▶ **FIGURE 25-3**

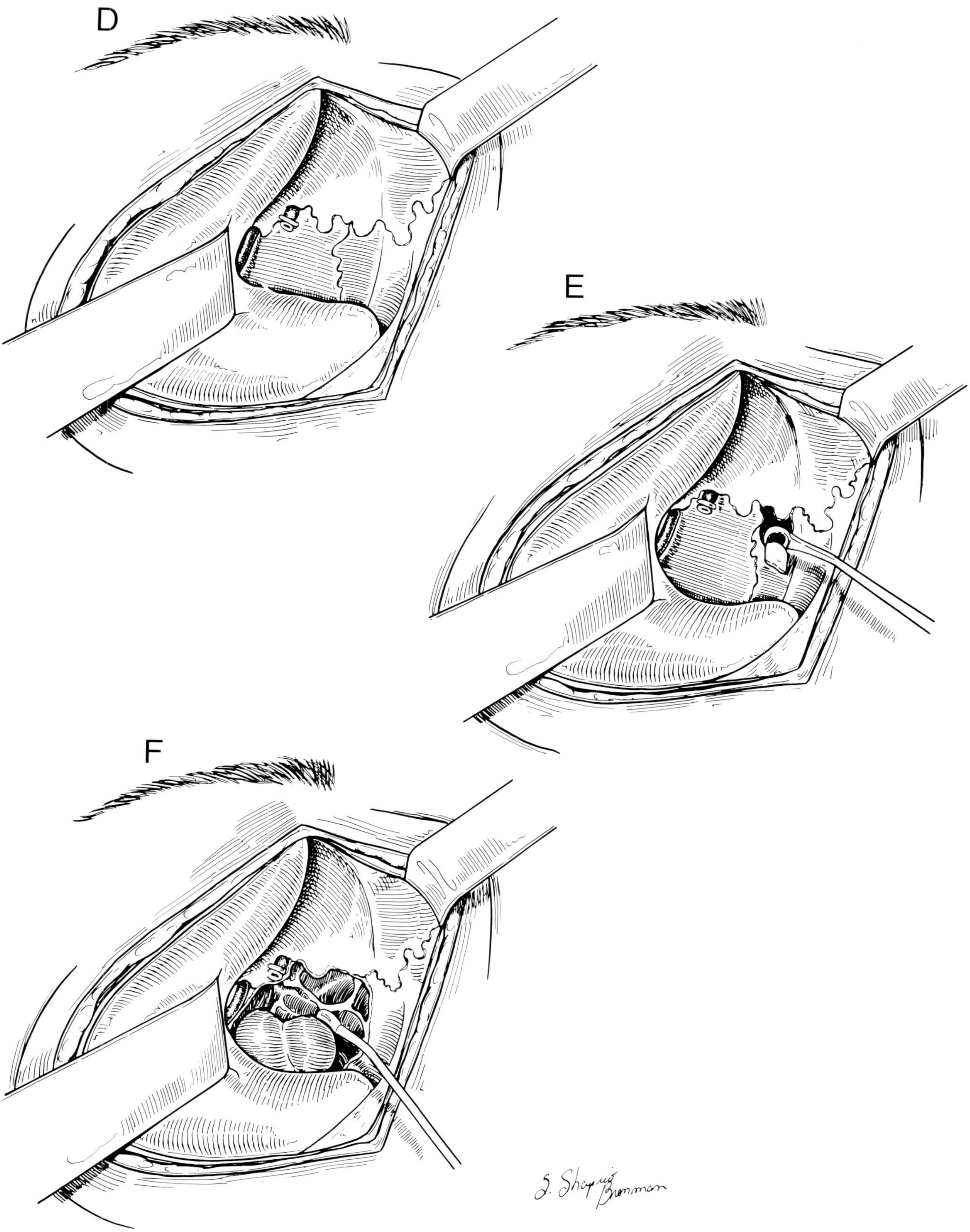


▶ **FIGURE 25-3**

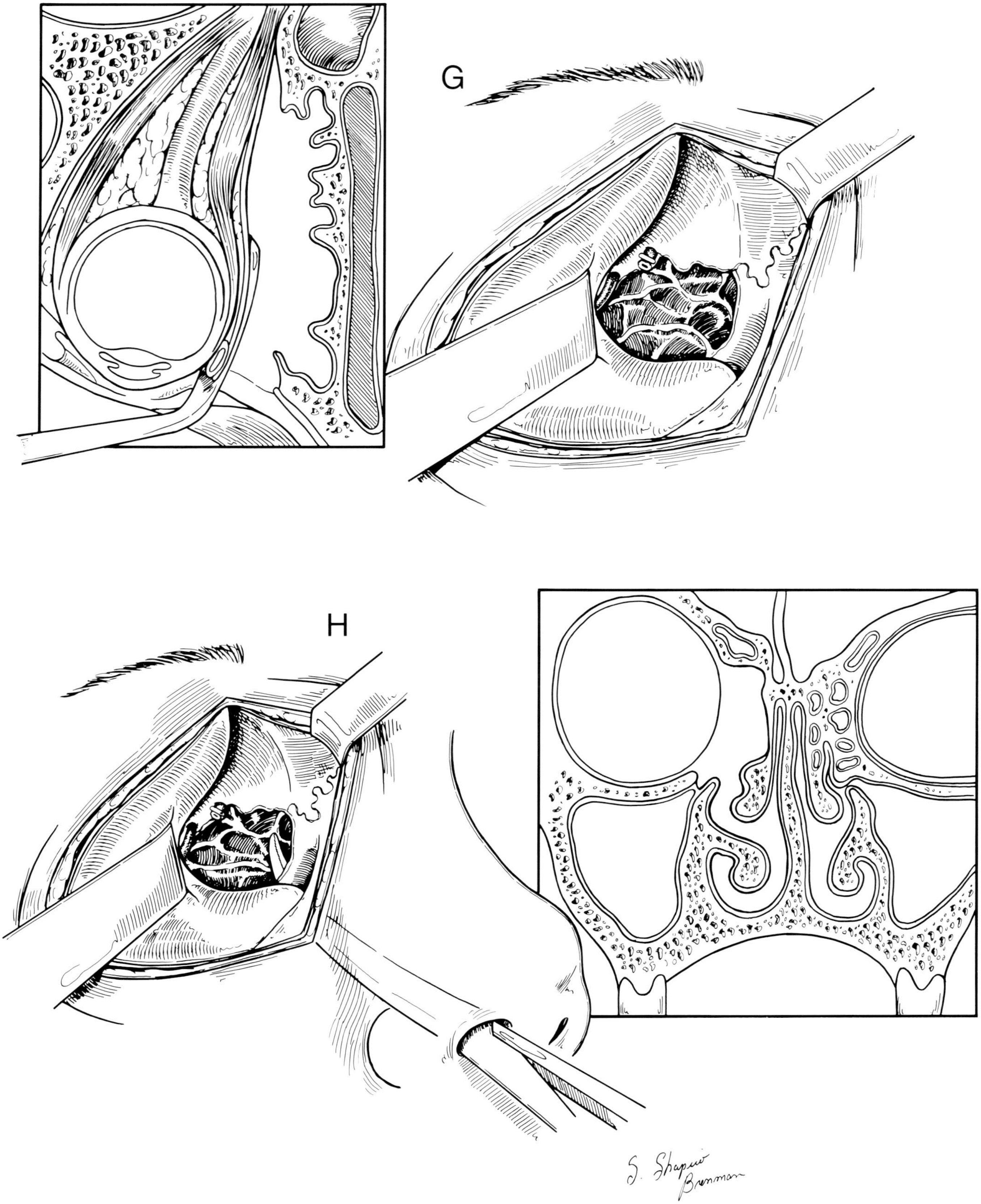


▶ **FIGURE 25-3**

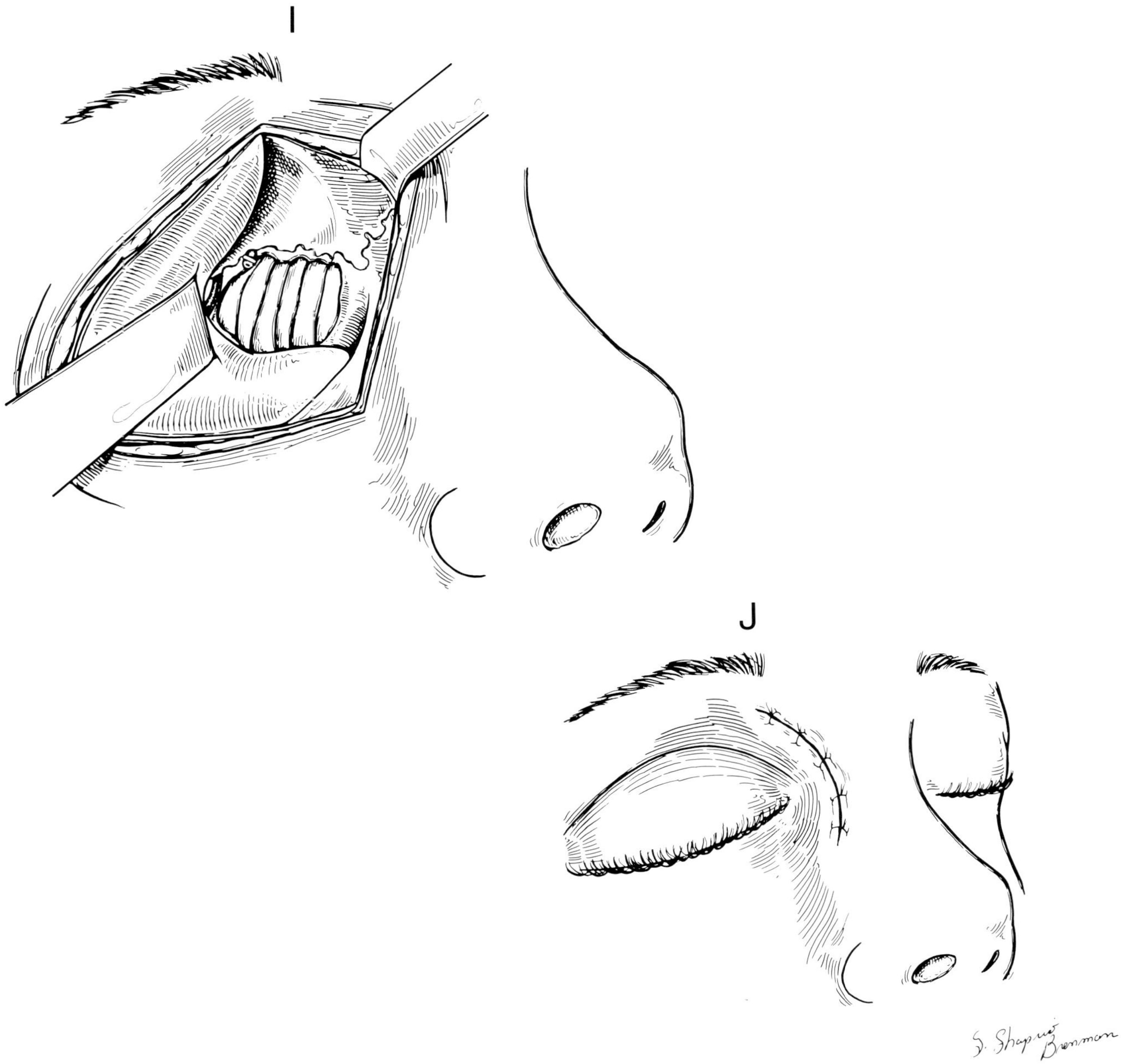


▶ **FIGURE 25-3**

# 26 ▸ Sphenoid Sinus

The sphenoid sinus, located behind the nasal cavity, is accessible by several routes. The approach is based on the disease process and associated findings.

## ▸ 26 - 1 TRANSNASAL PUNCTURE OF SPHENOID

Transnasal puncture of sphenoid is a procedure to provide acute drainage of the sphenoid sinus.

### Indications

Acute sphenoid sinusitis that is not responding to appropriate antimicrobial treatment is the indication for the procedure that provides the opportunity to aspirate and culture secretions, and to irrigate the sinus(es).

### Preoperative Evaluation

Sinus computed tomography (CT) scan is required prior to surgery.

### Operative Technique

1. General anesthesia is administered through an oral RAE endotracheal tube.
2. Cotton pledgets with 4% cocaine are placed in the inferior, middle, and superior meatus to aid in hemostasis and to facilitate visualization (alternately, any combination of a topical vasoconstrictor and local anesthetic may be used). One percent lidocaine with 1:100,000 epinephrine is injected into the inferior and middle turbinates and the nasal septal mucosa to supplement the topical cocaine.
3. A long nasal speculum is utilized to visualize the vomer and the face of the sphenoid (Fig. 26–1**A**).
4. A needle is placed on the face of the sphenoid (Fig. 26–1**B**). Appropriate placement is confirmed radiographically using fluoroscopic control. The needle can then be advanced into the sinus and material aspirated for culture (Fig. 26–1**C**). Irrigation of the sinus can also be performed, once again using radiographic control. Care must be taken to avoid the pituitary fossa superiorly and the cavernous sinus and the optic nerves laterally.

### Complications

1. CSF rhinorrhea
2. Cavernous sinus injury

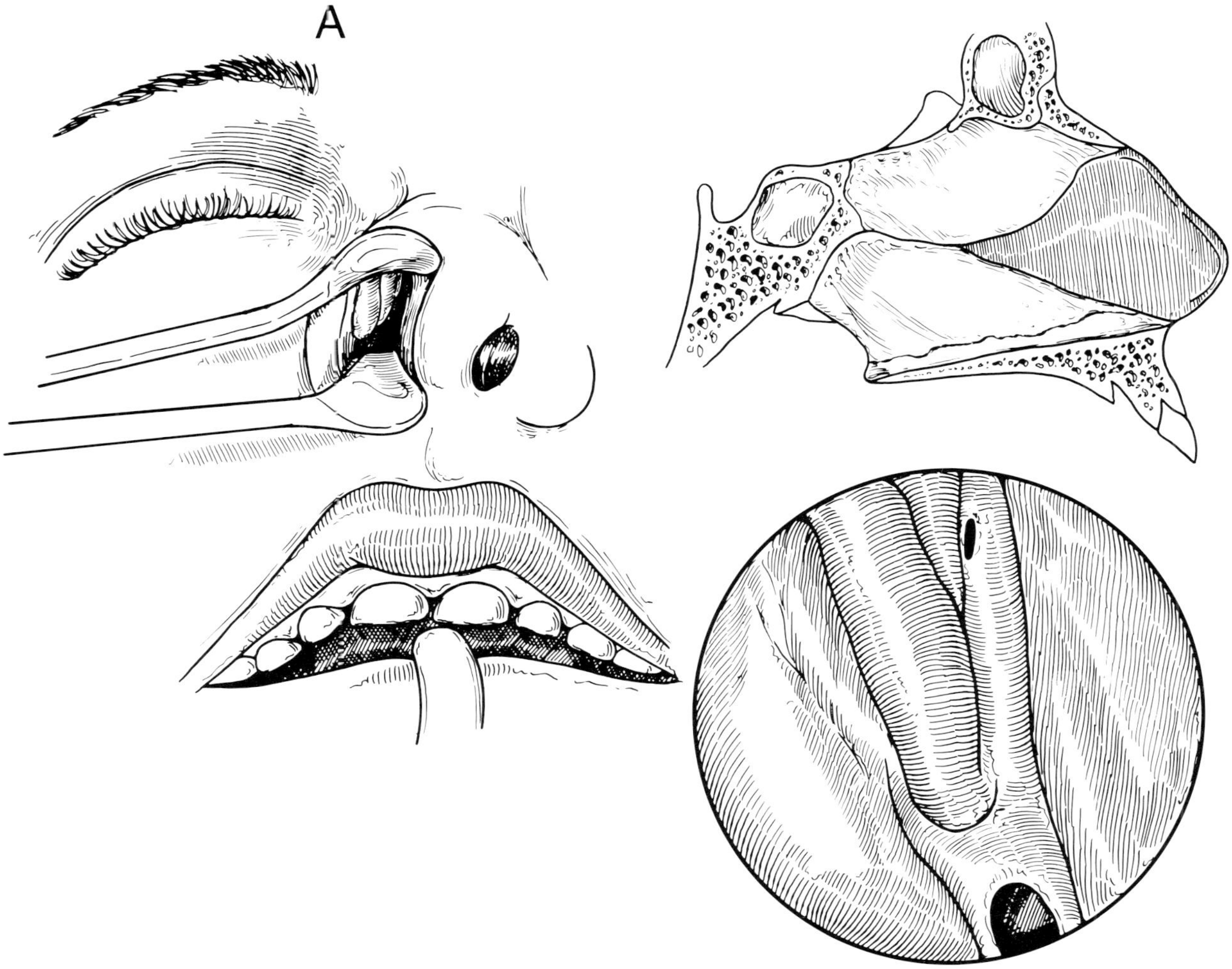


▸ **FIGURE 26-1**

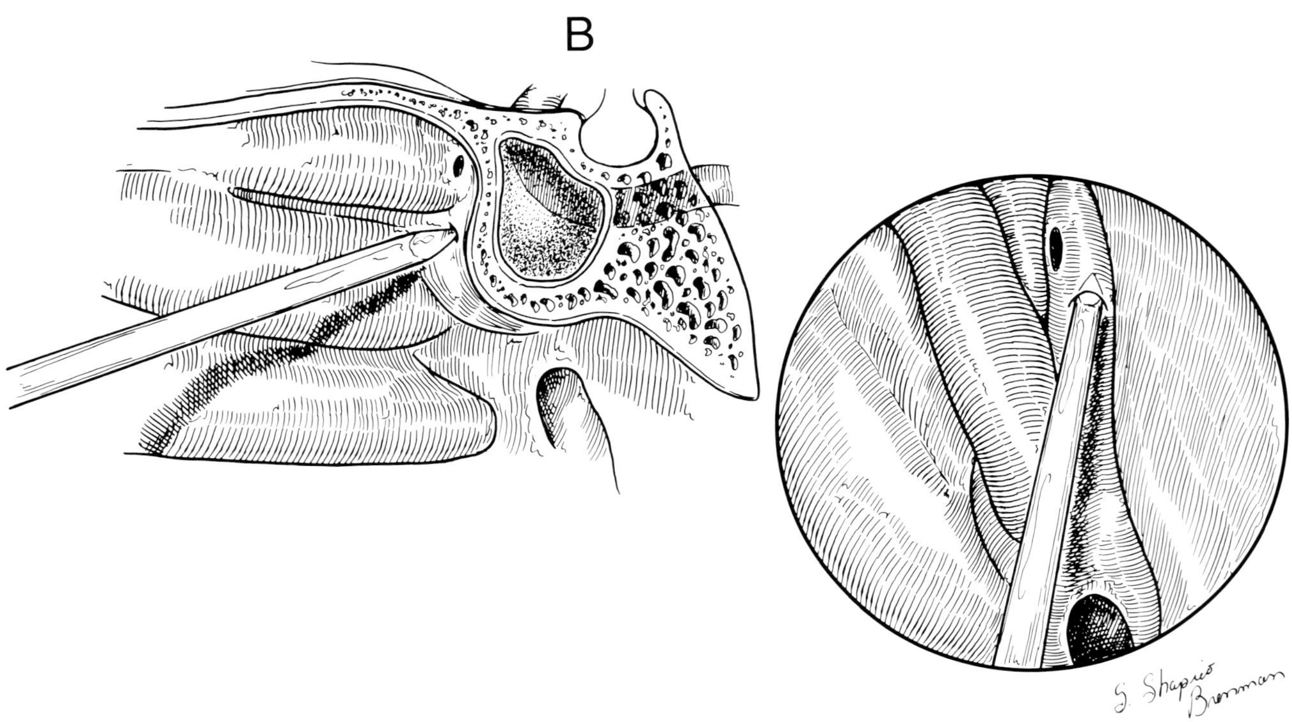


▶ **FIGURE 26-1**

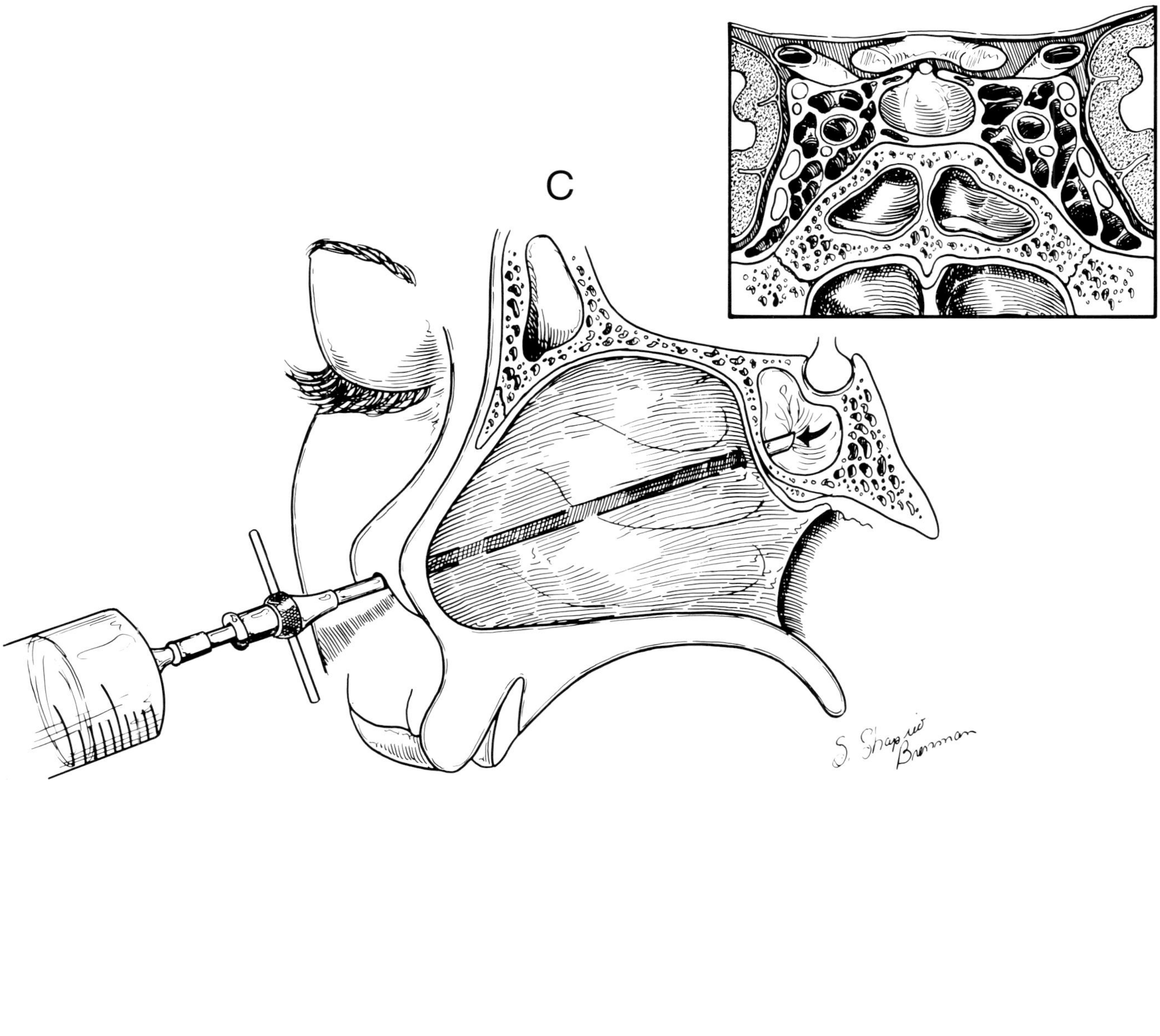


▶ **FIGURE 26-1**

## ▶ 26-2 TRANSEPTAL SPHENOIDECTOMY

### Indications

The transeptal approach is useful to obtain a biopsy specimen from the sphenoid sinus.

### Preoperative Evaluation

Sinus computed tomography (CT) scan is required prior to surgery.

### Operative Technique

1. General anesthesia is administered through an oral RAE endotracheal tube.
2. Cotton pledgets with 4% cocaine are placed in the inferior, middle, and superior meatus to aid in hemostasis and to facilitate visualization (alternately, any combination of a topical vasoconstrictor and local anesthetic may be used). One percent lidocaine with 1:100,000 epinephrine is injected in the inferior and middle turbinates and the nasal septal mucosa to supplement the topical cocaine (Fig. 26–2**A**).
3. A vertical incision is made in the septal mucosa just posterior to the junction of the quadrangular cartilage and the columella (Fig. 26–2**B**).
4. The mucosa, together with the periosteum of the vomer, is elevated laterally completely on one side (Fig. 26–2**C**).
5. The Cottle elevator is used to separate the quadrangular cartilage from the vomer so that nasal mucosa and periosteum can be elevated from the opposite side of the vomer (Fig. 26–2**D**).
6. Double-action biting rongeurs are used to bite away the superior aspect of the vomer taking care not to injure the mucosal flaps on either side (Fig. 26–2**E**).
7. As the end of the vomer is approached, the face of the sphenoid is identified. Once again, confirmation of position is obtained radiographically using fluoroscopic control. A drill or osteotome can be used to enter the face of the sphenoid (Fig. 26–2**F**).
8. The intersinus septum is identified and gently removed with biting forceps as is thickened mucosa and suspicious tissue (Fig. 26–2**G**).
9. An operating microscope may be useful in the most posterior dissection.
10. If the sphenoid sinus has been found to be free of infection or if there is possible CSF leak through the pituitary fossa, the nasal septal flaps are returned to their original position to seal off the sphenoid cavity. In the case of pituitary dissection, the sphenoid sinus is usually packed with muscle, fat, or fascia. If infection has been found in the sphenoid sinus, it is wise to incise the mucosal flap over one side of the sphenoid sinus to allow for adequate drainage of the sphenoid sinus and to prevent further mucocele formation.
11. A broad-spectrum antibiotic is administered for 7 to 10 days.

### Complications

1. Septal perforation
2. Saddle nose deformity
3. CSF rhinorrhea
4. Cavernous sinus puncture

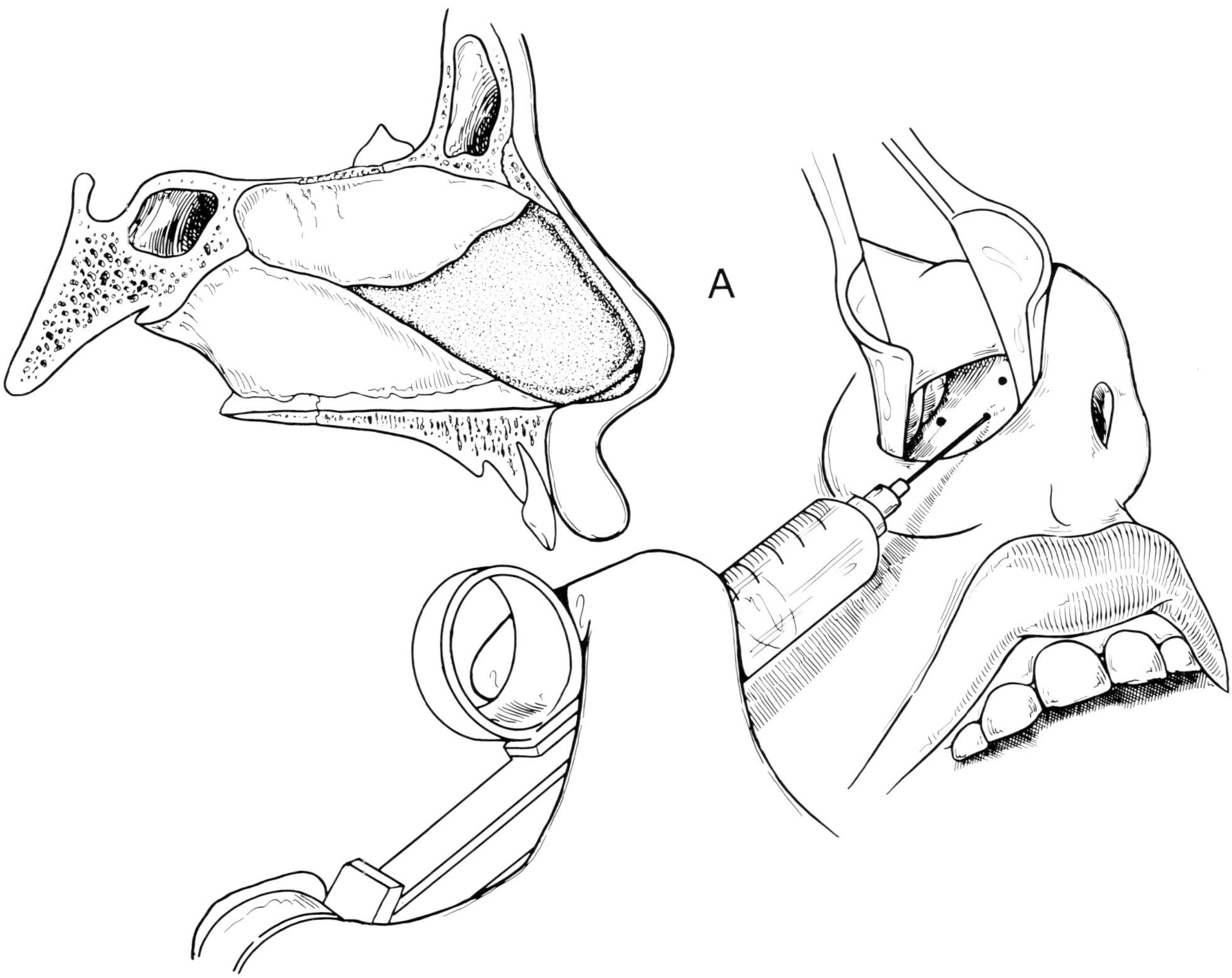


▶ **FIGURE 26-2**

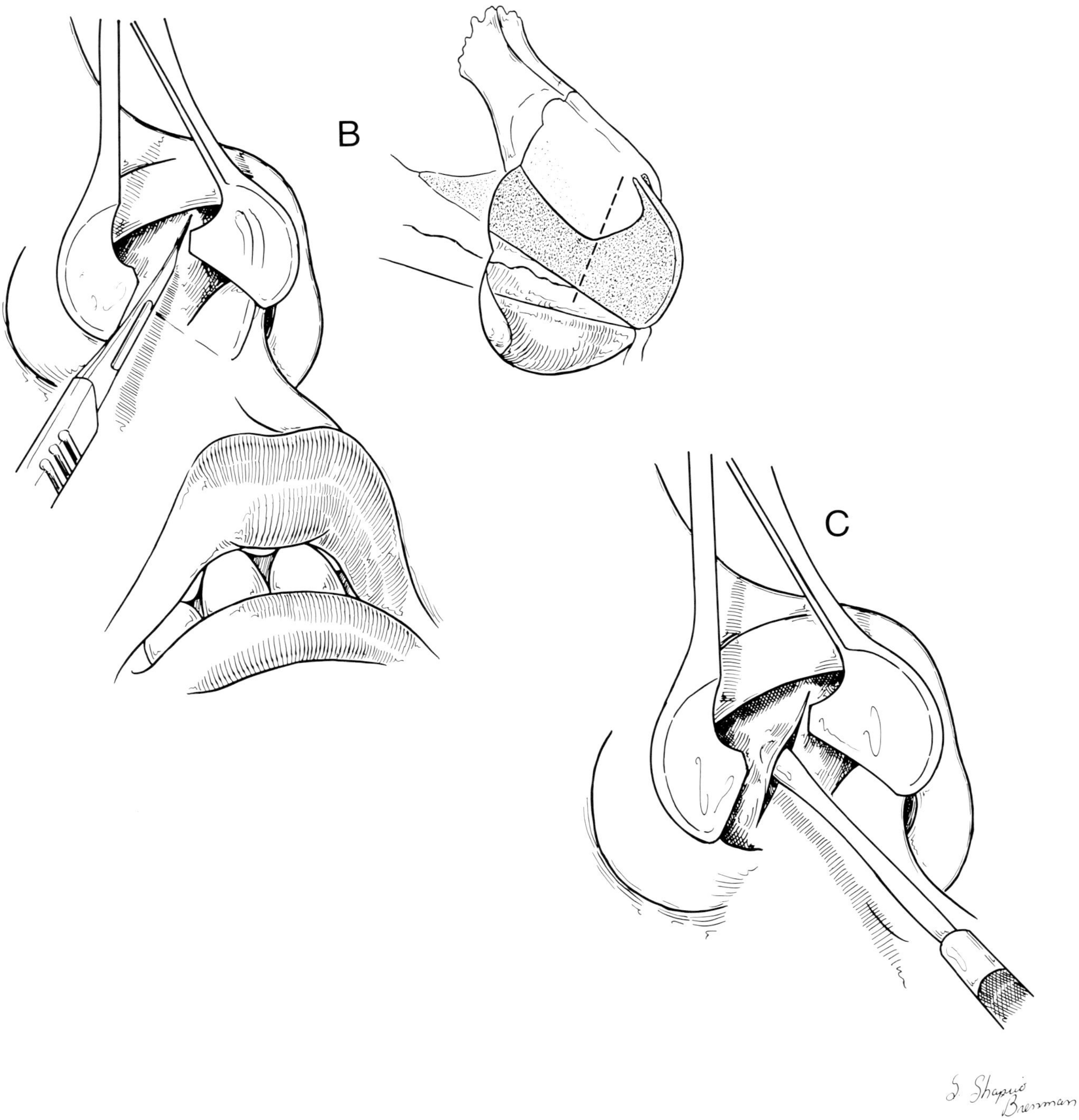


▶**FIGURE 26-2**

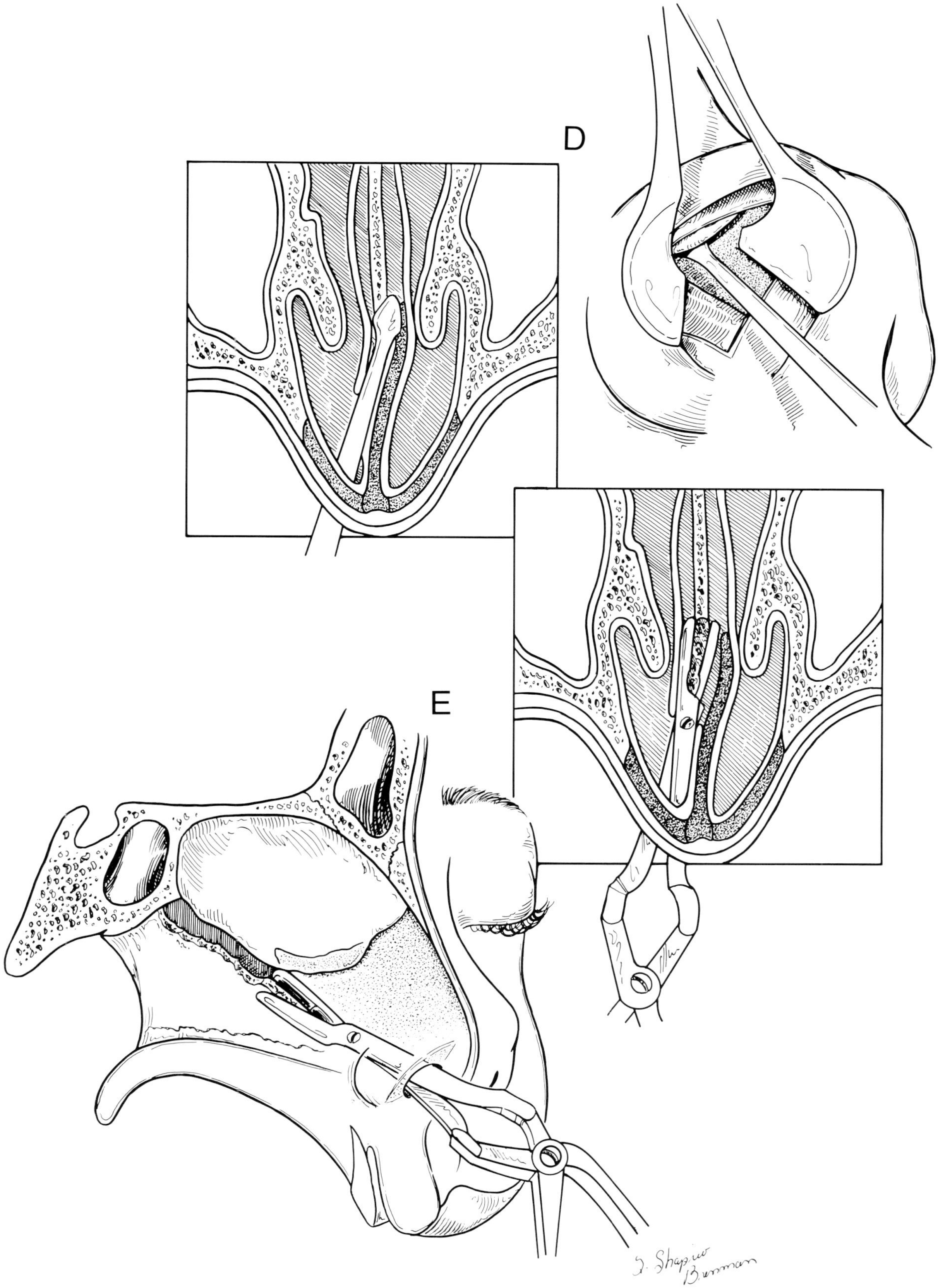


▶ **FIGURE 26-2**

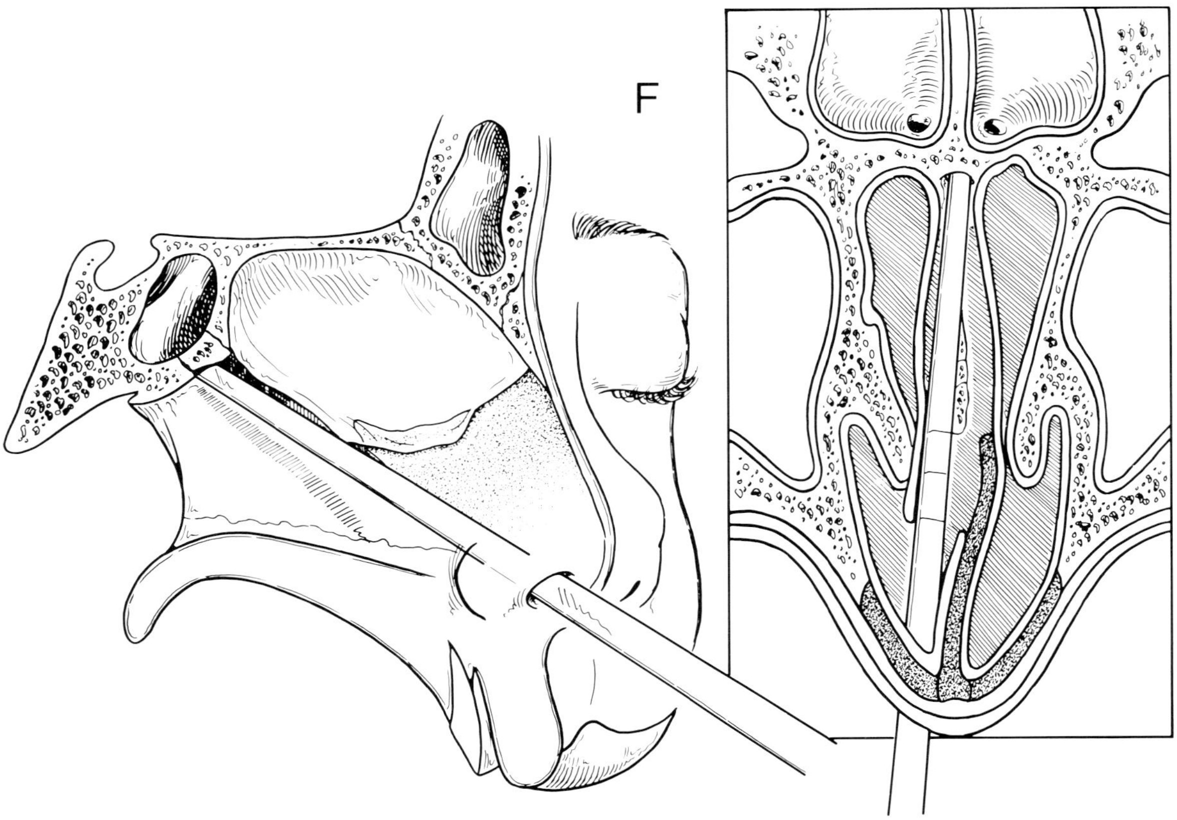


▶ **FIGURE 26-2**

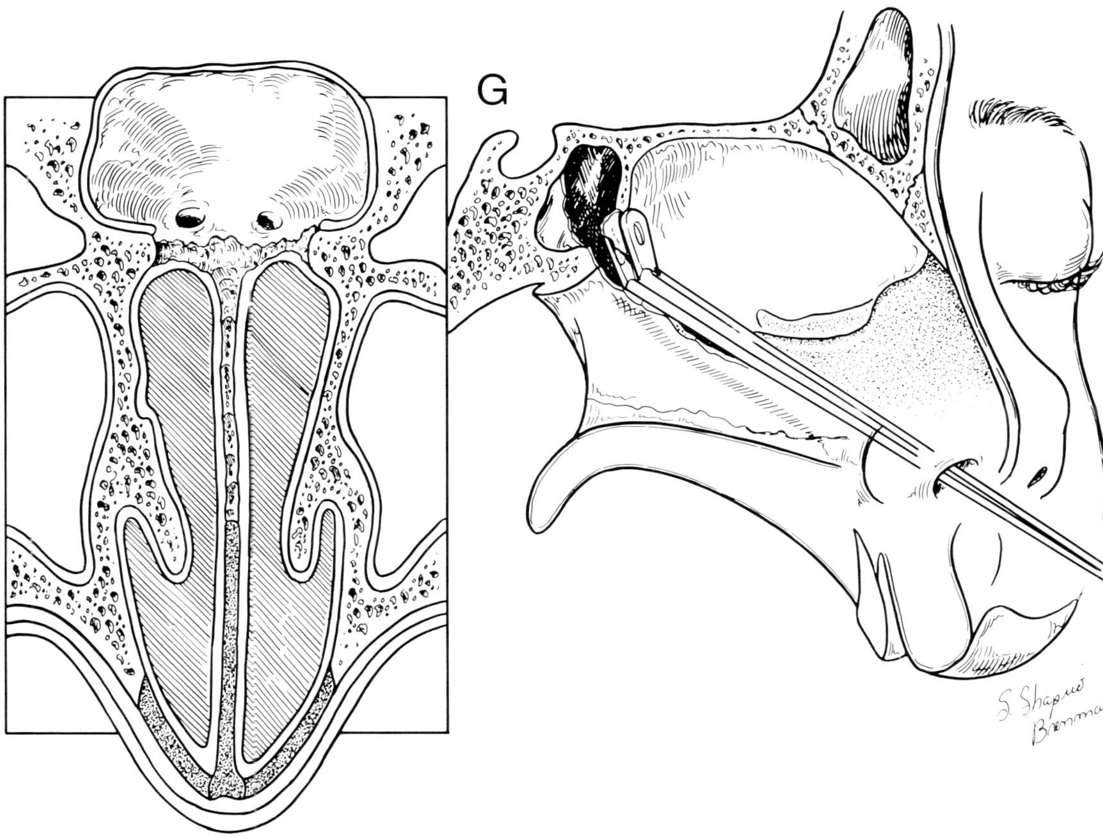


▶ **FIGURE 26-2**

## ▶ 26-3 TRANSEPTAL SUBLABIAL SPHENOIDECTOMY

The advantage of this approach is that it allows for greater visibility, especially in small children and permits a self-retaining retractor to be used for better stability during sphenoid and transphenoid pituitary procedures.

### Indications

The indication for this procedure is a patient with a pituitary lesion that is beneath the diaphragm sella and has a well-pneumatized sphenoid sinus.

### Preoperative Evaluation

Sinus computed tomography (CT) scan is required prior to surgery.

### Operative Technique

1. General anesthesia is administered through an oral RAE endotracheal tube.
2. Cotton pledgets with 4% cocaine are placed in the inferior, middle, and superior meatus to aid in hemostasis and to facilitate visualization (alternately, any combination of a topical vasoconstrictor and local anesthetic may be used). One percent lidocaine with 1:100,000 epinephrine is injected into the inferior and middle turbinates and the nasal septal mucosa to supplement the topical cocaine.
3. In addition, 1% lidocaine with 1:100,000 epinephrine is injected subcutaneously under the upper lip.
4. A gingival-buccal incision is made from canine to canine and taken down to the face of the pyriform aperture (Fig. 26–3**A**).
5. The soft tissues and periosteum of the floor of the nose are elevated bluntly as is the mucosa from one side of the cartilaginous nasal septum (Fig. 26–3**B**).
6. The anterior nasal spine is amputated with a chisel so that the whole septal cartilage and nasal spine can be deflected to the side of its remaining mucosal attachment (Fig. 26–3**C**).
7. The Cottle elevator is used to separate the quadrangular cartilage from the vomer so that dissection can now take place on the opposite side elevating the nasal mucosa and periosteum from the opposite side of the vomer (Fig. 26–3**C**).
8. Double-action biting rongeurs are used to bite away the superior aspect of the vomer taking care not to injure the mucosal flaps on either side (Fig. 26–3**D**).
9. As the end of the vomer is approached, the face of the sphenoid is identified. Once again, confirmation of position is obtained radiographically using fluoroscopic control. At this point, a self-retaining retractor may be placed in the incision to facilitate the remainder of the procedure. A drill or osteotome can be used to enter the face of the sphenoid (Fig. 26–3**E**).
10. The intersinus septum is identified and gently removed with biting forceps. Thickened mucosa and any suspicious-appearing tissue are also removed (Fig. 26–3**F**).
11. An operating microscope is often useful in the most posterior dissection.

12. The quadrangular cartilage and nasal spine are replaced in their normal anatomical position, and the nasal tissues are held in place with antibiotic-impregnated gauze. The sublabial incision is closed with interrupted 4-0 chromic sutures.
13. Antibiotic-impregnated gauze packing is placed and removed in 24 hours.
14. A broad-spectrum antibiotic is administered for 7 to 10 days.

## Complications

1. Septal perforation
2. Saddle nose deformity
3. CSF rhinorrhea
4. Cavernous sinus puncture

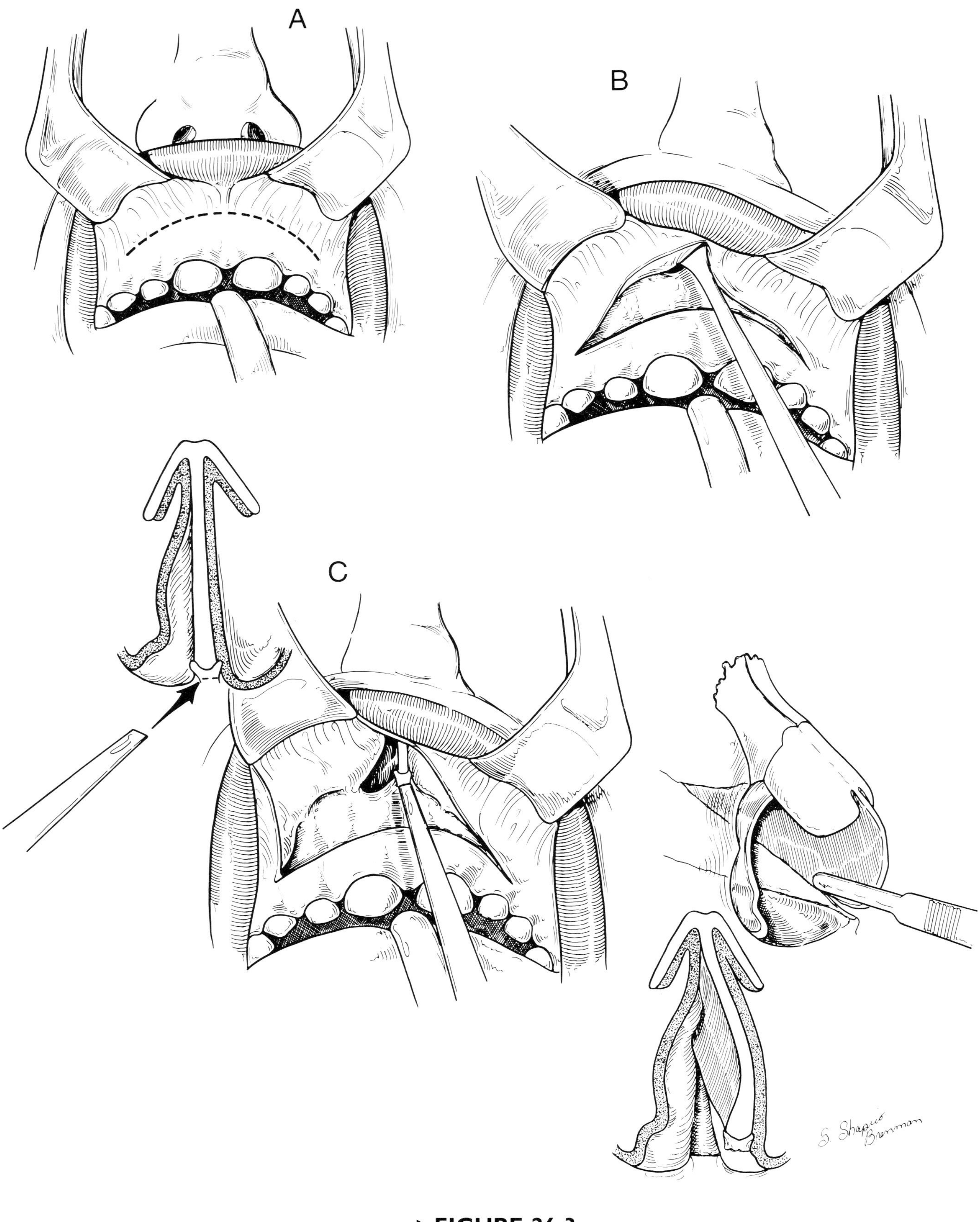


▶ **FIGURE 26-3**

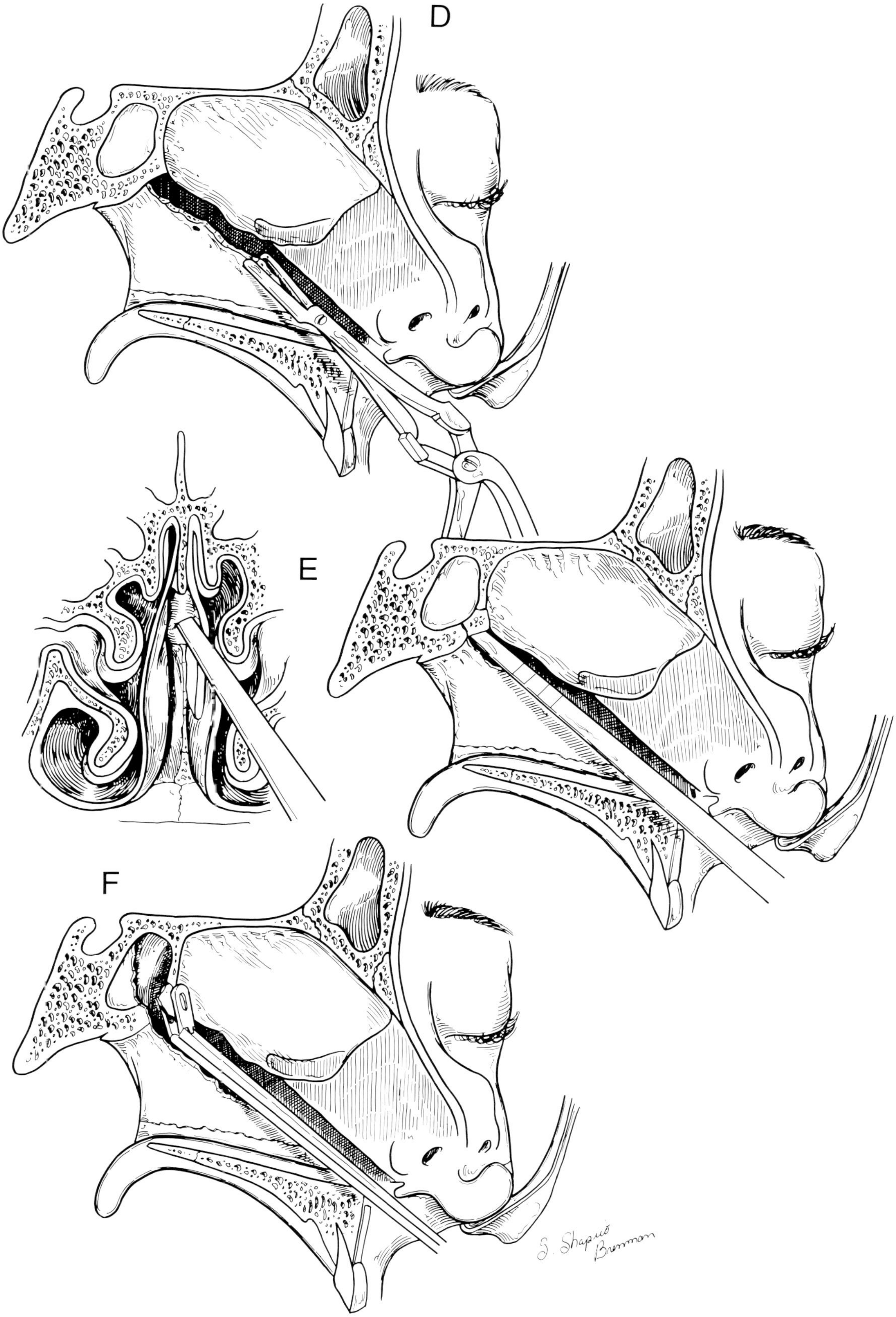


▶ **FIGURE 26-3**

## ▶ 26-4 TRANSETHMOID SPHENOIDOTOMY

### Indications

Transethmoid sphenoidotomy is indicated where there is chronic sphenoid disease associated with ethmoid disease and an external ethmoidectomy is being performed.

### Preoperative Evaluation

A complete nasal examination and sinus computed tomography (CT) scans are mandatory before sphenoid sinus surgery.

### Operative Technique

**1.** The standard external ethmoidectomy (see section 25–3) is performed (Fig. 26–4**A**).

**2.** The face of the sphenoid sinus is seen in the depth of the surgical field at the posterior aspect of the vomer. Occasionally, the ostium of the sphenoid sinus can be identified (if the ethmoid cavity is open to the nasopharynx). The mucosa from the face of the sinus is dissected from above downward to expose the bony wall (Fig. 26–4**B**).

**3.** The sinus is entered at its bony face using a sharp curette or small osteotome (Fig. 26–4**C**). The mucocele or suspicious tissue is then removed using a cup forceps.

**4.** The sphenoid septum (Fig. 26–4**D**) is removed to expose the entire sinus cavity (Fig. 26–4**E**).

**5.** Antibiotic-impregnated gauze is placed in the ethmoid cavity and into the sphenoid cavity. It is brought out through the anterior naris (Fig. 26–4**F**).

**6.** A broad-spectrum antibiotic is administered for 7 to 10 days.

**7.** The gauze is removed in 24 to 36 hours.

### Complications

1. Orbital trauma
2. CSF rhinorrhea
3. Nasolacrimal duct damage

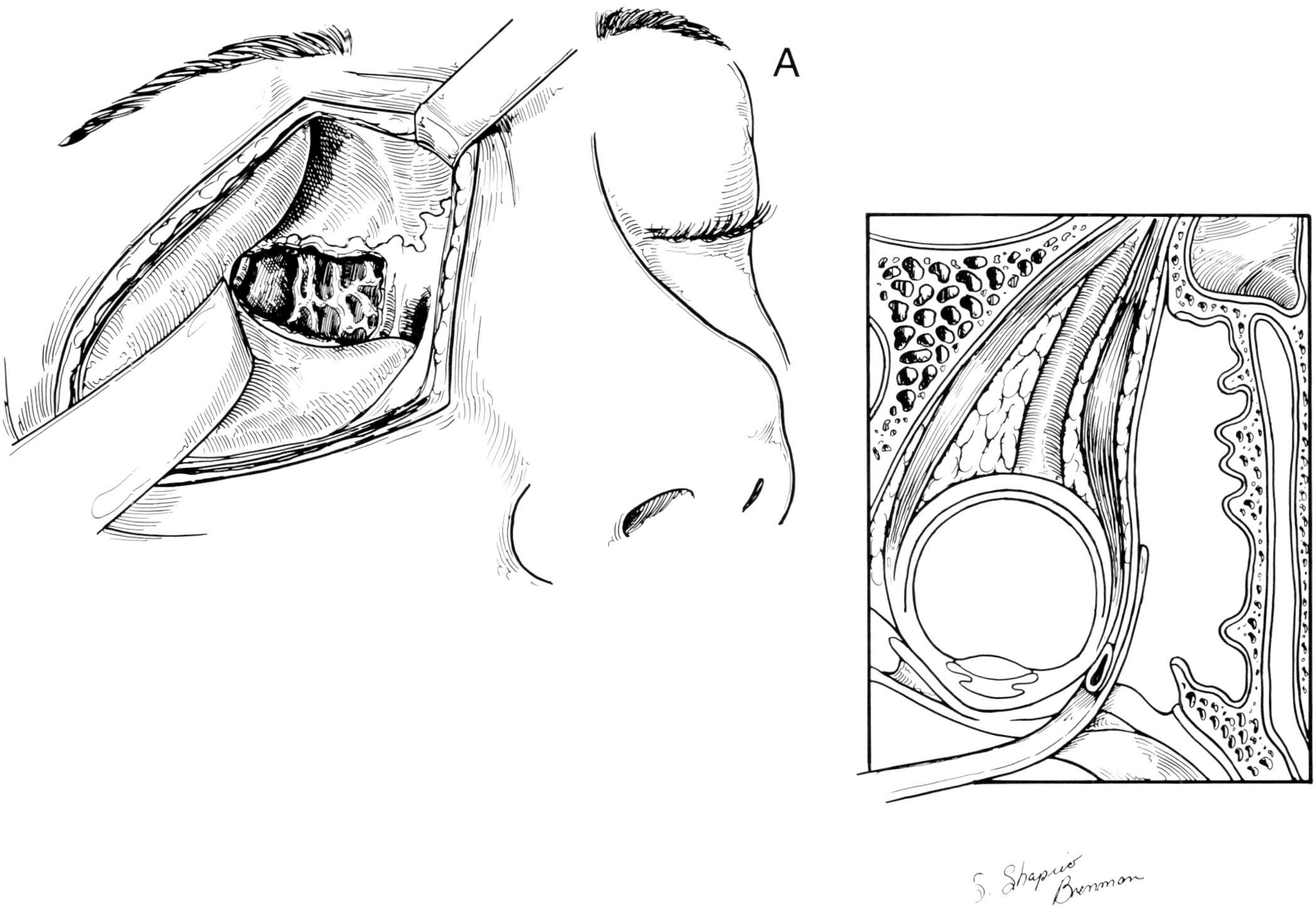


▶ **FIGURE 26-4**

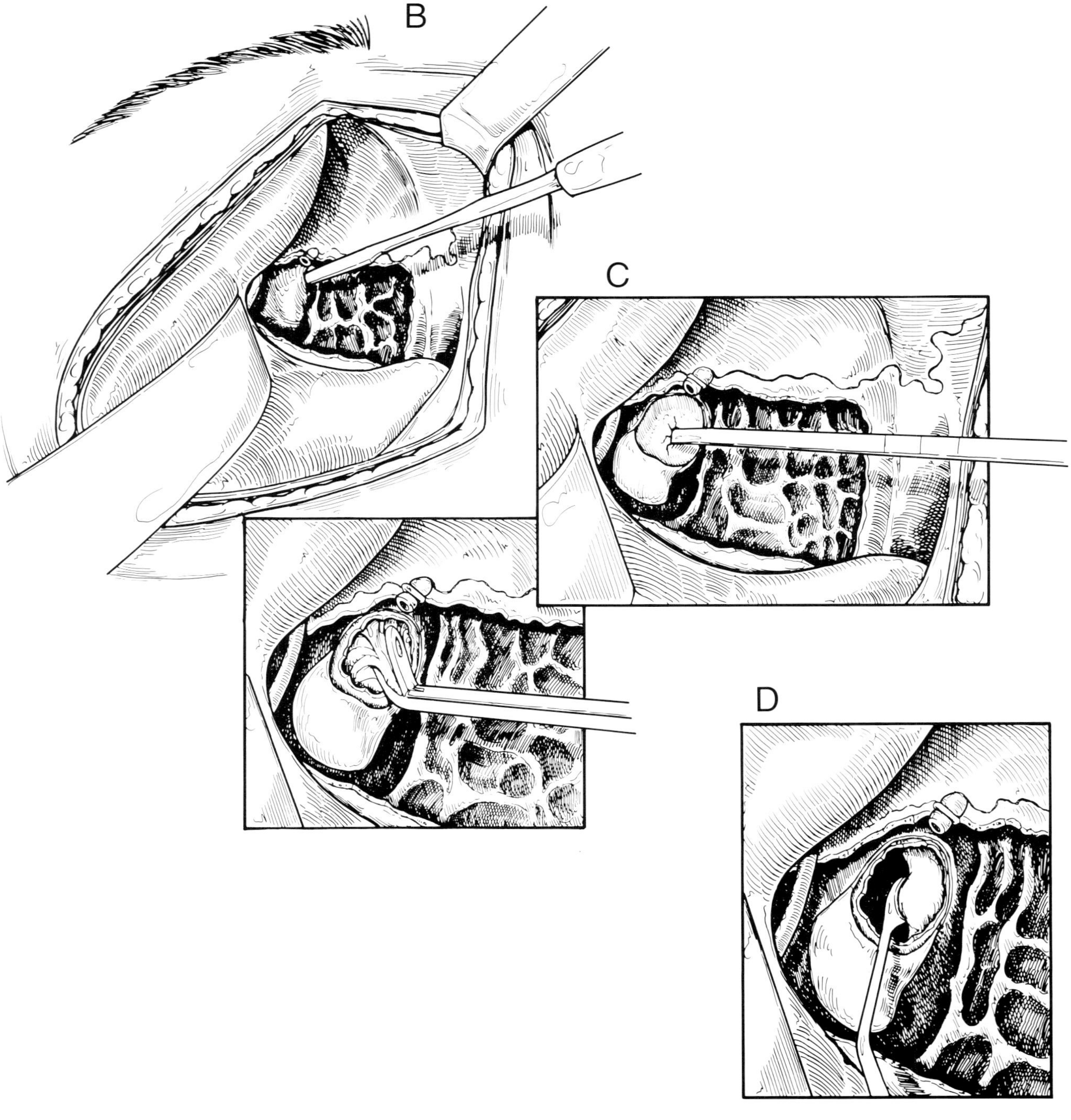


▶ **FIGURE 26-4**

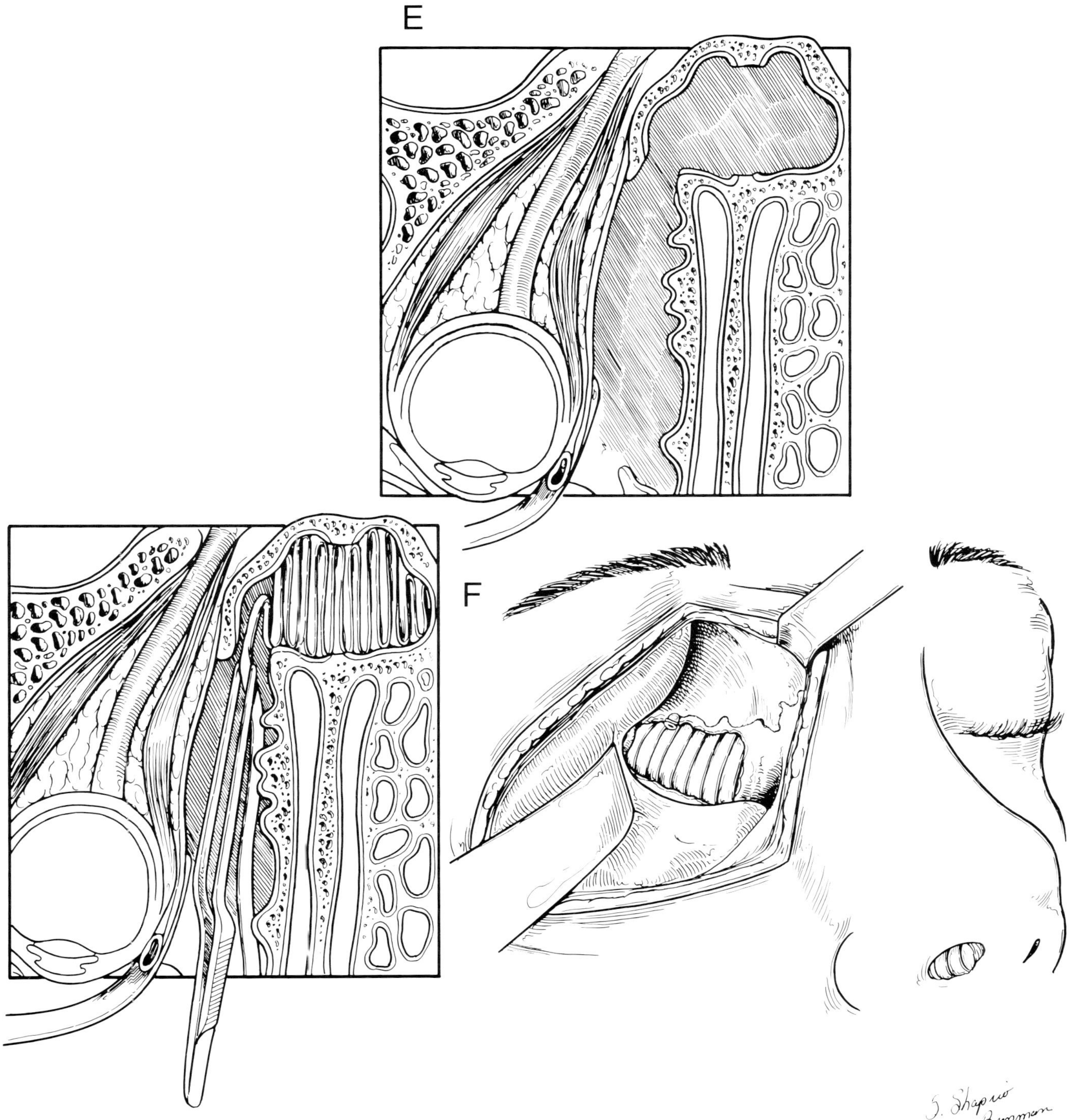

▶ **FIGURE 26-4**

# 27 ▶ Frontal Sinus

Frontal sinus infections are uncommon in young children because the frontal sinuses usually do not develop until the second decade of life.

## ▶ 27-1 FRONTAL SINUS TREPHINATION

Frontal sinus trephination is a procedure to drain the frontal sinus.

### Indications

Frontal sinus trephination is indicated in the treatment of acute frontal sinusitis that does not respond to medical management.

### Preoperative Evaluation

It is imperative to have computed tomograms of the frontal sinus to determine its exact location and extent.

### Operative Technique

1. Frontal sinus trephination is performed under general anesthesia.
2. One percent lidocaine with 1:100,000 epinephrine is injected subcutaneously and deep to the periosteum to help in hemostasis.
3. A curvilinear incision is outlined slightly below the eyebrow of the involved side and extending down to the level of the medial canthus (Fig. 27–1**A**).
4. The incision is carried through the skin, subcutaneous tissue, and periosteum with a #15 blade. Bleeding vessels are identified, clamped, and tied.
5. A periosteal elevator is used to elevate the periosteum superiorly and inferiorly so that the floor of the frontal sinus can be identified (Fig. 27–1**B**).
6. After careful consultation with the radiographs, the point of entry is determined as the floor of the frontal sinus is identified (Fig. 27–1**C**).
7. The sinus is entered using a small curette or bur until the sinus mucosa and secretions are identified (Fig. 27–1**D**). Care is taken not to damage the nasal frontal duct by perforating too medially and not to do any extensive dissection within the frontal sinus.
8. Secretions can be aspirated and sent for culture and sensitivity.
9. A 4 mm rubber or plastic catheter is placed through the trephination site (Figs. 27–1E and 27–1F).
10. The subcutaneous tissues are closed with 4-0 chromic suture and the skin is closed with interrupted 5-0 nylon sutures. The drain is sutured to adjacent skin and soft tissue.
11. The catheter is used to irrigate the sinus postoperatively until adequate drainage has been confirmed through the natural ostia of the nasal frontal duct. This can be confirmed by the patient tasting saline in his mouth or

seeing saline come out of the nose after it has been irrigated into the sinus through the irrigating catheter.

**12.** A broad-spectrum antibiotic is administered for 7 to 10 days.

## Complications

1. CSF leak
2. Nasofrontal duct injury

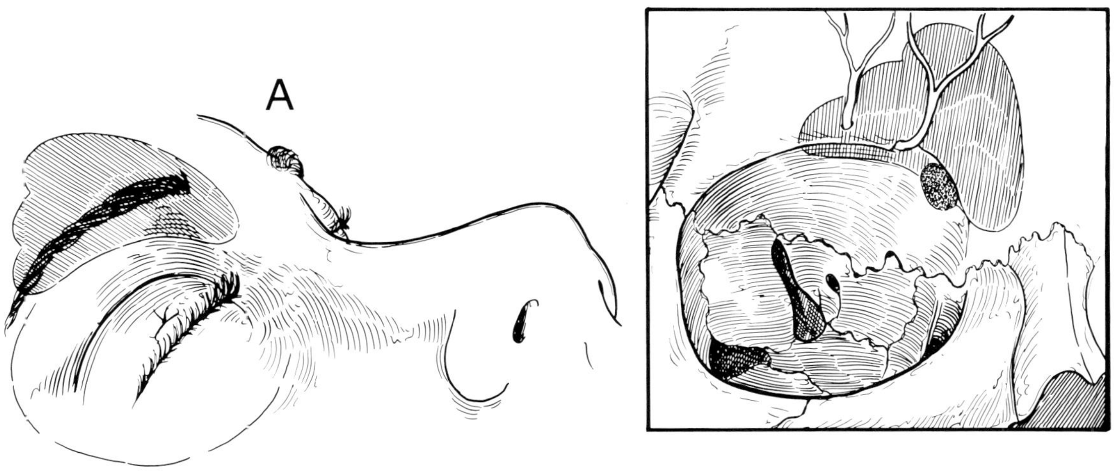


▶ **FIGURE 27-1**

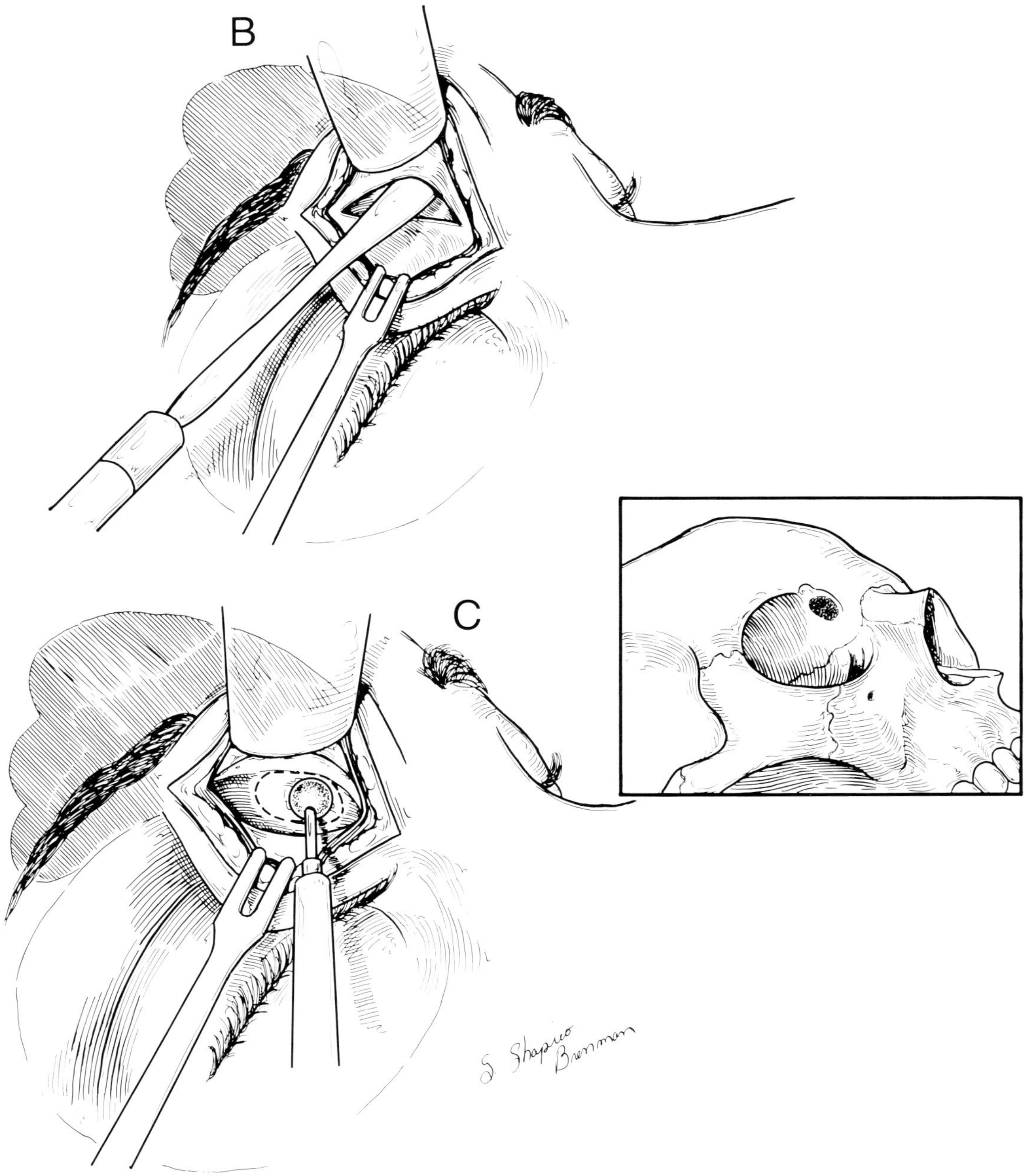


▶ **FIGURE 27-1**

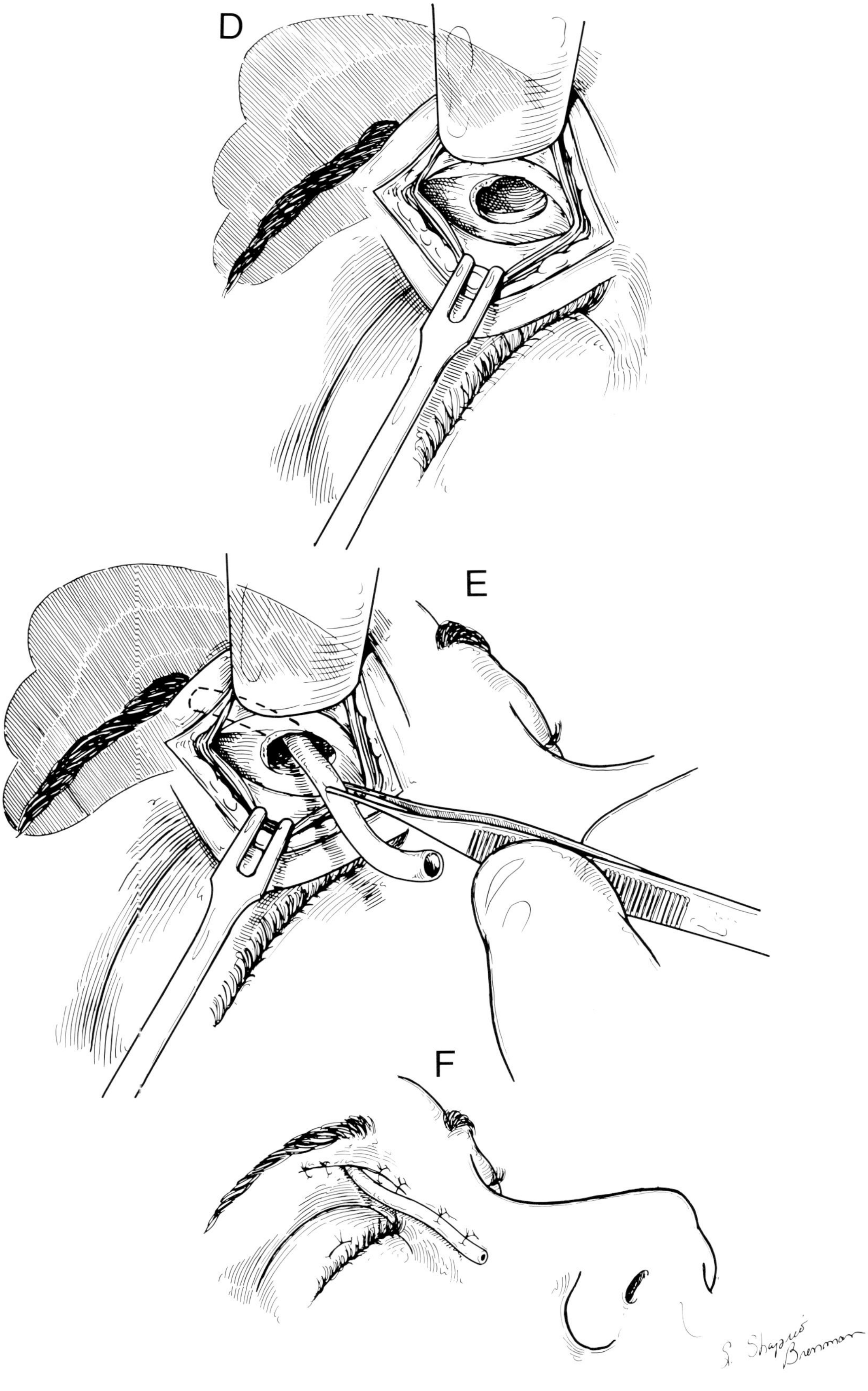


▶ **FIGURE 27-1**

## ▶ 27-2 FRONTAL SINUS OBLITERATION

Frontal sinus obliteration is a procedure used to treat chronic frontal sinusitis. The goal of this operation is to preserve cosmesis of the frontal bone while ensuring adequate treatment of chronic sinus disease by obliterating the sinus and the nasal frontal duct.

### Indications

Obliteration of the frontal sinus is indicated in the treatment of chronic frontal sinusitis with hypertrophic mucosal changes and mucocele. This technique is also very useful in the management of osteomas and fractures of the frontal sinus.

### Preoperative Evaluation

Sinus computed tomography (CT) scan is mandatory before frontal sinus surgery. A template of the frontal sinus is made from a standard Caldwell radiograph (Fig. 27–2**A**). This template is soaked in antiseptic solution to sterilize it.

### Operative Technique

1. The choice of coronal versus brow incision can be made depending upon the size of the frontal sinuses and the surgeon's preference (Fig. 27–2**B**). The coronal incision is most useful if the sinuses are large, but the incision in a male may be visible later as baldness progresses. The brow incision is adequate to approach the smaller frontal sinus but does involve a facial incision.
2. Frontal sinus obliteration is performed under general anesthesia. The anterior forehead and face are completely exposed, prepped, and draped. Bilateral tarsorrhaphy sutures are used to keep the lids closed and the corneas protected (Fig. 27–2**B**).
3. One percent lidocaine with 1:100,000 epinephrine is injected subcutaneously along the proposed incision site (either brow or coronal).
4. A #15 blade is used to incise the skin and subcutaneous tissue down to but not through the periosteum (Fig. 27–2**B**).
5. The skin and frontalis muscle are dissected from the underlying periosteum until the entire face of the frontal sinus is exposed (Fig. 27–2**C**). Hemostatic clamps may be placed on the skin edge to minimize blood loss.
6. When enough dissection of the subcutaneous tissue has been performed so that the sinus template can fit over the frontal bone, dissection is stopped. The template is placed over the periosteum and the outline of the sinus traced on the periosteum (Fig. 27–2**D**).
7. An incision through the periosteum is made approximately 5 mm superior to the edge of the sinus (Fig. 27–2**E**). This avoids the cosmetic depression that often accompanies the procedure when the bone and periosteal incisions lie on top of each other (Fig. 27–2**F** inset).
8. The periosteum overlying the frontal sinus is elevated inferiorly to approximately 1 cm past the superior margin of the sinus (Fig. 27–2**G, H**). Once again, the sinus x-ray template is used to determine the exact location of the superior margin of the sinus (Fig. 27–2**H**).

9. An oscillating saw or osteotome is used to make a beveled incision into the sinus superiorly and laterally (Fig. 27–2I). Care is taken to make sure the incision is into the sinus and not into the cranial cavity. It is also important to maintain an adequate periosteal connection inferiorly. A wide-blade chisel or elevator is used to elevate the anterior wall of the frontal sinus (Fig. 27–2J). Occasionally, it is necessary to use a chisel to sever its connection to an intersinus septum. The bone attached to its inferiorly based periosteal flap is elevated downward and the sinus exposed (Fig. 27–2K).
10. Treatment of the sinus can now proceed with removal of an osteoma, granulation tissue, or mucocele (Fig. 27–2K).
11. A cutting and diamond bur are used to remove all mucosa from the sinus (Fig. 27–2L). This is to ensure adequate mucosal removal and to prevent recurrence of sinus disease. Special attention is made to ensure complete cleansing around the area of the nasal frontal duct.
12. Abdominal fat from a left lower quadrant incision is used to fill the sinus cavity completely to prevent ingrowth of mucosa from the nose or nasal frontal duct (Fig. 27–2M).
13. The bony periosteal flap is replaced in its normal position. The periosteum is closed using interrupted 4-0 Vicryl suture (Fig. 27–2N). The coronal or brow incision is closed in two layers. The deep layer is closed with interrupted 4-0 chromic suture and the skin layer is closed with interrupted or running 4-0 nylon (for the coronal incision) or 5-0 nylon (for the brow incision) (Fig. 27–2O).
14. A drain is usually not required. However, a pressure dressing on the forehead area for 24 to 48 hours is recommended.
15. A broad-spectrum antibiotic is administered for 7 to 10 days.

## Complications

1. Dural laceration
2. CSF leak
3. Prominent visible scar
4. Recurrent mucocele

A

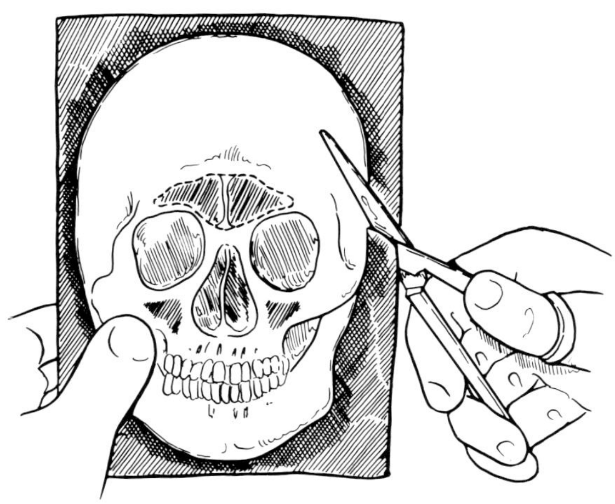

▶ **FIGURE 27-2**

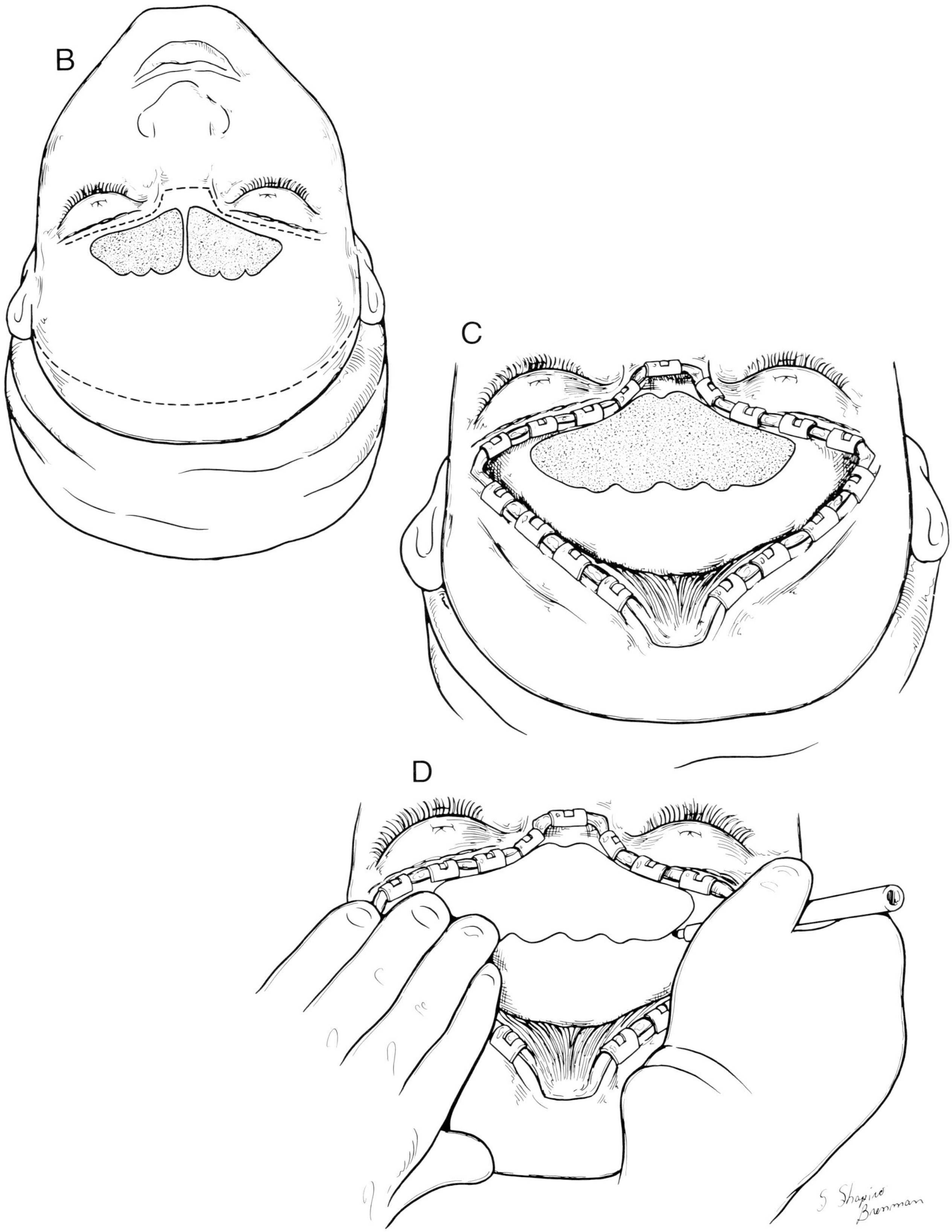


▶**FIGURE 27-2**

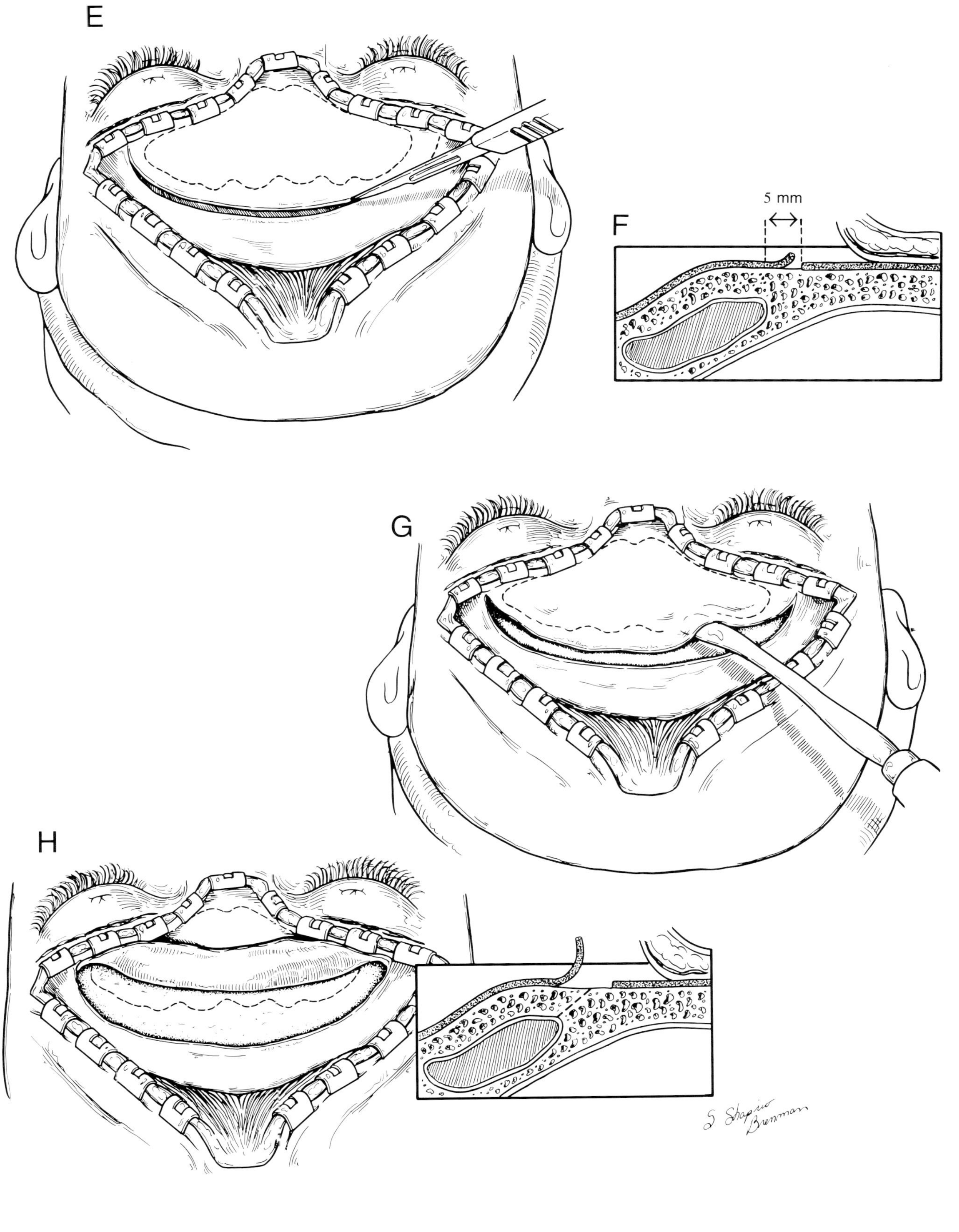


▶ **FIGURE 27-2**

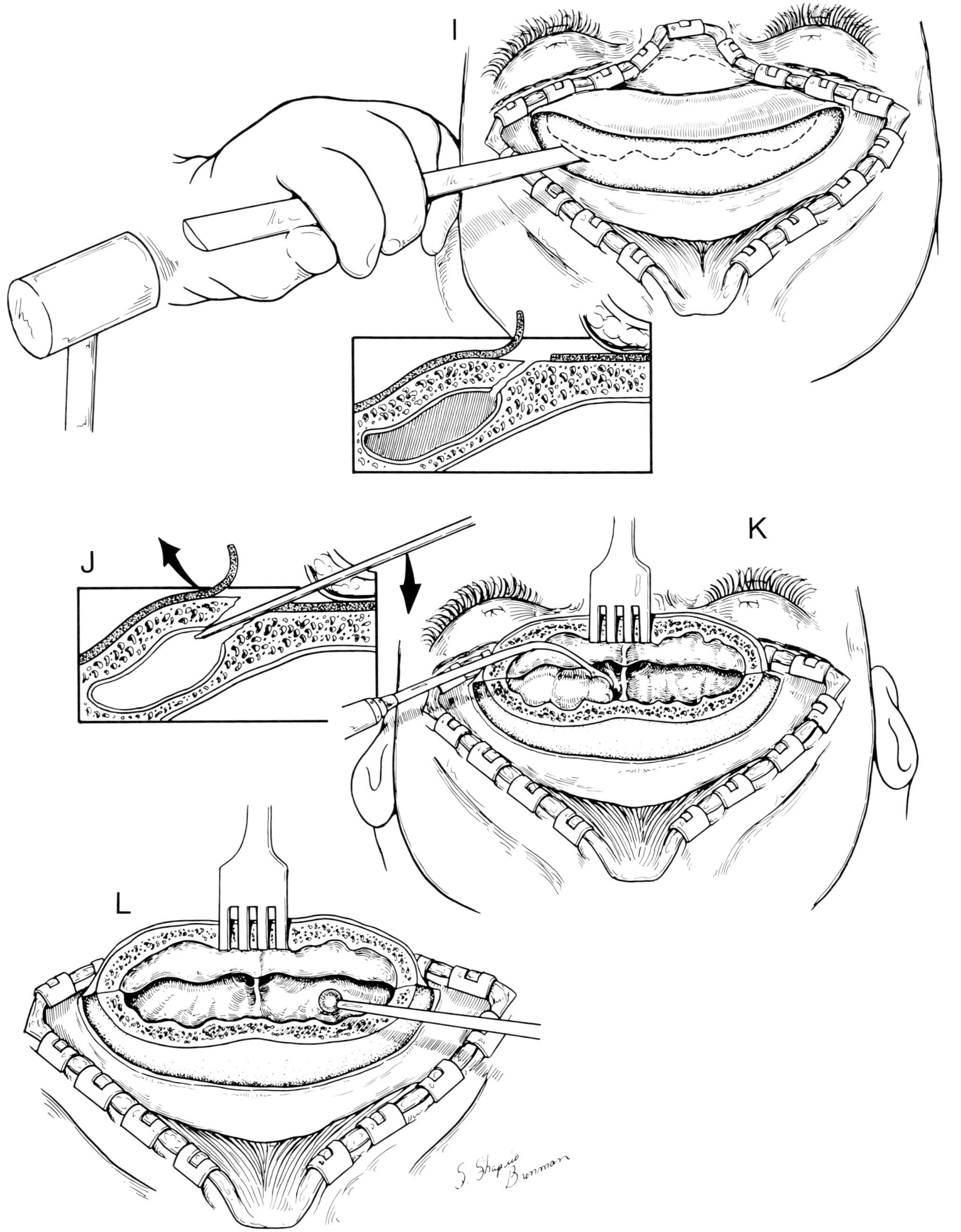


▶ **FIGURE 27-2**

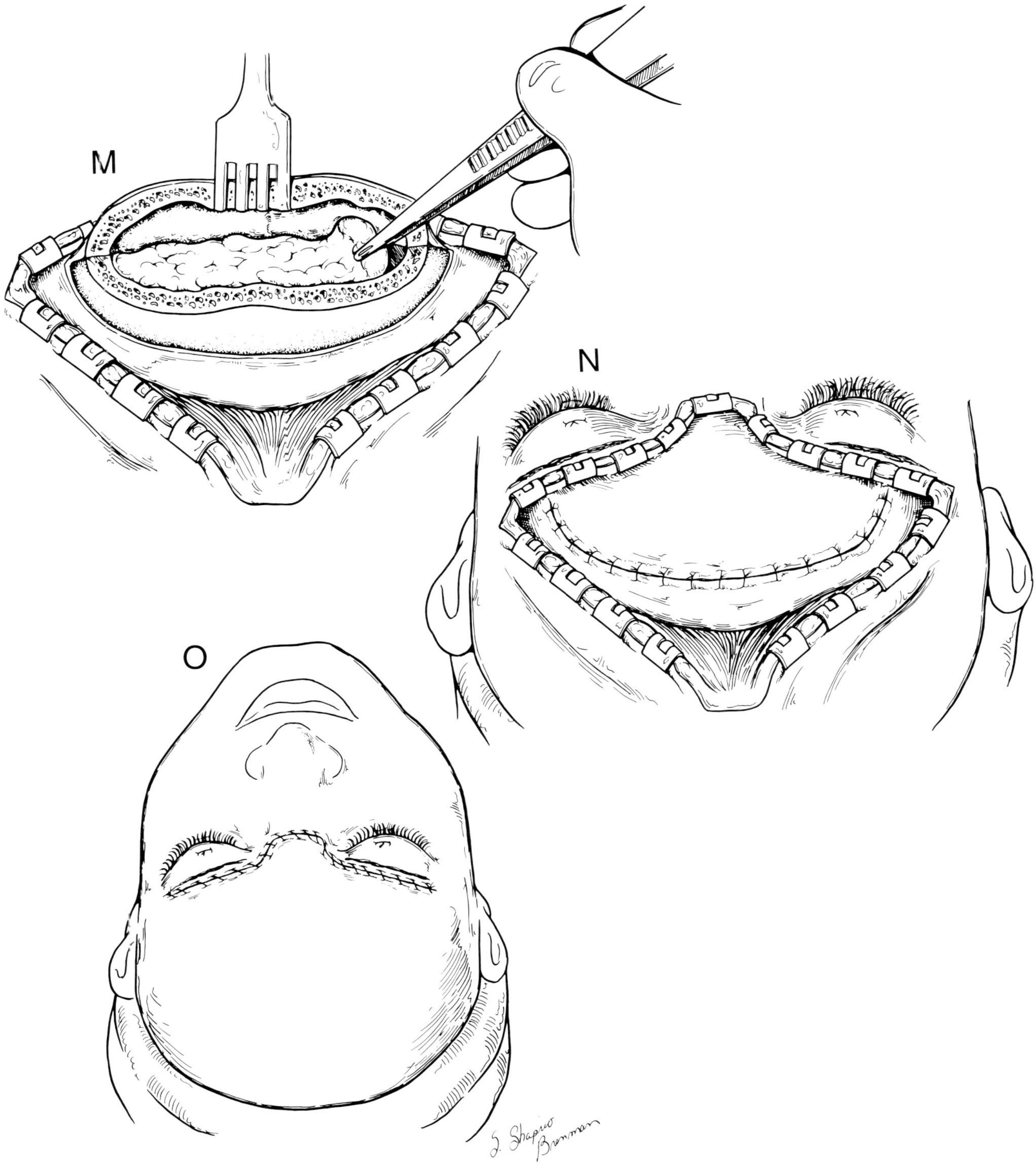


▶ **FIGURE 27-2**

# 28 ▸ Complications of Sinus Infection

The most common complication of sinus infection in children is a periorbital subperiosteal abscess. This is most often secondary to an ethmoid sinusitis, although sphenoid and frontal sinusitis can cause this condition.

## ▸ 28 - 1 DRAINAGE OF PERIORBITAL SUBPERIOSTEAL ABSCESS

### Indications

The presence of a periorbital subperiosteal abscess is the indication for surgical drainage. The presence of severe proptosis, restriction of extraocular motion, or changes in visual activity make drainage of the abscess urgent.

### Preoperative Evaluation

Computed tomography (CT) scan of the sinuses identifies involved sinuses and defines the location and size of the abscess. Magnetic resonance imaging (MRI) may be helpful to identify intracranial complications (e.g., cerebritis or abscess).

### Operative Technique

1. Under general anesthesia, the skin overlying the proposed incision is injected with 1% lidocaine with 1:100,000 epinephrine to reduce bleeding.
2. For a periorbital subperiosteal abscess in the frontal sinus region, the same incision described for frontal sinus trephination is used to drain the abscess and trephine the frontal sinus if desired (see section 27–1).
3. If the abscess is caused by ethmoid sinusitis, the incision and procedure described for external ethmoidectomy is employed (see section 25–3).
4. A drain may be placed in the abscess cavity and brought out through the incision. This is rarely required for an abscess caused by ethmoid disease because the abscess cavity is drained into the nose through the now widely opened ethmoid sinus system.
5. A broad-spectrum antibiotic is administered for 7 to 10 days.

### Complications

1. Recurrence of abscess
2. Complication of external ethmoidectomy (see section 25–3).

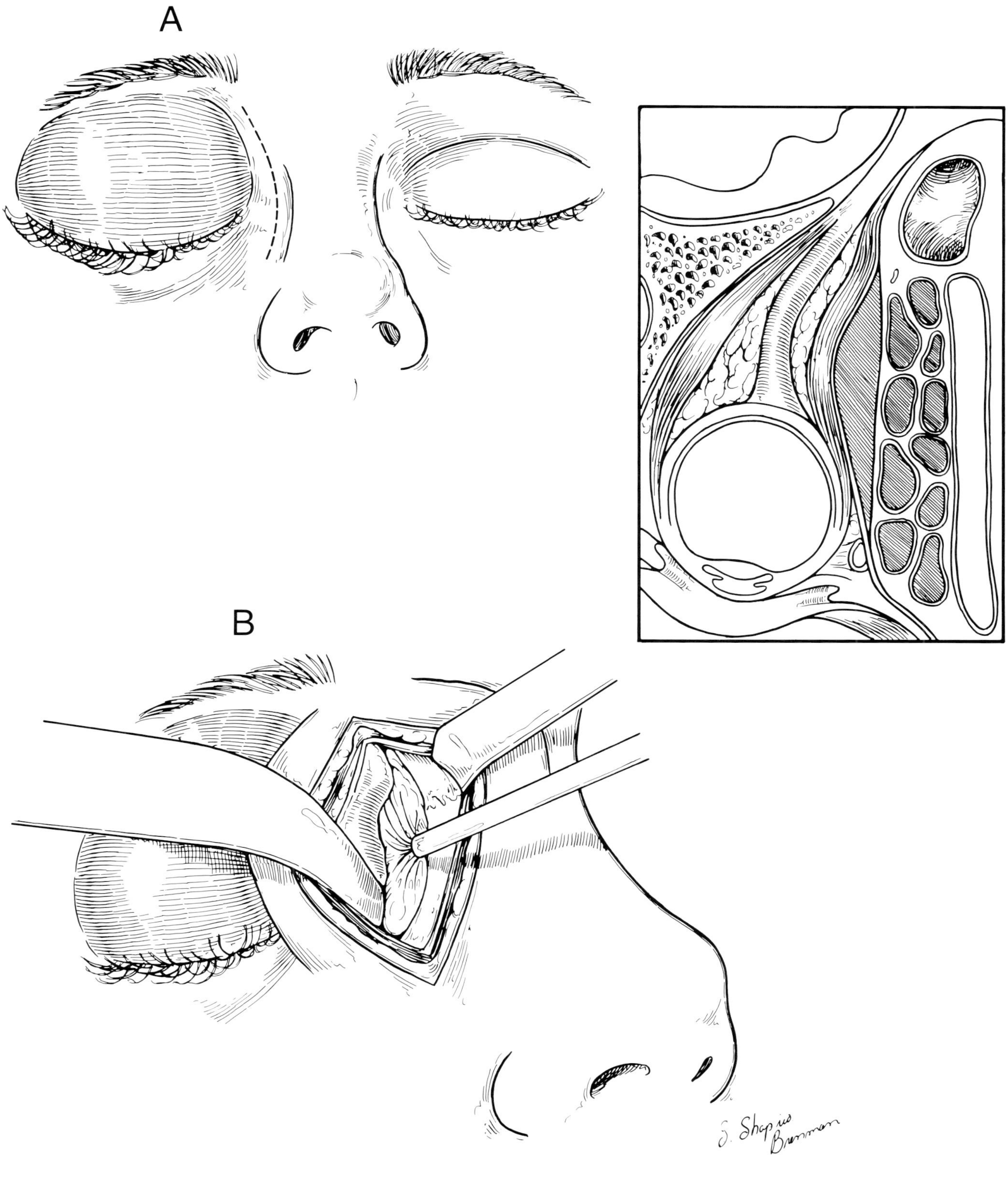


▶ **FIGURE 28-1**

# 29 ▶ Endoscopic Sinus Surgery (Rodney P. Lusk, M.D.)

## ▶ 29-1 ENDOSCOPIC MAXILLARY SINUSOTOMY AND ETHMOIDECTOMY

Endoscopic sinus surgery in children is an accepted option for treating chronic sinusitis. Availability of pediatric-sized instruments has facilitated the procedures in the small nasal cavities of children. The long-term effects are unknown and timing of the procedures remains controversial.

### Indications

Endoscopic sinus surgery is indicated for patients who have failed aggressive medical management with long-term broad-spectrum antibiotics and topical nasal steroid sprays. Patients should have sinus disease documented on computed tomography (CT) after 4 to 6 weeks of antibiotics. The effects of associated factors such as allergy, adenoidal hypertrophy, cystic fibrosis, gastroesophageal reflux, immune deficiency, and ciliary dyskinesia should be assessed and treated, if appropriate, prior to surgical intervention.

### Preoperative Evaluation

Preoperative examination includes outpatient anterior rhinoscopy with a telescope or an otoscope, and CT scan of the sinuses with coronal views to define the anatomy of the sinuses and extent of the sinus disease. The CT scan should be obtained after a course of at least 4 to 6 weeks of full-dose, broad-spectrum antibiotics therapy.

### Operative Technique

Endoscopic sinus surgery in children is best performed under general anesthesia. An oral RAE tube taped in the midline provides best access to the nose without distorting the face.

1. The patient is positioned with the head slightly elevated and turned to the right with the neck slightly extended. The patient is draped with eyes exposed. Lacri-Lube is placed in the eyes for protection (Fig. 29–1**A**).
2. The nasal cavity is vasoconstricted with 0.05% oxymetazoline (Afrin) on 3 × ½ inch neuropledgets on the side to be operated first (Fig. 29–1**B**). Care is taken to avoid mucosal abrasion when visually placing ½ × ½ inch pledgets into the middle meatus. The pledgets are left in place for 5 minutes.
3. The nasal cavity is examined with a 2.7-mm 0° telescope; a 30° telescope may also be used with care. The nasal cavity is examined all the way back to the nasopharynx (Figs. 29–1**C** and 29–1**D**); then the middle meatus is examined (Fig. 29–1**E**).
4. The middle turbinate may need to be reflected gently medially with a Freer elevator to introduce the telescope into the middle meatus (Fig. 29–1**F**).

5. The lateral wall of the nose, just anterior to the uncinate process, is injected under telescopic visualization with 1 to 2 cc of 1% lidocaine with 1:100,000 epinephrine using a retrobulbar needle bent 10° toward the bevel on a 3-cc syringe (Fig. 29–1G).

6. A ½ × ½ inch neuropledget with 0.05% oxymetazoline is then placed in the middle meatus for an additional 5 to 7 minutes.

7. The middle turbinate is again reflected medially with a Freer elevator exposing the middle meatus for complete examination with a 0° telescope (Fig. 29–1G).

8. The uncinate process and ethmoid bulla are identified. The uncinate process and the infundibulum are palpated with a Lusk seeker. The uncinate process moves with gentle pressure (Fig. 29–1H).

9. If a concha bullosa is present, the middle turbinate is injected with 1% lidocaine with 1:100,000 epinephrine (Figs. 29–1I and 29–1J), and an incision is made on the anterior face of the middle turbinate with a sickle knife.

10. The lateral wall of the bulla is removed with a scissors and sharp straight-biting forceps, taking care to preserve the medial mucosa of the remaining middle turbinate (Fig. 29–1K).

11. An incision is made with a sickle knife along the anterior lateral attachment of the uncinate process into the infundibulum. The incision extends through the uncinate process from its inferior limit to the break point just below the root of the middle turbinate. This prevents tearing of mucosa of the middle turbinate (Fig. 29–1L).

12. The uncinate process is removed with a small cup forceps exposing the ethmoid bulla (Fig. 29–1M). The uncinate process may also be removed by first cutting a window in the uncinate with a back bitter (Fig. 29–1La,b). The maxillary sinus ostium can be visualized and the remainder of the uncinate process is removed with the seeker (Fig. 29–1Lc).

13. The natural ostium of the maxillary sinus is identified with a seeker and a 30° telescope. The ostium lies in the anterior inferior part of the infundibulum. The uncinate process must be completely removed to see the ostium. The remaining mucosa may be removed along the uncinate with forceps or powered instrumentation (microdebrider) (Fig. 29–1N).

14. After the ostium is identified, if there is no mucosal disease, it is left alone.

15. If disease is present, the ostium is enlarged into the posterior fontanella.

16. The posterior fontanelle is cut with a scissors or through-biting forceps posteriorly and inferiorly. A small portion of the anterior fontanelle may be removed in revision cases, but care must be taken not to injure the nasolacrimal duct (Fig. 29–1O).

17. The bone and lateral nasal mucosa are removed with a forceps. The mucosa of the maxillary sinus is reflected over the inferior edge of the enlarged maxillary antrostomy and removed with forceps or a microdebrider (Fig. 29–1P). Care is taken not to perform a large antrostomy.

18. The anterior inferior medial portion of the ethmoid bulla is entered with a "J" curette. The bulla is further opened by moving the curette upward and anteriorly toward the surgeon (Fig. 29–1Q).

**19.** A 45° Blakesly or sharp-cutting forceps is used to remove the anterior face of the ethmoid bulla (Fig. 29–1**R**).

**20.** The medial wall of the bulla is then removed with cutting forceps to the sinus lateralis or its attachment to the middle turbinate. This identifies the basal lamella (Fig. 29–1**S**).

**21.** The remainder of the ethmoid bulla mucosa and cells are removed with a straight-cup forceps using a 30° telescope to identify the lamina papyracea (LP) (Fig. 29–1**T**). The lamina papyracea is smooth and has a yellow tint, and should not be penetrated.

**22.** The basal lamella is the anterior wall of the posterior ethmoid cells. The basal lamella is fractured with a "J" curette and dissection continues in the posterior ethmoid cells at the inferior medial region (Fig. 29–1**U**).

**23.** The posterior ethmoid cells are opened with a "J" curette by an inferior to superior dissection. Mucosa and septa are removed with an appropriate forceps (Fig. 29–1**V**).

**24.** The roof of the ethmoid sinus can be most easily identified in the posterior ethmoid cells. The dissection is carried anteriorly along the roof of the ethmoid sinus to the frontal recess. Mucosa is preserved along the roof of the ethmoid to promote better healing.

**25.** Dissection in the region of the frontal recess should be limited to avoid injury to the developing frontal sinus region.

**26.** If needed, the sphenoid sinus is entered through the natural ostium of the sphenoid sinus (Fig. 29–1**W**).

**27.** The sphenoid ostium may be visualized (occasionally, with some difficulty) by reflecting the middle and superior turbinate laterally with an elevator to establish the level of the sphenoid ostium. The inferior half of the superior turbinate can be removed to improve exposure to the natural ostium.

**28.** The opposite side, if necessary, is then operated on in the same fashion.

**29.** Nasal secretions are then suctioned clear from both nasal cavities.

**30.** A small roll of moistened Gelfilm may be placed in each middle meatus to prevent adhesion of the middle turbinate to the lateral wall of the nose (Fig. 29–1**X**).

**31.** The patient is maintained on antibiotics for 2 to 3 weeks and returned to the operating room to remove the Gelfilm endoscopically and to debride the healing cavities. Granulation tissue in the region of the frontal recess and maxillary ostium is removed with a forceps. Granulation tissue in the ethmoid cavity is left alone. Adhesions between the middle turbinate and lateral wall of the nose should be divided.

**32.** If indicated, a ½-sheet roll of Gelfilm may be placed in the middle meatus and left to dissolve spontaneously.

**33.** The patient remains on steroid nasal sprays, antibiotics, and saline nasal drops until seen in the office in 2 to 3 weeks, or until the cavities are adequately healed.

## Complications

1. Recurrence of disease
2. Intranasal complications
   Scarring of frontal recess

Scarring of maxillary sinus ostium
Adhesion between the middle turbinate and lateral wall of the nose

3. Orbital injury
   Diplopia
   Blindness
   Hematoma
   Infection
   Epiphora
4. Intracranial complications
   CSF rhinorrhea
   Intracranial trauma
   Meningitis

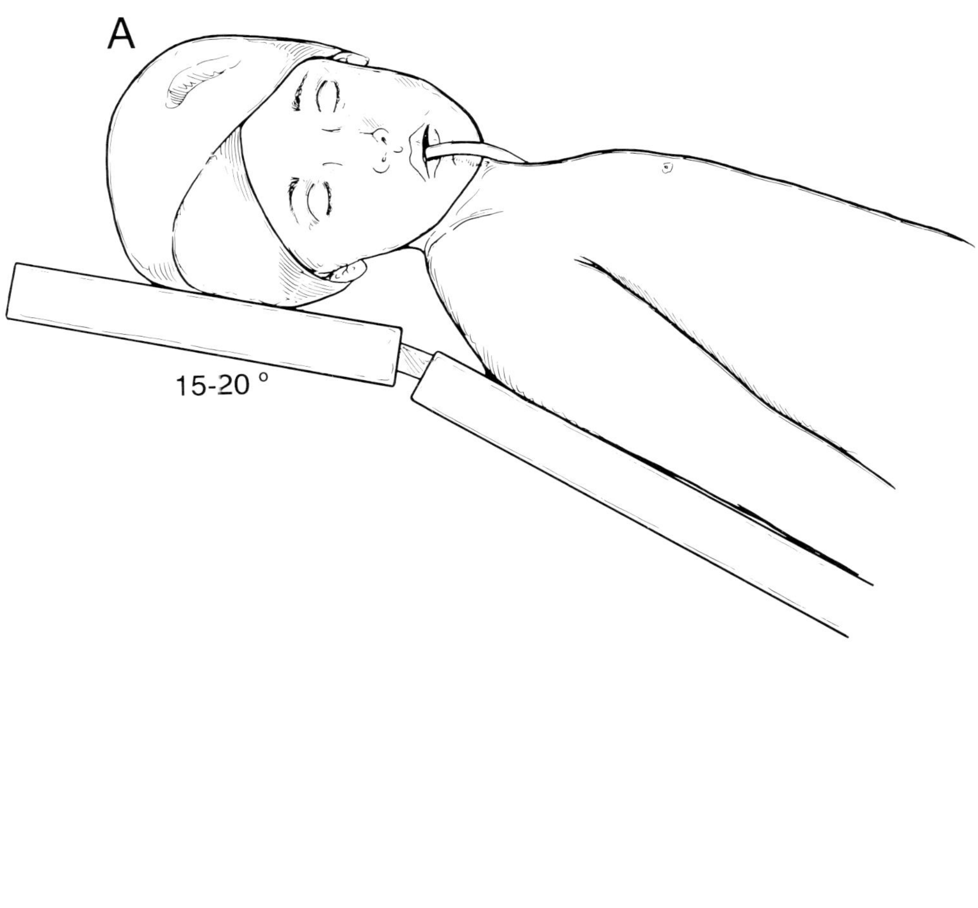


▶ **FIGURE 29-1**

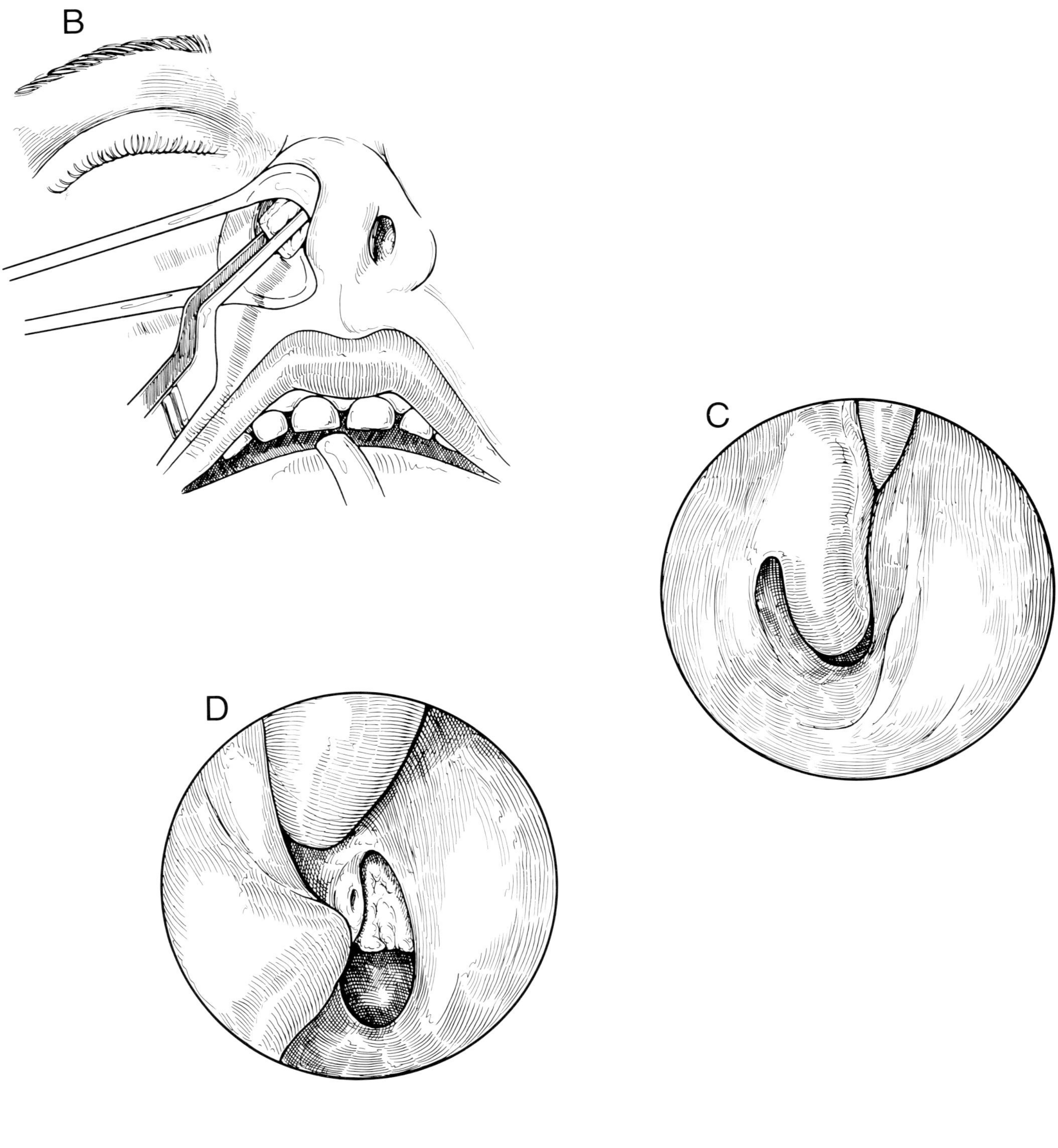


▶ **FIGURE 29-1**

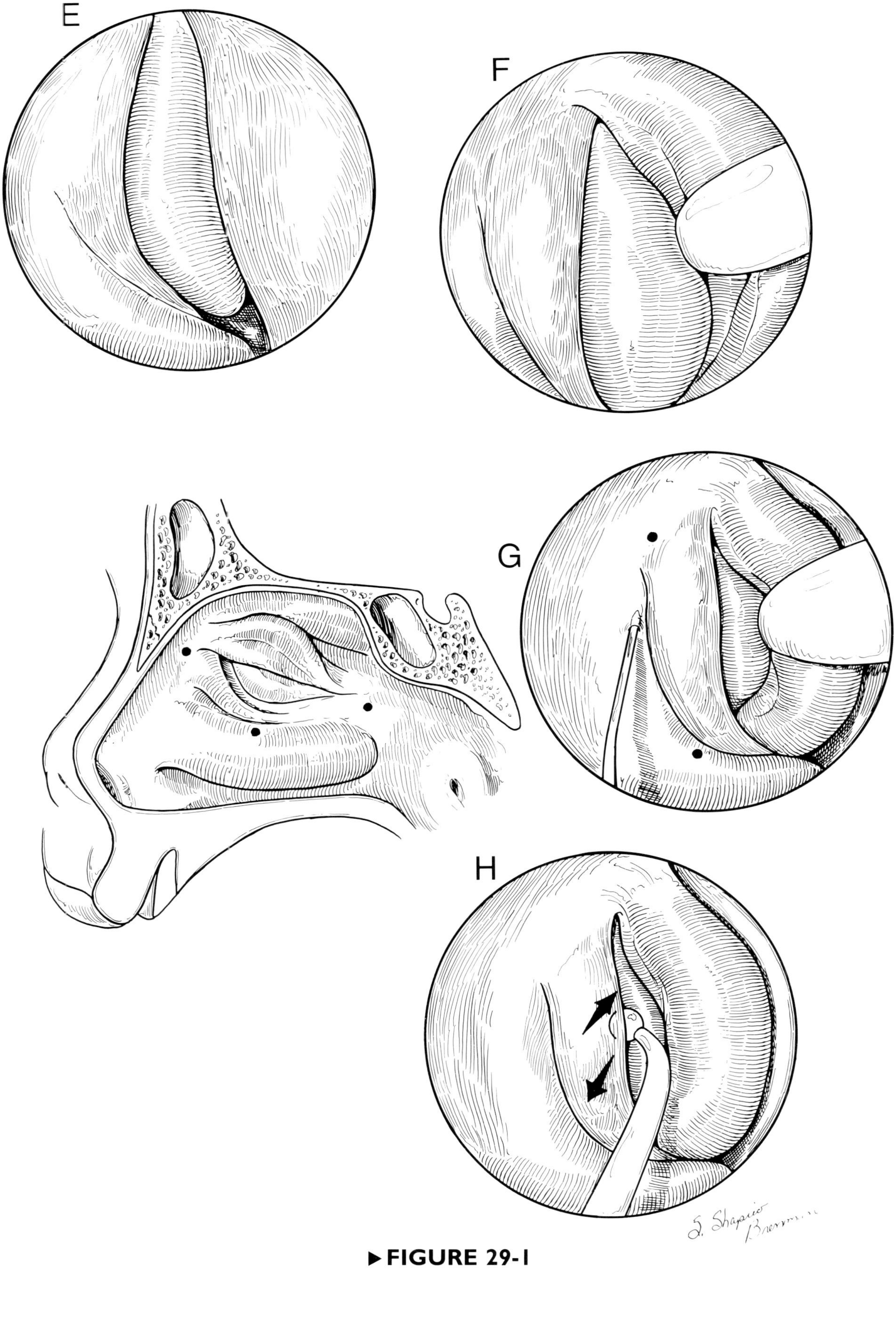


▶ **FIGURE 29-1**

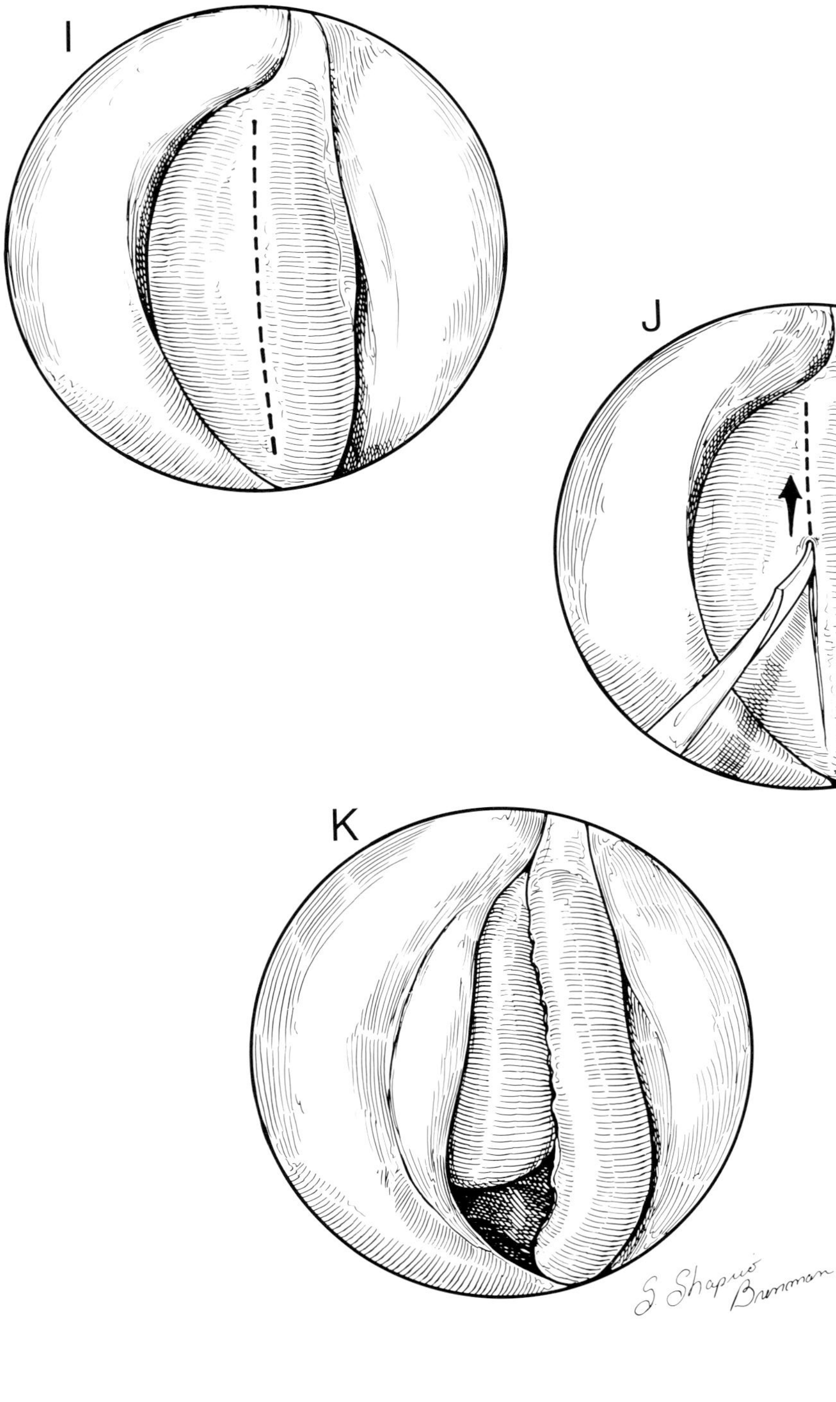


▶ **FIGURE 29-1**

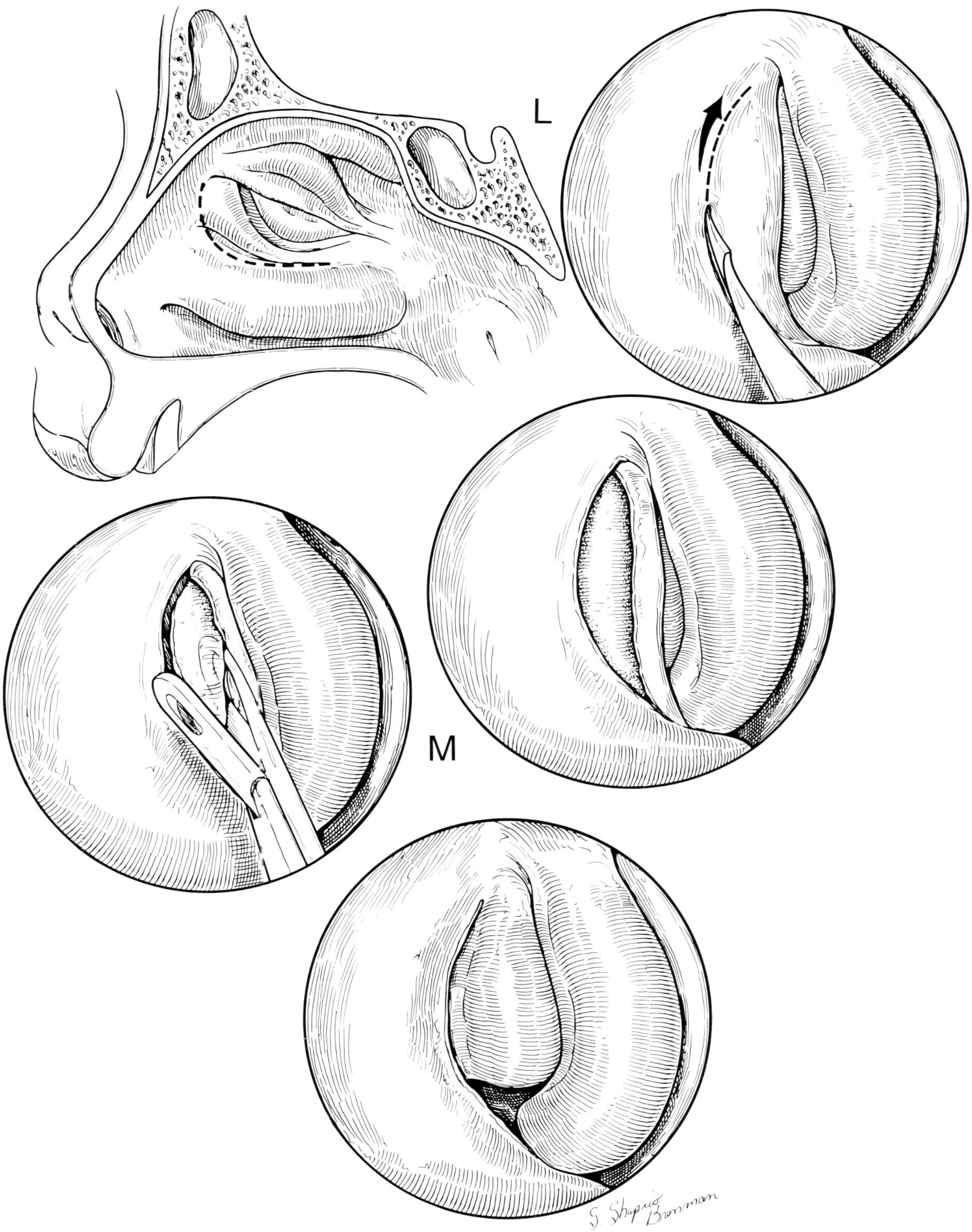


▶ **FIGURE 29-1**

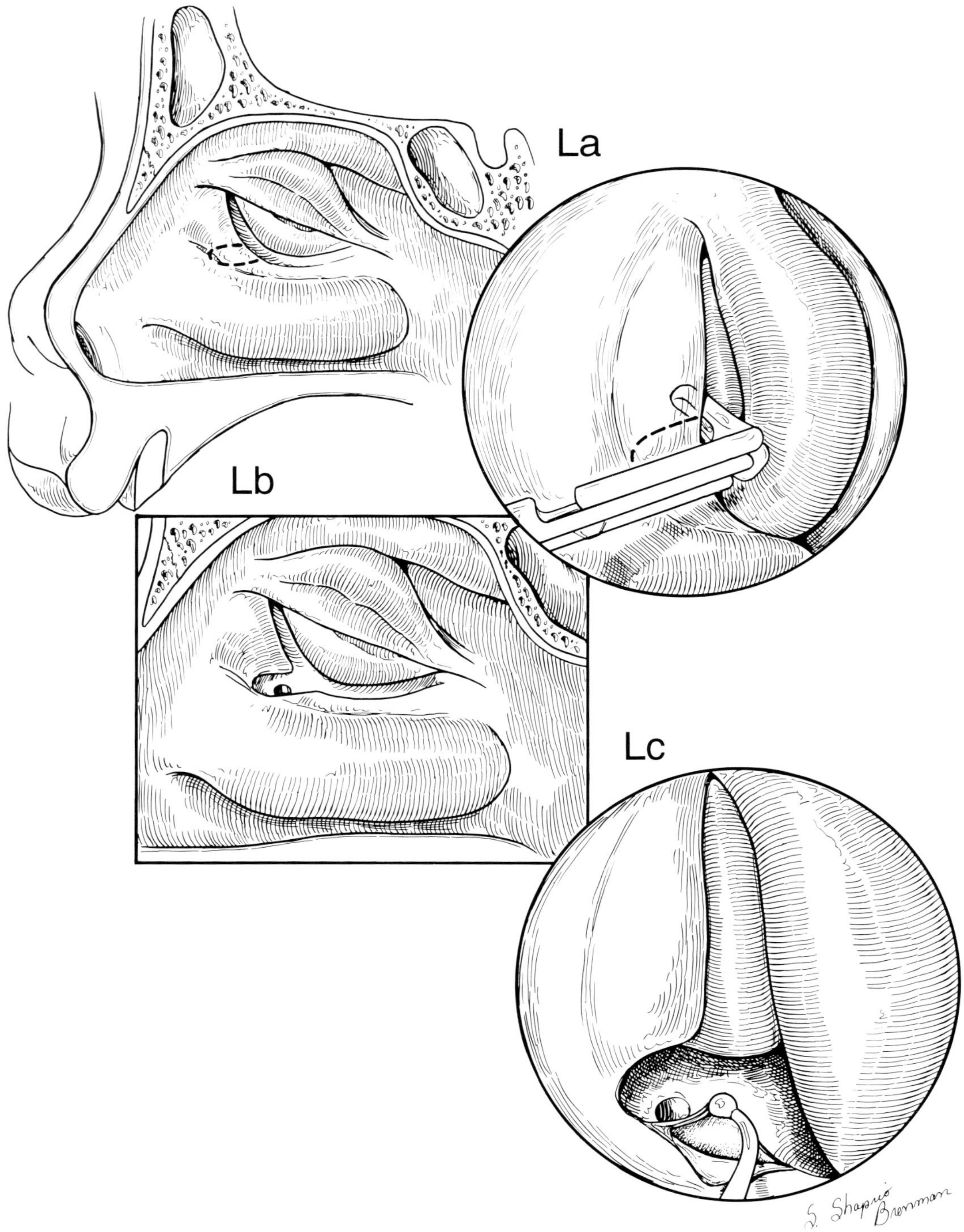


▶ **FIGURE 29-1**

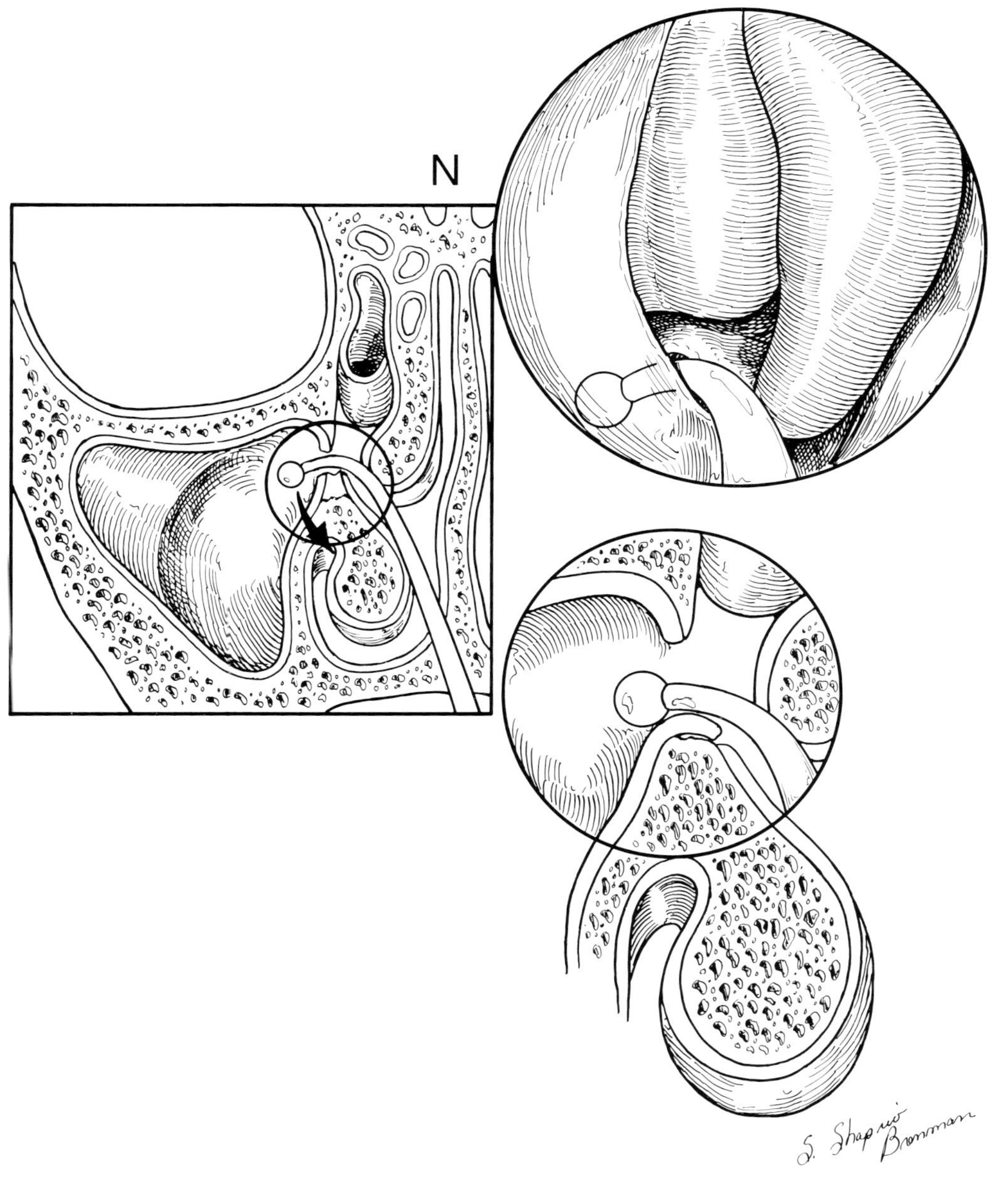


▶ **FIGURE 29-1**

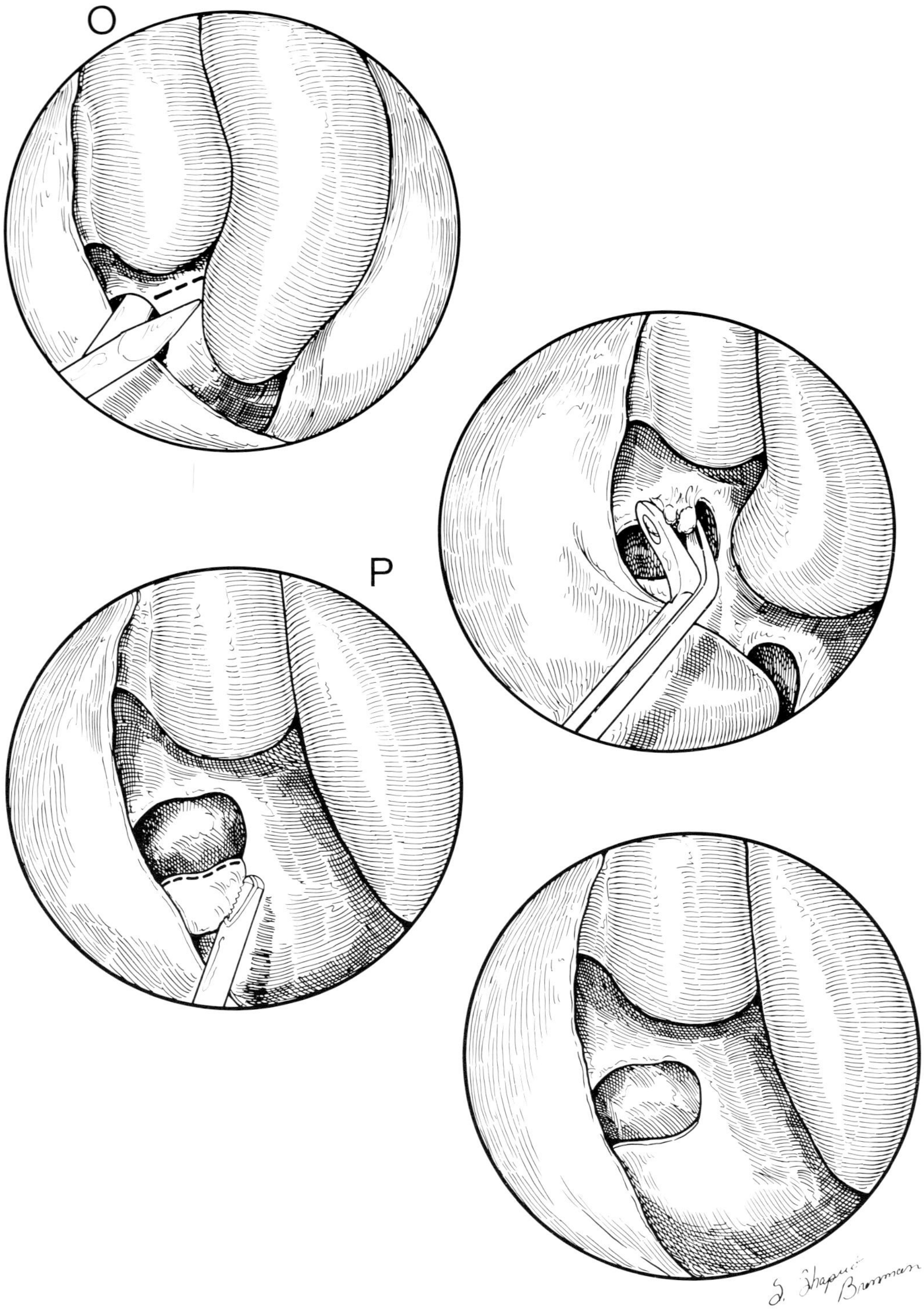


▶ **FIGURE 29-1**

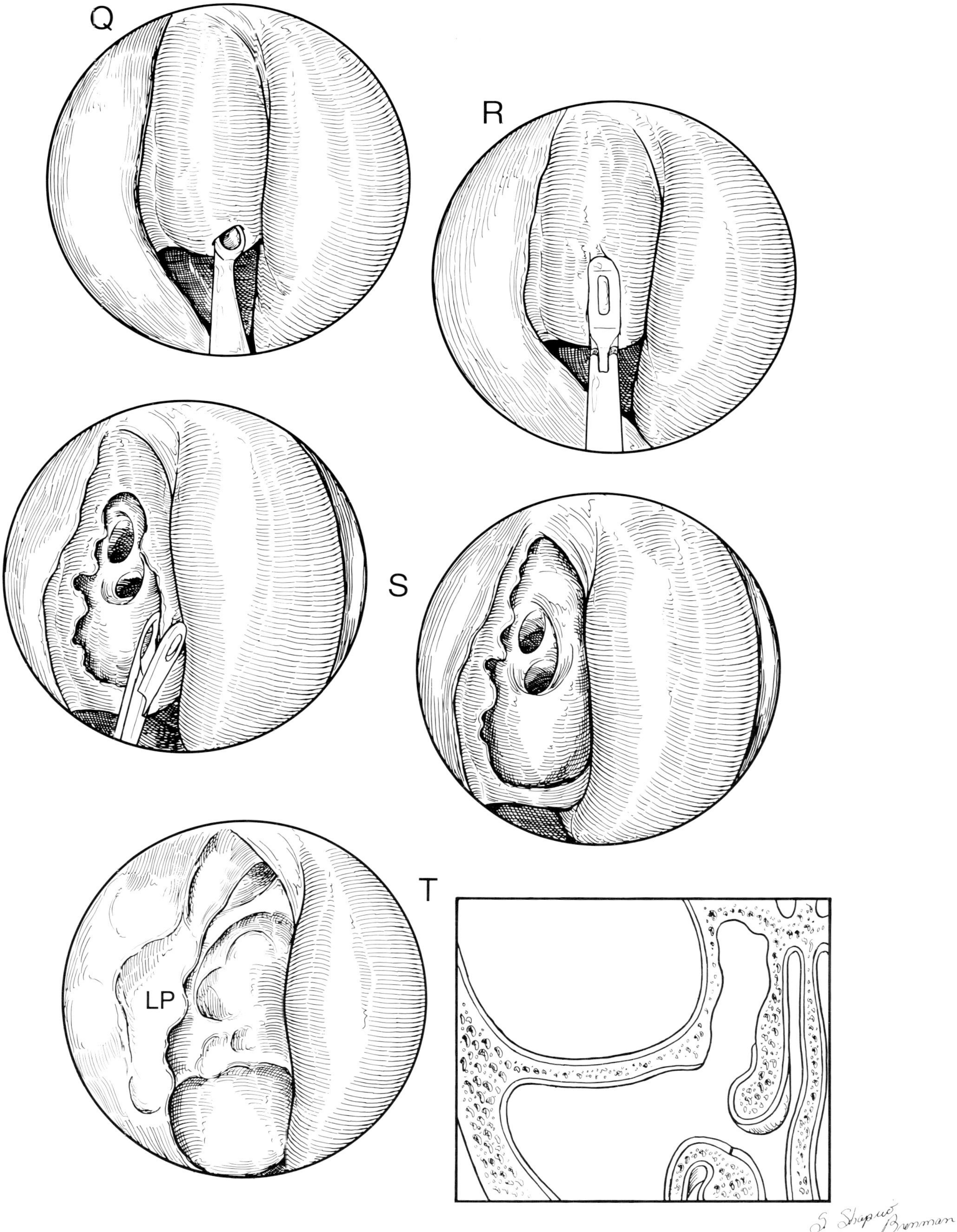


▶ **FIGURE 29-1**

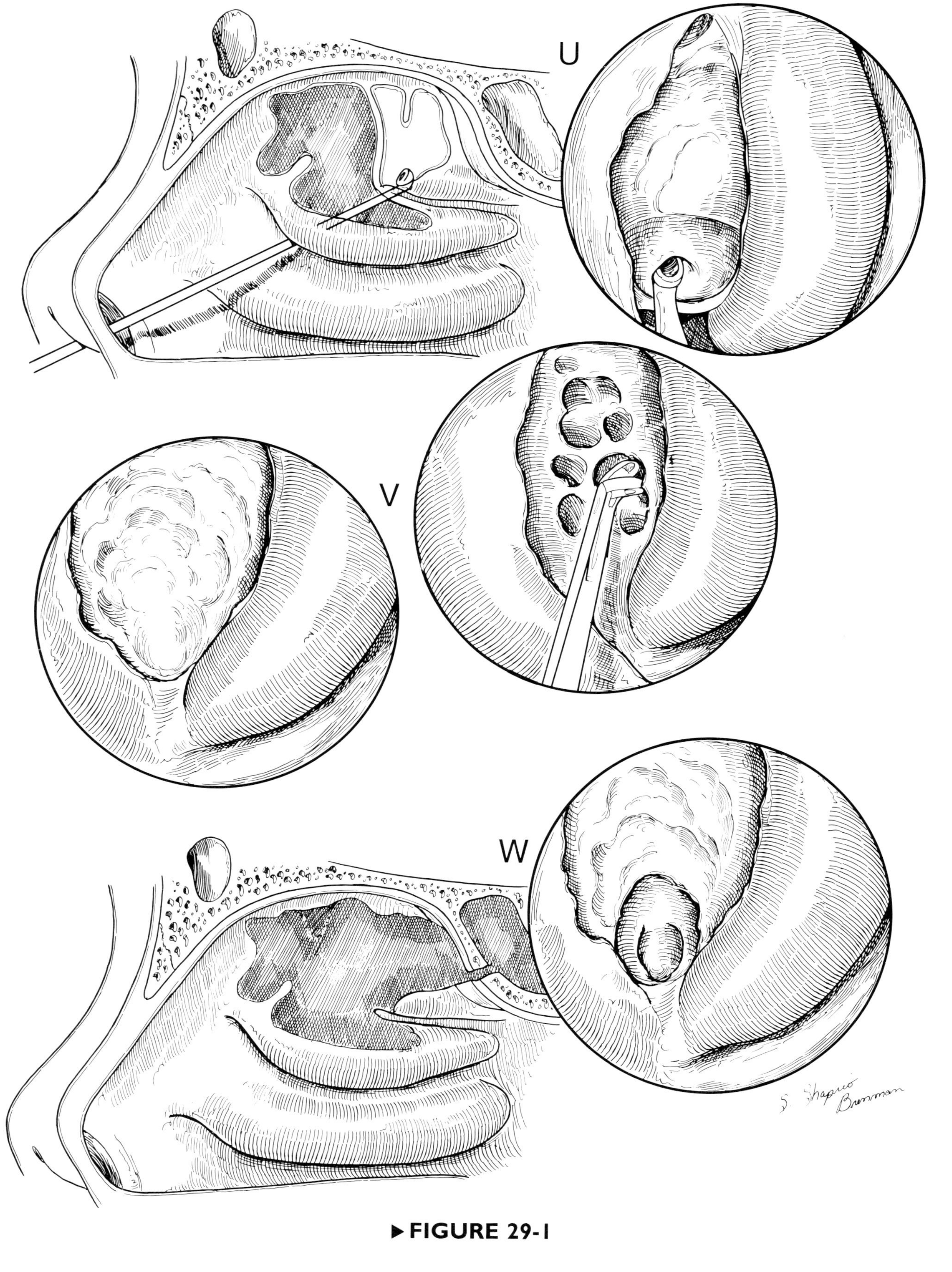


▶ **FIGURE 29-1**

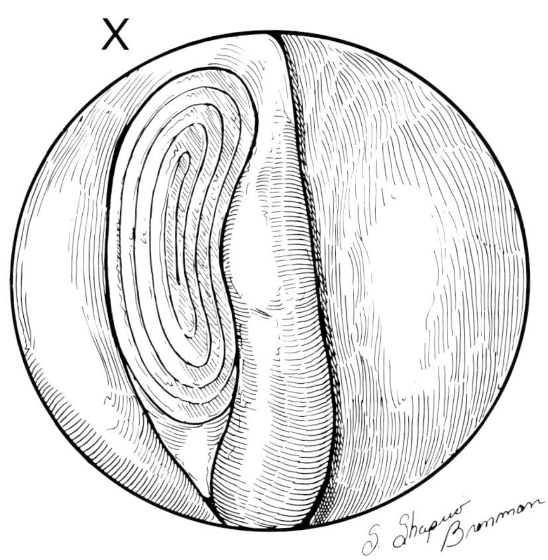


▶ **FIGURE 29-1**

# PART V

# The Neck

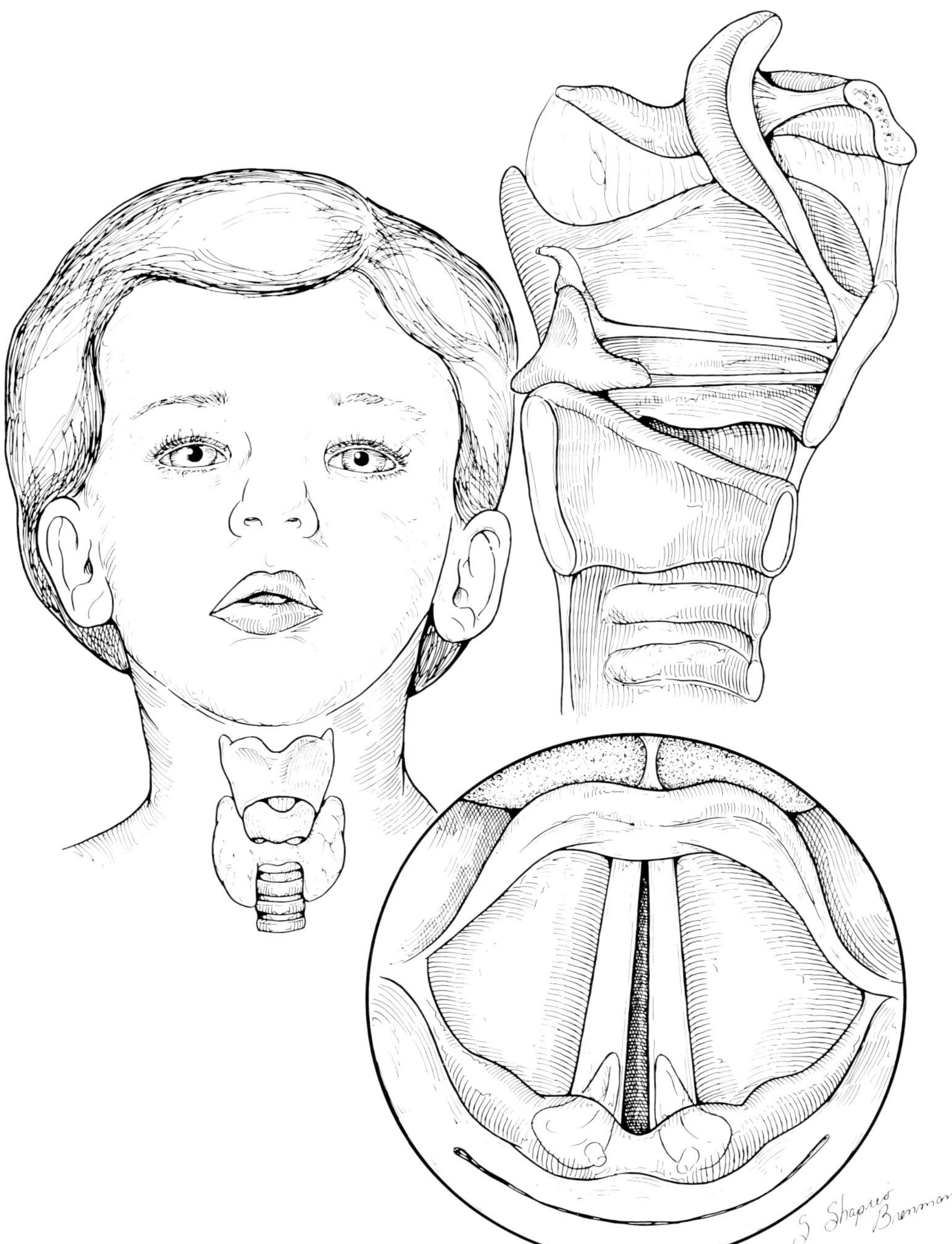

# 30 ▸ Trachea

## ▸ 30-1 TRACHEOTOMY

Tracheotomy is performed to provide access and ventilation through the trachea. In addition to bypassing the larynx, it allows easy clearing of secretions and a safe route for prolonged assisted ventilation.

### Indications

Tracheotomy is indicated to bypass the upper airway in conditions where upper airway obstruction causes inadequate ventilation. Tracheotomy permits a safe, comfortable route for prolonged, assisted ventilation and access to the airway to facilitate tracheobronchial toilet.

### Preoperative Evaluation

A preoperative chest radiograph is helpful to define the preoperative condition of the lungs and to compare to postoperative films.

### Operative Technique

1. Tracheotomy should be performed, if possible, with the patient intubated, under general anesthesia, and paralyzed.
2. If a bronchoscope is preferred, it is introduced after a satisfactory plane of anesthesia and relaxation is achieved (Fig. 30–1**A**,**B**).
3. If an endotracheal tube is in place and a bronchoscope is preferred, the bronchoscope is advanced into the trachea as the endotracheal tube is removed.
4. Nasogastric tubes and esophageal stethoscopes are removed prior to positioning the patient to avoid firm objects in the neck that may be confused with the trachea during palpation.
5. The child is positioned on a shoulder roll, with the neck extended and the occiput stabilized (Fig. 30–1**C**).
6. One percent lidocaine with 1:100,000 epinephrine is injected subcutaneously at the site of the incision to aid in hemostasis.
7. A horizontal skin incision is made halfway between the cricoid and the sternal notch (Fig. 30–1**D**).
8. Subcutaneous fat and tissue are reflected with a clamp, exposing the deep cervical fascia overlying the strap muscles, and ribbon retractors are placed to expose the field as well as to stabilize the trachea in the midline (Fig. 30–1**E**).
9. Vertical dissection with a scissors and clamp in the midline is carried out until the trachea is exposed (Fig. 30–1**E**,**F**).
10. Retractors are used to reflect the strap muscles and visualize the tracheal rings (Fig. 30–1**G**).

11. If the thyroid isthmus is encountered over the trachea, it may be reflected superiorly with a retractor or divided with a Bovie to provide better tracheal exposure (Fig. 30–1F).
12. Throughout the procedure, palpation of the trachea and laryngeal structures helps maintain the surgeon's orientation.
13. 4-0 nonabsorbable sutures are placed in the trachea on each side of the midline (Fig. 30–1G). These sutures are placed securely through the cartilage rings and are used for traction to expose the trachea should accidental decannulation occur before the tract is established.
14. The skin flaps are defatted with a Bovie (Fig. 30–1H).
15. The lateral retractors are removed and the trachea is elevated by traction on the stay sutures. A midline incision is made through 2 or 3 cartilage rings, opening the trachea (Fig. 30–1I). The bronchoscope or endotracheal tube can be seen in the tracheal lumen.
16. The skin flaps are sutured to the edges of the tracheotomy for safety in the event of accidental decannulation (Fig. 30–1J).
17. The endotracheal tube is withdrawn to just above the tracheal incision (Fig. 30–1K).
18. A suitably-sized age appropriate tracheostomy tube is inserted in the trachea (Fig. 30–1L).
19. After satisfactory ventilation is established through the tracheostomy tube, the bronchoscope is removed. If an endotracheal tube is used, it is left in place above the tracheostomy tube until a chest x-ray is later done to confirm the position of the tip of the tube and absence of a pneumothorax.
20. The stay sutures are clearly labelled for identification and taped to their respective side of the chest for use if decannulation occurs (Fig. 30–1M).
21. The tracheotomy tube is securely tied in place with tracheostomy tape while the head is in the neutral position (Fig. 30–1N).
22. A tracheostomy dressing is applied to the wound.
23. A postoperative AP chest radiograph is obtained to determine the position of the tip of the tube near the coria and to check for pneumothorax.

## Complications

1. Hemorrhage
2. Pneumothorax
3. Subcutaneous emphysema

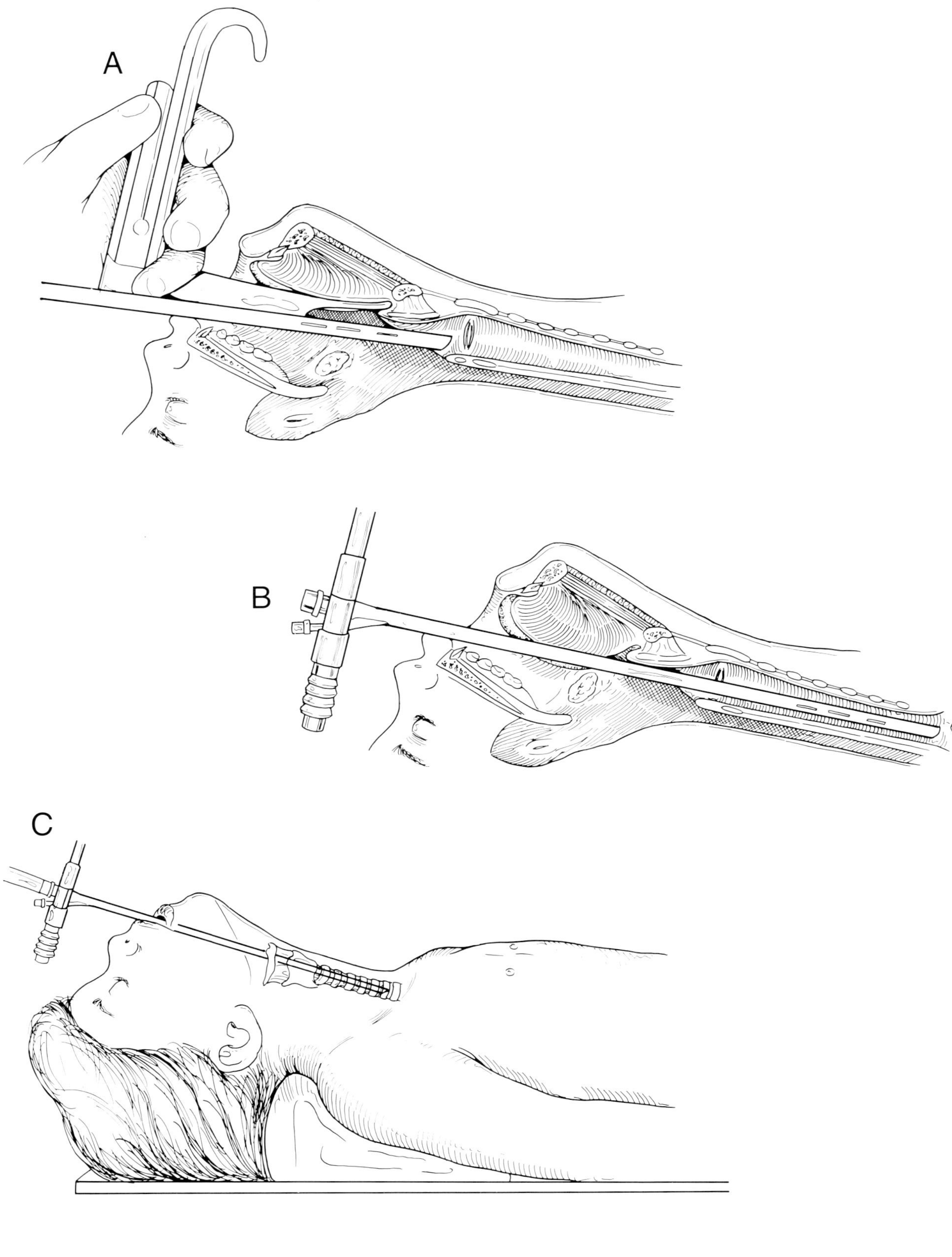


▸ **FIGURE 30-1**

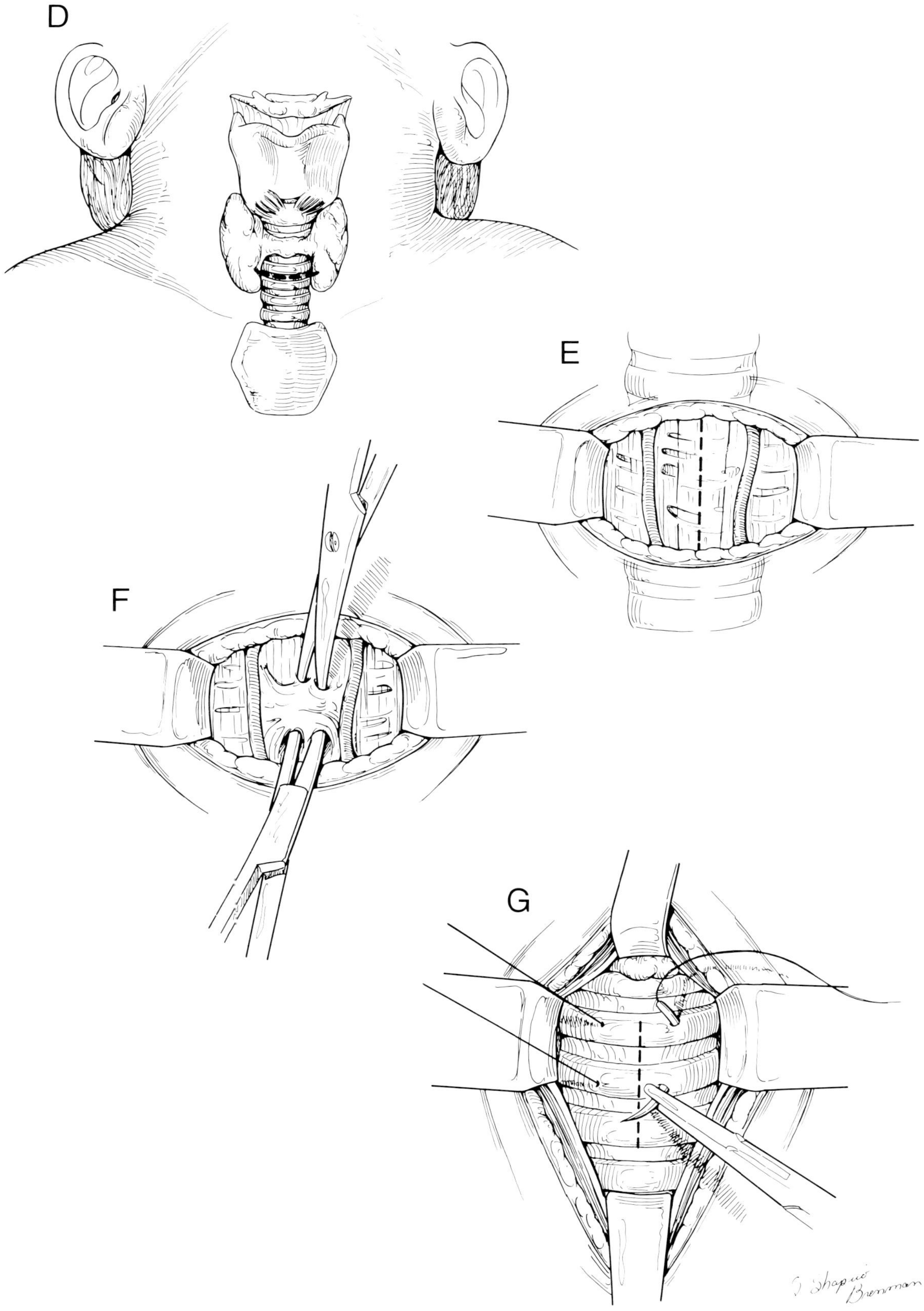


▶ **FIGURE 30-1**

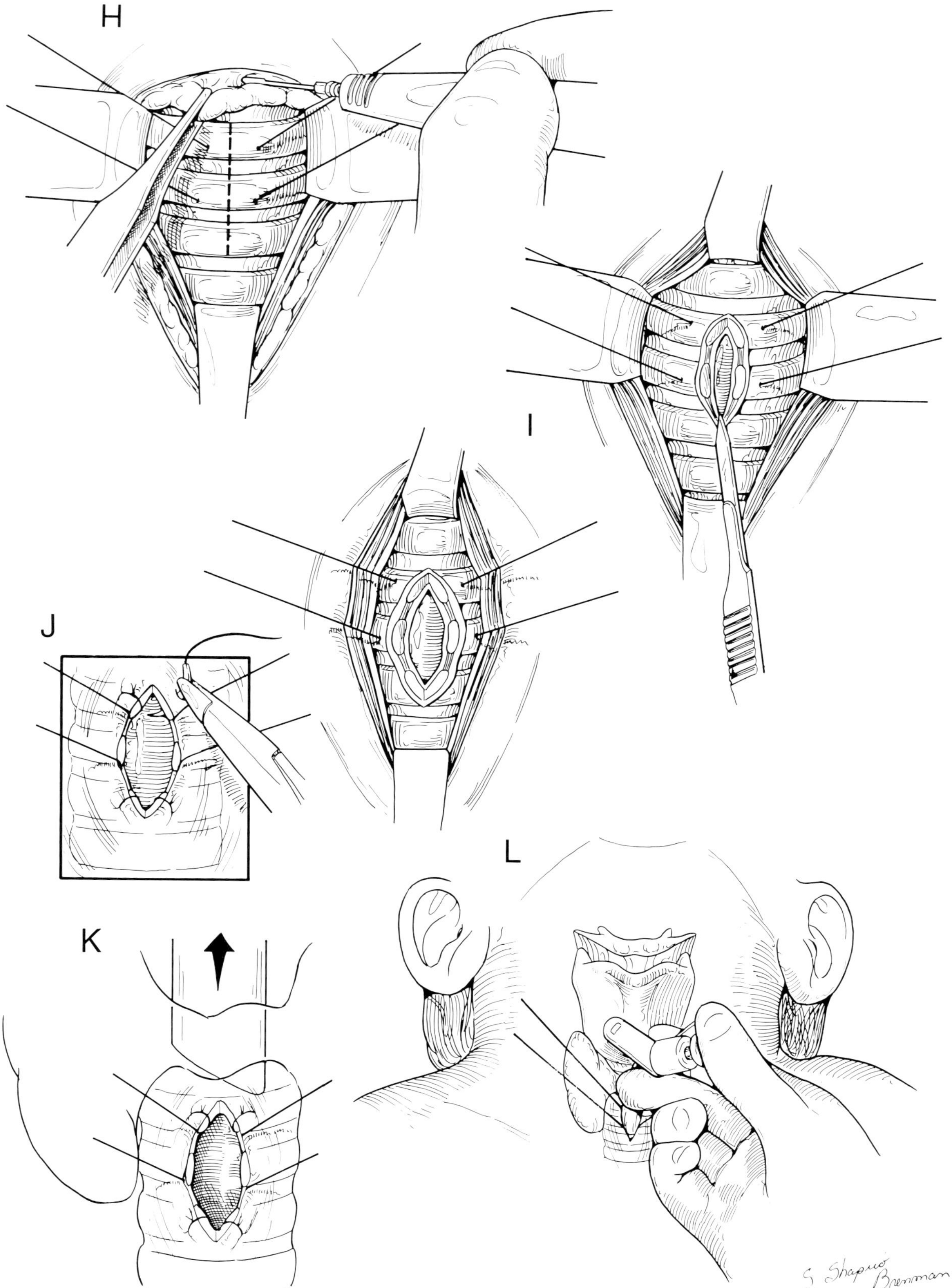


▶ **FIGURE 30-1**

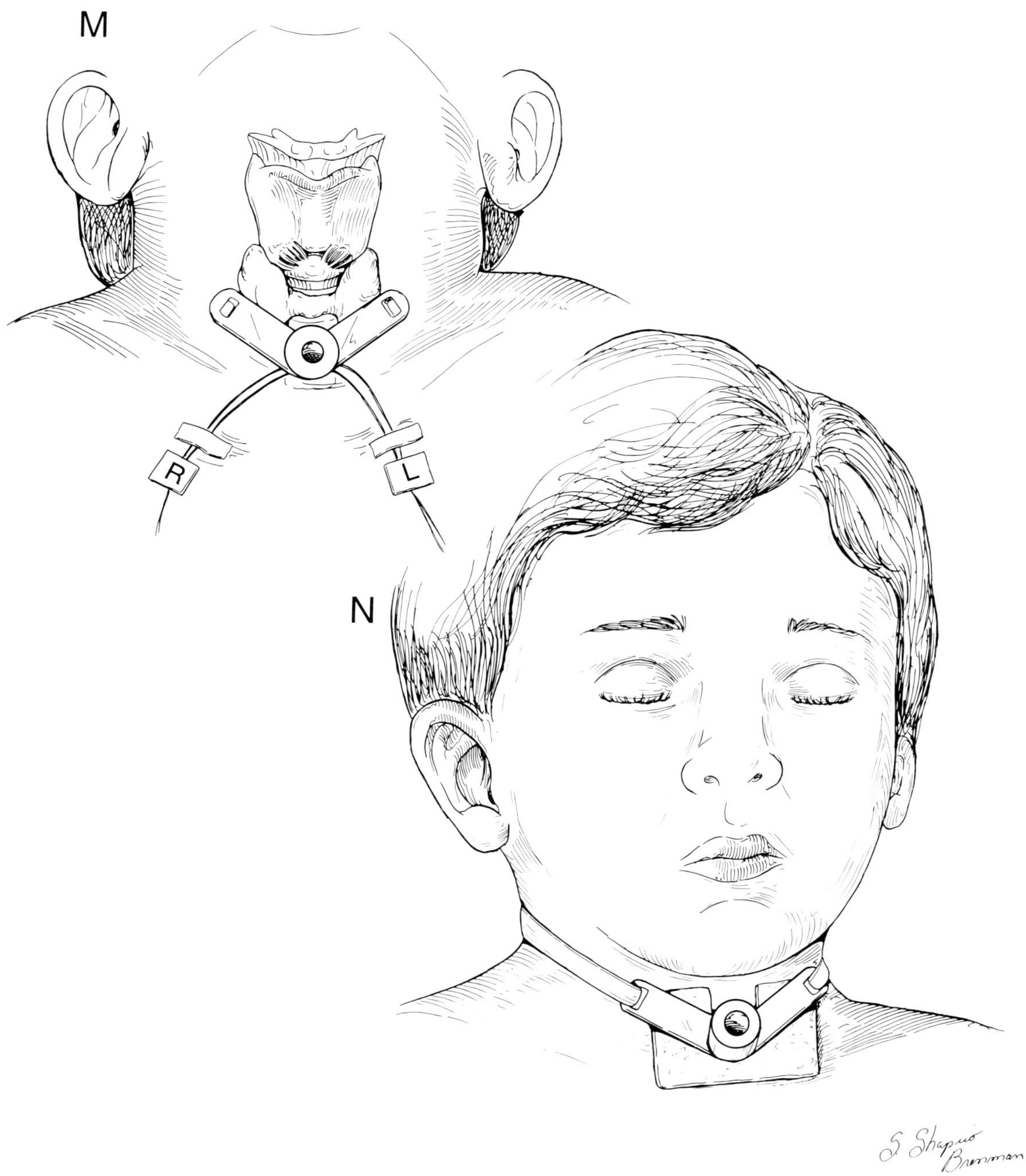


▶ **FIGURE 30-1**

## ▶ 30-2 TRACHEOCUTANEOUS FISTULA CLOSURE

A tracheocutaneous fistula may persist following removal of a tracheostomy tube. If it persists, it may permit aspiration of water while bathing or swimming. It may also be a nuisance, allowing mucous to exit the neck during coughing.

### Indications

Tracheocutaneous fistula closure is indicated when the fistula has persisted for one year after decannulation.

### Preoperative Evaluation

Direct laryngoscopy and bronchoscopy is necessary to be certain that no significant tracheal stenosis is present at or above the stoma. Closure of the stoma under these conditions could precipitate the need for reinserting the tracheotomy.

### Operative Technique

1. Tracheocutaneous fistula closure is done under general anesthesia with an endotracheal tube ½ size smaller than age appropriate.
2. One percent lidocaine with 1:100,000 epinephrine is injected in the line of the proposed incision to aid in hemostasis. A transverse elliptical incision is made in the neck, encompassing the fistula (Fig. 30–2**A**).
3. Small skin flaps are elevated above and below the incision (Fig. 30–2**B**).
4. The skin tract is dissected with scissors from its surrounding fibrous attachments down to its opening into the trachea (Fig. 30–2**C**).
5. The entire tract is removed from the tracheal mucosa with a knife (Fig. 30–2**D**).
6. A small opening in the trachea can be closed primarily with interrupted 4-0 Vicryl passed through the edges of the tracheal opening (Fig. 30–2**E**).
7. The strap muscles are then closed with 4-0 Vicryl after a rubber band drain is placed beneath the strap muscles and brought out through the wound (Fig. 30–2**F**). The drain is removed in 24 hours.
8. If the tracheal opening is large or the patient has compromised pulmonary function, the tracheal incision is not closed and a small tracheostomy tube is placed for 12–24 hours (Fig. 30–2**G**).
9. After the tracheostomy tube is removed, the fistula closes rapidly.

### Complications

1. Subcutaneous emphysema
2. Pneumothorax
3. Respiratory distress

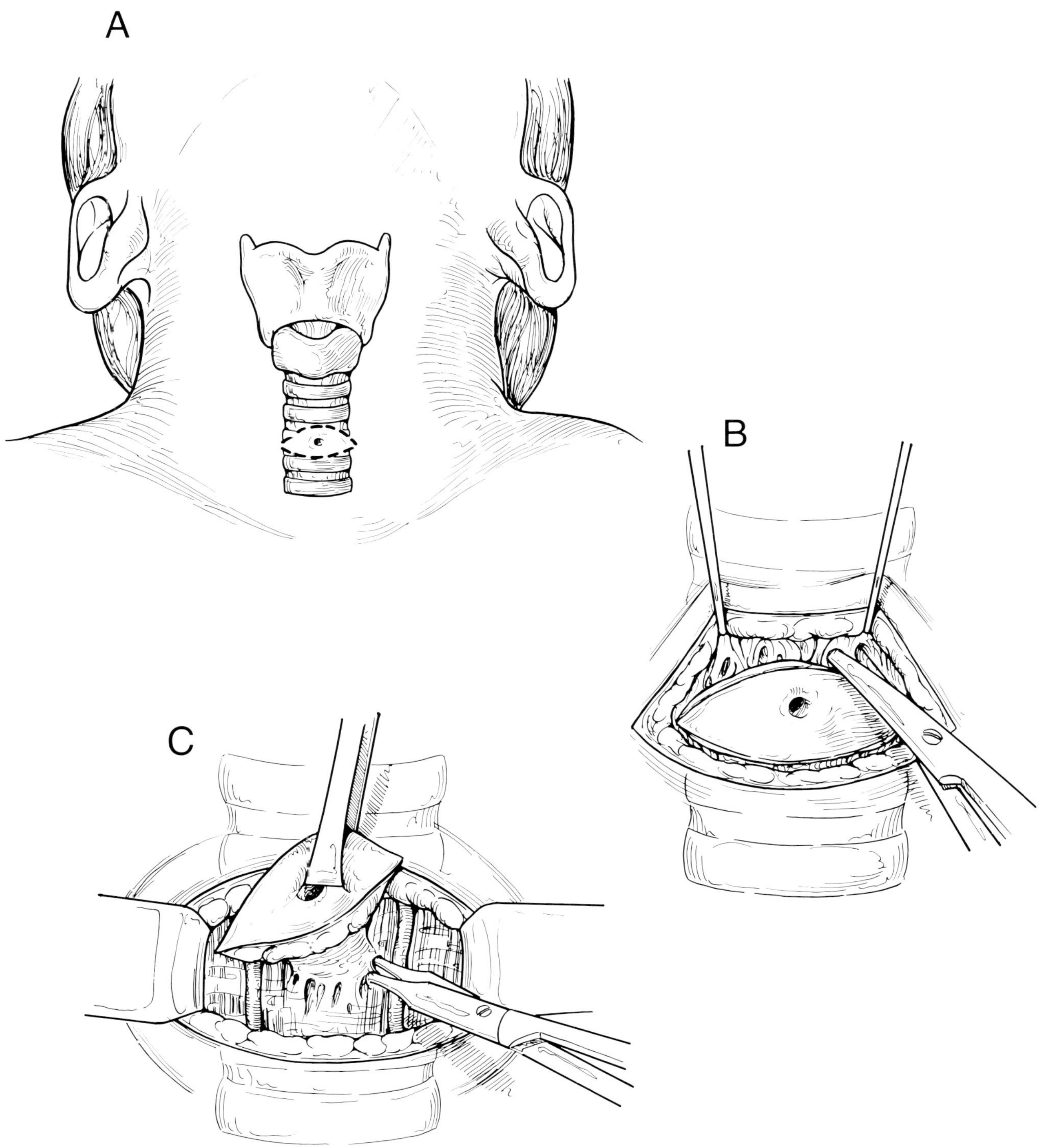


▶ **FIGURE 30-2**

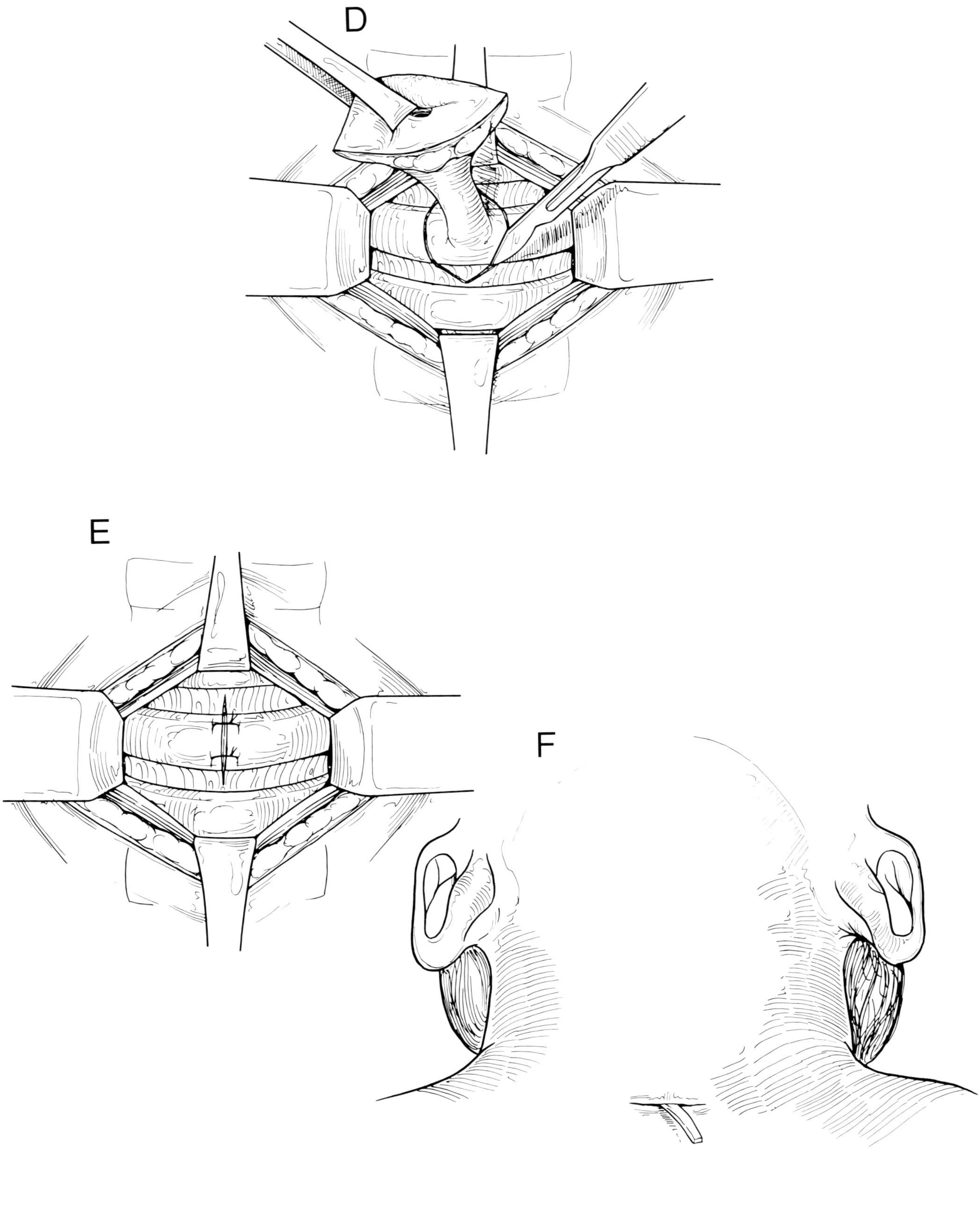


▶ **FIGURE 30-2**

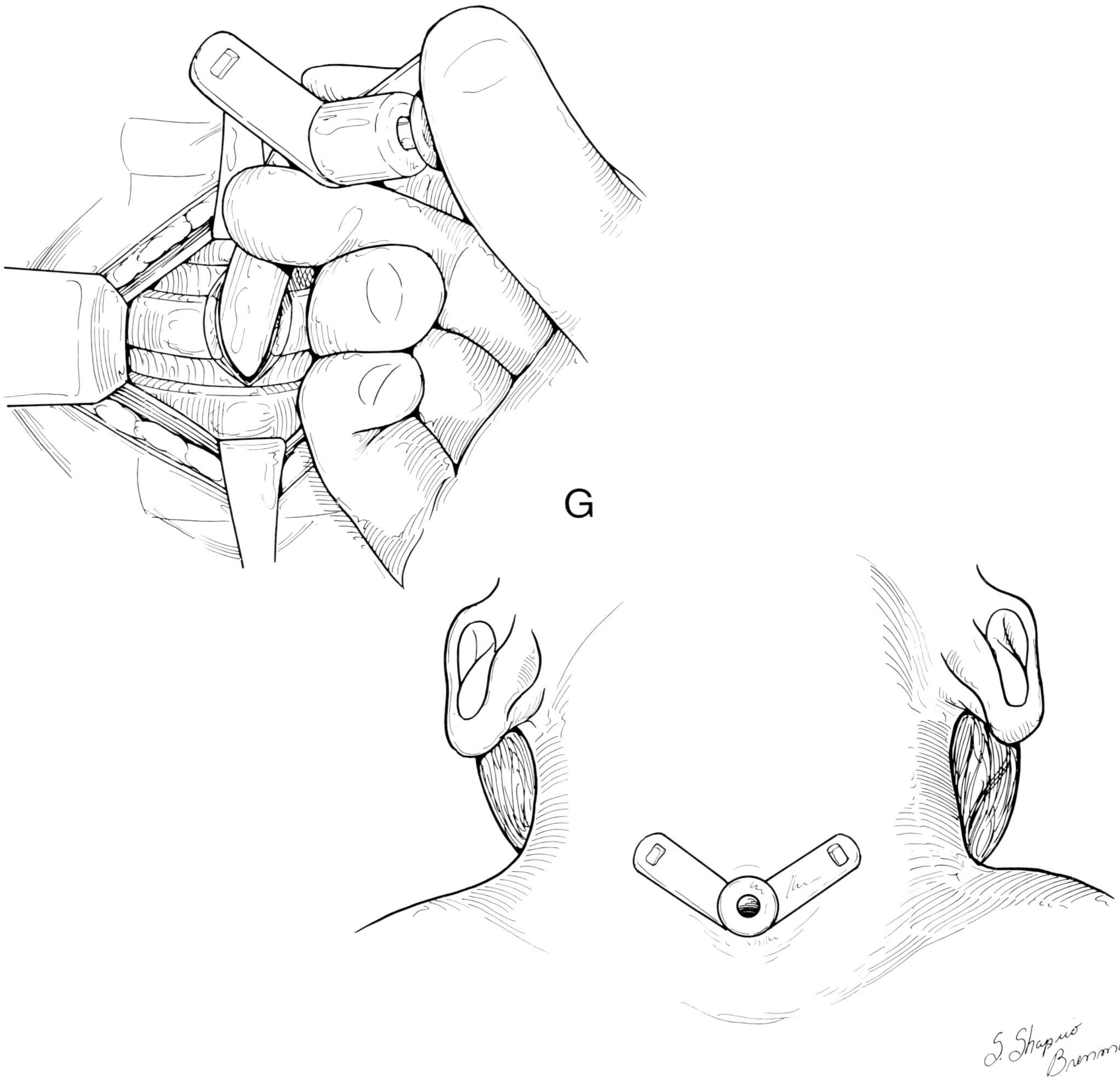


▶ **FIGURE 30-2**

# ▶ 30-3 TRACHEAL STENOSIS—END-TO-END ANASTOMOSIS

Resection of a portion of the cervical trachea with an end-to-end anastomosis is a useful technique in the armamentarium of repair of tracheal stenosis.

## Indications

Resection of a segment of trachea with end-to-end anastomosis is indicated for severe tracheal stenosis that involves no more than one-third of the cervical trachea.

## Preoperative Evaluation

Standard radiography may be helpful, but a CT scan or MRI of the tracheobronchial tree clearly outlines the length and shape of the stenosis. Direct laryngoscopy and bronchoscopy is essential to examine the intraluminal configuration.

## Operative Technique

1. Tracheal resection is performed under general endotracheal anesthesia. If the child has a tracheotomy tube in place, it is removed and an oral RAE tube is placed in the stoma.
2. The patient is placed on a shoulder roll with the neck extended as for tracheotomy (see section 30–1) and cricoid split (see section 31–5).
3. One percent lidocaine with 1:100,000 epinephrine is injected subcutaneously at the site of the incision to aid in hemostasis.
4. A transverse incision is made in the neck overlying the area of tracheal stenosis (Fig. 30–3**A**).
5. The incision is carried through the subcutaneous tissues through the deep cervical fascia, exposing the strap muscles. Superior and inferior subplatysmal skin flaps are created.
6. The strap muscles are divided in the midline and retracted laterally with 4-0 prolene sutures (Fig. 30–3**B**).
7. The pre-tracheal fascia is then incised with a scissors and reflected laterally exposing the trachea above and below the tracheal stenosis (Fig. 30–3**C**).
8. A vertical incision is made in the midline of the trachea through the stenotic segment identifying the limits of the stenosis (Fig. 30–3**D**).
9. The endotracheal tube is pulled back to a level above the stenosis and the lower segment of the trachea is intubated with a cut oral RAE tube as for LTP (see section 31–6, Fig. 31–6**E**).
10. The trachea is transected with a knife above the stenosis at the lower border of a normal tracheal ring (Fig. 30–3**E**). The incision includes the posterior tracheal wall, but the integrity of the esophagus is preserved (Fig. 30–3**F**). Care is taken to avoid injury to the recurrent laryngeal nerves.
11. The trachea is dissected away from the esophagus along the party wall with a scissors (Fig. 30–3**G**).
12. When the stenotic segment has been separated from the esophagus, the lower portion of the trachea is transected and the stenotic segment is removed (Fig. 30–3**H**).

**13.** The larynx is then released from its suprahyoid attachments.

**14.** A transverse incision is made just above the hyoid bone with cautery, releasing the geniohyoid and hyoglossal muscle from the hyoid bone (Fig. 30–3**I**).

**15.** The hyoid bone is divided at the insertion of the lesser cornu, which is the site of attachment of the digastric muscle (Fig. 30–3**J**). This releases the superior larynx, allowing it to move inferiorly.

**16.** The inferior portion of the trachea is released by careful dissection of soft tissue of the party wall to facilitate the anastomosis.

**17.** The trachea is reapproximated with interrupted 3-0 Vicryl suture beginning posteriorly and working anteriorly with the knots outside the trachea (Fig. 30–3**K**).

**18.** The cut RAE tube is removed and the patient is reintubated from above with an age-appropriate endotracheal tube.

**19.** The anastomosis is completed by placing a 2-0 prolene suture around the most superior tracheal rings (of the lower segment) and the most inferior tracheal rings (of the upper segment), working posteriorly to anteriorly (Fig. 30–3**L**) releasing tension the most at the anastomosis. If necessary, two or three additional tension-releasing sutures are placed encompassing two tracheal rings above and two below the anastomosis.

**20.** A penrose drain is placed in the wound, and the strap muscles are reapproximated over the trachea (Fig. 30–3**M**).

**21.** The subcutaneous tissues are closed with 3-0 interrupted Vicryl, and the skin is closed with 4-0 running subcuticular Vicryl.

**22.** Three sutures are placed from the skin of the chin to the skin of the chest with 0-prolene to keep the neck from extending (Fig. 30–3**N**).

**23.** The endotracheal tube is removed in 12 to 24 hours.

**24.** The drain is left in place 2 to 3 days.

**25.** Antibiotics are given for 2 weeks.

**26.** Ten days after the procedure, the chin stitches are removed and direct laryngoscopy and bronchoscopy are performed under general anesthesia. Granulation tissue, if present, is removed.

## Complications

1. Restenosis
2. Pneumothorax
3. Vocal cord paralysis
4. Esophageal perforation

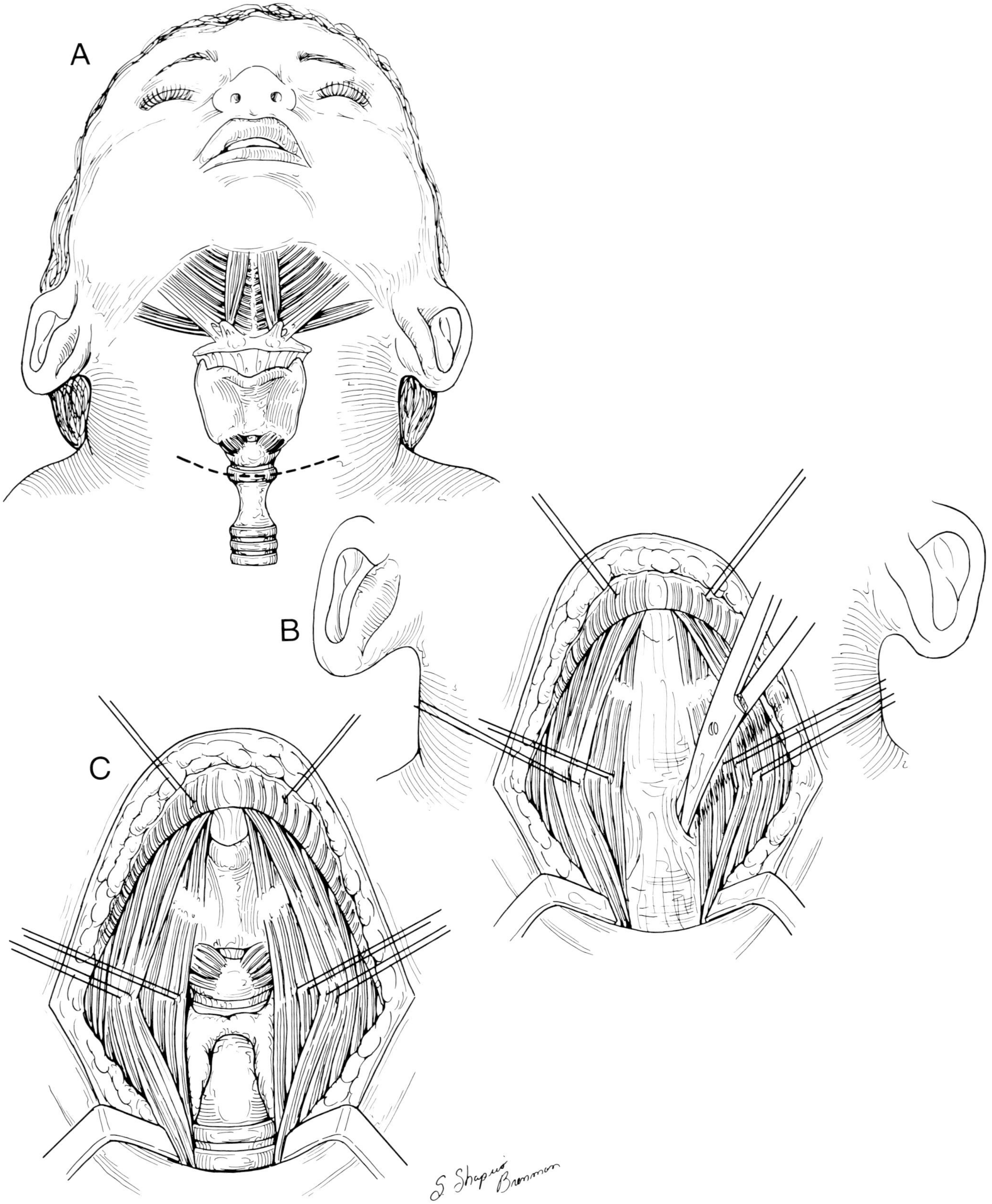


▶ **FIGURE 30-3**

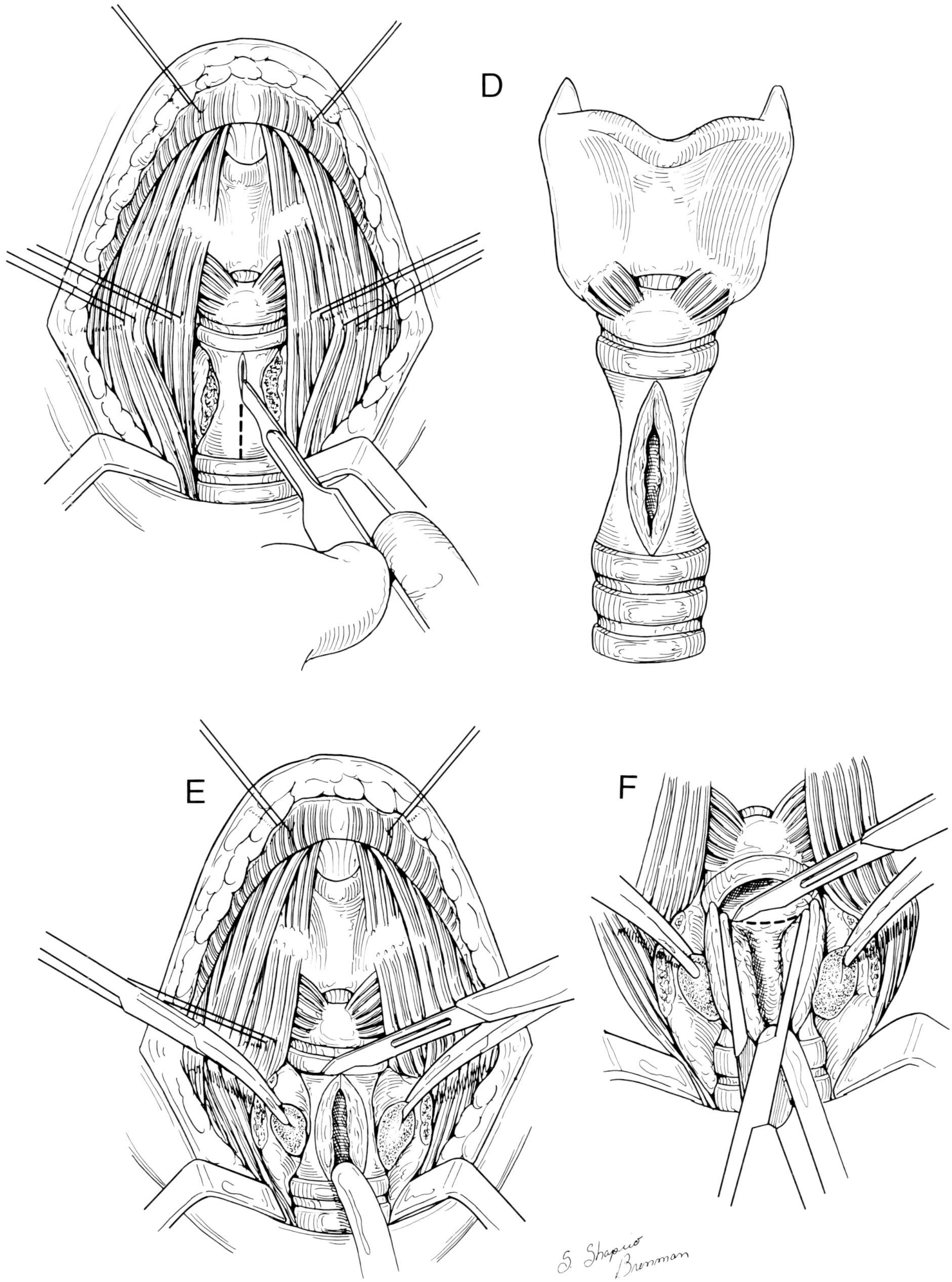


▸ **FIGURE 30-3**

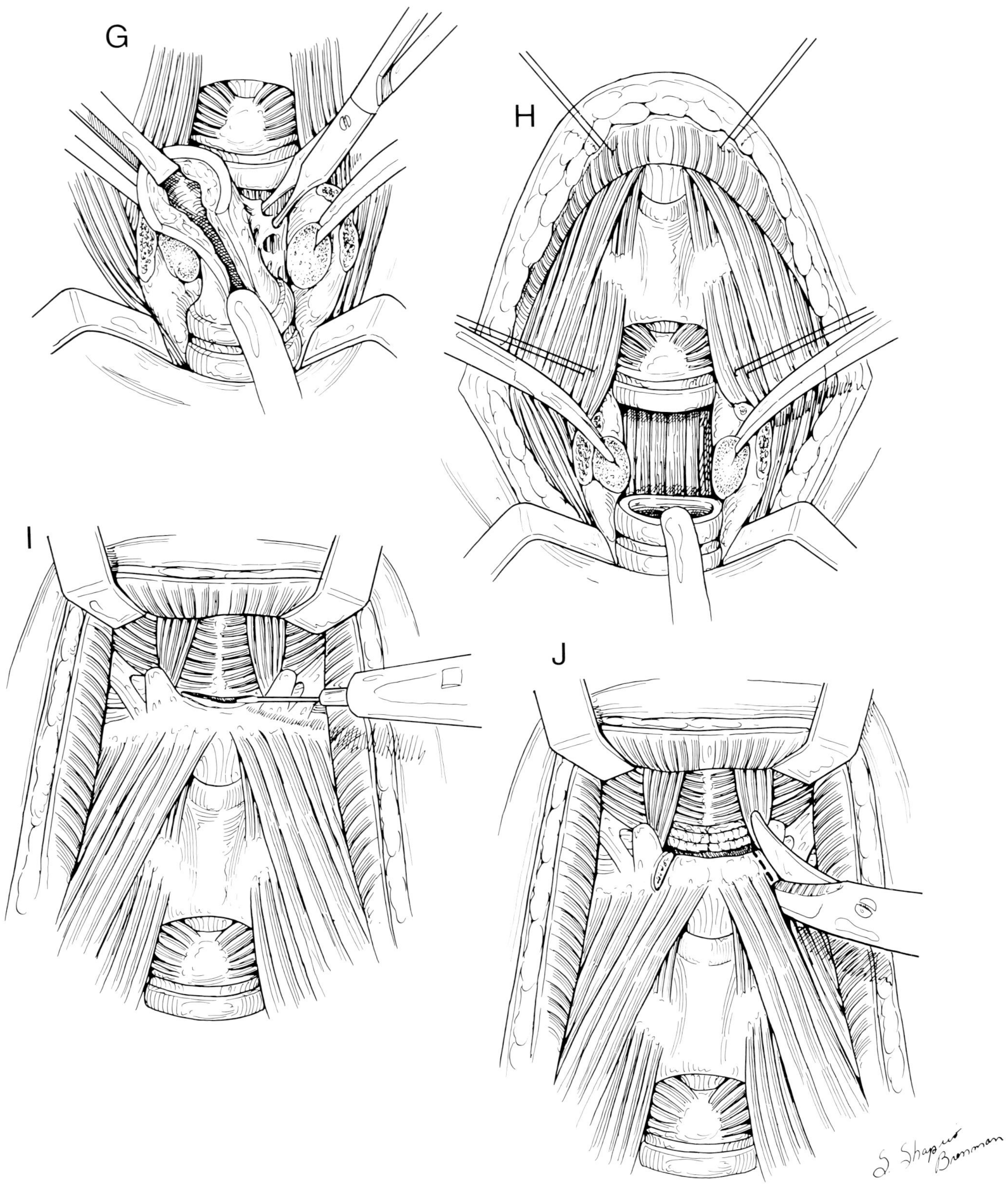


▶ **FIGURE 30-3**

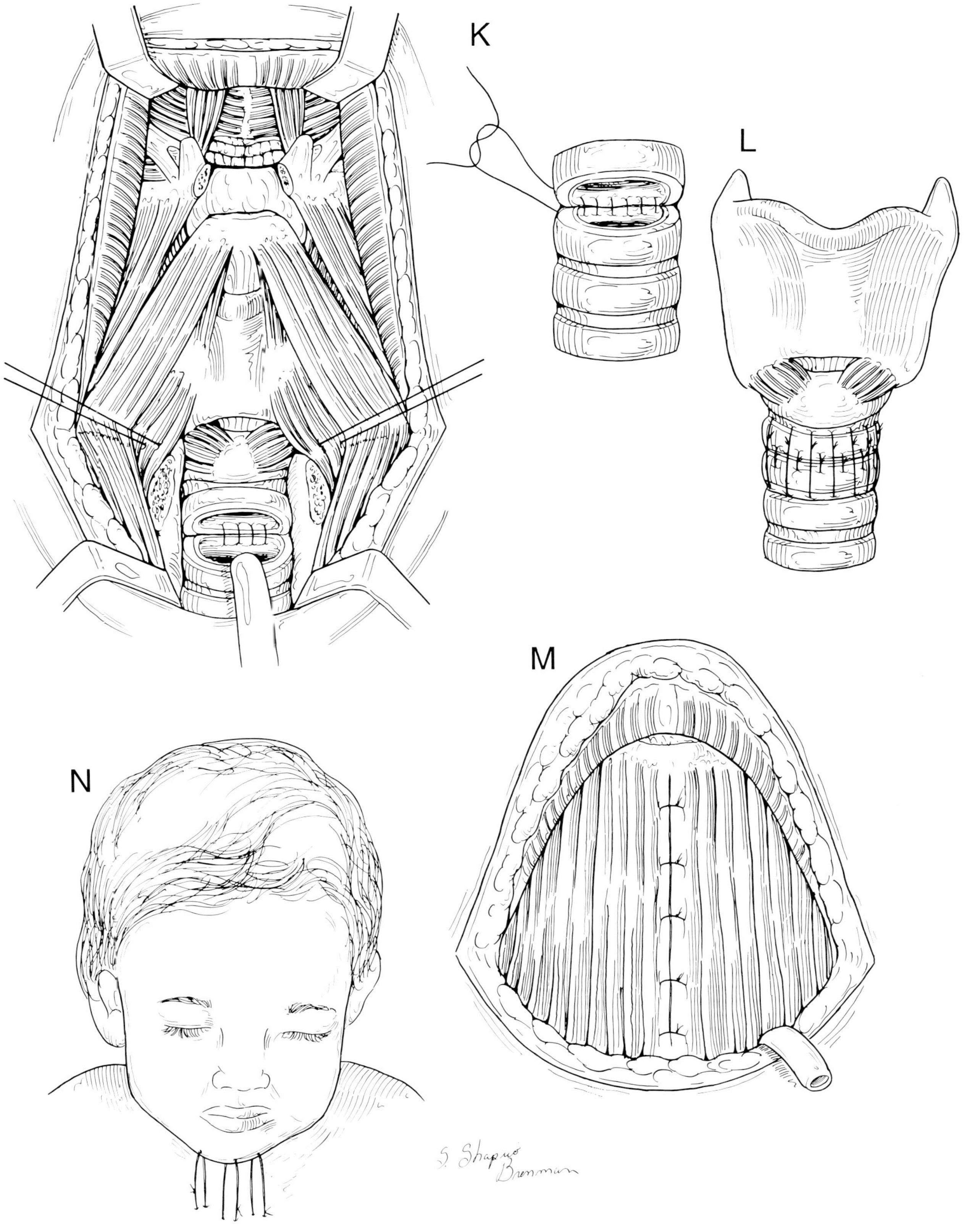


▶ **FIGURE 30-3**

## ▶ 30-4 THYROTRACHEAL ANASTOMOSIS (Subtotal Cricoid Resection with Thyrotracheal Anastomosis)

Tracheal atresia and severe high tracheal stenosis present a challenge for survival as well as reconstruction. Cricotracheal anastomosis is the treatment of choice for these conditions. An emergency tracheostomy is usually required shortly after birth.

### Indications

Cricotracheal anastomosis is indicated for severe high tracheal stenosis.

### Preoperative Evaluation

Standard radiography may be helpful, but a CT or MRI scan of the tracheobronchial tree clearly outlines the length and shape of the stenosis. Direct laryngoscopy and bronchoscopy is essential to examine the intraluminal configuration.

### Operative Technique

1. Tracheal resection is performed under general anesthesia administered through a cut oral RAE tube in the tracheostomy site (Fig. 30–4**A**).
2. The patient is placed on a shoulder roll with the neck extended as for tracheotomy (see section 30–1) and cricoid split (see section 31–5).
3. One percent lidocaine with 1:100,000 epinephrine is injected subcutaneously at the site of the incision to aid in hemostasis.
4. A transverse incision is made in the neck overlying the lower border of the cricoid (Fig. 30–4**A**).
5. The incision is carried through the subcutaneous tissues and through the deep cervical fascia, exposing the strap muscles. Superior and inferior subplatysmal skin flaps are created.
6. The strap muscles are divided in the midline and retracted laterally with 4-0 prolene sutures (Fig. 30–4**B**).
7. The pretracheal fascia is incised providing exposure of the trachea as well as the cricoid and thyroid cartilages (Fig. 30–4**C**).
8. A vertical incision is made through the cricoid and atresia segment extending to the normal trachea below (Fig. 30–4**D**).
9. The trachea is transected below the atresia with a knife, preserving the integrity of the esophagus (Fig. 30–4**D**). The recurrent laryngeal nerves should be identified and protected. The inferior border of the cricoid cartilage is resected with a knife (Fig. 30–4**E**). The portion of larynx and trachea resected is shown in Figure 30–4**E.**
10. The larynx is then released from its suprahyoid attachments (Fig. 30–4**F**). A transverse incision is made just above the hyoid bone with a cautery, releasing the geniohyoid and hyoglossal muscle from the hyoid bone.
11. The hyoid bone is divided with a scissors at the insertion of the lesser cornu, which is the site of attachment of the diagnostic muscle (Fig. 30–4**G**). This releases the larynx, allowing it to move inferiorly.

12. The inferior portion of the trachea is released by careful dissection of soft tissue of the party wall to facilitate the anastomosis (Fig. 30–4H).
13. The mucosa of the trachea and cricoid are reapproximated with interrupted 3-0 Tevdec suture beginning posteriorly and working anteriorly (Fig. 30–4I).
14. The cut RAE tube is removed and the patient is reintubated from above with an age-appropriate endotracheal tube.
15. The anastomosis is completed by placing 2-0 prolene sutures around the cricoid cartilage and inferior tracheal rings, working posteriorly to anteriorly (Fig. 30–4J) releasing tension at the anastomosis.
16. Two or three additional tension-releasing sutures are placed between the cricoid and the tracheal rings below the anastomosis (Fig. 30–4J).
17. A penrose drain is placed in the wound, and the strap muscles are reapproximated over the larynx and trachea (Fig. 30–4K).
18. The subcutaneous tissues are closed with 3-0 interrupted Vicryl, and the skin is closed with 4-0 running subcuticular Vicryl.
19. Three sutures are placed from the skin of the chin to the skin of the chest with 0-prolene to keep the neck from extending (Fig. 30–4L).
20. The endotracheal tube is removed in 12 to 24 hours.
21. The drain is left in place 2 to 3 days.
22. Antibiotics are given for 2 weeks.
23. Ten days after the procedure, the chin stitches are removed and a direct laryngoscopy and bronchoscopy are performed under general anesthesia. Granulation tissue, if present, is removed.

## Complications

1. Restenosis
2. Pneumothorax
3 Vocal cord paralysis

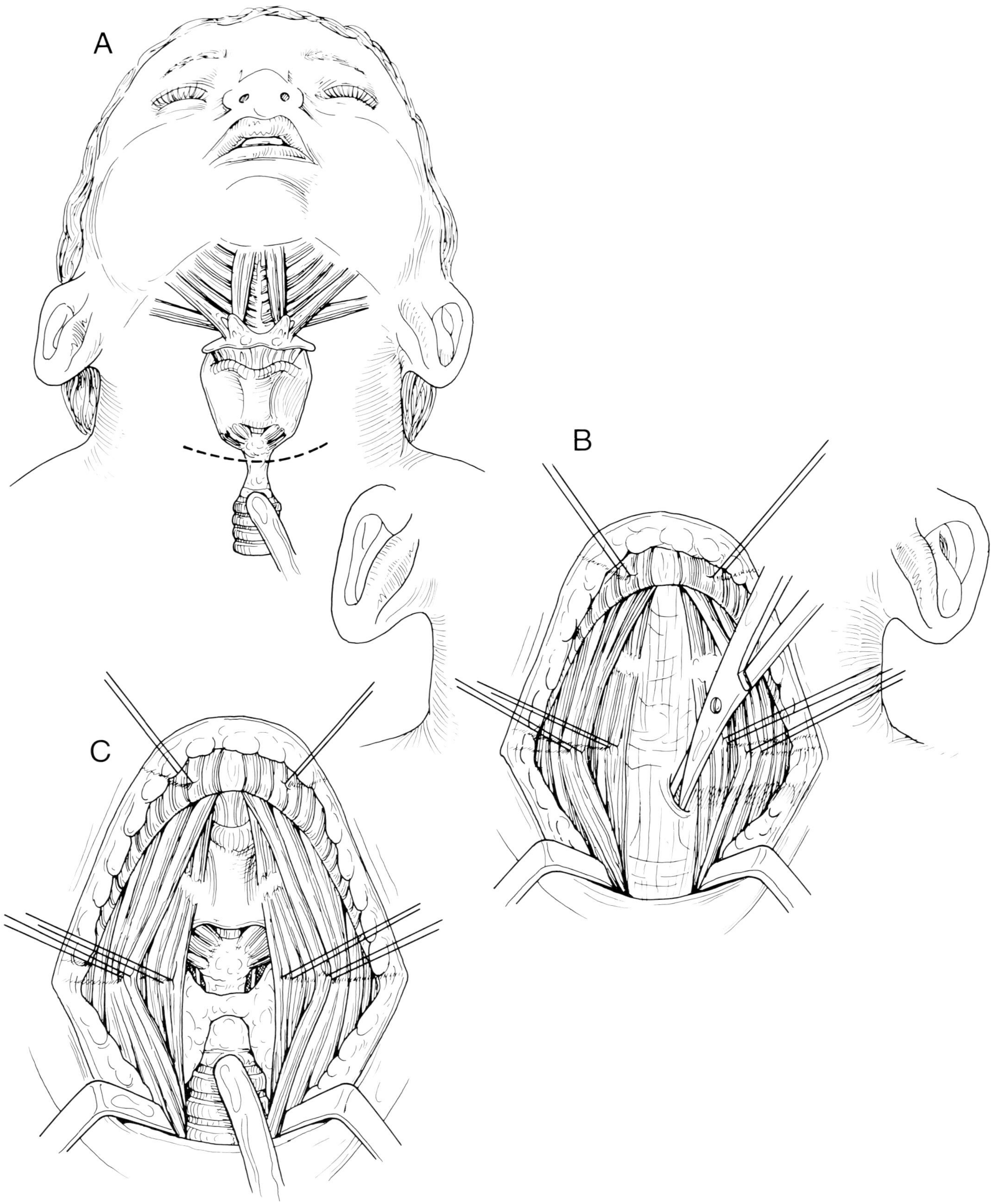


▶ **FIGURE 30-4**

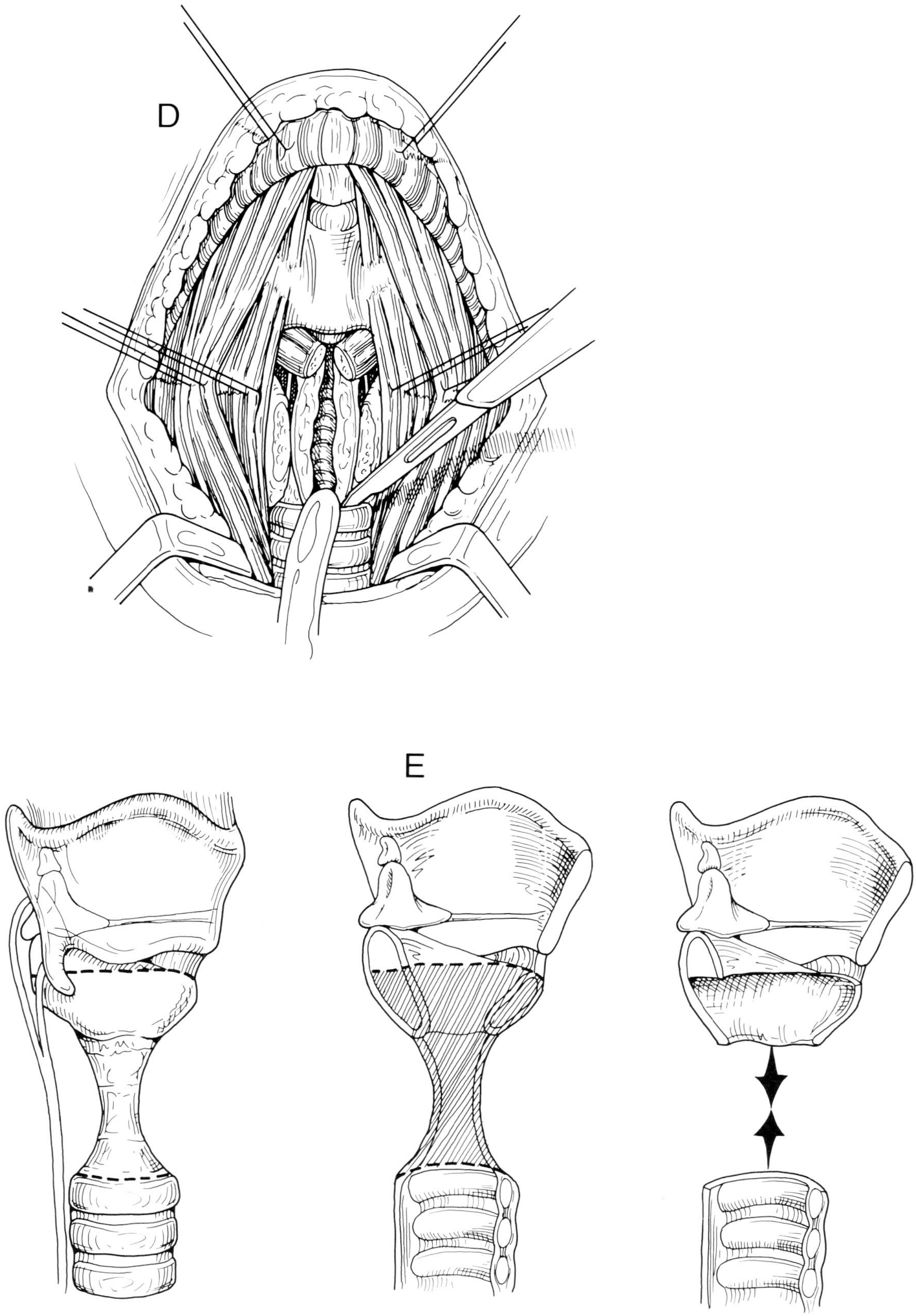


▶ **FIGURE 30-4**

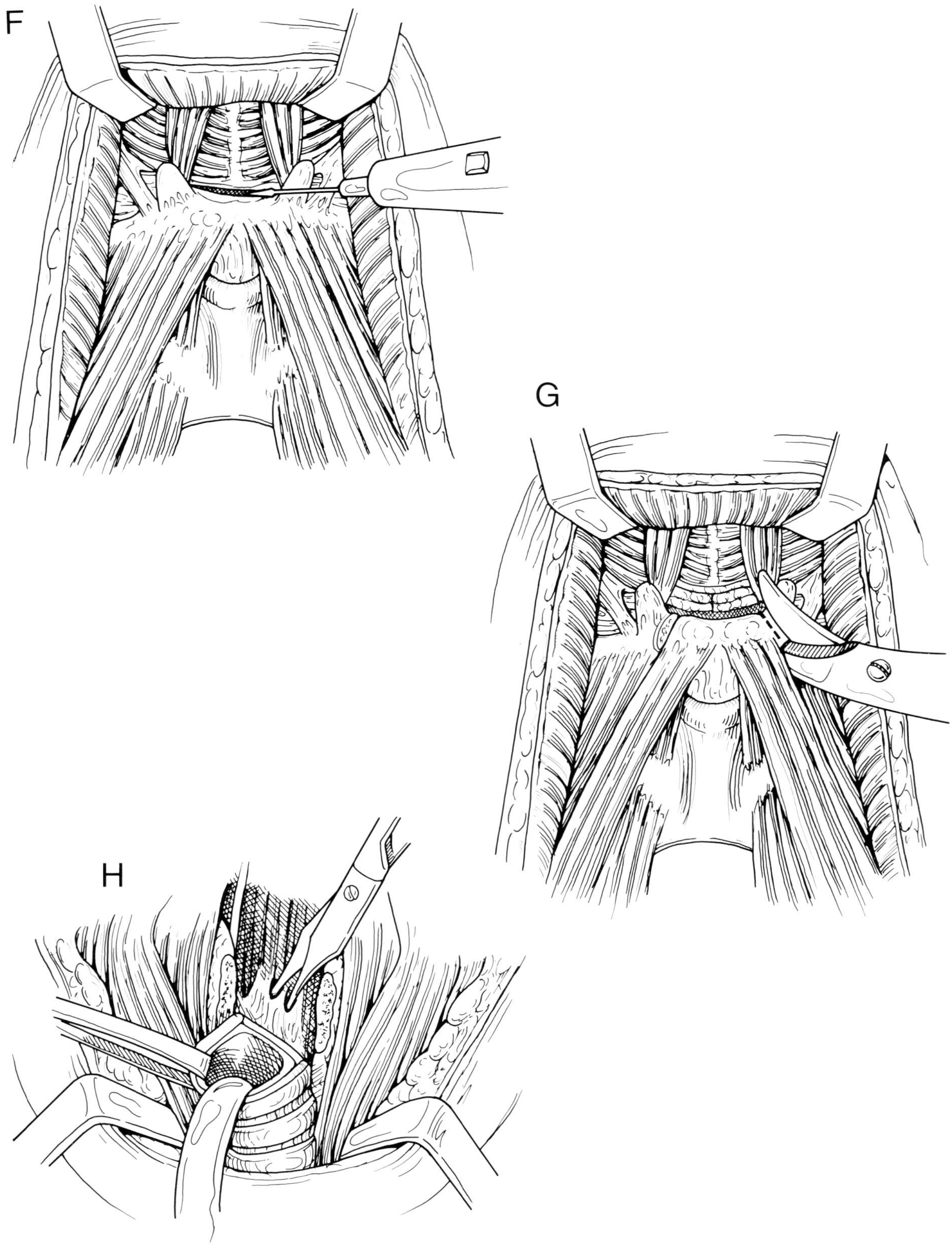


▶ **FIGURE 30-4**

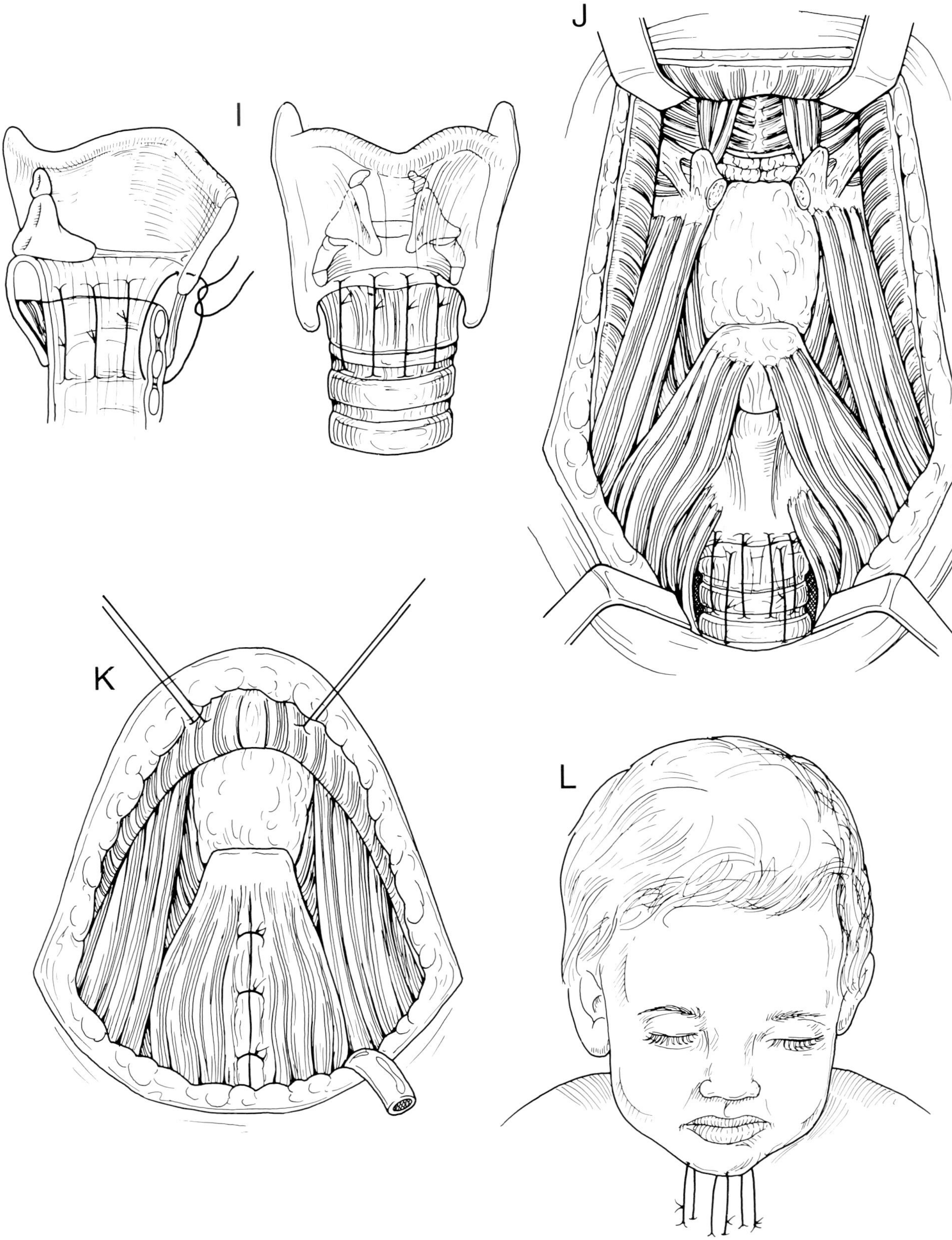


▶ **FIGURE 30-4**

## ▸ 30-5 REPAIR OF COMPLETE TRACHEAL RINGS

Complete tracheal rings is a congenital disorder that causes tracheal stenosis and may result in severe respiratory distress.

### Indications

The repair of tracheal stenosis resulting from complete tracheal rings is indicated when respiratory distress is sufficient to interfere with growth and development or the child presents with a life-threatening obstruction.

### Preoperative Evaluation

Preoperative evaluation includes a magnetic resonance imaging (MRI) scan of the tracheobronchial tree to demonstrate the anatomy of the trachea, the length of the stenosis, the surrounding soft tissue anatomy, and any abnormal vessels. If severe tracheal stenosis from complete tracheal rings is suspected, laryngoscopy and bronchoscopy is deferred until the time of the definitive procedure, which is done on cardiopulmonary bypass.

### Operative Technique

1. Correction of tracheal stenosis from complete tracheal rings is performed under general anesthesia and cardiopulmonary bypass. The patient is intubated with a 2mm endotracheal tube which is impacted into the upper portion of the stenotic segment or positioned just above the stenosis. The patient is then placed on cardiopulmonary bypass and a bronchoscopy is performed to evaluate the stenotic segment (Refer to Section 8.8, Bronchoscopy).
2. A collar neck incision is made to expose the trachea (Fig. 30–5**A**). A vertical incision is made to connect to the sternal incision. One percent lidocaine with 1:100,000 epinephrine is injected subcutaneously at the site of the incision to aid in hemostasis of the neck incision.
3. A midline sternotomy is performed by a cardiothoracic surgeon. The innominate artery and vein are identified and retracted to avoid injury to the vessels. The area of stenosis of the trachea is identified. The patient is placed on cardiopulmonary bypass.
4. A vertical incision is made through the stenotic segment. The lower trachea is suctioned frequently to prevent blood from entering the bronchial tree below (Fig. 30–5**B**).
5. An age-appropriate (or one size smaller) endotracheal tube is placed with the tip below the stenotic segment (Fig. 30–5**C**). The tracheal defect is closed with a free pericardial patch and that is sewn in place with a continuous suture of 5-0 monofilament PDS (Fig. 30–5**D**). A metal clip is placed at the lower end of the stenosis to evaluate the position of the endotracheal tube by x-ray later prior to chest closure by the thoracic surgeon. The neck incision is closed with running subcuticular 4-0 Vicryl sutures.
6. Bronchoscopy is performed to assure adequate repair of the lower end of the stenosis and the patient is then reintubated with a nasotracheal tube.
7. The endotracheal tube is left in place for 2 days. The patient remains on antibiotics for 6 weeks. Chest tubes remain in place as long as is needed to re-expand the lungs.
8. The patient is extubated in the ICU and maintained on nasal CPAP.

### Complications

1. Restenosis
2. Tracheomalacia
3. Mediastinitis
4. Complications of cardiopulmonary bypass

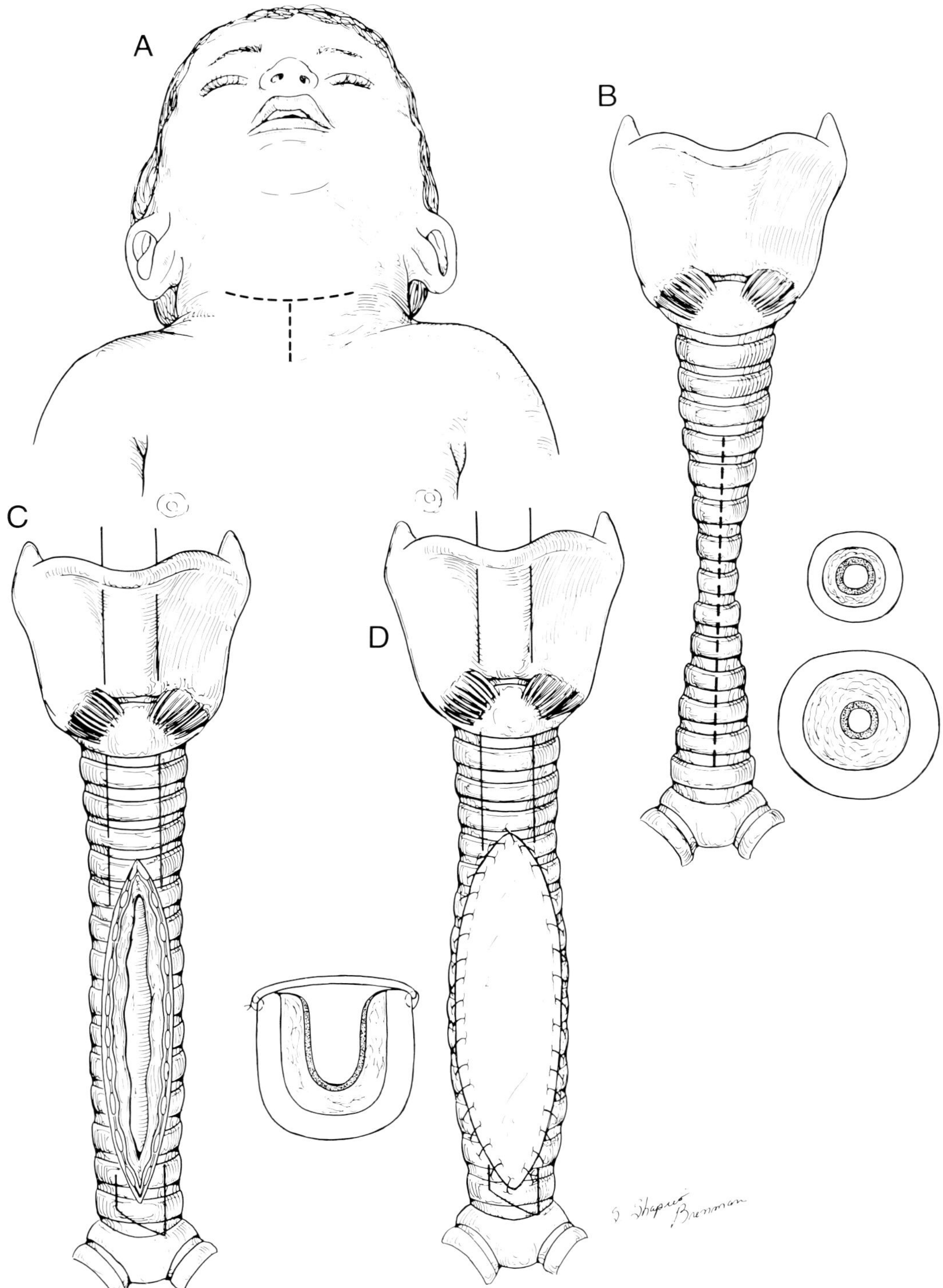


▶ **FIGURE 30-5**

## ▶ 30-6 REMOVAL OF A SUPRASTOMAL FIBROMA

Granulation tissue, suprastomal depression and suprastomal fibroma formation at the anterior-superior edge of the tracheostomy site are common occurrences with a pediatric tracheostomy.

### Indications

Removal of a suprastomal fibroma is indicated when it occludes the trachea. This creates a critical airway, prevents phonation around the tracheostomy tube, and precludes decannulation.

### Preoperative Evaluation

Direct laryngoscopy and bronchoscopy are sufficient to evaluate a stomal fibroma. Radiography is not helpful.

### Operative Technique

1. The suprastomal fibroma is visualized directly with an open bronchoscope under general anesthesia (Fig. 30–6**A**). The tracheostomy tube is removed.
2. A curved Kerrison or sphenoid punch is placed in the tracheal stoma and the fibroma is removed with the punch under direct vision (Fig. 30–6**B**). Alternatively, the granuloma/fibroma may be pulled out of the tracheostoma with a skin hook and severed with a knife, scissors, or cautery.
3. The tracheostomy tube is replaced. If the patient is a candidate for decannulation, the tracheostomy tube may be removed the next day with the child fully awake.

### Complications

1. Stenosis at stoma site
2. Reformation of granuloma

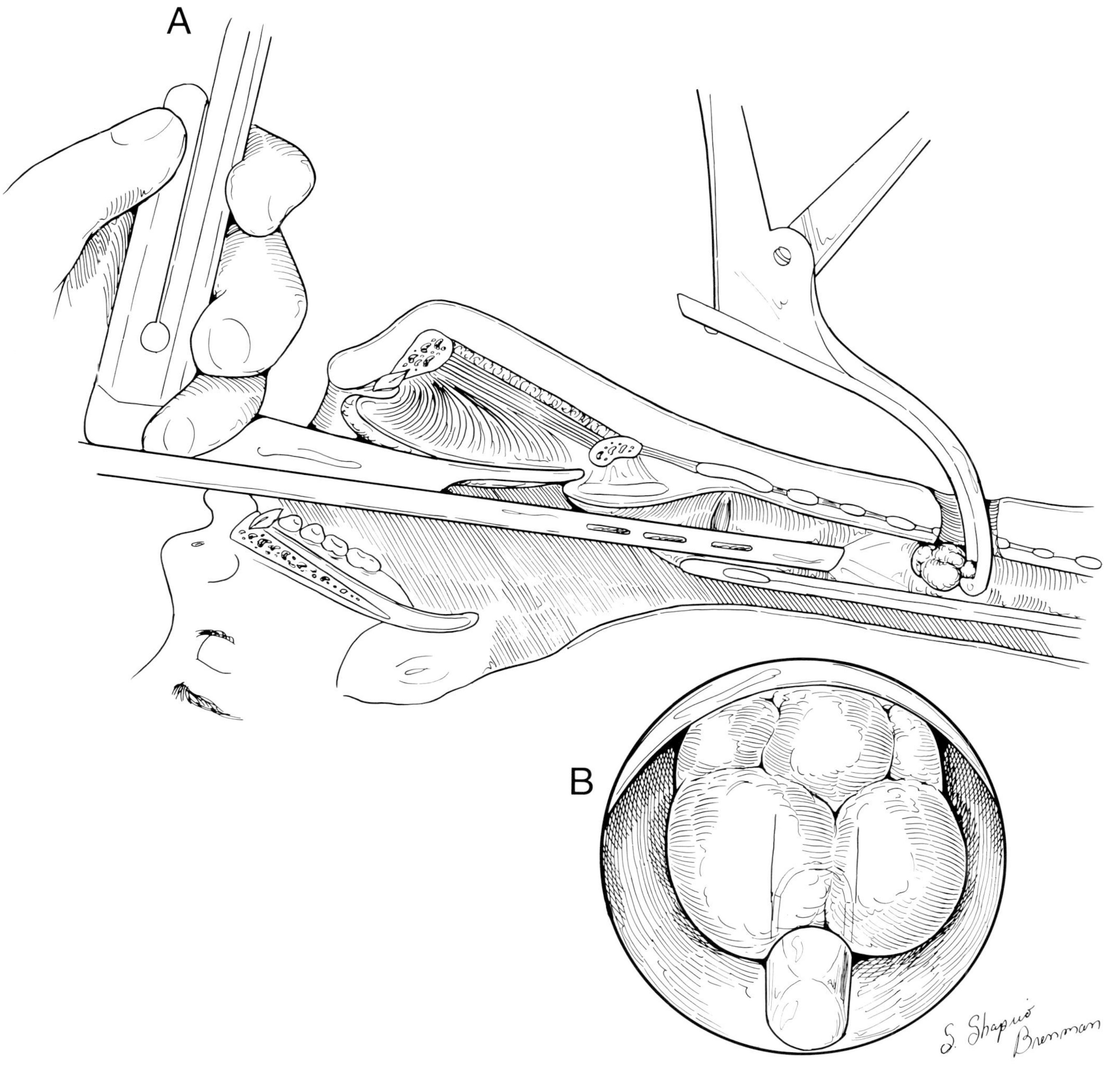


▶ **FIGURE 30-6**

# 31 ▶ Larynx

## ▶ 31-1 VOCAL CORD MEDIALIZATION FOR UNILATERAL VOCAL CORD PARALYSIS (GELFOAM-TEFLON INJECTION)

Vocal cord medialization is a technique to treat chronic aspiration and/or a breathy voice secondary to unilateral vocal cord paralysis.

### Indications

Vocal cord medialization to control chronic aspiration is indicated if the child demonstrates progressive pulmonary disease or recurrent pneumonias. Procedures to control aspiration are attempted only after medical and/or surgical treatment have reduced pharyngeal secretions. This may include procedures such as bilateral submandibular gland resection and parotid duct ligation. Surgical treatment of a breathy voice is indicated if the patient has not responded to a 3- to 6-month trial of voice therapy.

### Operative Technique

1. With the patient breathing spontaneously under general anesthesia, a Jako microlaryngoscope is placed (Fig. 31–1**A**).
2. The anesthetic is maintained by insufflating anesthetic gas delivered through the side light port of the laryngoscope.
3. A laryngeal injection needle is inserted through the ventricle between the vocalis muscle and the thyroid ala at the midpoint of the vocal cord (Fig. 31–1**B**).
4. Approximately 1 cc of Gelfoam paste is injected (Fig. 31–1**C**) until the vocal fold is determined to be in the midline (Fig. 31–1**D**).
5. If the Gelfoam injection is successful in reducing aspiration, a Teflon injection is performed in a similar fashion 4 to 6 weeks later.

### Complications

1. Continued aspiration and/or breathy voice
2. Edema with airway obstruction

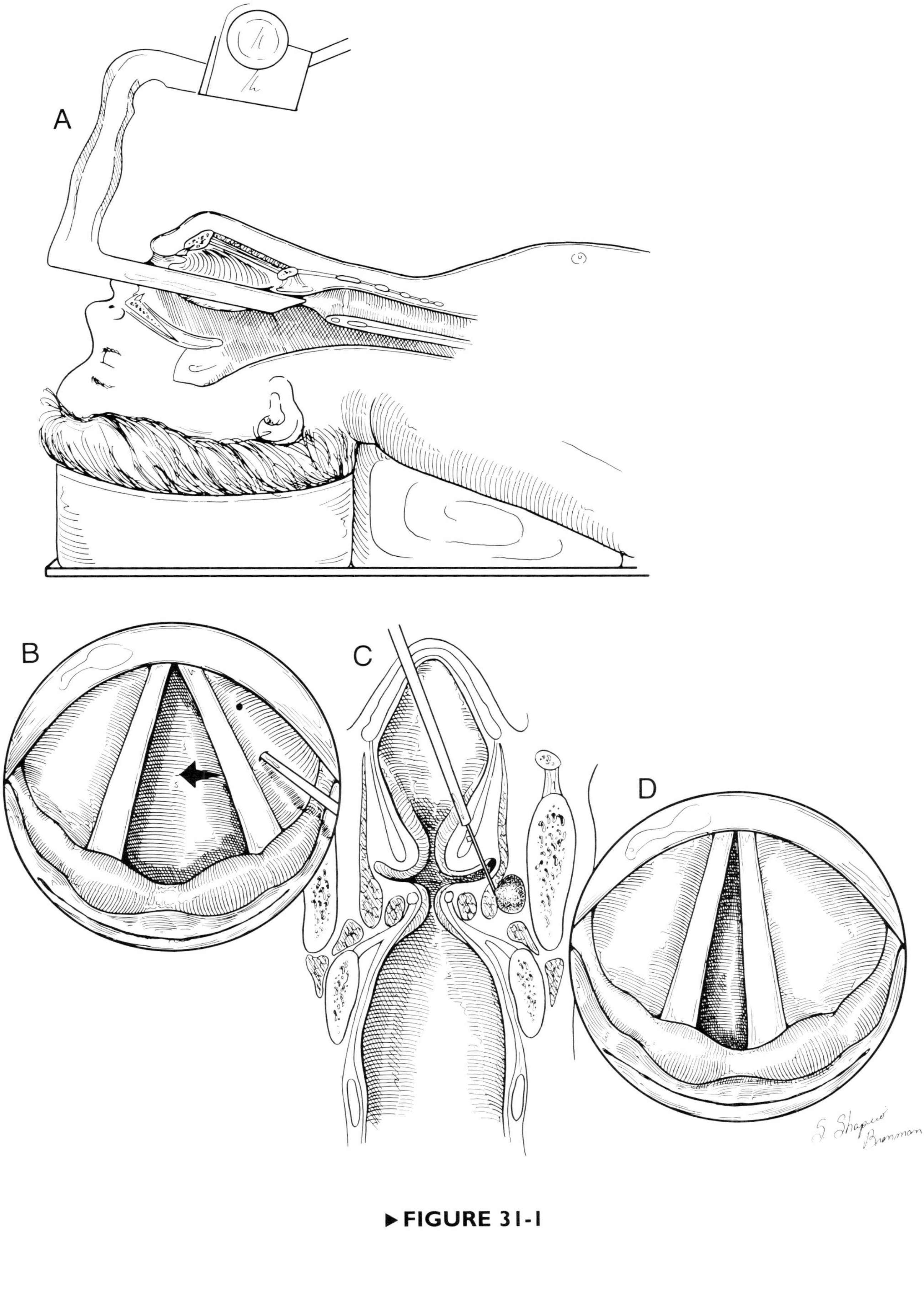


▶ **FIGURE 31-1**

## ▶ 31-2 LARYNGEAL DIVISION

Laryngeal division is a procedure to manage severe aspiration secondary to laryngeal incompetence.

### Indications

Laryngeal division is indicated for severe life-threatening aspiration and progressive pulmonary complications after other procedures to control aspiration have failed to provide protection for the airway.

### Preoperative Evaluation

A gastrograffin swallow is essential to demonstrate the severity of the aspiration. Pulmonary function studies are also obtained if the patient is able to cooperate.

### Operative Technique

1. Laryngeal diversion is performed using general anesthesia with an endotracheal tube in place.
2. The patient is positioned on a shoulder roll with the neck extended as for tracheotomy (see section 30–1).
3. A horizontal skin incision is made halfway between the cricoid and the sternal notch (Fig. 31–2**A**). One percent lidocaine with 1:100,000 is injected subcutaneously at the site of the incision to aid in hemostasis.
4. Subcutaneous fat and tissue are reflected with a clamp, exposing the deep cervical fascia overlying the strap muscles, and ribbon retractors are placed to expose the field as well as stabilize the trachea in the midline (Fig. 31–2**B**). Superior and inferior sub-platysmal skin flaps are elevated. 3.0 silk sutures may be used to stabilize the superior flap.
5. Vertical dissection with a scissors and clamp in the midline is carried out until the trachea is exposed. After the trachea is exposed, the strap muscles are separated in the midline to expose the cricoid and thyroid cartilage (Fig. 31–2**C**).
6. The trachea is transected between the 4th and 5th rings horizontally, sloping the incision superiorly (Fig. 31–2**D**).
7. The oral endotracheal tube is removed and a cut RAE tube is placed in the tracheostoma to facilitate ventilation during the completion of the operation (Fig. 31–2**E**).
8. The trachea is mobilized inferiorly from the tracheoesophageal septum (Fig. 31–2**E**).
9. The anterior edge of the trachea is sutured to the inferior edge of the skin incision with 4-0 prolene suture (Fig. 31–2**F**).
10. The upper stump of the trachea is then mobilized from the tracheoesophageal septum and then closed with 3-0 prolene suture, creating a blind pouch (Fig. 31–2**G**).
11. A penrose drain is placed in the wound.
12. The subcutaneous tissues are closed with 4-0 interrupted Vicryl, and the skin is closed with 4-0 running subcuticular Vicryl. The central portion of

the upper skin is sutured to the posterior tracheostoma with 4-0 interrupted prolene (Fig. 31–2**H**).

13. The RAE tube is removed and an appropriate-sized tracheostomy is secured in place (Fig. 31–2**I**).
14. The drain is left in place 2–3 days.

## Complications

1. Fistula between proximal tracheal stump and skin incision.
2. Continued aspiration through fistula to tracheal stoma.

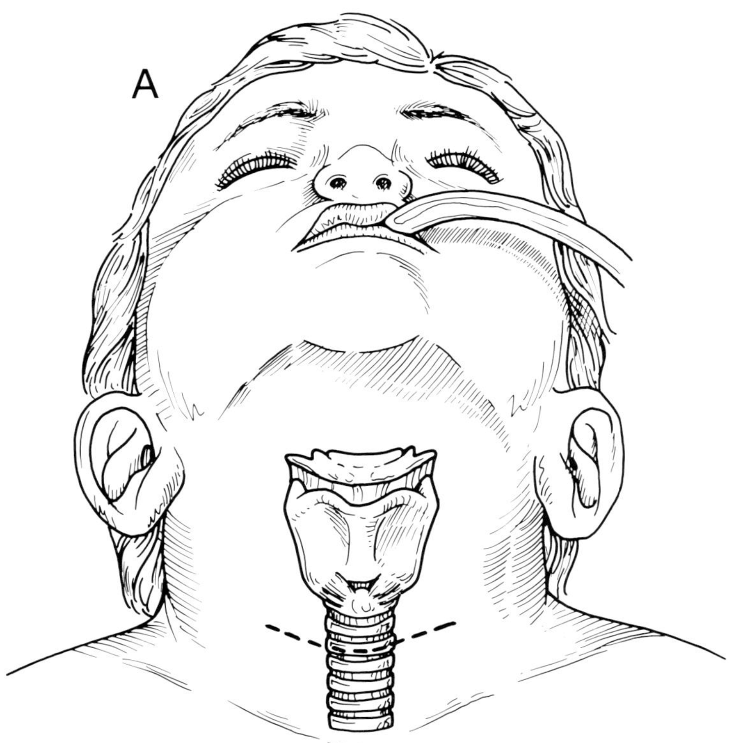


▶ **FIGURE 31-2**

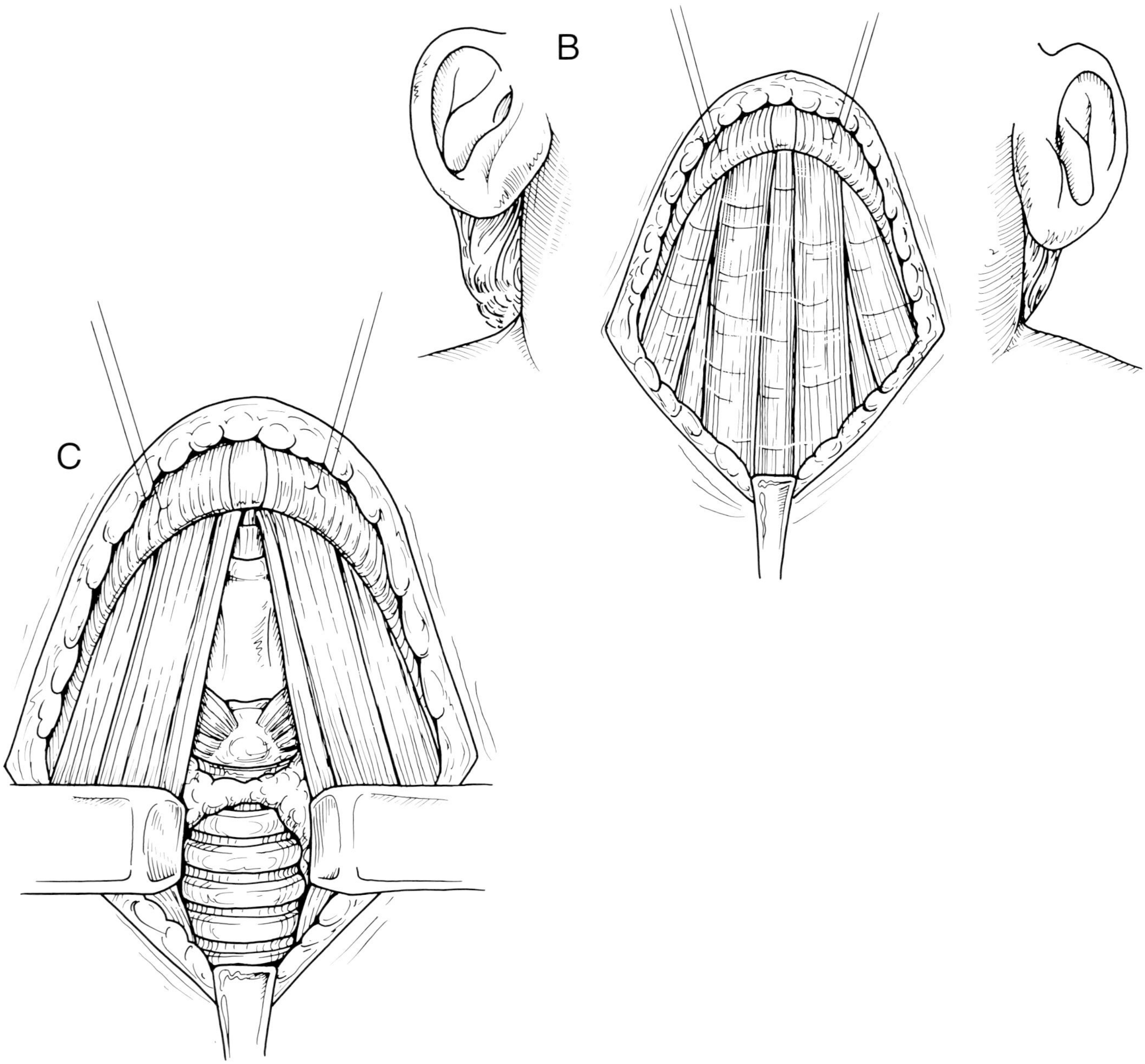


▶ **FIGURE 31-2**

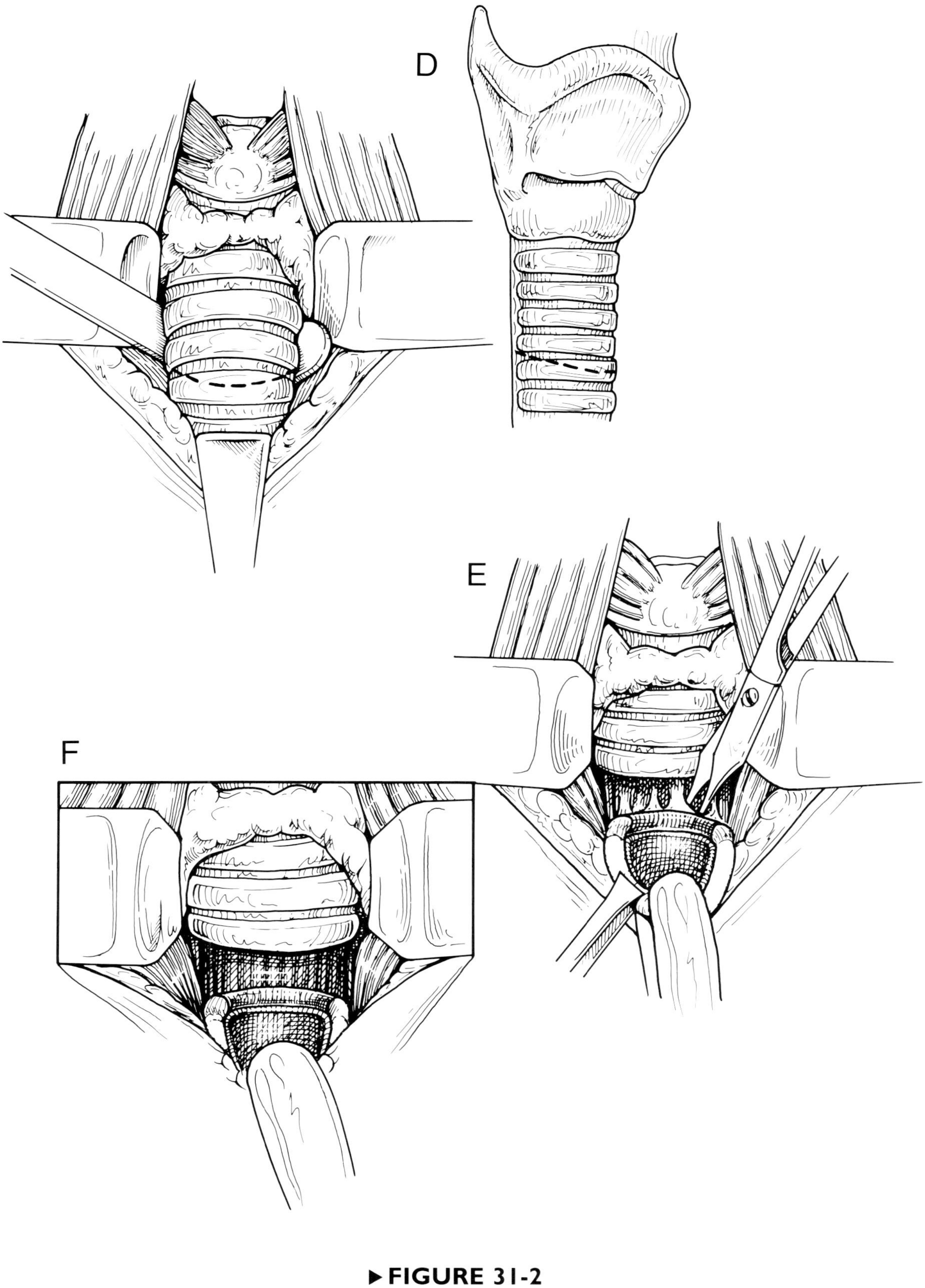


▶ **FIGURE 31-2**

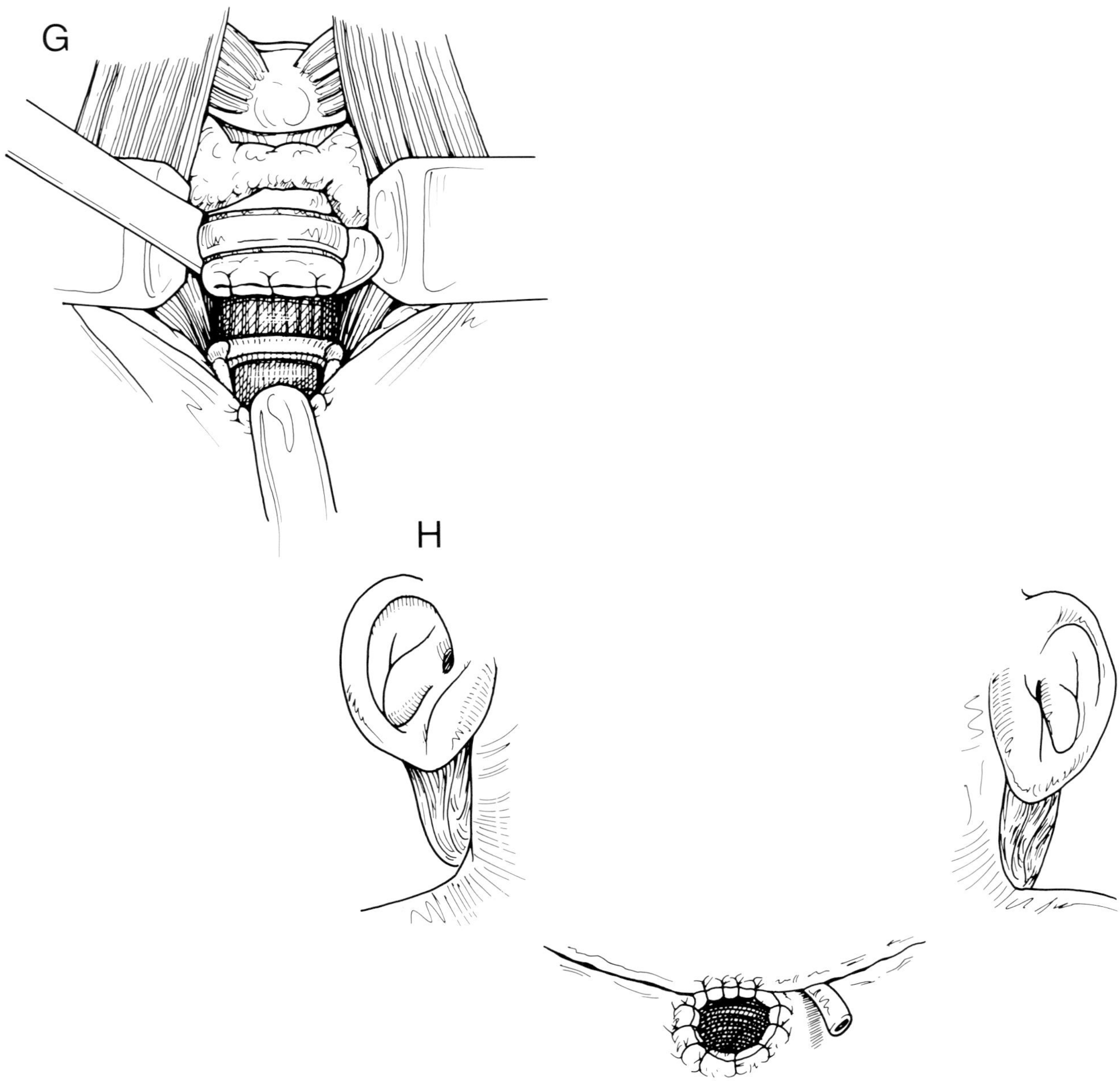


▶ **FIGURE 31-2**

I

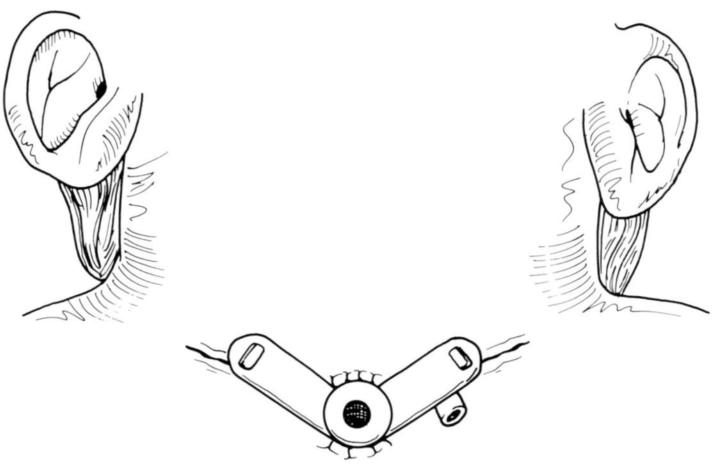

▶ **FIGURE 31-2**

## ▶ 31-3 EXCISION OF LARYNGEAL NODULES, POLYPS, AND GRANULOMAS

Vocal cord nodules are common in children and develop from vocal misuse and abuse.

### Indications

Vocal cord nodules are excised in postpubescent patients who have persistent hoarseness after failure of voice therapy. Younger children may need surgery if their signs and symptoms are severe and no response to voice therapy is detected after 6 months to 1 year. Granulomas and polyps usually occur secondary to some trauma, such as intubation or gastroesophageal reflux.

### Preoperative Evaluation

Direct laryngoscopy with a flexible laryngoscope or open laryngoscope is required to assess vocal cord function and identify the laryngeal lesion. Vocal nodules should not be removed until sufficient time has passed in voice therapy to expect significant improvement.

### Operative Technique

1. Using insufflation general anesthesia through a Jako laryngoscope with the patient breathing spontaneously, the larynx is exposed (see section 42–1) (Fig. 31–3**A**). For subglottic lesions, a subglottiscope is used.
2. The nodules, polyps or granulomas are vaporized with a $CO_2$ laser, taking care to preserve the underlying normal tissue (Fig. 31–3**B**). A metal suction protector may be used to avoid tissue damage in the surrounding area.
3. The remaining eschar is removed with a suction.
4. Alternatively, the lesion may be removed with small cup forceps.

### Complications

1. Laryngeal scar
2. Nodule recurrence

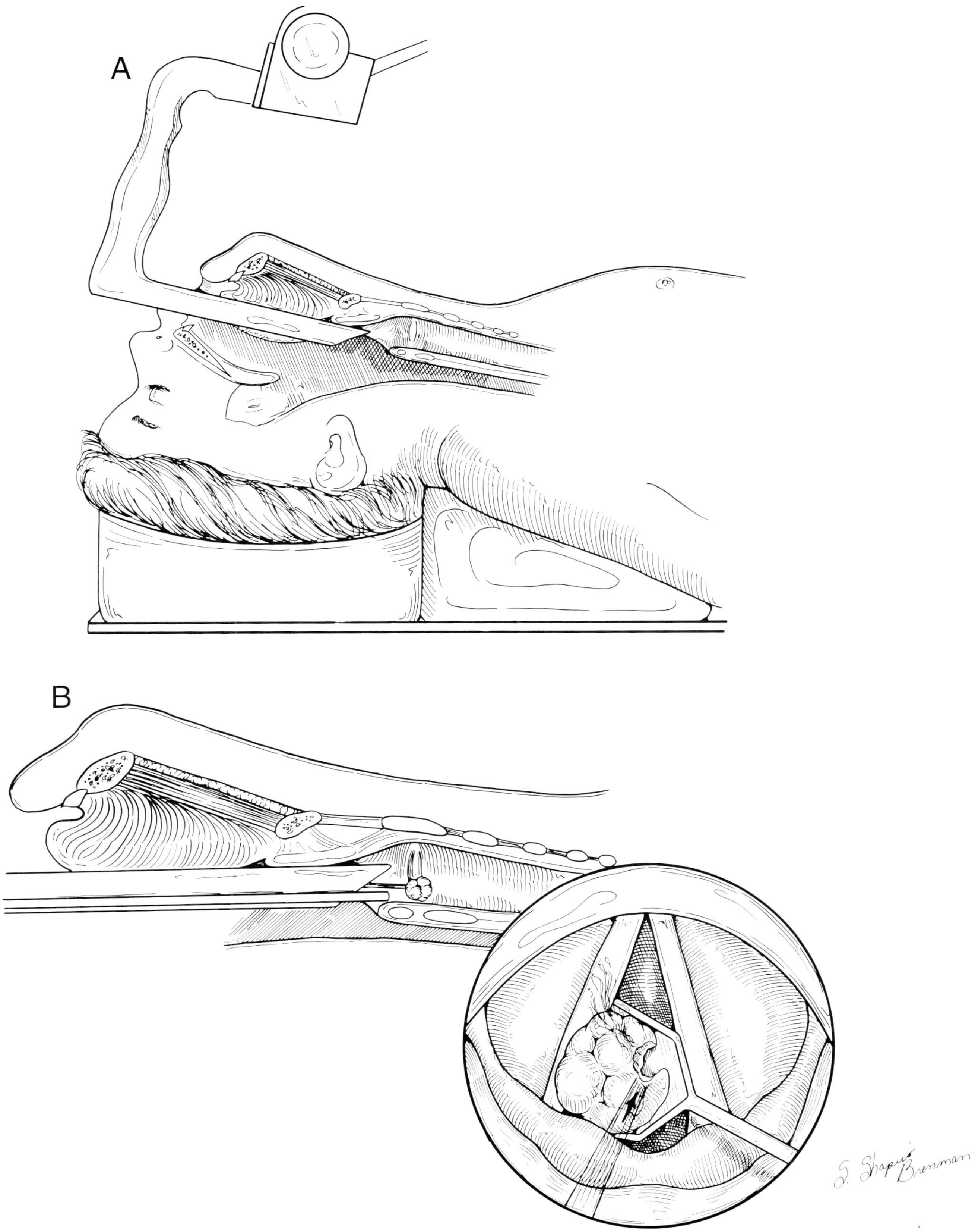


▶ **FIGURE 31-3**

## ▶ 31-4 REPAIR OF LARYNGEAL FRACTURE

Laryngeal fractures in children usually occur from a direct blow to the neck as a result of a "clothesline injury" or a motor vehicle accident. These patients usually arrive at the emergency department intubated with an endotracheal tube or a tracheostomy in place.

### Indications

Displaced laryngeal fractures require reduction to avoid laryngeal stenosis and airway obstruction.

### Preoperative Evaluation

Standard cervical and chest radiographs are obtained to rule out associated injuries. Computed tomography (CT) scan of the larynx will help to delineate the fractures. Direct laryngoscopy and bronchoscopy will define the configuration of the lumen and identify other laryngeal pathology, e.g., vocal cord paralysis, hematoma, and arytenoid dislocation.

### Operative Technique

1. Reduction of a laryngeal fracture is performed under general anesthesia administered through an endotracheal tube or an oral RAE tube placed in a tracheostoma.
2. One percent lidocaine with 1:100,000 epinephrine is injected subcutaneously at the site of the incision to aid in hemostasis.
3. A transverse incision is made at the level of the cricothyroid membrane down to the strap muscle (Fig. 31–4**A**).
4. A superior skin flap is elevated with a scissors to the level of the hyoid bone. An inferior skin flap is elevated exposing the strap muscles over the upper trachea (Fig. 31–4**B**).
5. The midline fascia is divided with a scissors, and the strap muscles are retracted with 4-0 prolene suture clamped with a hemostat exposing the thyroid, lamina, cricoid cartilage, and trachea (Fig. 31–4**B**).
6. Depressed thyroid cartilage fragments are aligned with a Cottle elevator (Fig. 31–4**C**).
7. The cartilage fragments are sutured in place with 4-0 prolene suture (Fig. 31–4**D**).
8. If the thyroid lamina is ossified, small holes can be drilled to hold the sutures.
9. The strap muscles are reapproximated in the midline with 4-0 Vicryl suture (Fig. 31–4**E**).
10. A Penrose drain is placed in the wound, and the subcutaneous tissue is closed with 4-0 Vicryl suture (Fig. 31–4**F**).
11. The skin is closed with 4-0 running subcuticular Vicryl.
12. If the child does not have a tracheostomy tube in place, the patient remains intubated with an endotracheal tube for 7 days. If there is a tracheotomy, the oral RAE tube is removed and replaced with a tracheostomy tube. An age-appropriate size Aboulker or Cotton-Lorenz stent is placed in the larynx

(Fig. 31–4D). The stent is secured with 2-0 prolene suture (see section 31–8, step 11, Fig. 31–8G).

**13.** Intravenous broad-spectrum antibiotics are continued for 14 days.

**14.** Seven days after the fracture reduction, the endotracheal tube or Aboulker stent (see section 31–8, step 14) is removed in the operating room, and direct laryngoscopy and bronchoscopy is performed.

**15.** If the cricoid cartilage is fractured, displaced, and comminuted, it is resected as described for severe high tracheal stenosis and tracheal atresia (see section 30–4).

**16.** The tracheostomy tube, if present, may be removed when the upper airway lumen is sufficient to permit normal respiration.

## Complications

1. Laryngeal stenosis
2. Dysphagia

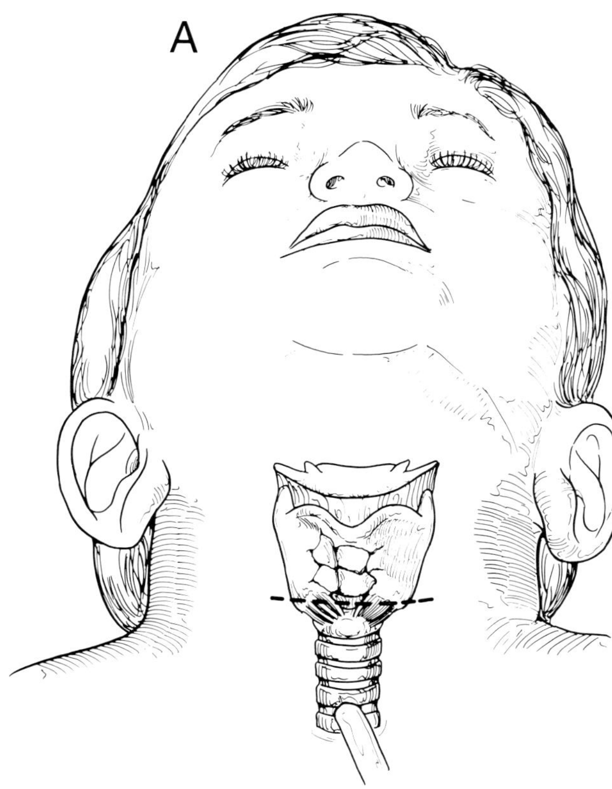


**▸ FIGURE 31-4**

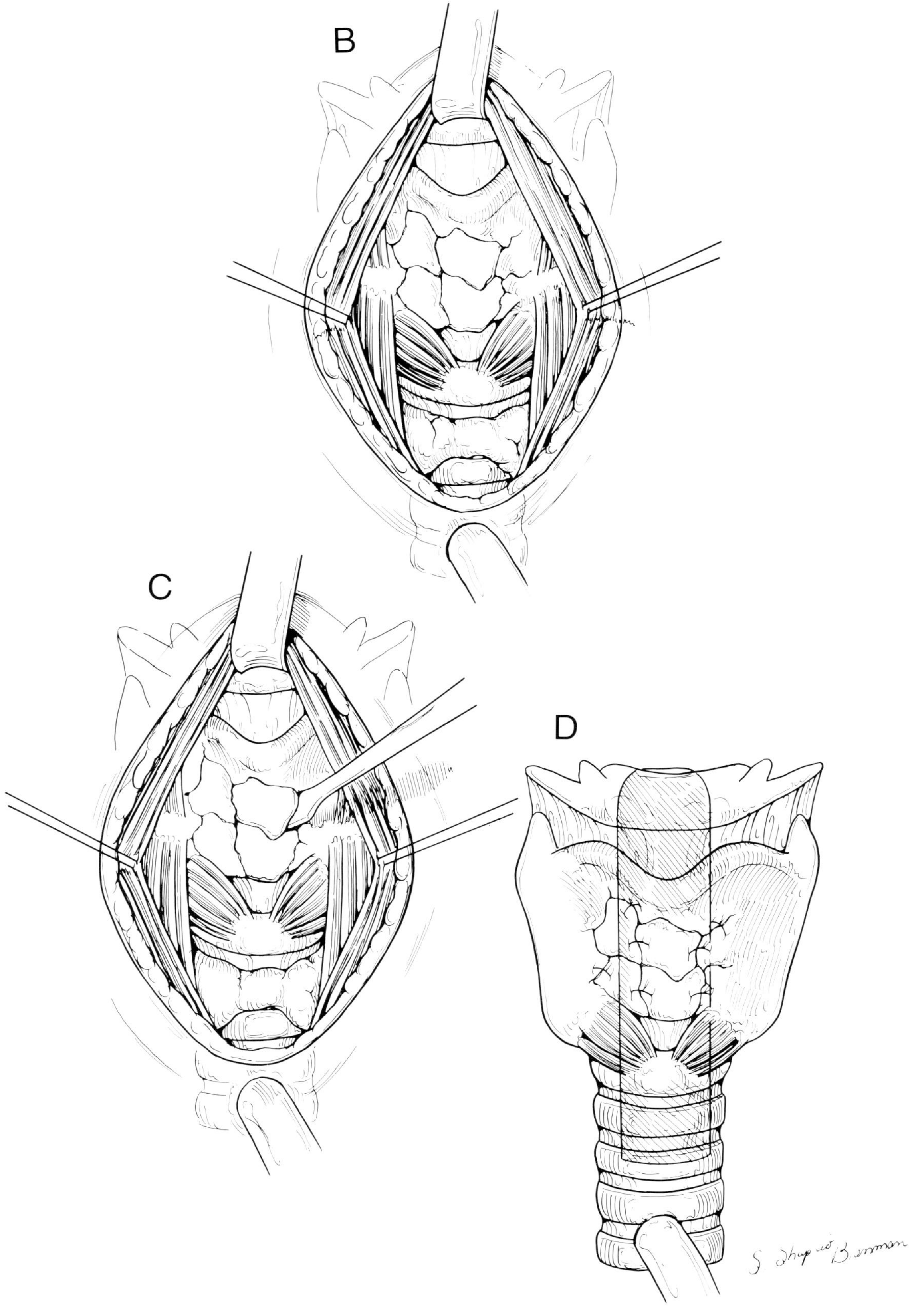


▶ **FIGURE 31-4**

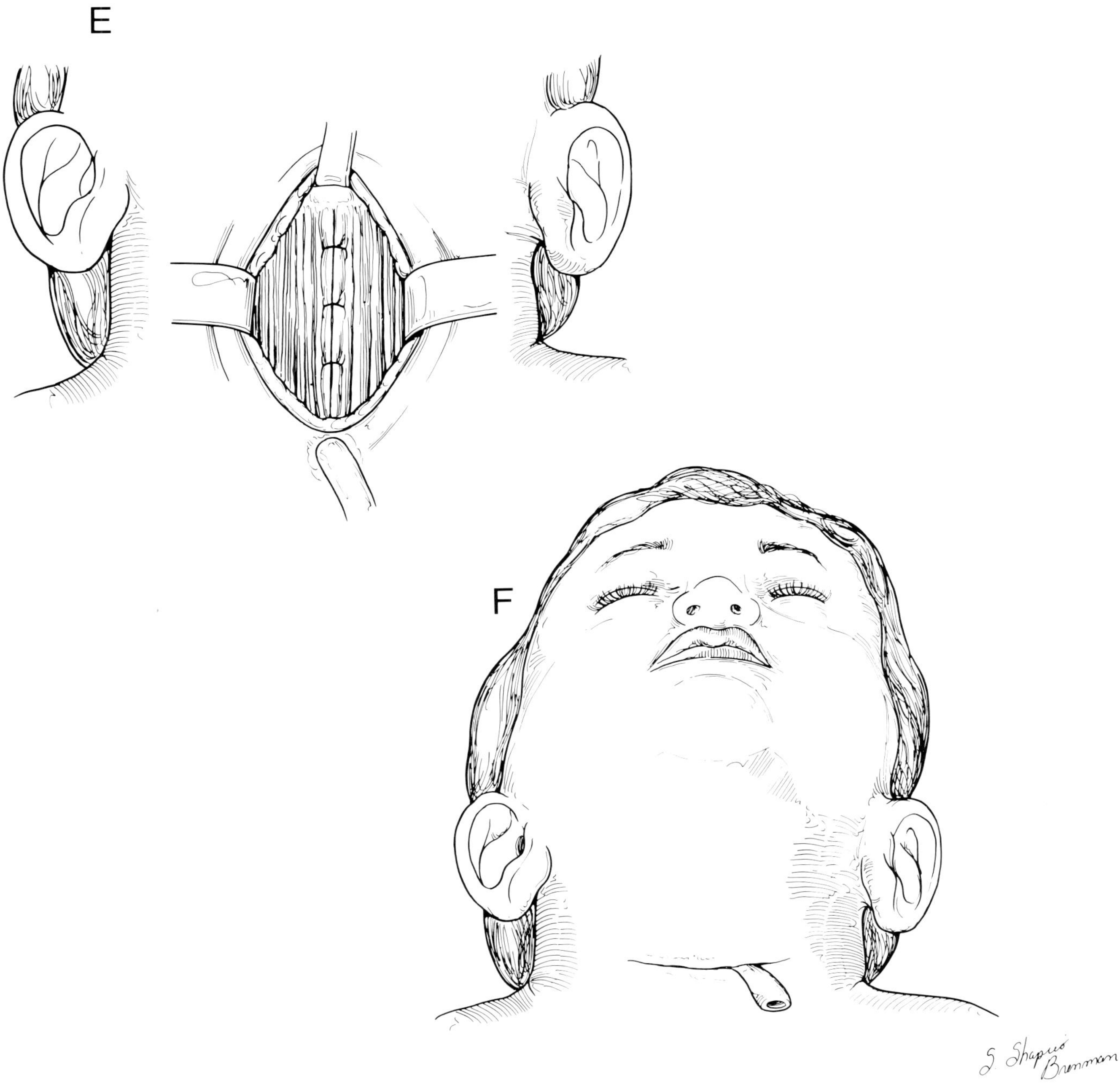


▶ **FIGURE 31-4**

## ▶ 31-5 CORRECTION OF SUBGLOTTIC STENOSIS—CRICOID SPLIT

Cricoid split is a procedure to enlarge the subglottic space. Early congenital and acquired subglottic stenosis can be treated with this procedure, avoiding the need for a tracheotomy. This procedure is especially helpful in facilitating extubation in a child who is difficult to extubate.

### Indications

The indication for a cricoid split is the inability to extubate a child under 2 years of age after a period of extended intubation.

The following criteria must be filled:

1. Extubation has failed on at least two occasions.
2. The child's weight is greater than 1,500 g.
3. Extubation failure is due only to laryngeal pathology.
4. No assisted ventilation is required for 10 days prior to consideration of a cricoid split.
5. Supplemental oxygen requirement is less than 35%.
6. No congestive heart failure has been present for one month prior to evaluation.
7. No acute upper or lower respiratory tract infection is present at the time of evaluation.
8. No antihypertensive medication is required for 10 days prior to evaluation.

### Preoperative Evaluation

The preoperative evaluation for a cricoid split includes a direct laryngoscopy and bronchoscopy. Radiographic studies are not helpful.

### Operative Technique

1. A cricoid split is performed under general anesthesia with the patient intubated with a bronchoscope or an endotracheal tube.
2. One percent lidocaine with 1:100,000 epinephrine is injected subcutaneously at the site of the incision to aid in hemostasis.
3. A horizontal incision is made over the cricoid cartilage through the skin and subcutaneous tissues (Fig. 31–5**A**).
4. The hyoid, thyroid, and cricoid cartilages are palpated through the incision.
5. The cervical fascia is divided horizontally, exposing the strap muscles (Fig. 31–5**B**). Superior and inferior skin flaps are elevated.
6. The fascia between the strap muscles is divided vertically, exposing the hyoid, thyroid, cricoid cartilage, and upper two tracheal rings (Fig. 31–5**C**).
7. A vertical incision is made through the cricoid cartilage and mucosa of the larynx, and extended inferiorly into the trachea through the upper two tracheal rings (Fig. 31–5**D**).
8. The incision is extended superiorly to within 2 mm of the thyroid notch, being certain to stay in the midline. Care must be taken to avoid cutting the hyoid bone (Fig. 31–5E), which may overlap the upper portion of the thyroid cartilage in infants.

**9.** A 5-0 prolene traction suture is placed through the cricoid cartilage, on each side of the incision, and the cricoid split is held open. These sutures assist in intubation of the trachea in the event of accidental extubation of the endotracheal tube (Fig. 31–5E).

**10.** An appropriate-sized endotracheal tube is passed from the nose into the trachea (Fig. 31–5F):

| | |
|---|---|
| <2,000 g | 3.0-mm endotracheal tube |
| 2,000–3,000 g | 3.5-mm endotracheal tube |
| 3,001–4,000 g | 4.0-mm endotracheal tube |

The endotracheal tube is secured with tape or suture to the nose

**11.** The strap muscles are not closed. The subcutaneous fat is closed loosely with 5-0 chromic suture.

**12.** A rubber band drain is placed in the wound and secured with a loose suture in the subcutaneous tissues. The skin is not sutured (Fig. 31–5F). The traction sutures are labeled "R" and "L" and taped to the chest.

**13.** No dressing is applied to the wound.

**14.** The drain is left in place 3 days while the patient is observed in the intensive care unit for airway obstruction.

**15.** The patient is extubated 10 days after the cricoid split. Dexamethasone 1 mg/kg per day is given 12 hours prior to extubation and is continued for 3 days.

## Complications

1. Emphysema
   - Subcutaneous
   - Mediastinal
2. Pneumothorax
3. Persistent subglottic stenosis
4. Endotracheal tube complications
   - Accidental extubation
   - Mucus plugging

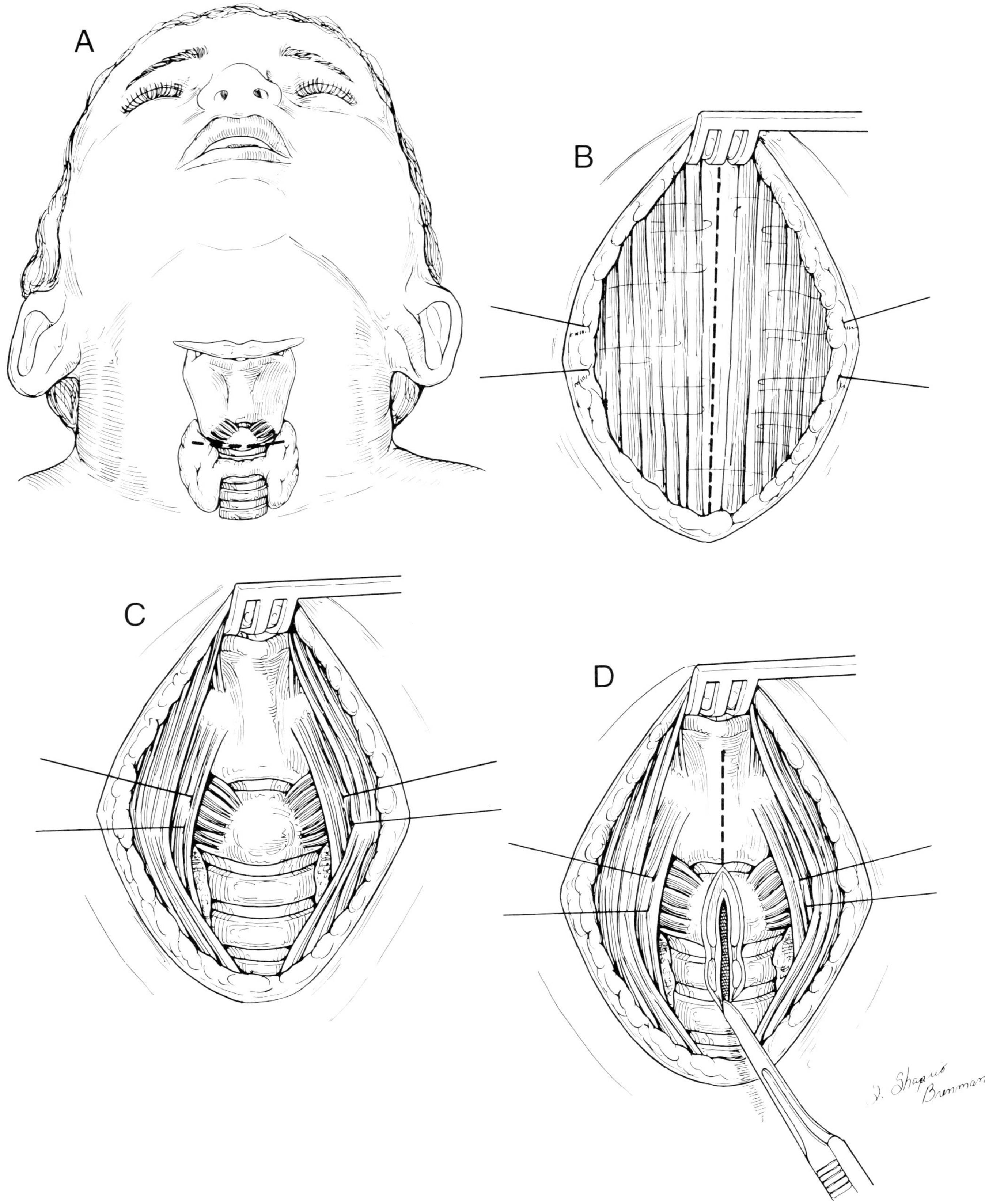


▶ **FIGURE 31-5**

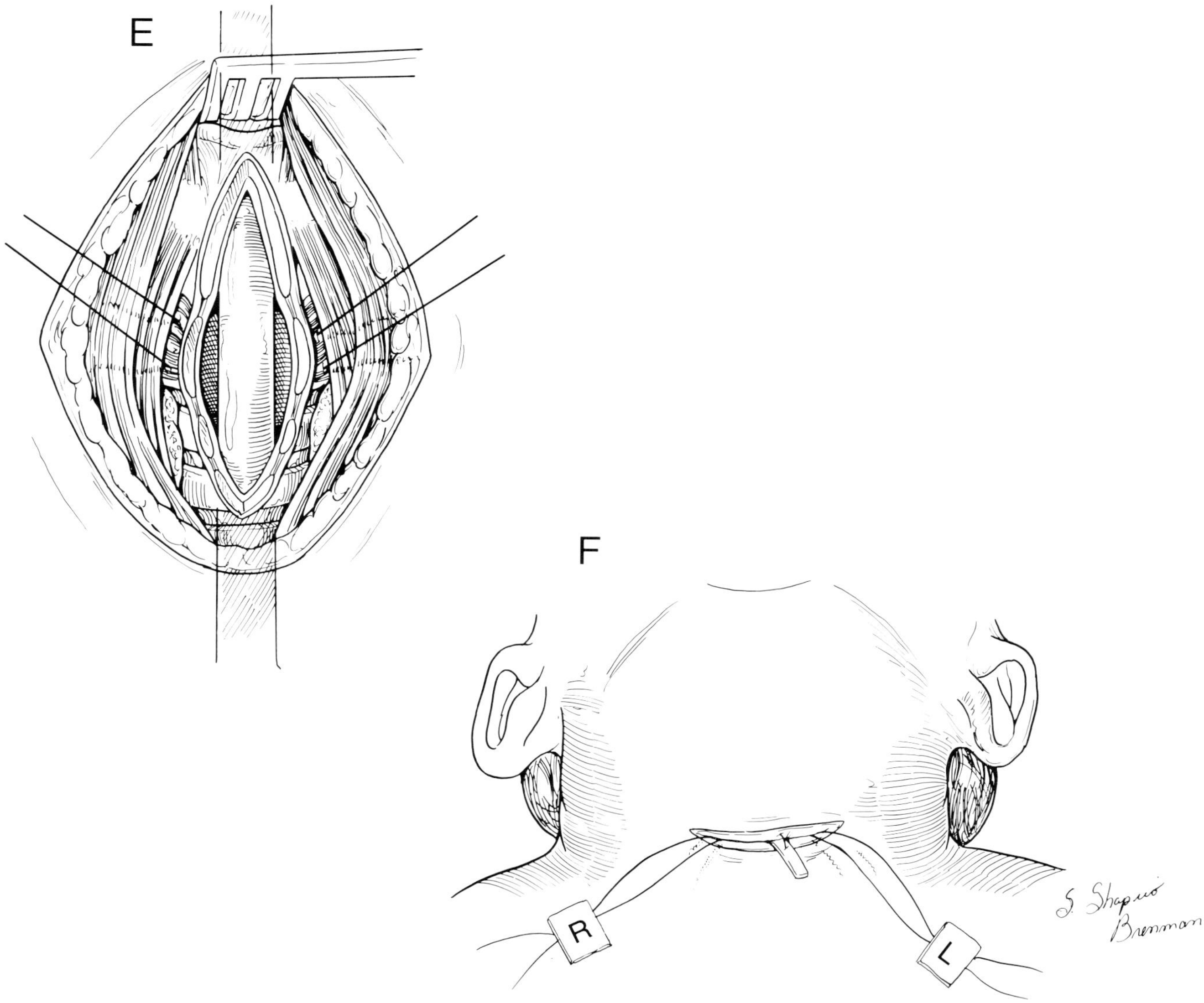


▶ **FIGURE 31-5**

## ▶ 31-6 LARYNGOTRACHEOPLASTY (LTP) (ANTERIOR GRAFT)

LTP with cartilage graft is a procedure that is used in the management of subglottic stenosis.

### Indications

The indication for LTP is anterior subglottic stenosis that is most often acquired. This includes patients who have not had any surgical treatment for their subglottic stenosis and those who may have failed other procedures. These patients usually have a tracheotomy in place.

### Preoperative Evaluation

The preoperative evaluation includes direct laryngoscopy, bronchoscopy, and esophagoscopy. A 24-hour double-lumen pH probe study is needed to rule out gastroesophageal (GE) reflux, and a milk scan may be obtained. A speech evaluation should be obtained for children who are speaking.

A pulmonary evaluation is required to be certain the patient does not require supplemental oxygen therapy. Uncontrolled GE reflux or pulmonary disease requiring supplemental oxygen must be corrected prior to LTP.

### Operative Technique

LTP is performed using general anesthesia.

1. The patient is positioned on a shoulder roll with the neck extended as for tracheotomy. The neck and right chest are prepped to facilitate taking the cartilage graft. The upper edge of the drape is placed on the lower lip to provide access to the oral cavity for laryngoscopy during the procedure. A sticky bi-drape is best for this exposure.
2. A cut oral RAE tube is placed in the tracheostoma and sutured to the chest (Fig. 31–6**A**).
3. One percent lidocaine with 1:100,000 epinephrine is injected subcutaneously at the site of the incision to aid in hemostasis.
4. A horizontal incision is made above the tracheostoma through the platysma to the cervical fascia (Fig. 31–6**A**).
5. The flap is elevated superiorly with a knife to the level of the thyroid notch and is sutured to the drape to provide exposure (Fig. 31–6**B**).
6. The strap muscles are divided in the midline and retracted laterally with prolene sutures in the muscle, exposing the larynx and trachea (Fig. 31–6**B**).
7. A midline incision is made in the cricoid and extended inferiorly to a point just above the tracheostoma without entering the stoma (Figs. 31–6**B** and 31–6**C**).
8. The incision is extended superiorly into the thyroid cartilage to a level just below the anterior commissure. Care is taken not to violate the anterior commissure.
9. A neurosurgical pledget soaked with oxymetazoline is placed in the larynx to decongest the mucosa in the region of the laryngeal pathology.

10. Wet 4 × 4 sponges are placed over the neck and a cartilage graft is taken from the previously prepped right chest (see section 31–11). The surgeon re-gowns and -gloves, and separate instruments are used for the cartilage graft. Because the laryngotracheal exposure is completed, the size of graft can be determined prior to harvesting the costal cartilage.
11. The cartilage graft is shaped with a knife to create a boat-shaped piece with a beveled edge that fits into the anterior tracheal wall defect (Fig. 31–6D).
12. The side of the cartilage graft with the perichondrium intact is placed in the larynx (Fig. 31–6E).
13. The graft is sutured in place with 5-0 prolene suture on a cutting needle using the minimum of sutures needed to hold the graft in place (Fig. 31–6E).
14. Laryngoscopy and tracheoscopy is performed to assess the lumen in the subglottic region.
15. The wound is closed approximating the strap muscles with 4-0 Vicryl around the graft to provide vascularity. A Penrose drain is placed in the wound.
16. The subcutaneous tissues are closed with 4-0 Vicryl and the skin closure is completed with 4-0 running subcuticular Vicryl sutures (Fig. 31–6F). A minimal gauze dressing is applied. The oral RAE tube is removed and the tracheotomy tube is replaced.
17. A chest x-ray is obtained in the OR or in the recovery room.
18. Broad-spectrum antibiotics are administered for 10 days. The drain is removed in 24 to 36 hours.
19. The patient is placed on dexamethasone 1 mg/kg/day with a maximum of 20 mg for 48 hours before stent removal and every other day for 2 weeks. At the end of 2 weeks, the patient returns for another laryngoscopy and bronchoscopy. Residual granulation tissue is removed as needed.
20. When the airway is adequate as determined by direct laryngoscopy and bronchoscopy, decannulation can be attempted.

## Complications

1. Pneumothorax
2. Restenosis
3. Failure to extubate

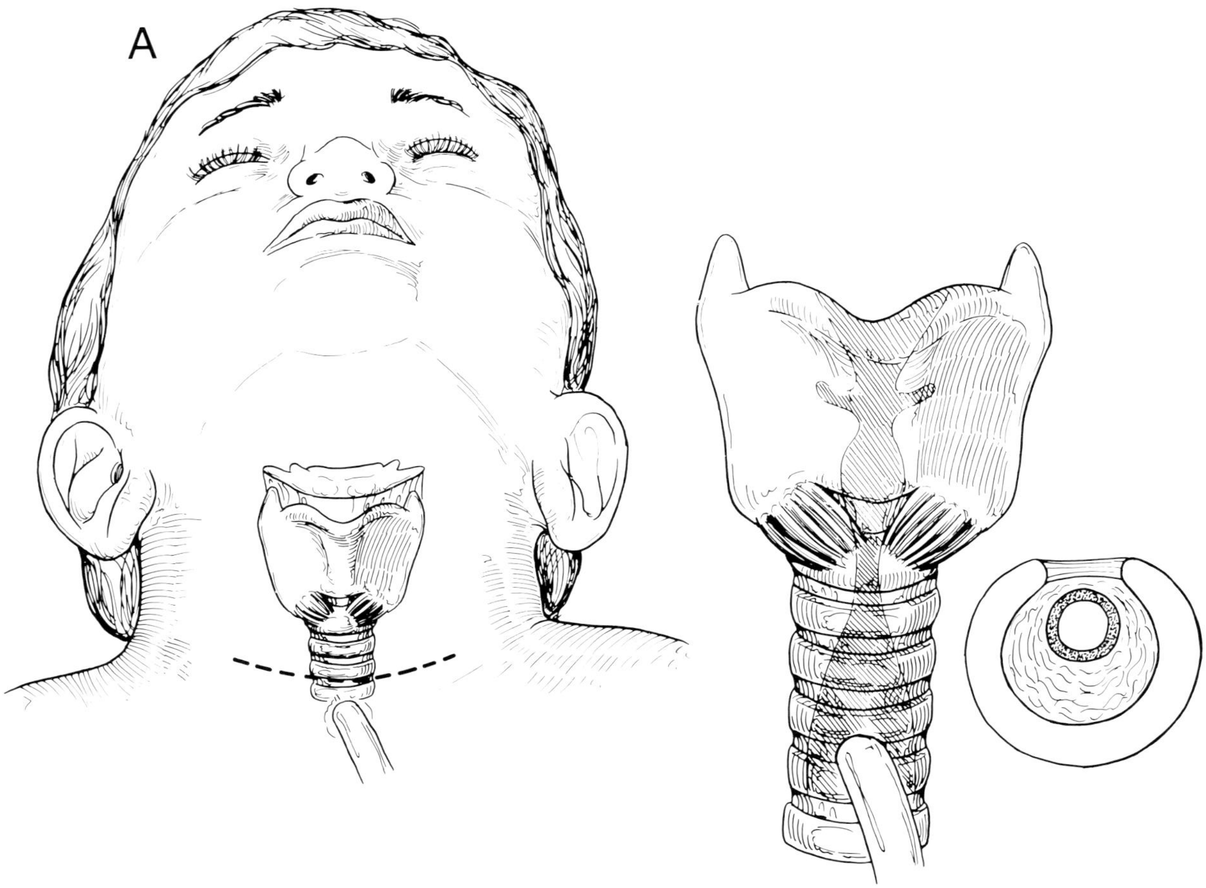


▶ **FIGURE 31-6**

B

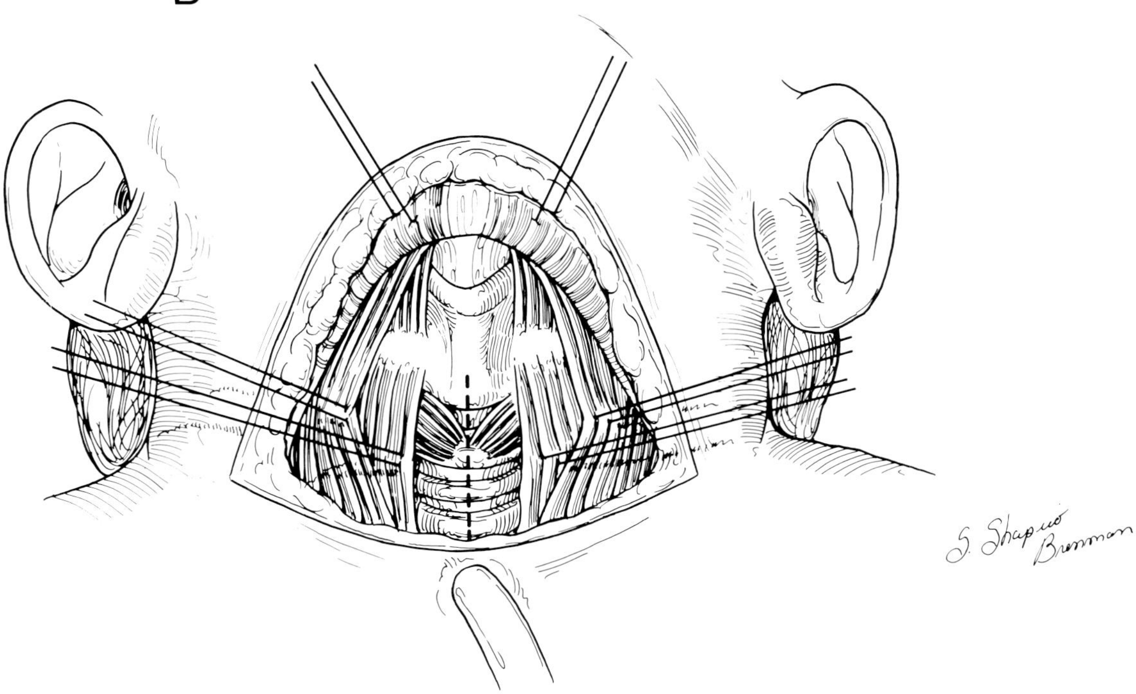

▶ **FIGURE 31-6**

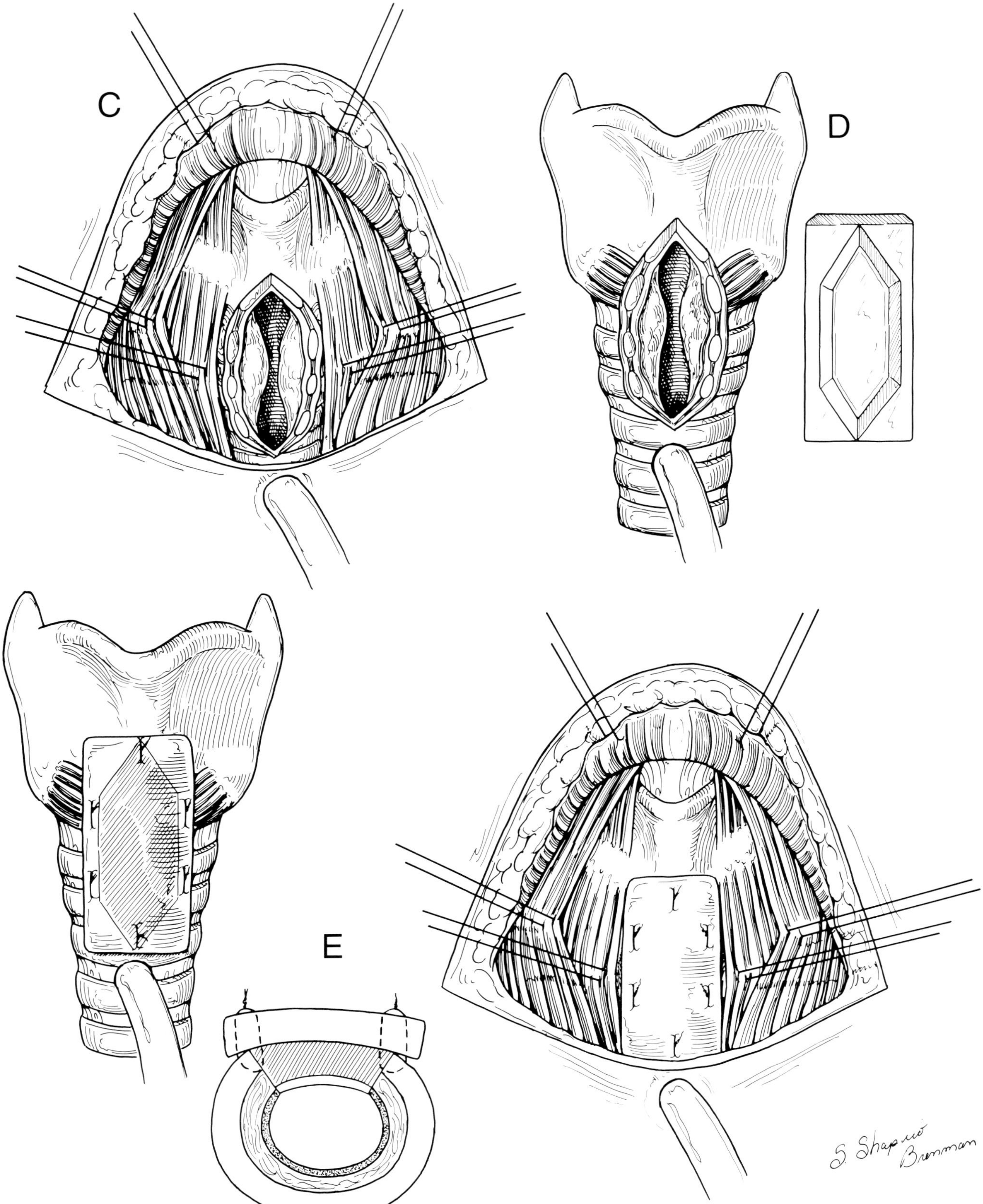


▶ **FIGURE 31-6**

F

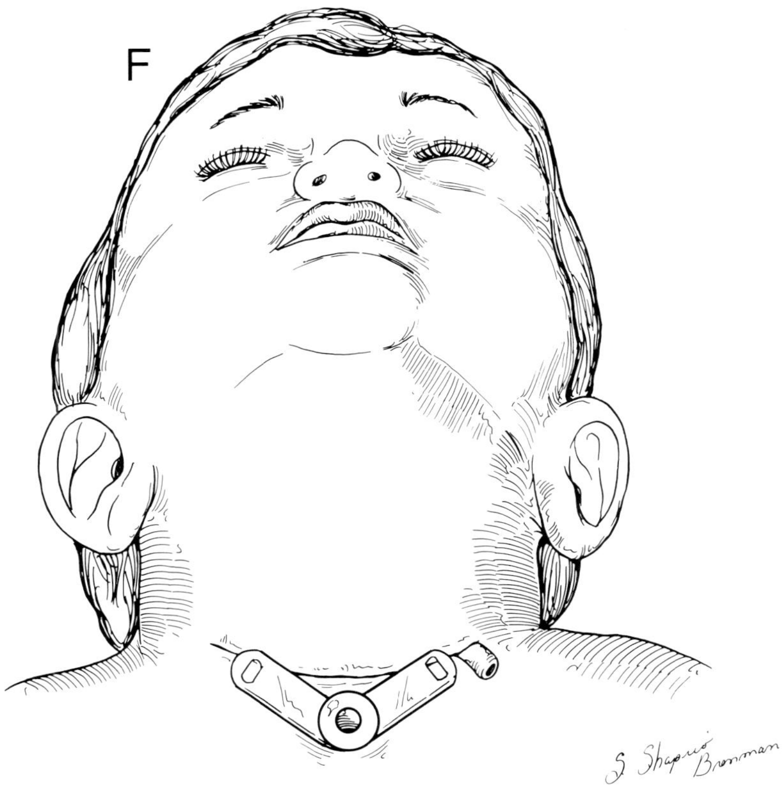

▶ **FIGURE 31-6**

## ▶ 31-7 LARYNGOTRACHEOPLASTY (LTP) (SINGLE-STAGE)

### Indications

The indication for single-stage LTP is moderate anterior subglottic stenosis where prolonged stenting is judged not to be necessary.

### Preoperative Evaluation

The preoperative evaluation includes direct laryngoscopy, bronchoscopy, and esophagoscopy. A 24-hour double-lumen pH probe study is needed to rule out gastroesophageal (GE) reflux, and a milk scan may be obtained. A speech evaluation should be obtained for children who are speaking.

A pulmonary evaluation is required to be certain the patient does not require supplemental oxygen therapy. Uncontrolled GE reflux or pulmonary disease requiring supplemental oxygen must be corrected prior to LTP.

### Operative Technique

LTP is performed using general anesthesia.

1. The patient is positioned on a shoulder roll with the neck extended as for tracheotomy. The neck and right chest are prepped to facilitate taking the cartilage graft. The upper edge of the drape is placed on the upper lip to provide access to the oral cavity for laryngoscopy during the procedure. A sticky bi-drape is best for this exposure.
2. A cut oral RAE tube is placed in the tracheostoma and sutured to the chest.
3. One percent lidocaine with 1:100,000 epinephrine is injected subcutaneously at the site of the incision to aid in hemostasis.
4. A horizontal incision is made above the tracheostoma through the platysma to the cervical fascia (Fig. 31–7**A**).
5. The flap is elevated superiorly with a knife to the level of the thyroid notch and is sutured to the drape to provide exposure. The strap muscles are divided in the midline and retracted laterally with prolene sutures in the muscle, exposing the larynx and trachea (Fig. 31–7**A**).
6. A midline incision is made in the cricoid and extended inferiorly to include the tracheostoma (Fig. 31–7**B**).
7. The incision is extended superiorly into the thyroid cartilage to a level just below the anterior commissure. Care is taken not to violate the anterior commissure.
8. The oral RAE tracheostomy tube is removed and an endotracheal tube is placed through the nose into the larynx to facilitate ventilation and postoperative stenting (Fig. 31–7**C**).
9. Wet 4 × 4 sponges are placed over the neck and a cartilage graft is taken from the previously prepped right chest (see section 31–11). The surgeon regowns and -gloves, and separate instruments are used for the cartilage graft. Because the laryngotracheal exposure is completed, the size of grafts can be determined prior to harvesting the costal cartilage.
10. The cartilage is cut into two pieces to create the grafts needed for reconstruction (Fig. 31–7**D**). A knife is used to shape the first piece into a boat-

shaped graft with beveled edges. Note that the bottom of the main graft is flat (Figs. 31–7C and 31–7D) to accommodate the second graft that will cover the tracheostoma (Fig. 31–7D).

**11.** The side of the cartilage graft with the perichondrium intact is placed in the larynx (Fig. 31–7D).

**12.** The graft is sutured in place with 5-0 prolene suture on a cutting needle using the minimum of sutures needed to hold the graft in place (Fig. 31–7E).

**13.** The second cartilage graft that has been cut in a stair-step fashion to accommodate the vertical graft is placed over the tracheostoma (Figs. 31–7D and 31–7E). This piece of cartilage is buried laterally in pockets under the strap muscles.

**14.** The wound is closed approximating the strap muscles with 4-0 Vicryl around the grafts to provide vascularity. A Penrose drain is placed in the wound (Fig. 31–7F).

**15.** The subcutaneous tissues are closed with 4-0 Vicryl and the skin closure is completed with 4-0 running subcuticular Vicryl sutures (Fig. 31–7A). A minimal gauze dressing is applied.

**16.** A chest x-ray is obtained in the operating room or the recovery room.

**17.** The endotracheal tube is secured with tape or suture to the nose (Fig. 31–7G). The tube remains in place 7 to 10 days and is removed in the operating room.

**18.** If the airway is determined to be satisfactory by endoscopy, the patient is reintubated with a ½ size smaller tube and then extubated when fully awake in the intensive care unit the next day.

**19.** The drain is removed in 24 to 36 hours.

**20.** Broad spectrum antibiotics are administered for 10 days.

## Complications

1. Pneumothorax
2. Restenosis
3. Failure to extubate

A

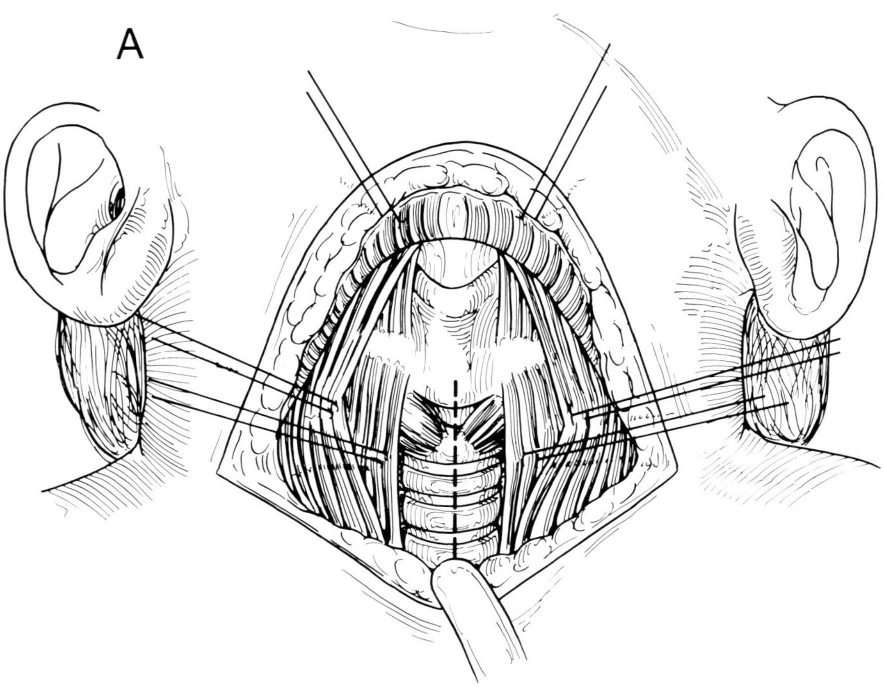

▶ **FIGURE 31-7**

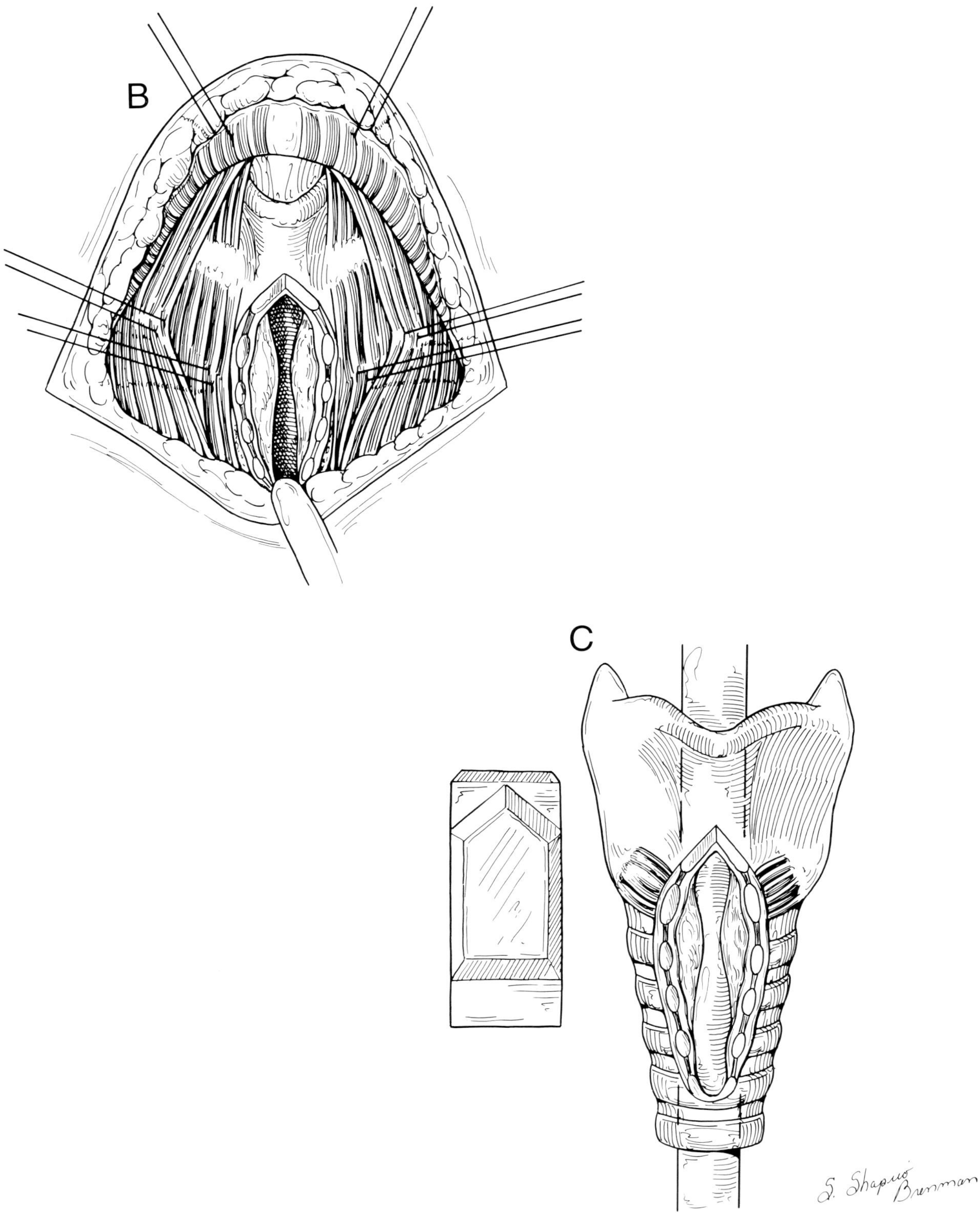


▶ **FIGURE 31-7**

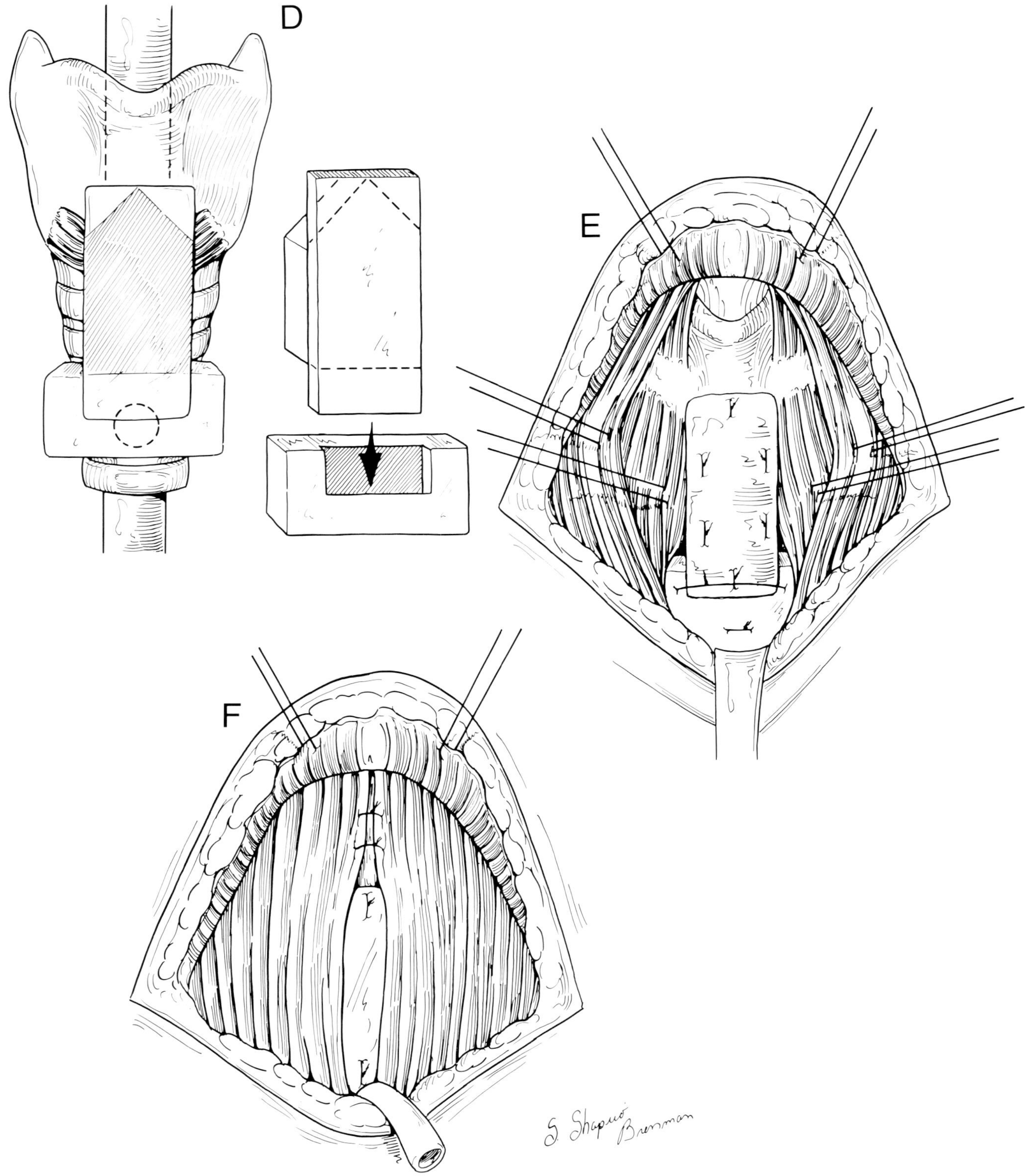


▶ **FIGURE 31-7**

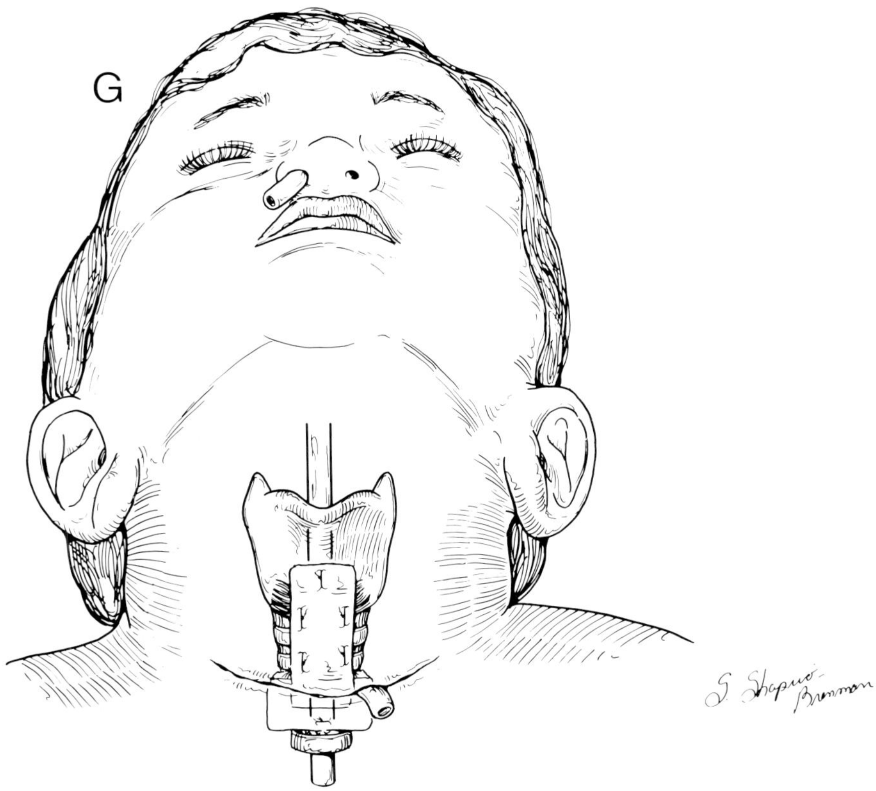


▶ **FIGURE 31-7**

## ▶ 31-8 LARYNGOTRACHEOPLASTY (LTP) (POSTERIOR GRAFT)

### Indications

Posterior costal cartilage grafting is indicated for posterior laryngotracheal stenosis with or without anterior stenosis. It is also effective in the treatment of a congenital elliptical cricoid stenosis as well as a glottic or interarytenoid web. Posterior graft may be used with or without an anterior graft (see section 31–6).

### Preoperative Evaluation

The preoperative evaluation includes laryngoscopy, bronchoscopy, and esophagoscopy. A 24-hour double-lumen pH probe study to rule out gastroesophageal (GE) reflux is needed and a milk scan may be obtained. A speech evaluation should be obtained for children who are speaking.

A pulmonary evaluation is required to be certain the patient does not require supplemental oxygen therapy. Uncontrolled GE reflux or pulmonary disease requiring supplemental oxygen therapy must be corrected prior to LTP.

### Operative Technique

1. The same procedure is used for LTP with a posterior graft as for anterior graft LTP (see section 31–6) with a cut oral RAE tube in the tracheostoma.
2. One percent lidocaine with 1:100,000 epinephrine is injected subcutaneously at the site of the incision to aid in hemostasis.
3. The incision is extended superiorly through the thyroid cartilage to within 2 mm of the thyroid notch, but the anterior commissure is kept intact if possible (Fig. 31–8**A**).
4. The thyroid and cricoid cartilages are retracted with 4-0 prolene suture, exposing the posterior interarytenoid region (Fig. 31–8**B**).
5. One percent lidocaine with 1:100,000 epinephrine is injected submucosally in the posterior midline of the larynx and trachea (Fig. 31–8**B**).
6. A neurosurgical pledget soaked with oxymetazoline is placed in the posterior cricoid region to decongest the mucosa and is left in place for 3 to 4 minutes.
7. A vertical incision is made through the mucosa, posterior lamina of the cricoid cartilage, and posterior perichondrium with a #69 Beaver blade. The incision extends from the interarytenoid muscles to approximately 1 cm below the inferior border of the cricoid cartilage and is taken down to the tracheoesophageal septum (Fig. 31–8**C**). Care should be taken not to enter the epipharyngeal mucosa.
8. If the incision is not in the midline, the posterior cricoarytenoid muscle fibers will guide the surgeon back to the midline.
9. The posterior cricoid is distracted laterally by placing the boat-shaped cartilage with a carved ledge overlapping posteriorly (Fig. 31–8**D**).
10. The graft is sutured in place with 5-0 Vicryl suture on a $P_2$ needle using a minimum of six sutures to hold the graft in place. The suture passes through mucosa, costal cartilage, and back out through the mucosa as a mattress suture tied in the laryngeal side (Figs. 31–8**D** and 31–8**E**).

11. An Aboulker or Cotton-Lorenz stent is placed through the larynx and secured in place with a suture. The stent size is selected to match the external diameter of the age-appropriate endotracheal tube for that child. The stent is cut to extend from just above the true vocal cords to 1 cm above the tracheostoma (Fig. 31–8F). A 2-0 prolene suture is passed through strap muscle on one side of the larynx, the cricoid cartilage, the stent, the cricoid cartilage on the other side, and the opposite strap muscle. The suture is threaded through a 16-gauge angiocath and tied with a knot of 10 to 15 throws, so it can be felt easily through the skin for later removal (Fig. 31–8G).
12. An anterior rib graft, if needed, may be placed at this time (see section 31–6).
13. The tracheotomy tube is replaced in the tracheostoma (Figs. 31–8F and 31–8H).
14. The stent is left in place for 6 weeks.
15. If a single-stage LTP is done with a posterior graft, no stent is placed. An age-appropriate endotracheal tube is left in place 7 to 10 days.
16. When the stent is removed in 6 weeks, an incision is made over the knot, and the suture is cut, permitting the suture and angiocath to be removed.
17. Direct laryngoscopy and tracheoscopy are performed and any exuberant granulation tissue is removed.
18. The patient is placed on dexamethasone 1 mg/kg/day (with a maximum of 20 mg) for 48 hours before stent removal and then every other day for 2 weeks. At the end of 2 weeks, the patient returns for another laryngoscopy and bronchoscopy. Residual granulation tissue, if present, is removed.
19. The patient remains on broad-spectrum antibiotics from the time of the initial procedure until the surgeon deems them no longer necessary.
20. When the airway is adequate as determined by direct laryngoscopy and bronchoscopy, decannulation can be attempted.

## Complications

1. Pneumothorax
2. Failure to decannulate
3. Restenosis

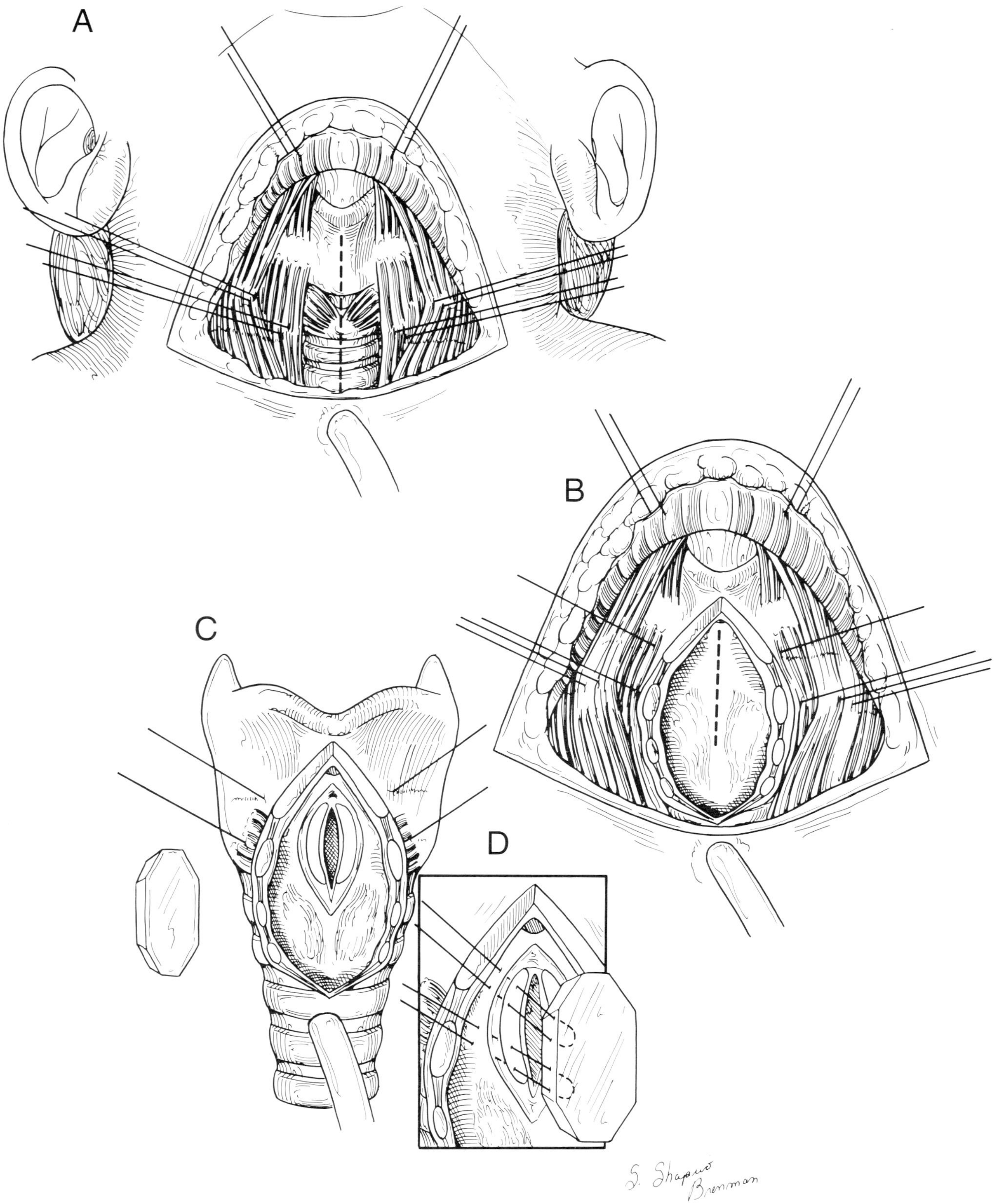


▶ **FIGURE 31-8**

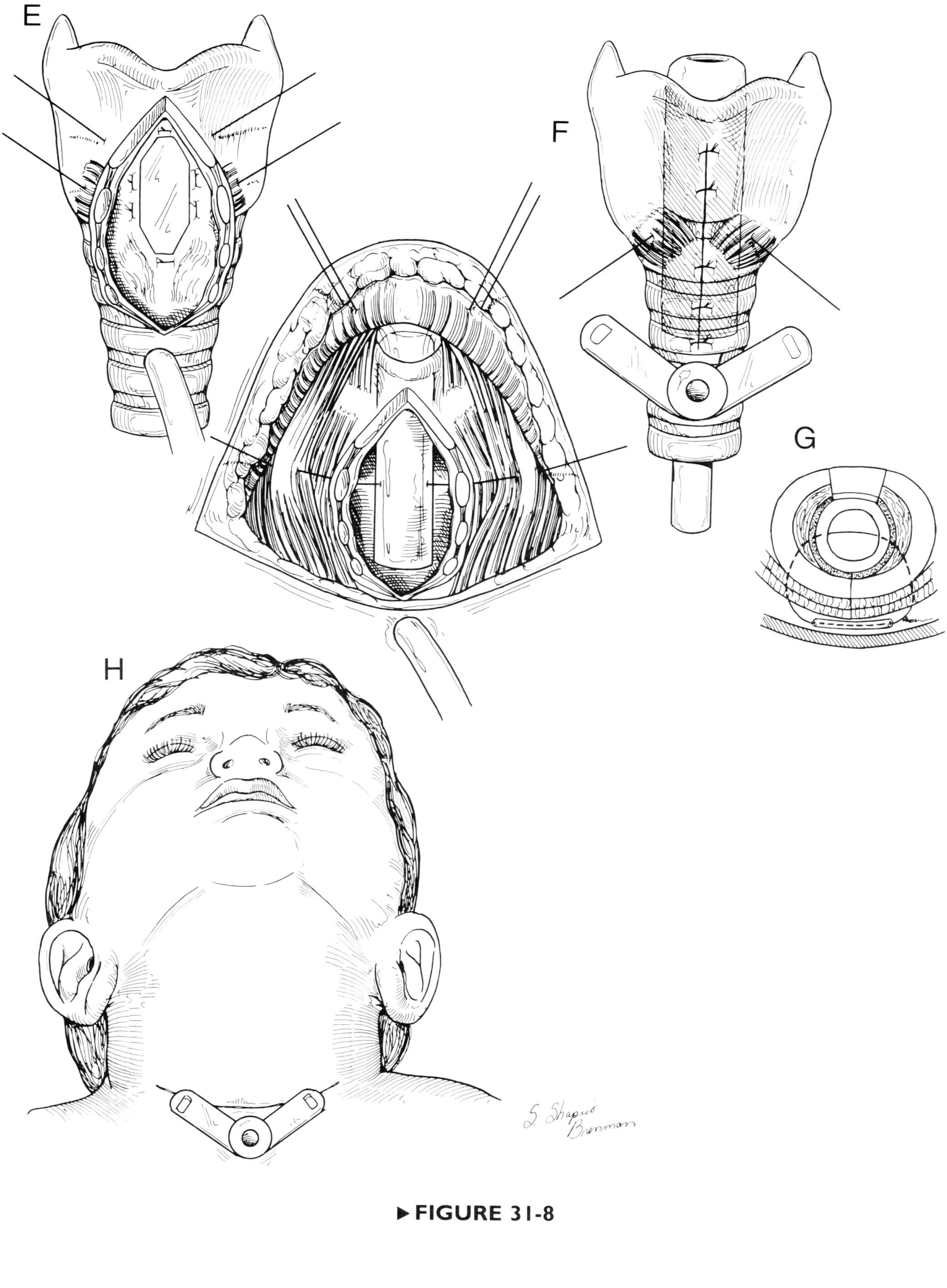


▶ **FIGURE 31-8**

## ▶ 31-9 LARYNGOTRACHEOPLASTY (LTP) (LATERAL CUTS)

### Indications

Lateral cuts are indicated in the management of severe laryngeal stenosis and complete or nearly complete laryngeal atresia not amenable to management with anterior and/or posterior grafts.

### Operative Procedure

1. After completion of exposure for an anterior (see section 31–6) and posterior (see section 31–8) costal cartilage graft (Fig. 31–9**A**), an incision is made at 3 and 9 o'clock into the lateral cricoid ring through the lateral periochondrium with a sickle-shaped Beaver knife without entering the soft tissue lateral to the cartilage (Figs. 31–9**B** and 31–9**C**). This avoids injury to the recurrent laryngeal nerves.
2. No cartilage grafts are placed in the lateral cuts.
3. The posterior and anterior costal cartilage grafts are placed (Fig. 31–9**D**) as needed with an Aboulker or Cotton-Lorenz stent in the larynx. If complete cricoid atresia is present, and there is only sufficient room for an anterior graft, the stent is left in place 6 to 12 months and is secured to a metal tracheostomy tube to avoid tracheal stenosis (Fig. 31–9**E**).
4. The extubation procedure used for all LTPs with stents is followed (see section 31–8).

### Complications

1. Pneumothorax
2. Breakage of stent at the attachment to the metal tracheostomy tube
3. Failure to decannulate
4. Restenosis

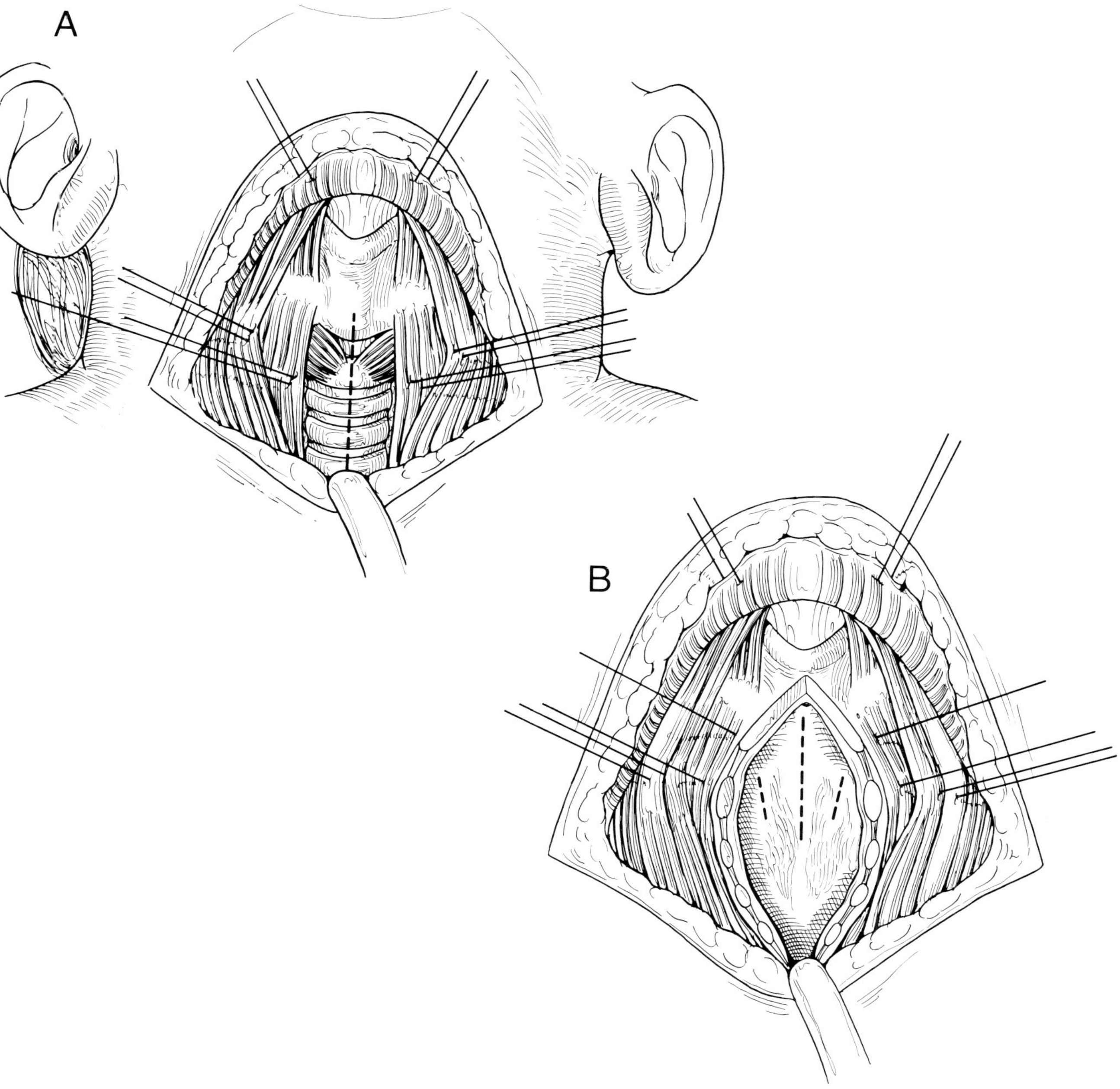

▶ **FIGURE 31-9**

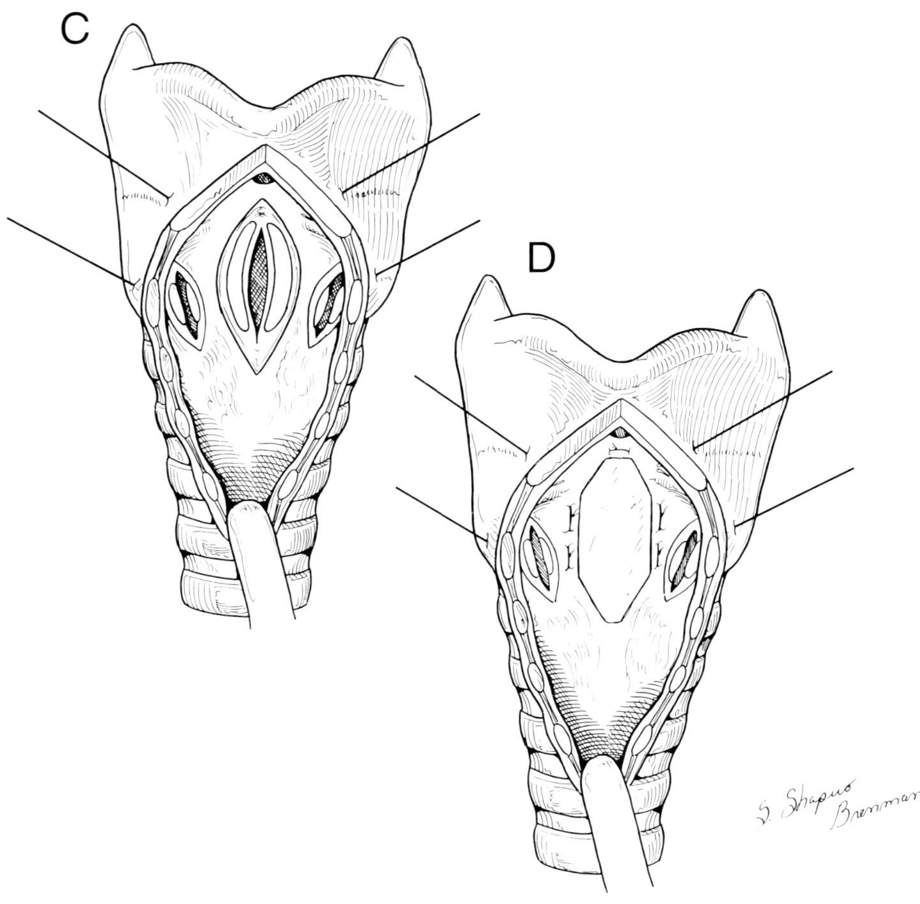


▶ **FIGURE 31-9**

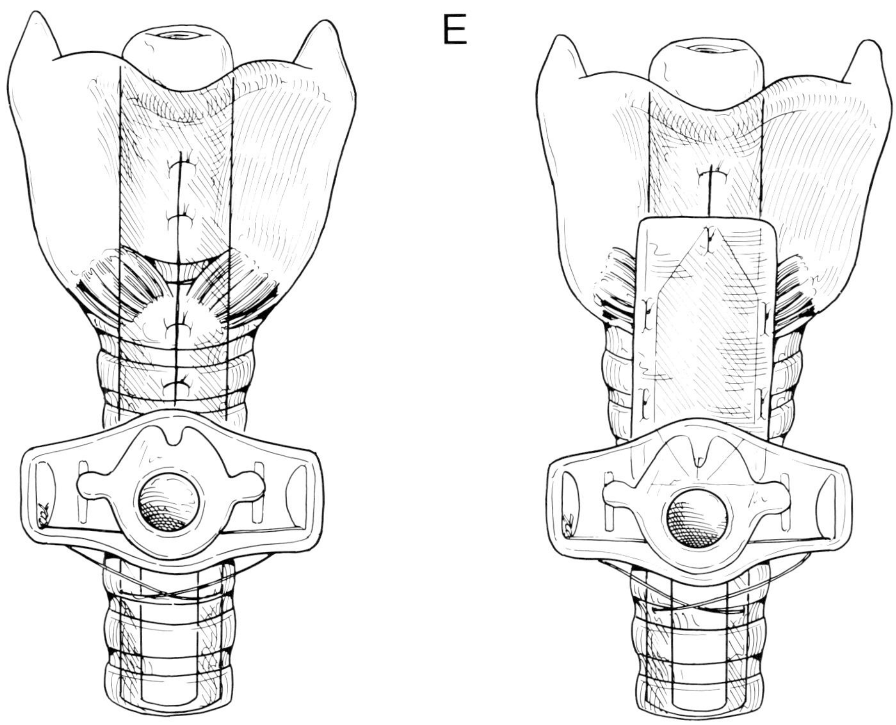


▶ **FIGURE 31-9**

## ▶ 31-10 TRACHEOPLASTY (REPAIR OF TRACHEAL STENOSIS AT TRACHEOSTOMY SITE)

Tracheoplasty may be required to correct malacia or stenosis that develops as a result of a long-term tracheostomy.

### Indications

Tracheoplasty is indicated in the management of tracheal stenosis or tracheomalacia at a tracheostomy stoma site that is preventing decannulation.

### Preoperative Evaluation

Direct laryngoscopy and bronchoscopy are required to assess the stomal site. Radiographic studies are not helpful.

### Operative Technique

1. Tracheoplasty is performed using general anesthesia using a cut oral RAE tube placed in the tracheostomy site.
2. The patient is positioned as for tracheostomy.
3. One percent lidocaine with 1:100,000 epinephrine is injected subcutaneously at the site of the incision to aid in hemostasis.
4. A transverse elliptical neck incision is made encompassing the tracheostoma (Fig. 31–10**A**).
5. The incision is carried through subcutaneous and fibrous tissue down to the trachea.
6. The strap muscles are released and retracted laterally with 4-0 prolene sutures clamped with a hemostat (Fig. 31–10**B**).
7. The tracheocutaneous fistula is dissected with a scissors down to the trachea and then resected (Fig. 31–10**C**).
8. The trachea is opened vertically with a knife, exposing the tracheal pathology (Fig. 31–10**D**).
9. The vertical incision is extended from normal trachea above, through the stenosis or malacic segment, to normal trachea below (Fig. 31–10E).
10. An age-appropriate size endotracheal tube is placed through the nose and into the trachea and the cut oral RAE tube is removed.
11. The surgeon covers the wound and regowns and -gloves. A costal cartilage graft is taken as described for anterior costal cartilage graft (see section 31–11).
12. The cartilage graft is shaped as described for anterior costal cartilage graft (see section 31–6).
13. The graft is sutured in place with the periochondrial-covered side in the tracheal lumen using 4-0 prolene passed through the tracheal rings and sutured to the costal cartilage graft (Fig. 31–10F).
14. The strap muscles are closed over the graft with 4-0 Vicryl to make it as airtight as possible and to provide additional vascularity to the graft (Fig. 31–10G).

**15.** A Penrose drain is placed in the wound from the level of the strap muscles through the skin closure.

**16.** The subcutaneous tissues are closed with 4-0 interrupted Vicryl and the skin is closed with running subcuticular Vicryl (Fig. 31–10H).

**17.** The drain is left in place for 2 to 3 days. The patient remains intubated for 7 to 10 days.

**18.** Seven to ten days later, the patient is extubated in the operating room and a direct laryngoscopy and bronchoscopy is done. If the airway is determined to be satisfactory by endoscopy, the patient is re-intubated with a ½-size smaller tube and then extubated when fully awake in the intensive care unit the next day.

**19.** Follow-up laryngoscopy and bronchoscopy is performed 10 days later and granulation tissue, if present, is removed.

## Complications

1. Restenosis
2. Pneumothorax
3. Complications of anterior costal cartilage graft (see section 31–6)

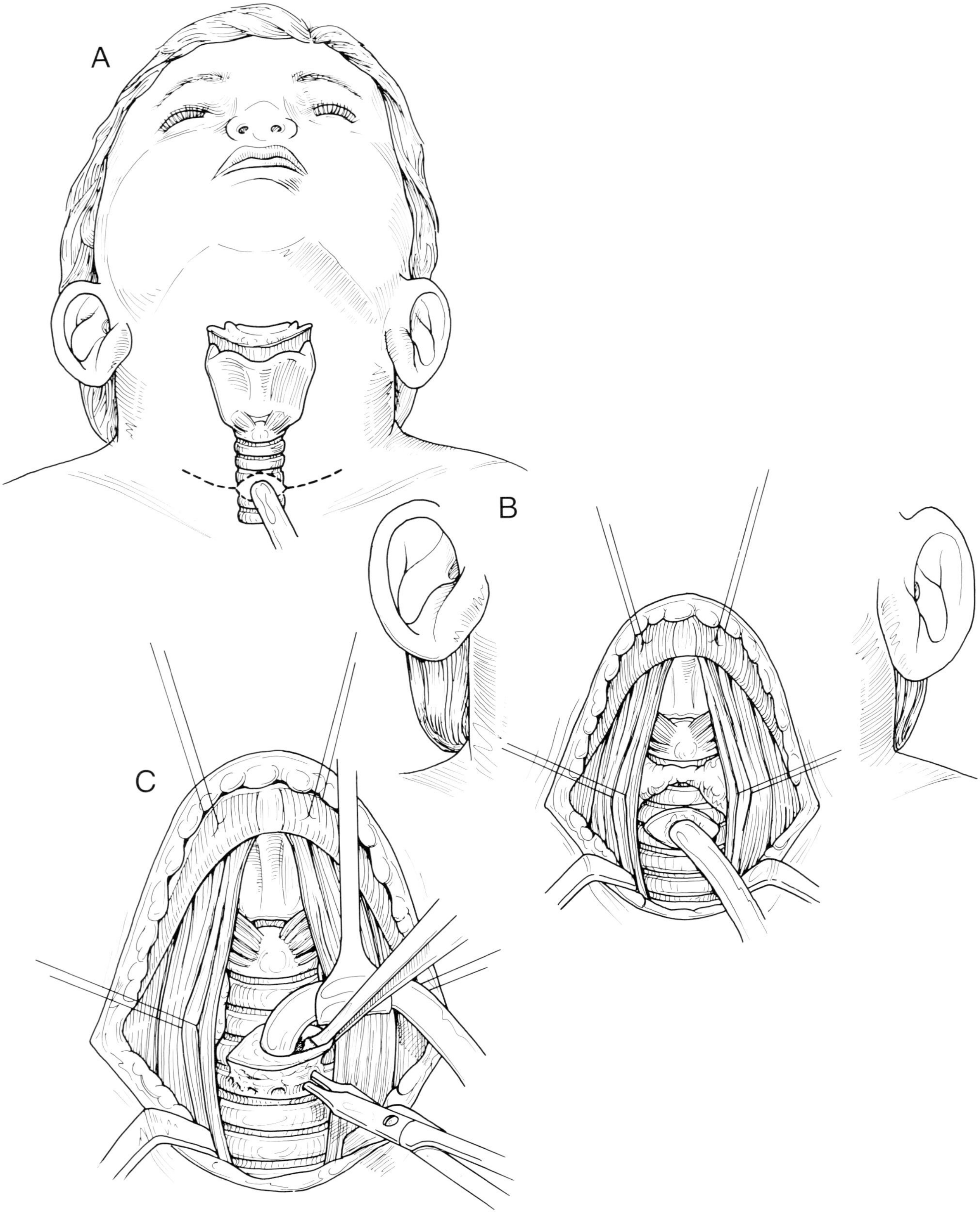


▶ **FIGURE 31-10**

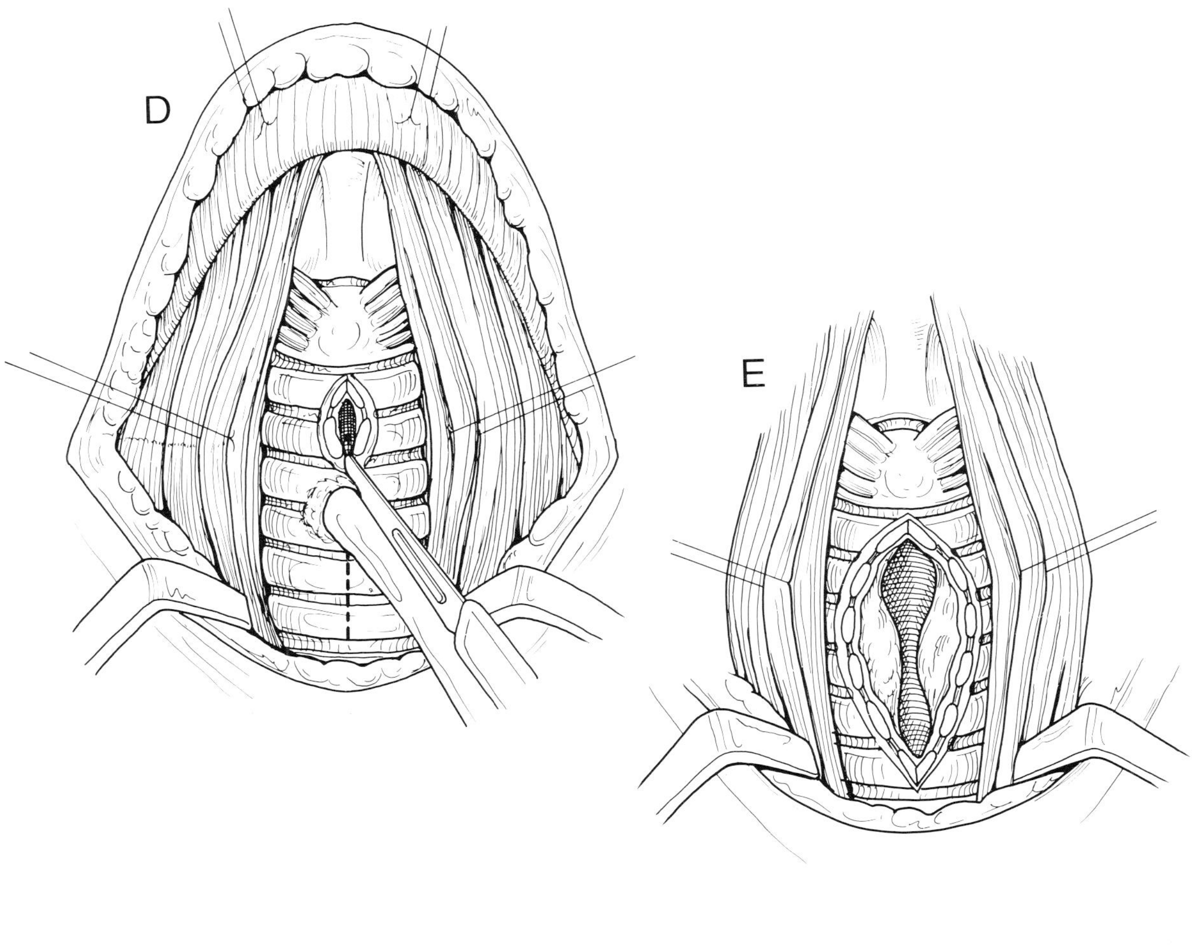


▶ **FIGURE 31-10**

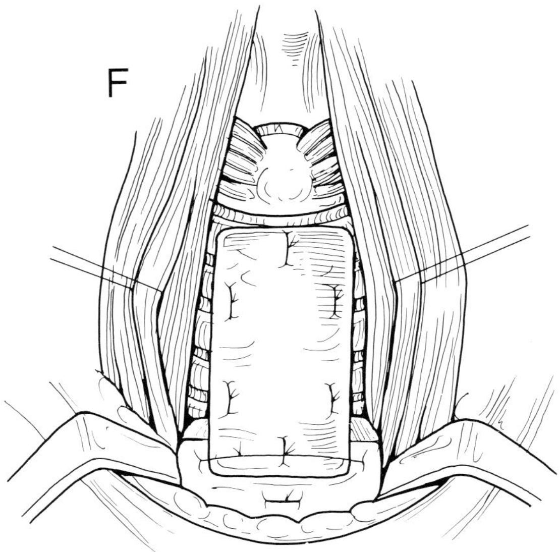


▶ **FIGURE 31-10**

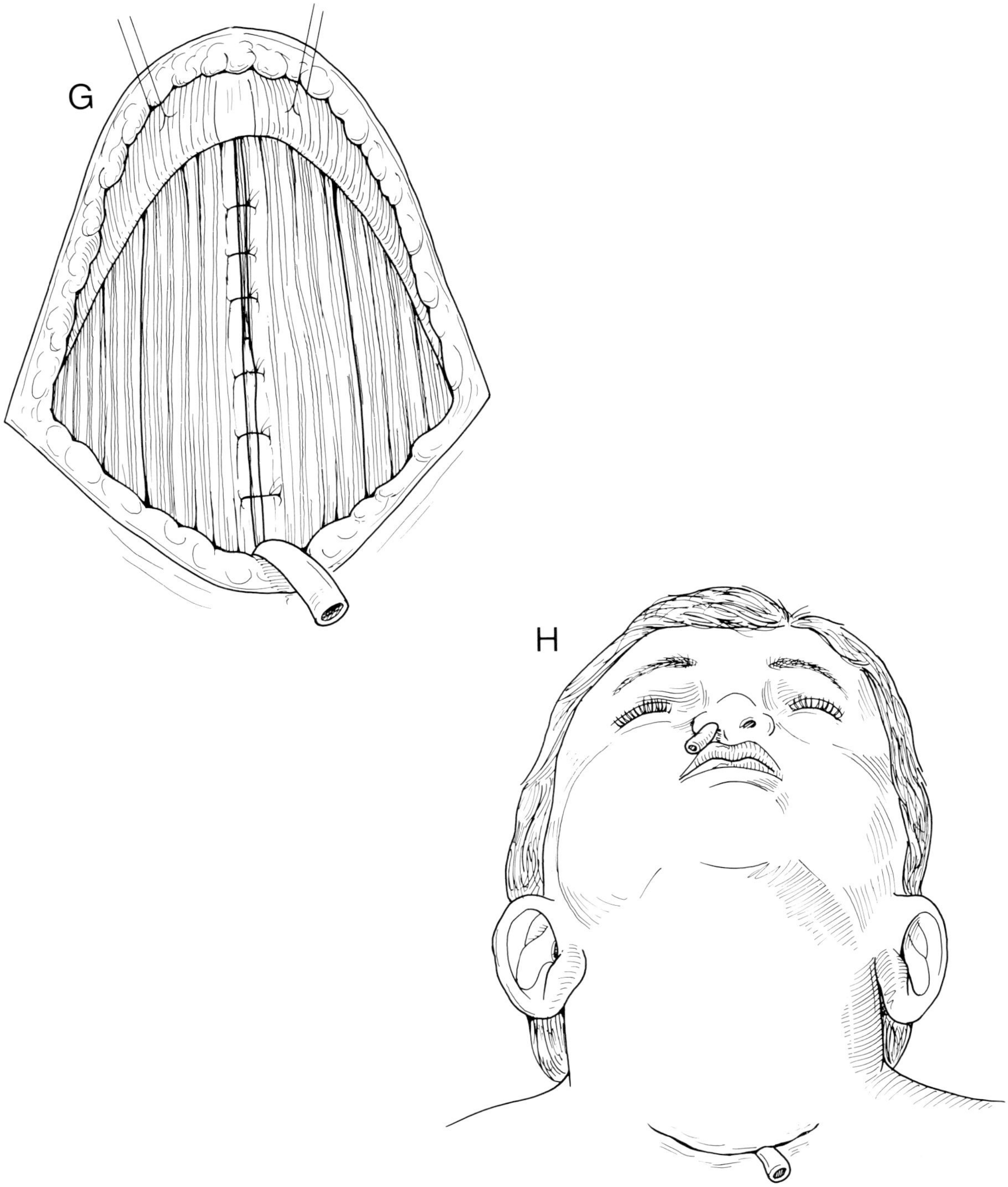


▶ **FIGURE 31-10**

## ▶ 31-11 HARVESTING THE COSTAL CARTILAGE GRAFT

Costal cartilage has been the mainstay of graft material for managing moderate to severe laryngotracheal stenosis. The graft is usually taken after the laryngeal pathology is exposed. This provides the information necessary to determine how much cartilage is needed.

### Indications

A posteroanterior and lateral chest x-ray should be obtained prior to harvesting a costal cartilage graft.

### Operative Technique

1. After the larynx has been exposed, the surgeon regowns and -gloves to harvest the costal cartilage graft. This avoids contamination of the sterile chest wound.
2. An incision is made over the 4th or 5th rib where the inframammary crease would be expected (Fig. 31–11**A**).
3. The incision is carried through the subcutaneous tissues and muscle to the rib cartilage perichondrium (Fig. 31–11**B**).
4. The rib is exposed by releasing the overlying fibrous attachments with a scissors, taking care to keep the perichondrium intact.
5. The rib perichondrium is cut at the upper and lower border with a Bovie or Cottle elevator, releasing the intercostal muscles (Fig. 31–11**C**).
6. The deep perichondrium is dissected off the rib using a periosteal elevator, taking care to leave it intact to avoid a pneumothorax. The dissection is completed with a Doyan rib elevator (Figs. 31–11**D** and 31–11**E**).
7. The rib is cut at the costochondral junction with a knife and then as far medially as possible. It is placed in a saline-soaked sponge until needed (Fig. 31–11**F**).
8. Saline is placed in the wound, and the lung is expanded to be certain there is no air leak (e.g., pneumothorax).
9. If a laceration of the parietal pleura is encountered, the defect is closed with 3-0 interrupted chromic suture.
10. The wound is closed with 3-0 interrupted chromic in the subcutaneous tissues and a Penrose drain is placed (Fig. 31–11**G**).
11. The skin is closed with 4-0 running subcuticular Vicryl or prolene suture. A small gauze dressing is applied.
12. A postoperative chest x-ray is taken after completing the laryngotracheoplasty.
13. The drain is removed in 24 to 36 hours.

### Complications

1. Pneumothorax
2. Atelectasis

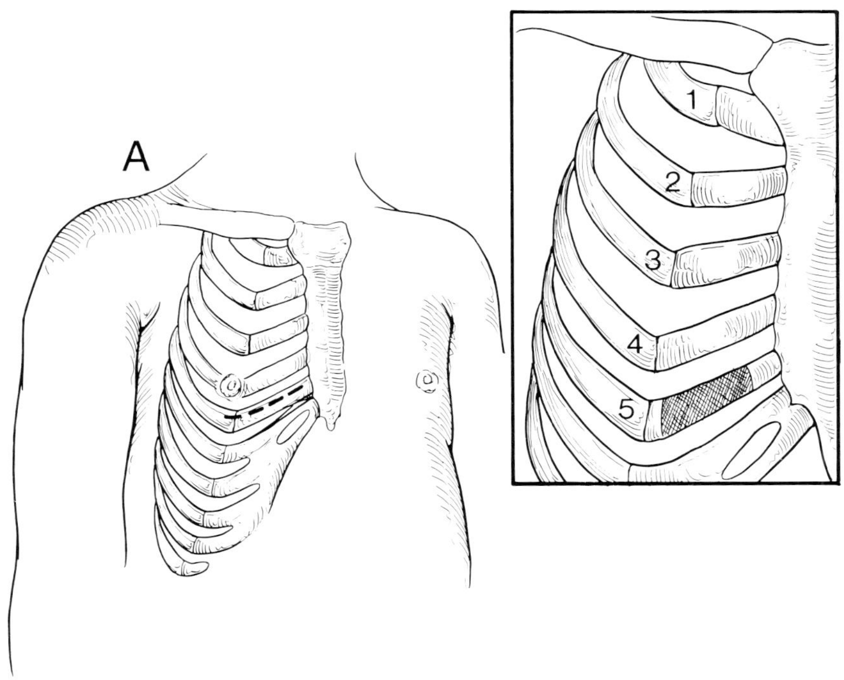


▶ **FIGURE 31-11**

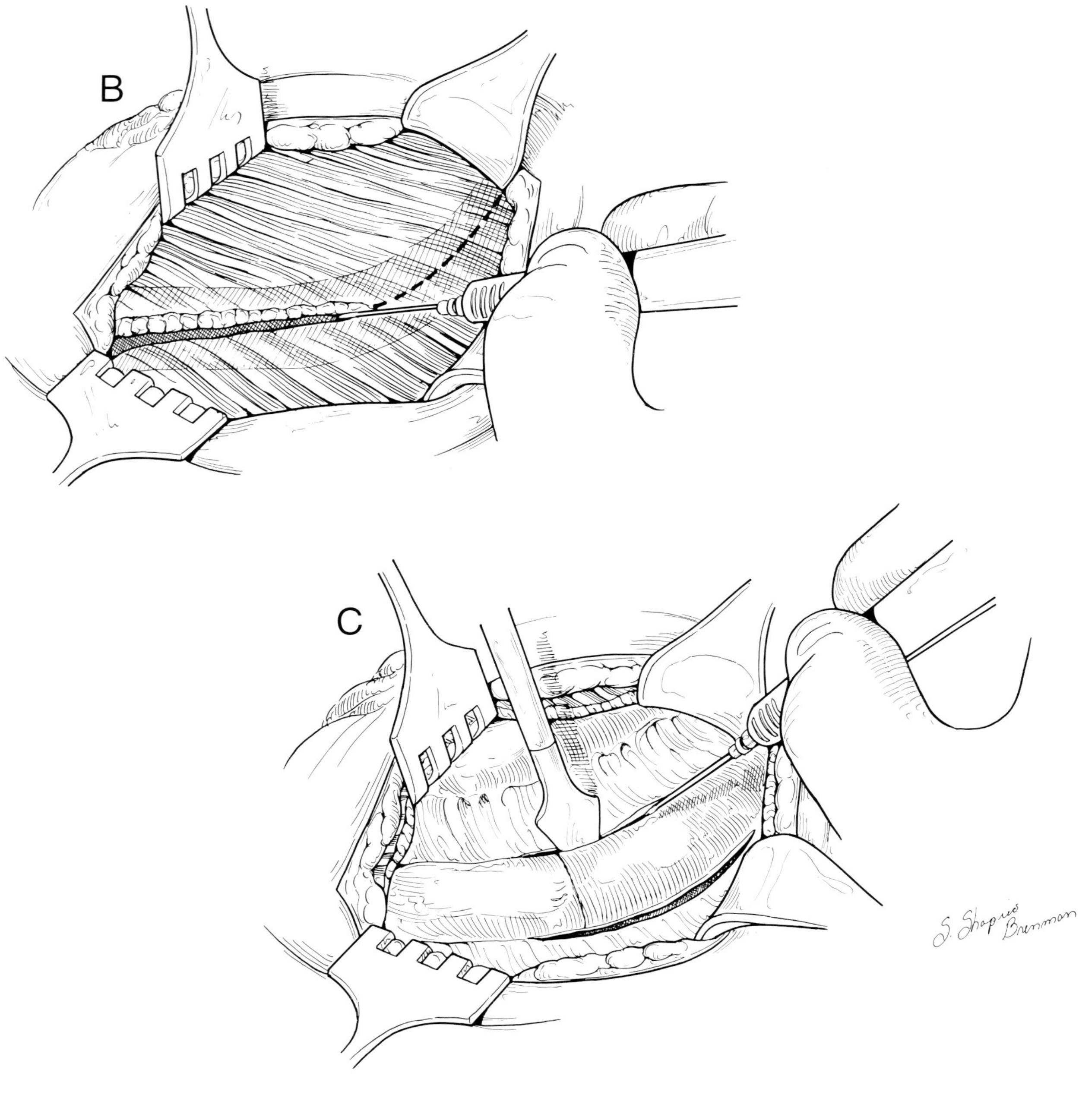


▶**FIGURE 31-11**

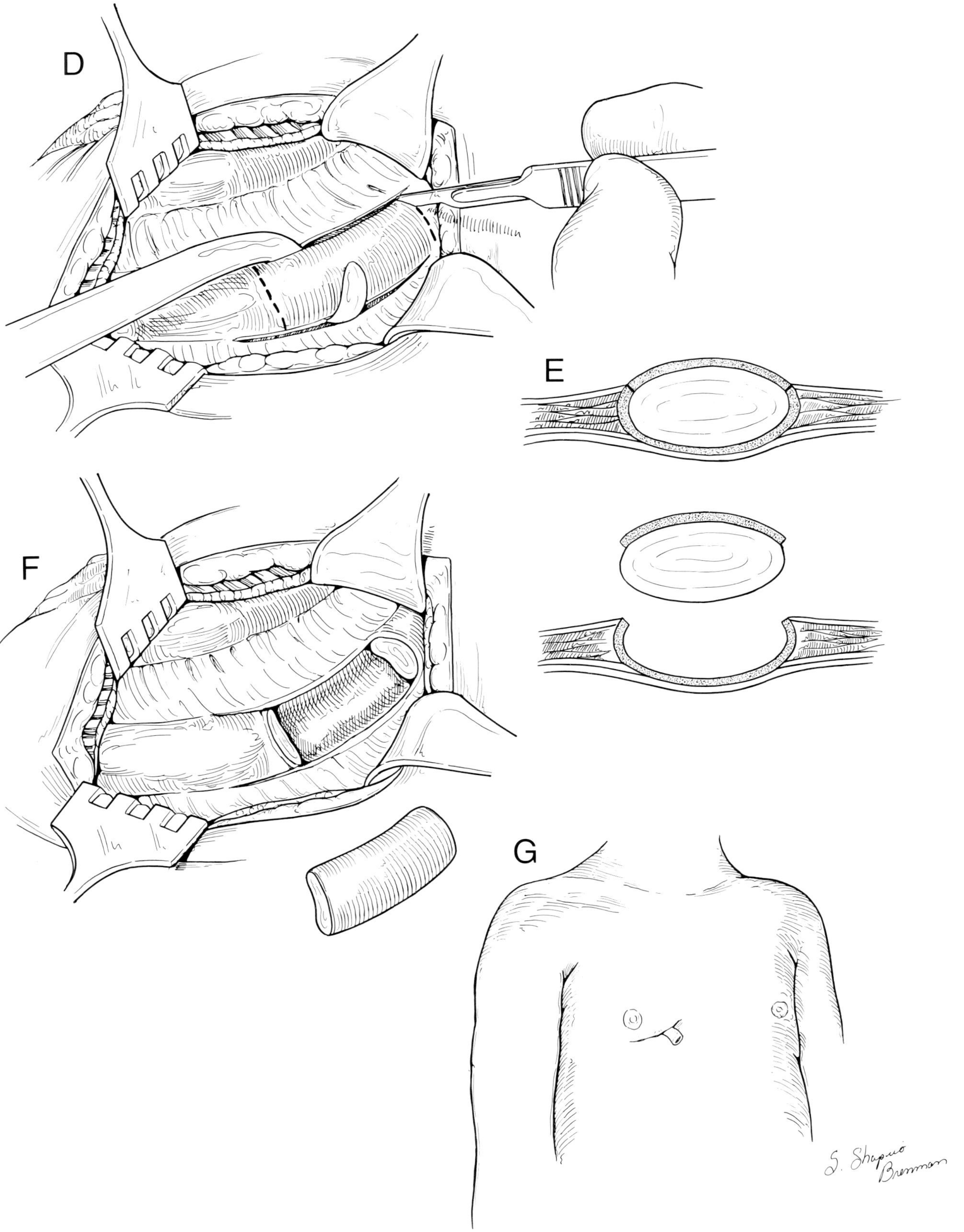


▶ **FIGURE 31-11**

## ▶ 31-12 REPAIR OF CLEFT LARYNX AND LARYNGOTRACHEOESOPHAGEAL CLEFT

A cleft larynx is a congenital deformity that may vary in severity from a small notch in the interarytenoid region to a complete cleft through the posterior lamina of the cricoid and into the cervical esophagus.

### Indications

Repair of a cleft larynx is indicated when the cleft causes debilitating aspiration or airway obstruction from the lack of support of the arytenoid cartilages.

### Preoperative Evaluation

Preoperative evaluation includes barium swallow, direct laryngoscopy, bronchoscopy, and esophagoscopy.

### Operative Technique

1. Closure of a laryngeal cleft is performed under general anesthesia. Laryngotrachoesophageal clefts entering the chest are repaired through a midline sternotomy incision with the child on cardiopulmonary bypass (see section 30–5).
2. A tracheotomy is performed in the standard fashion (see section 30–5). A cut oral RAE tube is placed in the tracheostoma and sutured to the chest (Fig. 31–12**A**).
3. A horizontal neck incision is made over the cricoid cartilage after infiltrating the area with 1% lidocaine with 1:100,000 epinephrine (Fig. 31–12**E**).
4. A superior skin flap is developed to the level of the hyoid bone and an inferior skin flap is elevated to expose the upper area of the trachea as described for laryngotracheoplasty (see section 31–6).
5. The strap muscles are separated by cutting the midline fascia with a scissors and the muscles are retracted laterally with 4-0 prolene sutures (Fig. 31–12F).
6. A midline incision is made with a knife through the cricoid and thyroid cartilages as well as the underlying mucosa. Care is taken to be certain that the incision is in the anterior commissure (Fig. 31–12**F**).
7. The endolarynx is exposed by retracting the laryngeal cartilages laterally with 4-0 prolene sutures (Fig. 31–12**G**).
8. The midline incision may be extended inferiorly in the trachea if the cleft extends below the cricoid.
9. An esophageal bougie is passed through the mouth into the esophagus to improve exposure of the cleft.
10. The margins of the cleft are injected with 1% lidocaine with 1:100,000 epinephrine.
11. The margins of the cleft are excised with a scissors taking care to preserve as much laryngeal mucosa as possible (Fig. 31–12**H**).
12. The shelf of the cleft is then divided with a knife and scissors to facilitate a two-layer closure (Fig. 31–12**I**).

**13.** Starting inferiorly, the esophageal closure is performed with 4-0 Vicryl interrupted suture placing the knots in the esophageal and hypopharyngeal lumen (Fig. 31–12**I**). The inferior suture is used for traction before each additional suture is placed. The laryngeal and tracheal mucosa is closed in a similar fashion with 4-0 interrupted chromic placing the knots in the lumen (Fig. 31–12**J**).

**14.** The superior limit of the closure is approximately 2 mm above the level of the vocal process of the arytenoids (Fig. 31–12**K**).

**15.** The laryngofissure is closed with 4-0 Vicryl in the laryngeal perichondrium and tracheal tissues (Fig. 31–12**L**).

**16.** The strap muscles are reapproximated in the midline with 4-0 Vicryl suture, and subcutaneous tissues are closed with 4-0 Vicryl as well.

**17.** The skin is closed with 4-0 interrupted prolene suture.

**18.** The oral RAE tube is removed and the tracheotomy tube is replaced (Fig. 31–12**M**).

**19.** The patient is maintained on intravenous antibiotics with a nasogastric (N-G) tube and the tracheotomy in place.

**20.** The N-G tube is removed in 1 week, but the tracheotomy remains until the larynx is healed.

**21.** A barium swallow is performed prior to resuming oral feedings at 4 weeks.

**22.** If feeding is adequate and there is no aspiration at 4 weeks, a direct laryngoscopy is performed.

**23.** If the larynx is healed, decannulation is attempted 12 to 24 hours later.

## Complications

1. Persistent aspiration
2. Recurrence of the laryngeal cleft
3. Laryngotracheal stenosis

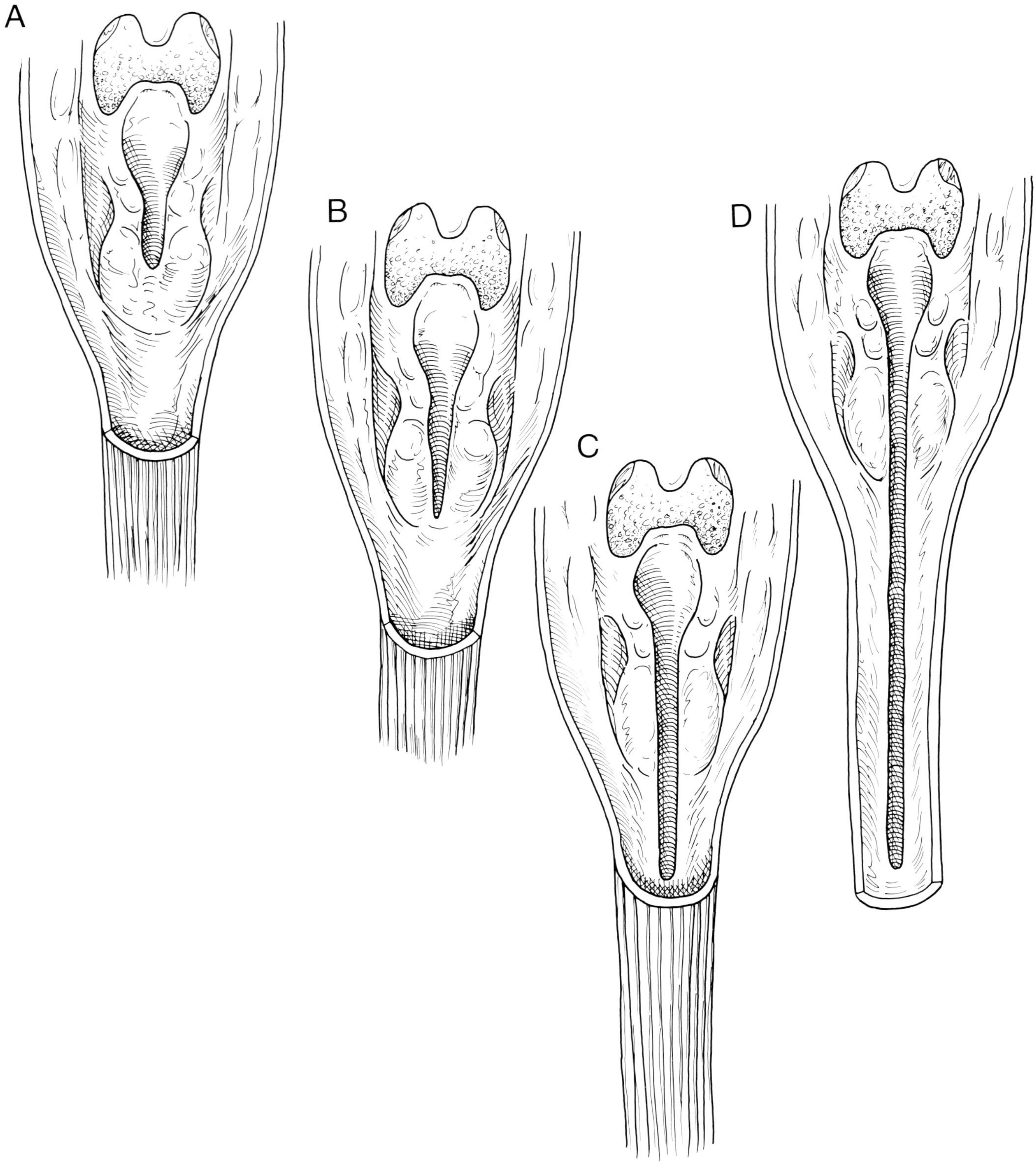


▶ **FIGURE 31-12**

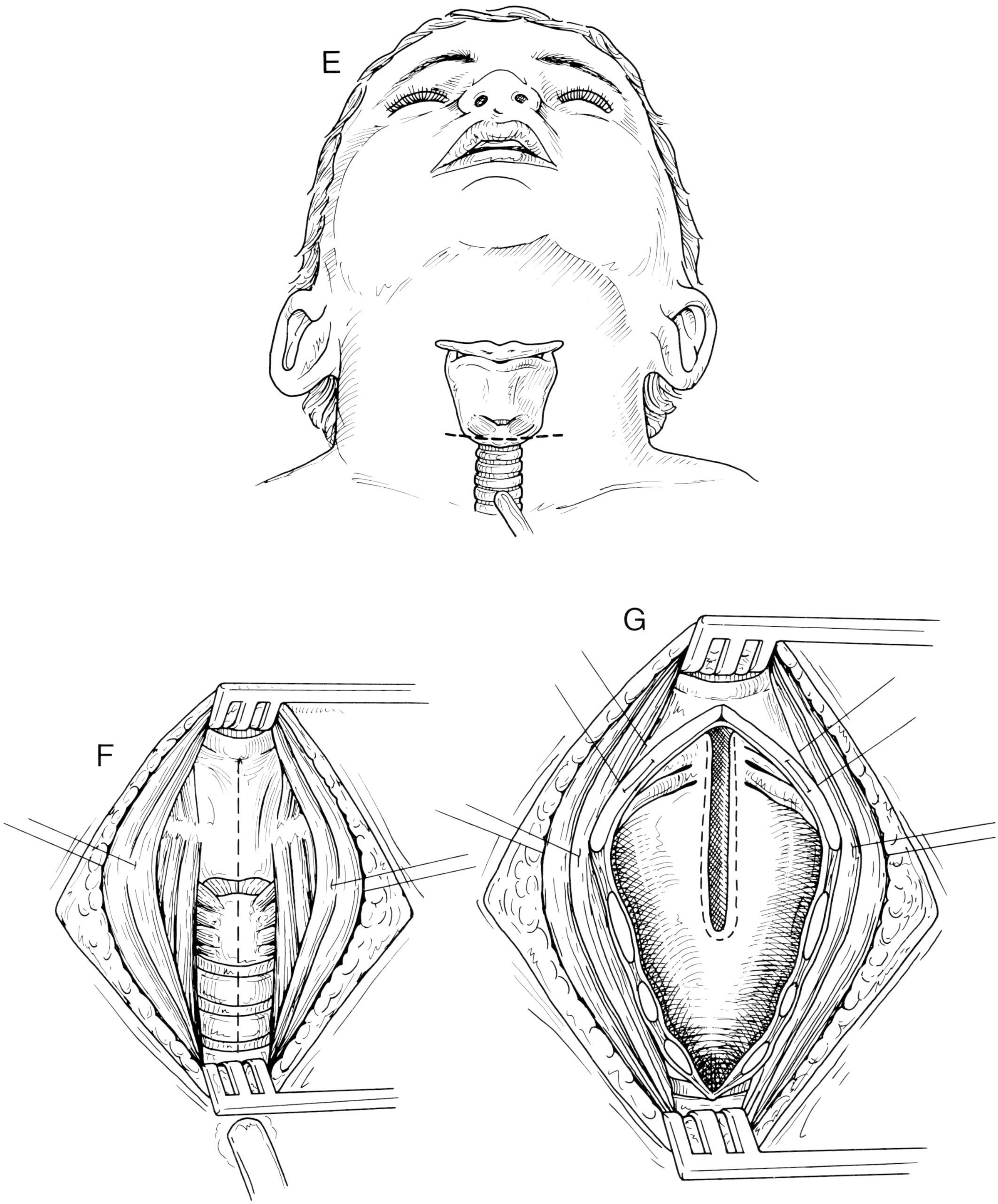


▶ **FIGURE 31-12**

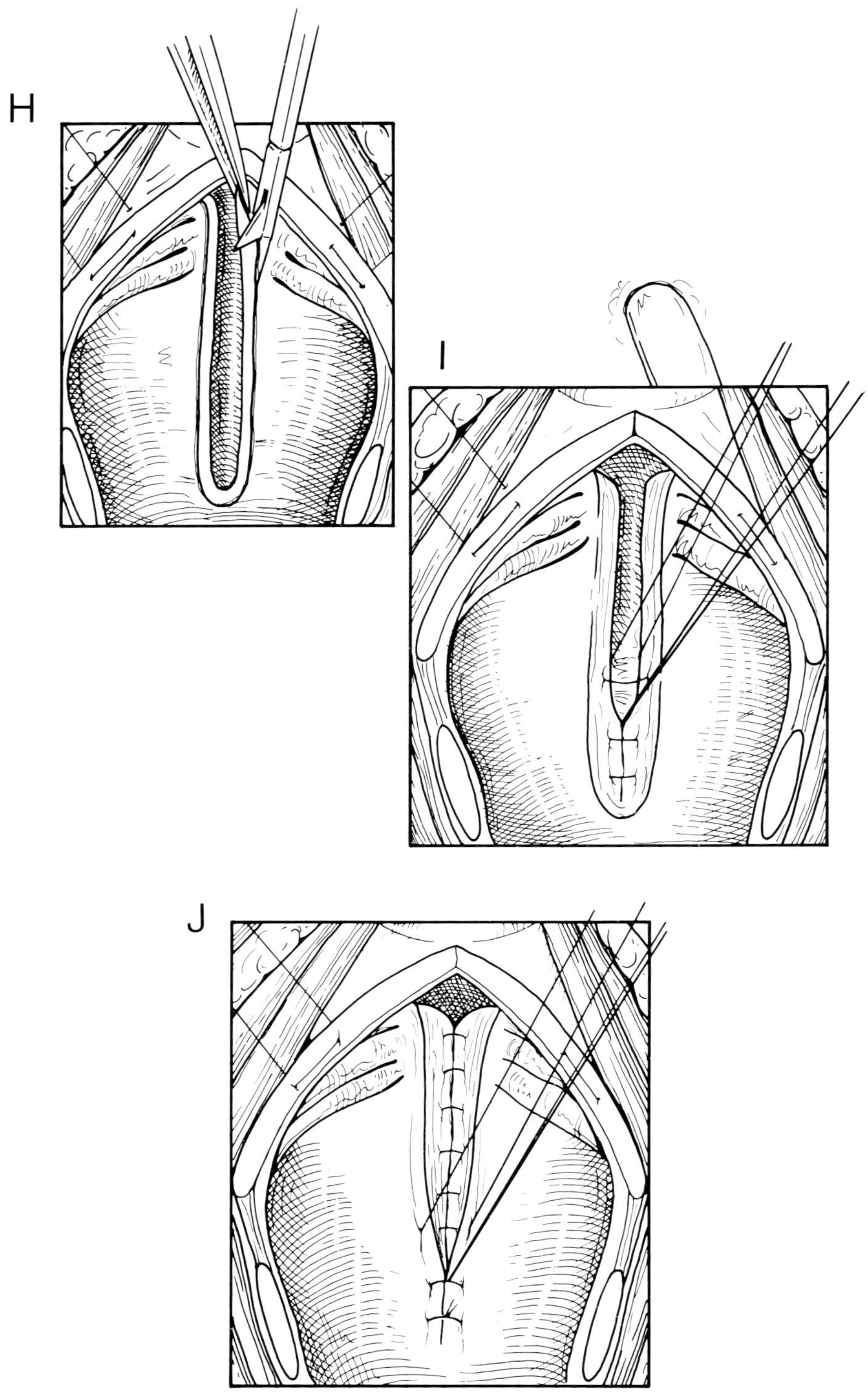


▶ **FIGURE 31-12**

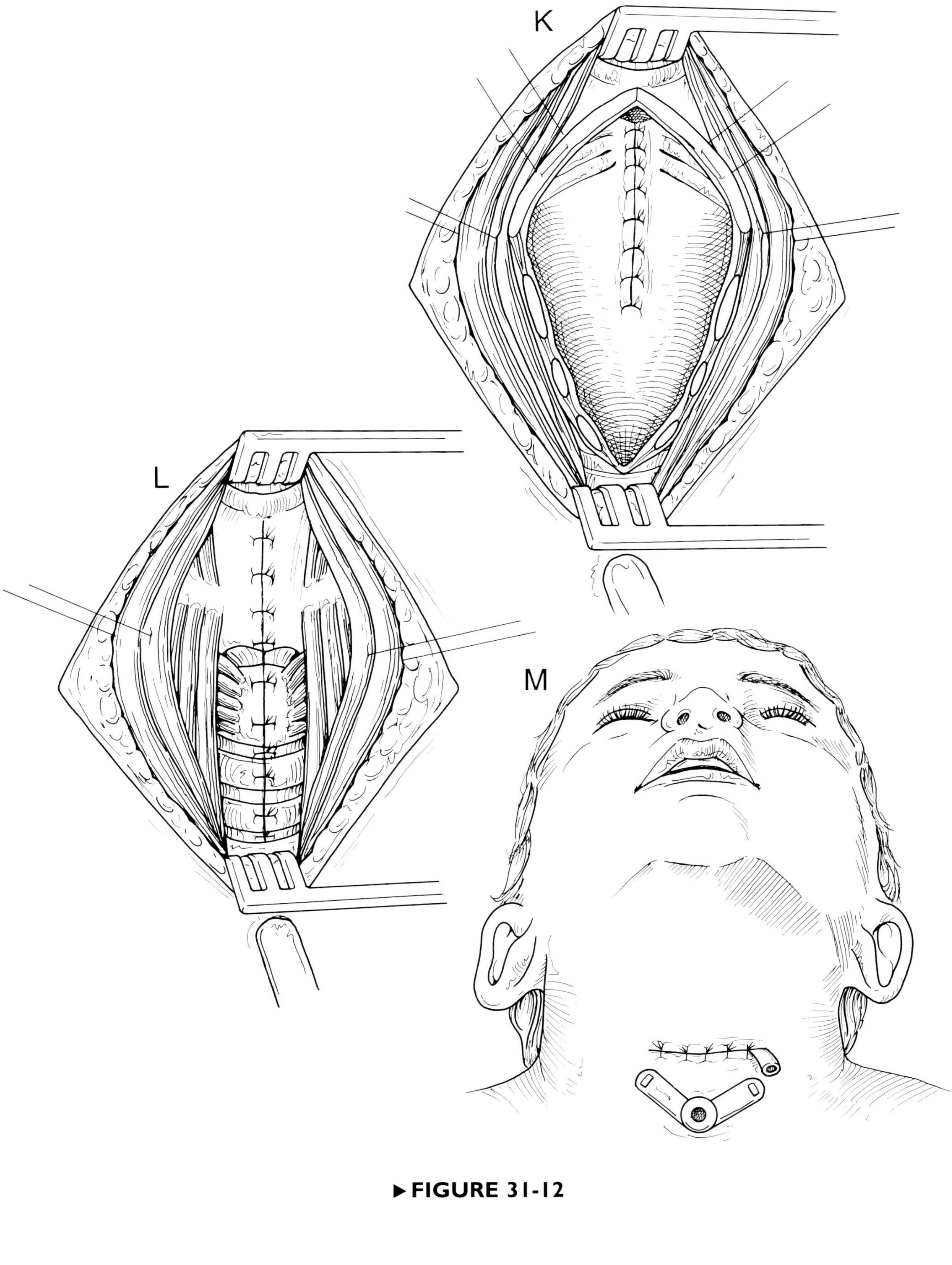


▶ **FIGURE 31-12**

## ▶ 31-13 DIVISION OF LARYNGEAL WEB

A laryngeal web occurs when there is fusion of all or part of the vocal cords. This most often presents as a congenital anomaly, although it can be acquired from laryngeal trauma. Small anterior webs may have no presenting symptoms. Larger webs are associated with varying degrees of respiratory distress, as the laryngeal lumen is compromised, and vocal alteration (usually high-pitched).

### Indications

Small asymptomatic laryngeal webs require no treatment. Treatment is directed toward relieving airway obstruction and to improve vocal quality.

### Preoperative Evaluation

Flexible and rigid laryngoscopy and bronchoscopy are required in the preoperative evaluation of a laryngeal web. Bronchoscopy is indicated to determine the thickness of the web and its potential response to simple division. Thin webs are not well seen in conventional radiographs. Computed tomography (CT) or magnetic resonance imaging (MRI) may demonstrate the presence and extent of thicker webs. Pulmonary function studies may be used to determine the degree of preoperative airway obstruction and the necessity for surgery.

### Operative Technique

1. Thin webs are incised endoscopically under a general anesthetic with a small endotracheal tube in place. If a laser is used to divide the web, a laser-resistant tube must be used.
2. A Jako laryngoscope is placed in the larynx, exposing the anterior commissure and full extent of the web (Fig. 31–13**A**).
3. The web is divided all the way to the anterior commissure with a laryngeal knife, scissors or a laser, taking care not to cut into the substance of the true vocal cords (Fig. 31–13**B**).
4. The child is left intubated for 24 hours to keep the vocal cords apart to help prevent reformation of the web.
5. If the web is thick or has recurred after simple division, it is best treated with an open procedure utilizing a keel. If the child does not already have a tracheotomy tube in place, one will be required during the time that the laryngeal keel is in place, usually around three weeks (Refer to Section 6.1).
6. The patient is positioned on a shoulder roll with the neck extended as for a tracheotomy.
7. A cut oral RAE tube is placed in the tracheostoma and sutured to the chest. A horizontal incision is made above the tracheostomy stoma through the platysma to the cervical fascia (Fig. 31–13**C**). The skin flap is elevated superiorly to the level of the thyroid notch and sutured to the upper drape to provide exposure. The strap muscles are divided in the midline and retracted laterally with sutures to expose the thyroid and cricoid cartilages and upper trachea (Fig. 31–13**C**).
8. A midline laryngofissure incision is made in the midline of the thyroid cartilage starting at its inferior border. The incision is continued superiorly until the level of the vocal cords is reached, just below the thyroid notch (Fig. 31–13**C**). The web is divided with a knife, taking care not to injure the vo-

cal cords themselves. If the web is thick, the incision may need to be extended inferiorly through the anterior portion of the cricoid cartilage (Fig. 31–13D).

9. A commercially available laryngeal keel (Fig. 31–13E) may be used or one may be created using a sheet of Silastic (Fig. 31–13F).
10. The laryngeal keel is placed so that the intra-laryngeal portion is between the cut edges of the anterior portion of the vocal cords (Fig. 31–13G). The external flanges are sutured to the external surface of the thyroid cartilage with 4-0 silk suture. The laryngofissure incision is closed with 4-0 Vicryl sutures (Fig. 31–13G) and the overlying strap muscles are approximated with 4-0 chromic sutures (Fig. 31–13H). A penrose drain is placed in the wound.
11. The subcutaneous tissues are closed with interrupted 4-0 Vicryl sutures and the skin is approximated with subcuticular 4-0 chromic sutures (Fig. 31–13I).
12. The RAE tube is removed and the standard tracheostomy tube replaced in the tracheostoma (Fig. 31–13I). The drain is removed in 24 to 36 hours.
13. In three weeks, sufficient epithelialization of the medial surfaces of the vocal cords should have occurred to prevent reformation of the web.
14. The child is reanesthetized and the tracheostomy tube replaced by a cut oral RAE tube.
15. The central portion of the neck incision is opened by using a #15 blade until the lateral external flanges of the keel are identified. The silk sutures securing the keel to the thyroid cartilages are cut and the keel is removed (Fig. 31–13J). Endoscopy is then performed and granulation tissue, if present, is removed with cup forceps. The incision is closed as described in steps 10 to 12 above, except no penrose drain is used.
16. Flexible and rigid endoscopy may be performed in 3 to 4 weeks to determine the adequacy of the airway before decannulating the child.

## Complications

1. Reformation of web
2. Laryngeal/subglottic stenosis
3. Poor vocal quality—hoarseness, breathiness
4. Laryngeal incompetence

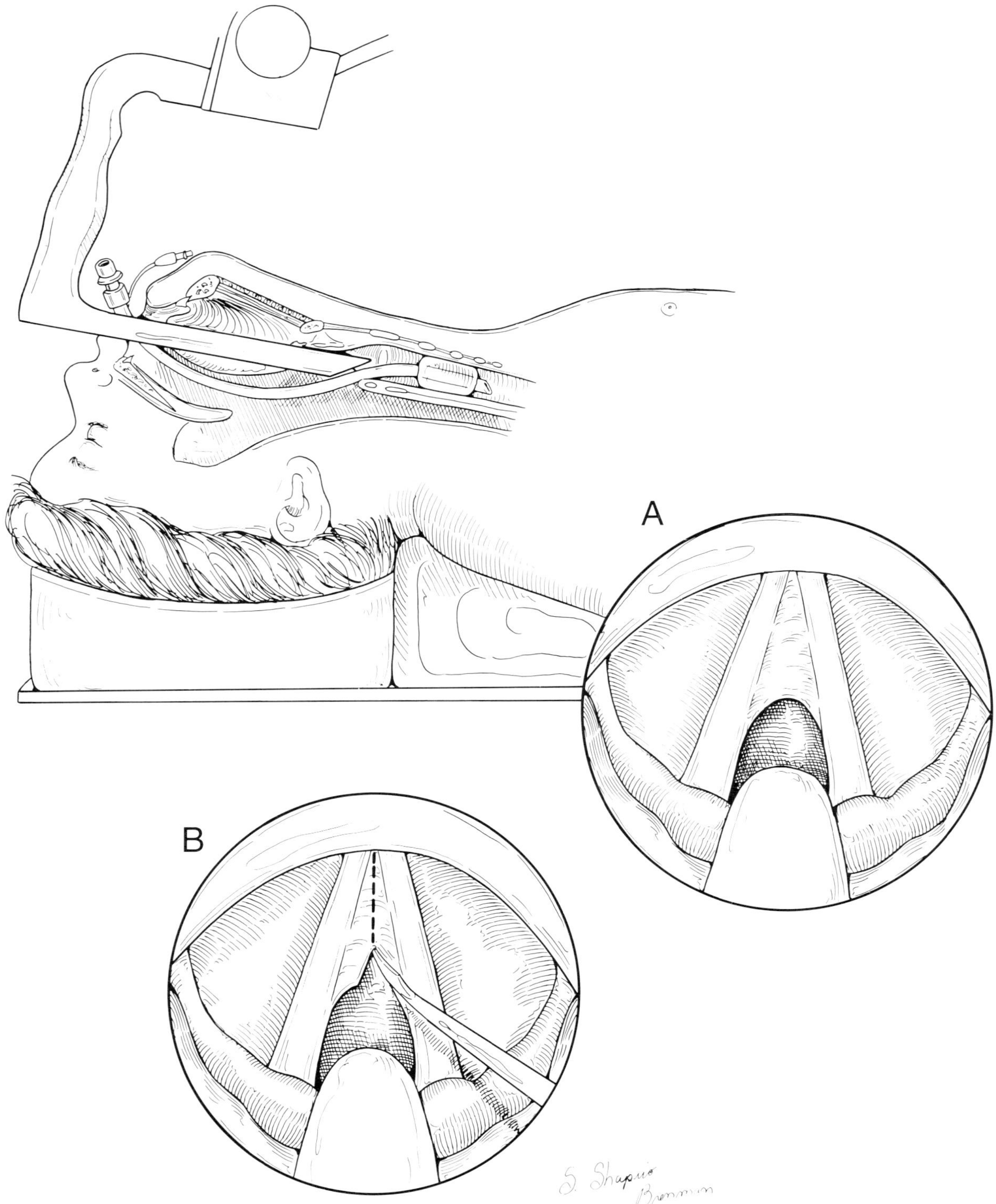


▶ **FIGURE 31-13**

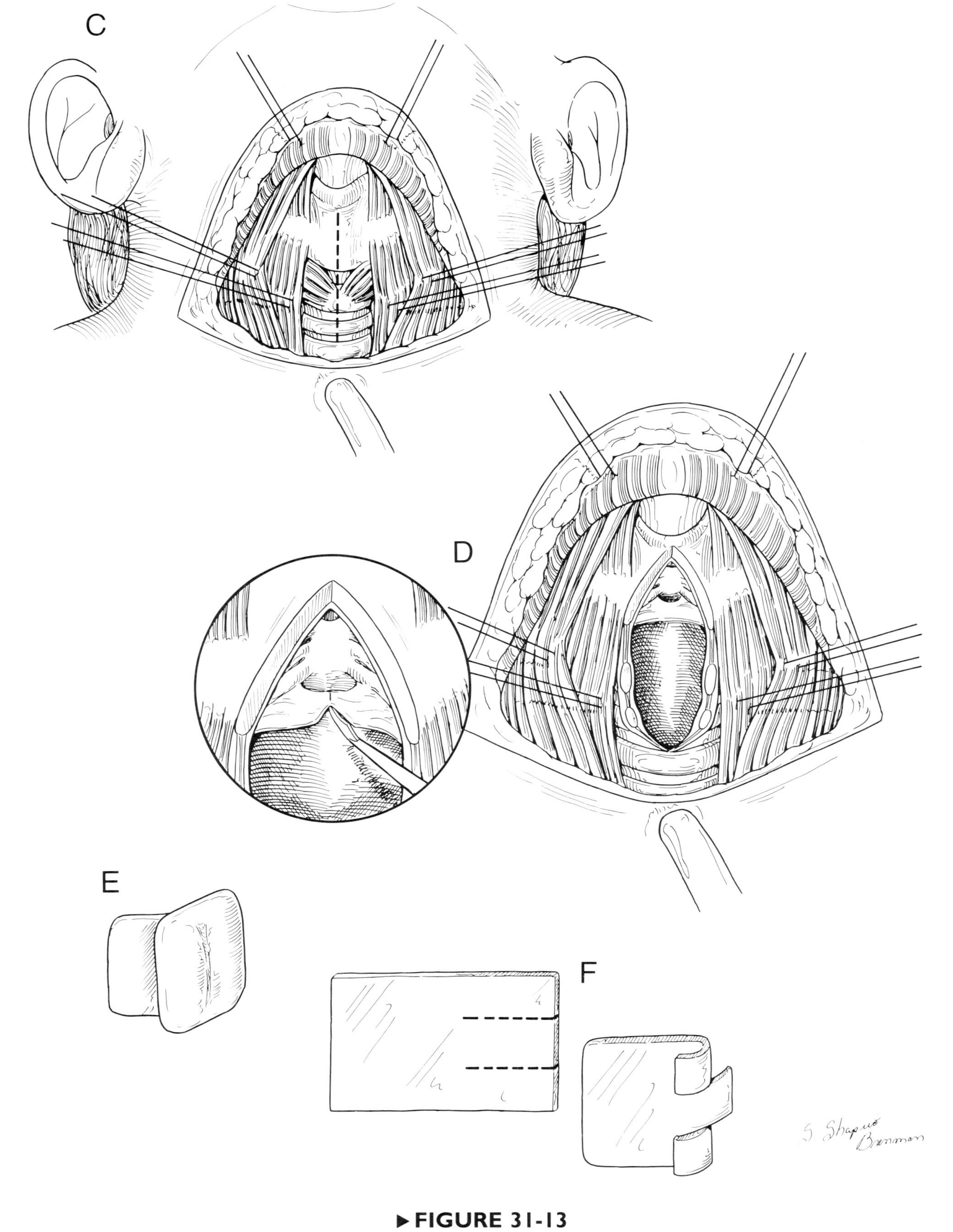


▶ **FIGURE 31-13**

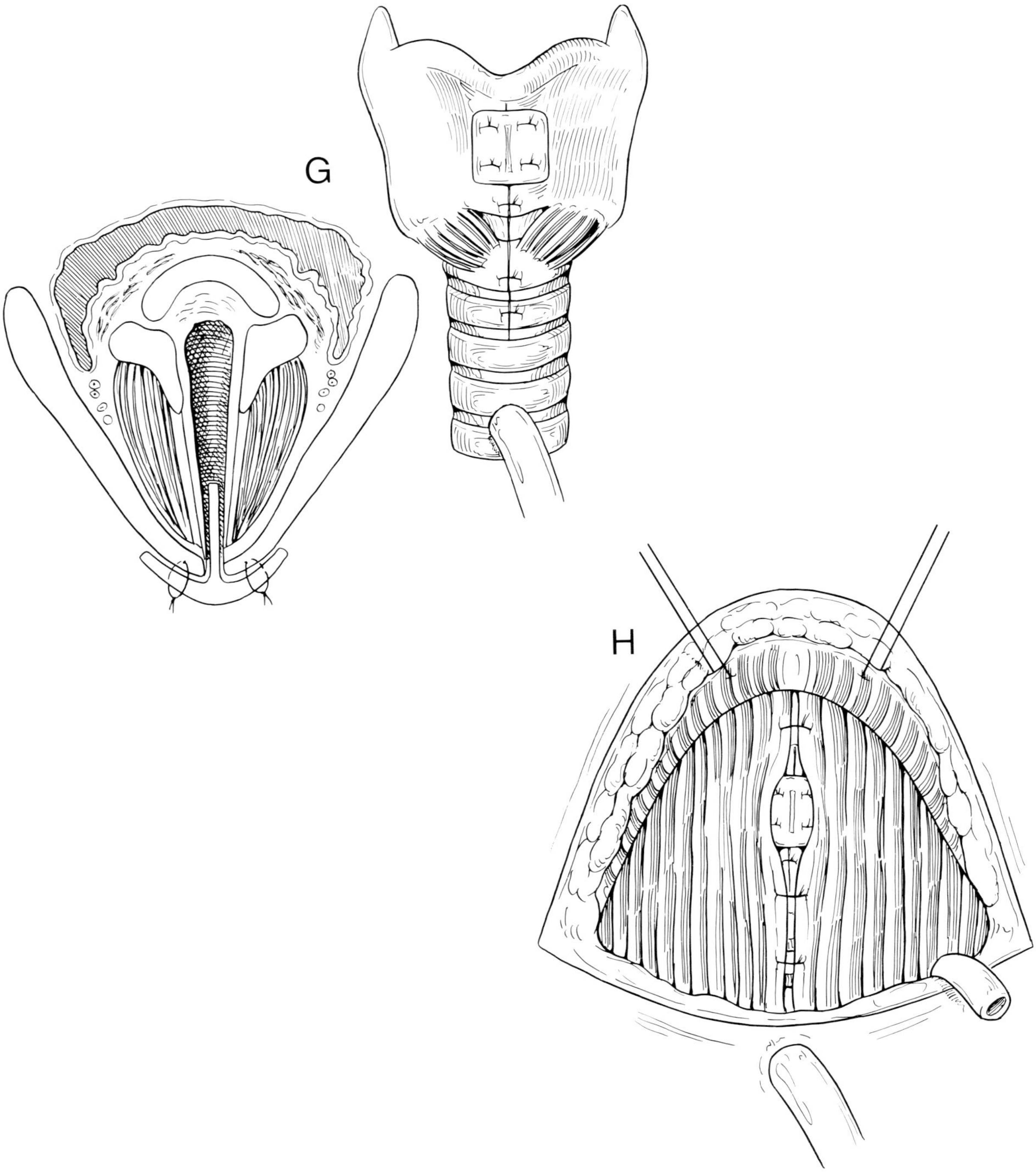


▶ **FIGURE 31-13**

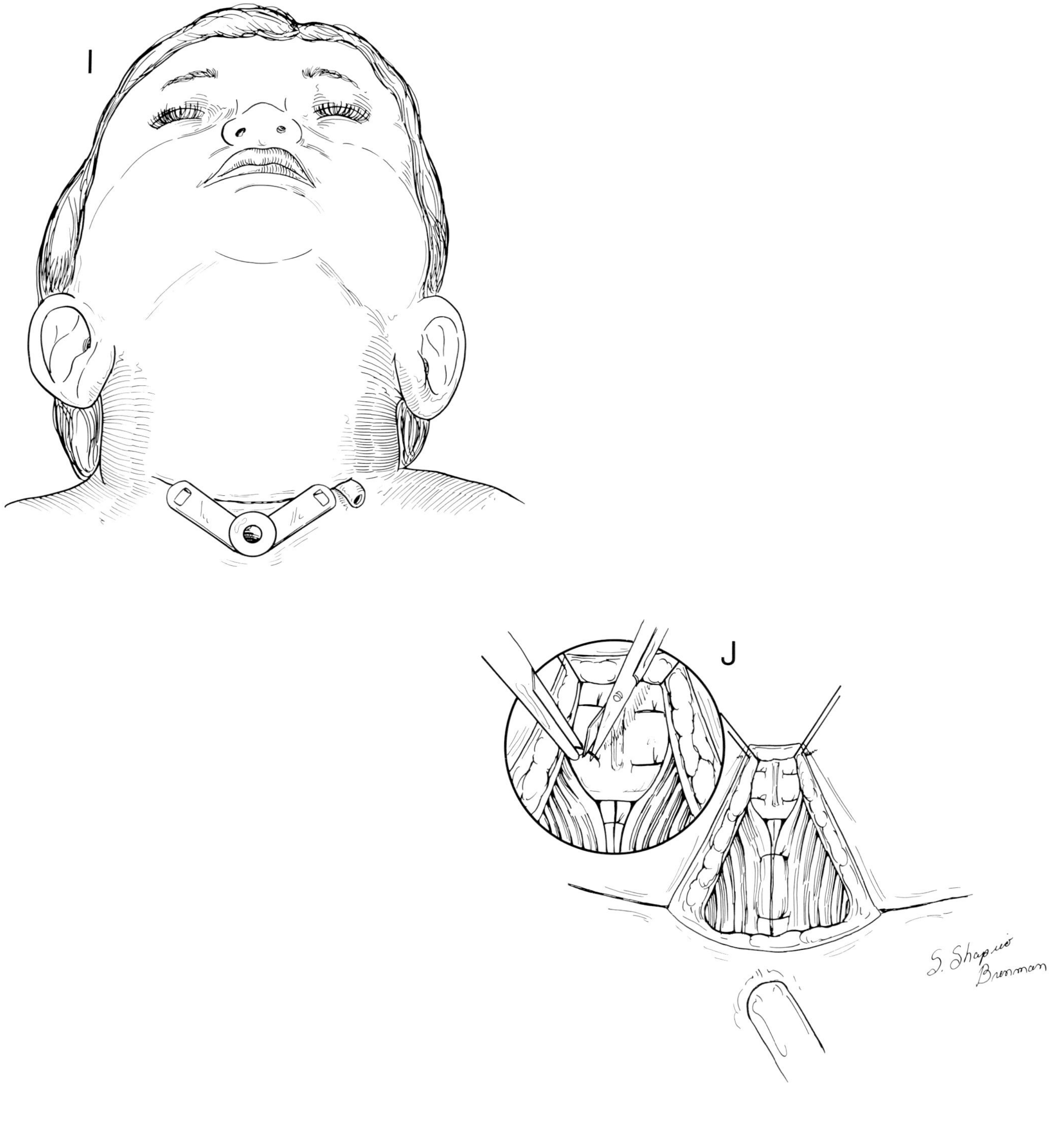


▶ **FIGURE 31-13**

## ▶ 31-14 EXCISION OF LARYNGEAL PAPILLOMAS

Laryngeal papillomatosis is a disease that may range from a small isolated lesion that is "cured" after one excision to rapidly recurring lesions that grow on all areas of the larynx. The lesion may present at any age with the onset of hoarseness with or without airway obstruction.

### Indications

Excision of laryngeal papillomas is indicated to maintain an adequate airway and voice.

### Preoperative Evaluation

The diagnosis of laryngeal papillomas is usually made by direct laryngoscopy in the office or in the operating room. Anteroposterior and lateral neck radiographs may be of help prior to endoscopy and/or surgical excisions.

### Operative Technique

1. Laryngeal papillomas are excised under general insufflation anesthesia with spontaneous ventilation. No inflammable anesthetic agents are used.
2. A Jako laryngoscope is placed in the larynx exposing the papillomas (Fig. 31–14**A**). The laryngoscope is suspended to free the operating surgeon's hands.
3. A $CO_2$ laser with a 400-mm microscopic attachment and micromanipulator is used to remove the papillomas (Fig. 31–14**B**).
4. After each mass of papilloma is charred, the eschar is removed with a suction (Fig. 31–14**B**).
5. An attempt is made to remove as much papilloma as possible without producing scarring that can lead to permanently hoarse voice or laryngeal stenosis.
6. If papillomas are present in the subglottic space, these are removed in a similar fashion through a subglottiscope.
7. Four percent cocaine on small pledgets is placed on the raw surface of the larynx to reduce swelling, prevent hemorrhage, and provide some postoperative pain relief.
8. Steroids and antibiotics are administered to prevent swelling and resultant airway obstruction.

### Complications

1. Laryngeal edema
2. Laryngeal stenosis
3. Hoarseness

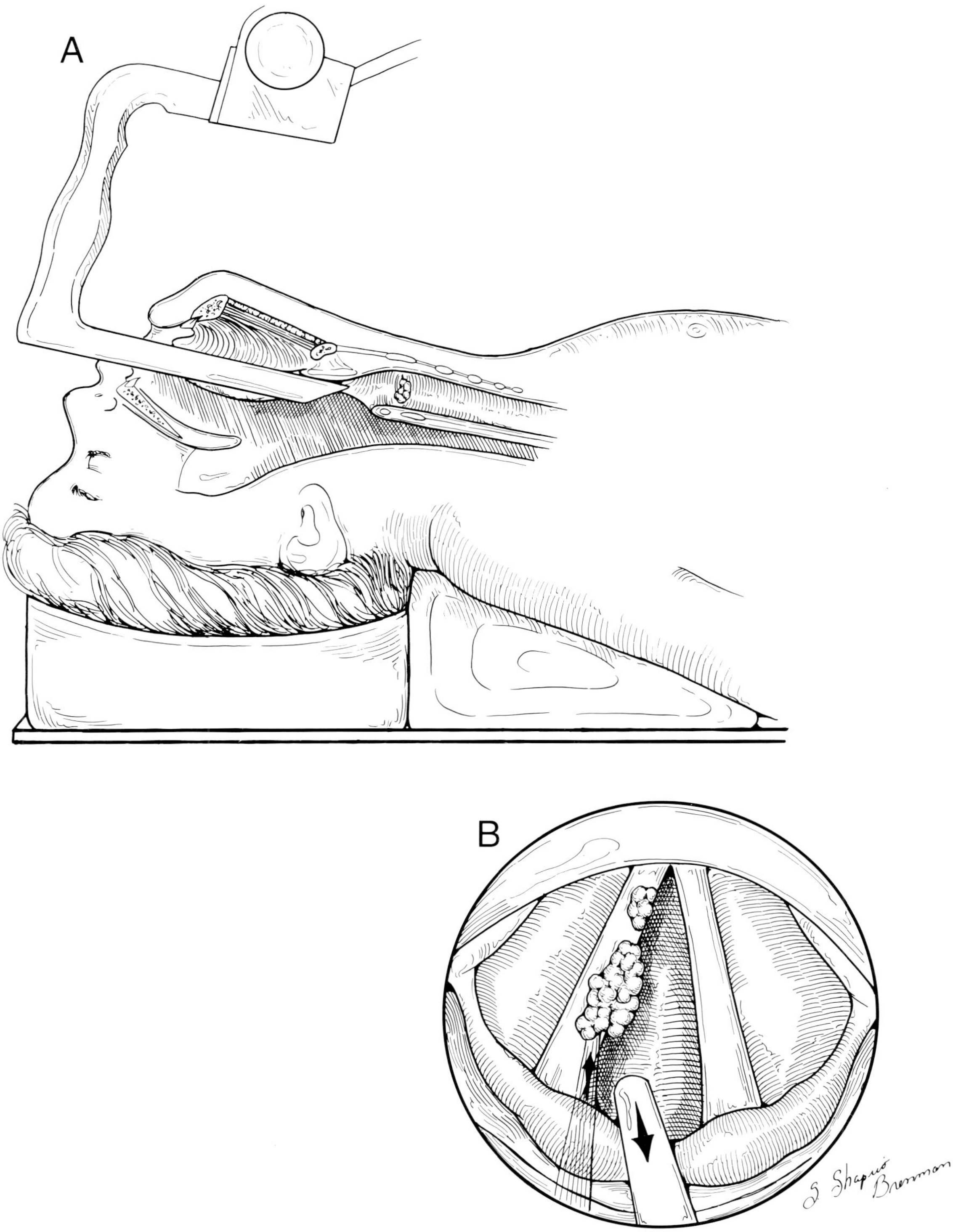


▶ **FIGURE 31-14**

## ▶ 31 - 15 ARYTENOIDECTOMY: EXTERNAL ARYTENOIDECTOMY—EXTERNAL APPROACH

Arytenoidectomy is an operation to improve the airway of a child with bilateral vocal cord paralysis. The paralysis may be congenital or acquired. It may be associated with other central nervous system anomalies such as Arnold-Chiari malformation. Traditionally, arytenoidectomy has been performed via an external approach through a neck incision. However, endoscopic laser arytenoidectomy has become the preferred method of performing arytenoidectomy in children.

### Indications

External arytenoidectomy is indicated in the patient with persistent bilateral vocal cord paralysis who is unable to be decannulated because of airway obstruction or significant exertional dyspnea.

### Preoperative Evaluation

Direct laryngoscopy while the child is breathing spontaneously is required to document vocal cord paralysis. The arytenoids must be palpated to make sure that they are mobile and that the paralysis is not related to arytenoid fixation or glottic scarring.

### Operative Technique

1. An external arytenoidectomy is performed under general anesthesia administered through an oral RAE tube in the tracheostomy site.
2. A horizontal incision in made over the thyroid cartilage (Fig. 31–15**A**). One percent lidocaine with 1:100,000 epinephrine is injected subcutaneously at the site of the incision to aid in hemostasis.
3. Inferior and superior skin flaps are created. The strap muscles are divided in the middle and retracted laterally with silk sutures (Fig. 31–15**B**).
4. An anterior thyrotomy is performed cutting through cartilage, mucosa, and the anterior commissure (Fig. 31–15**B** and **C**).
5. An incision is made over the body of the arytenoid, which is then removed leaving the vocal cord process attached to the vocal cord (Figs. 31–15**D** and 31–15**E**).
6. Two 4-0 prolene sutures are passed through the thyroid cartilage and vocal process to secure the vocal process of the arytenoid to the lateral aspect of the thyroid alae, thus lateralizing the cord (Figs. 31–15**F** and 31–15**G**).
7. The mucosal incisions are closed with 5-0 chromic suture and the thyroid alae are approximated with 4-0 Vicryl in the periochondrium (Fig. 31–15**H**).
8. The strap muscles are re-approximated in the midline with 4-0 Vicryl suture, and subcutaneous tissues are closed with 4-0 Vicryl as well.
9. A Penrose drain is placed in the wound. The skin is closed with 4-0 interrupted chromic subcuticular sutures (Fig. 31–15**I**). Steri-strips are placed to help approximate the skin edge.

**10.** The oral RAE tube is removed and the tracheotomy tube is replaced (Fig. 31–15**I**).

**11.** The drain is removed in 24 to 36 hours.

**12.** The child is given a 7 day course of antibiotics.

**13.** Follow-up endoscopy is performed approximately one month later to assess the result. If the airway is satisfactory, the child may be decannulated.

## Complications

1. Failure to lateralize the cord sufficiently

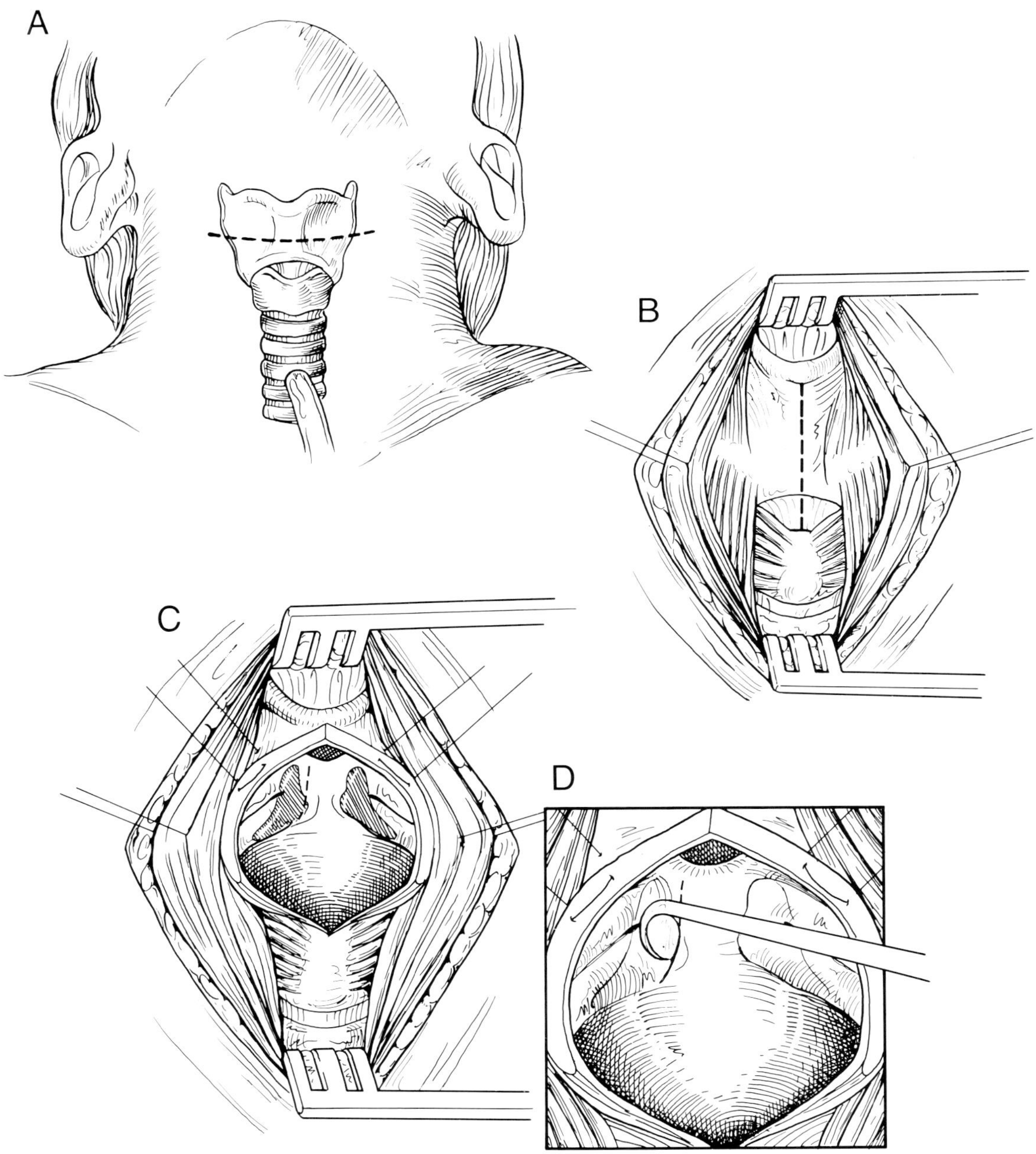


▶**FIGURE 31-15**

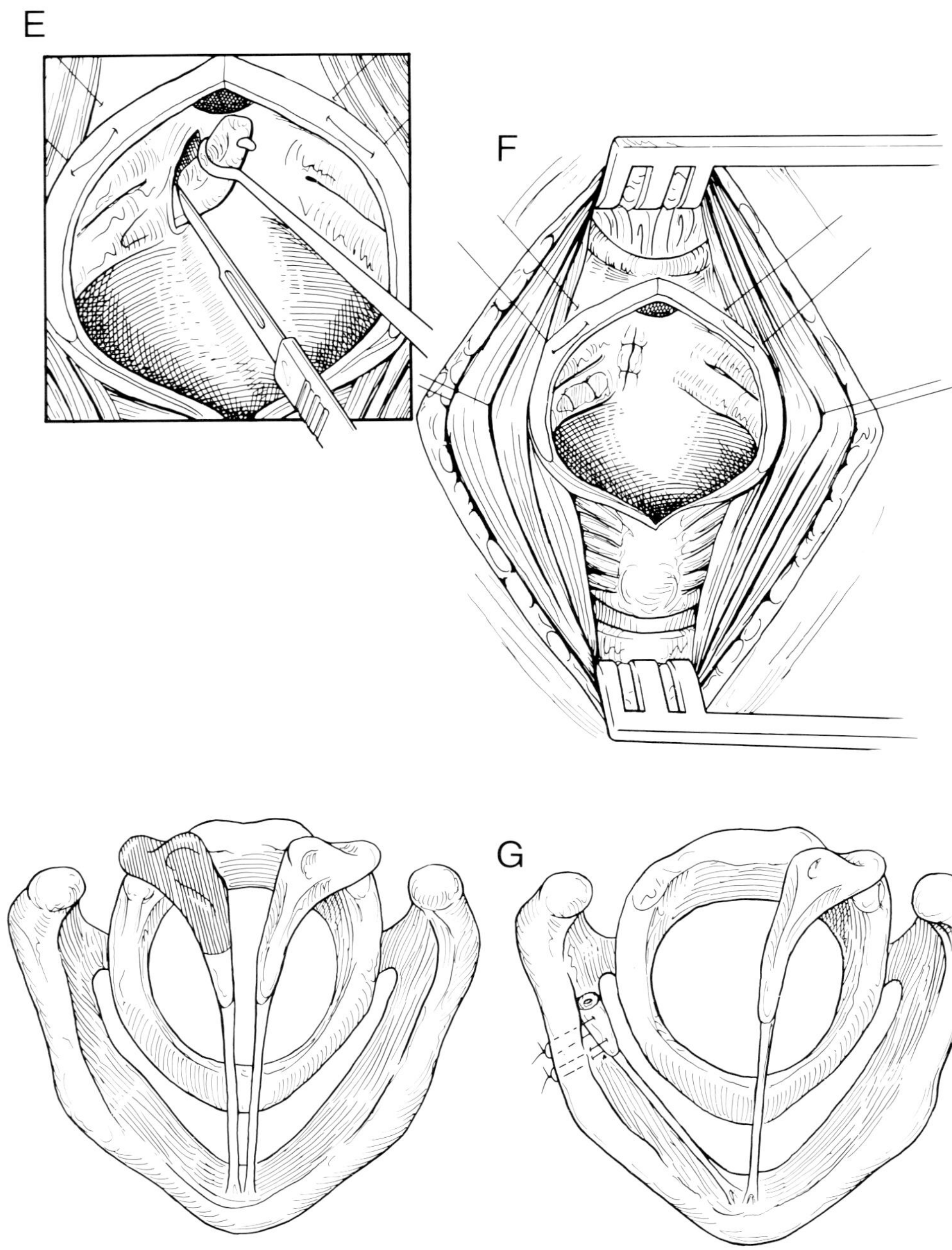


▶ **FIGURE 31-15**

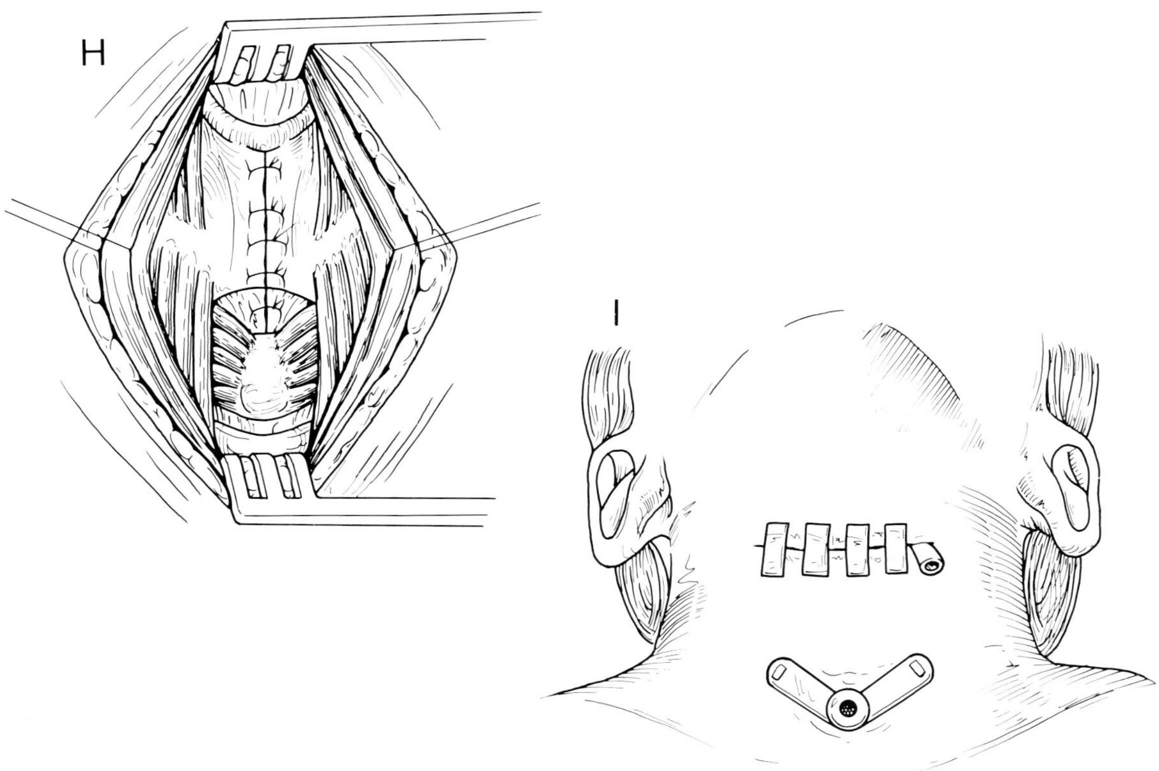


▸ **FIGURE 31-15**

## ▶ 31-16 ARYTENOIDECTOMY (LASER)

### Indications

Arytenoidectomy is indicated in the patient with persistent bilateral vocal cord paralysis who is unable to be decannulated because of airway obstruction or significant exertional dyspnea.

### Preoperative Evaluation

Direct laryngoscopy while the child is breathing spontaneously is required to document vocal cord paralysis. The arytenoids must be palpated to make sure that they are mobile and that the paralysis is not related to arytenoid fixation or glottic scarring.

### Operative Technique

1. Arytenoidectomy is performed under general anesthesia administered through the tracheotomy tube that is already in place or by jet ventilation.
2. A Jako laryngoscope is advanced into the larynx exposing the region of the vocal process and arytenoid cartilage (Figs. 31–16**A** and 31–16**B**).
3. Using a $CO_2$ laser, the vocal process and base of the arytenoid are removed creating a sufficient posterior glottic opening (Fig. 31–16**C**).
4. No attempt is made to completely remove the entire arytenoid cartilage. Care is taken to avoid damage to the interarytenoid area.
5. The patient is given intravenous antibiotics for 10 days.
6. If a tracheotomy tube is in place, the cannula remains for 2 weeks, at which time a direct laryngoscopy and bronchoscopy is performed. If the larynx is healed, a decannulation is attempted 12 to 24 hours later.
7. If no tracheotomy tube is in place, an age-appropriate size of endotracheal tube is left in place for 4 days, and the patient is extubated in the operating room where a direct laryngoscopy and bronchoscopy are performed.
8. If the airway is adequate, the endotracheal tube is replaced and then removed 12 to 24 hours later with the child fully awake in the intensive care unit.

### Complications

1. Persistent inadequate airway
2. Posterior glottic web/scarring

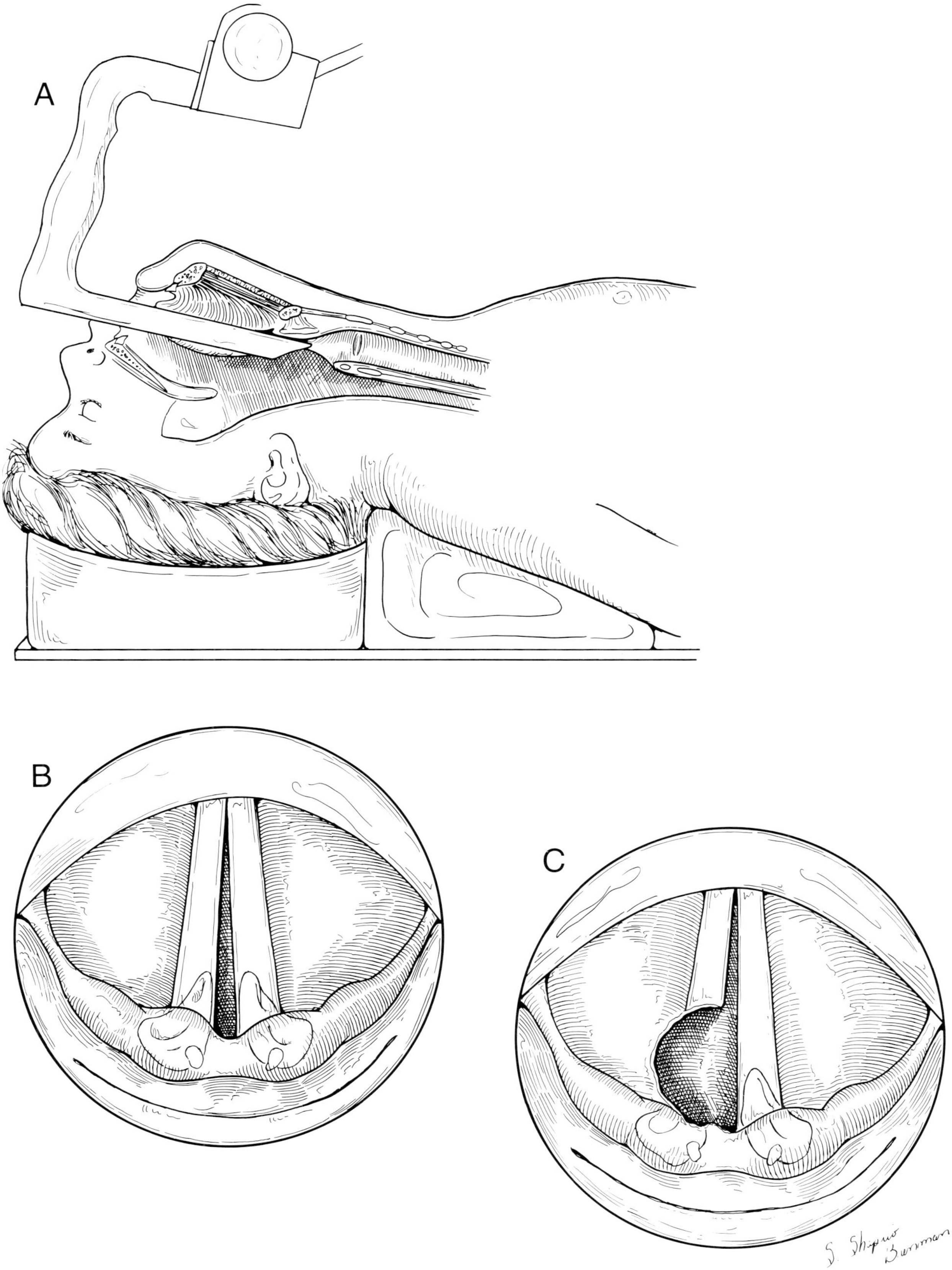


▶ **FIGURE 31-16**

## ▶ 31-17 ARYEPIGLOTTOPLASTY (LARYNGOMALACIA)

Laryngomalacia is the most common cause of stridor in children. While the majority of these patients only have noisy breathing, a small number have severe respiratory obstruction that requires surgical intervention.

### Indications

The indication for aryepiglottoplasty is severe airway obstruction secondary to laryngomalacia that compromises growth and development or results in significant oxygen desaturation.

### Preoperative Evaluation

Direct laryngoscopy and bronchoscopy, both flexible and rigid, with the patient breathing spontaneously is required to localize the region of the larynx that is flaccid and causing obstruction. Airway fluoroscopy is rarely helpful.

### Operative Technique

1. Flexible laryngoscopy is performed during spontaneous respiration (Fig. 31–17**A**, inspiration, Fig. 31–17**B**, expiration) to determine the soft tissue(s) responsible for the obstruction during inspiration. The most common offenders are the lateral aryepiglottic folds, the corniculate and cuneiform regions of the aryepiglottic fold, and, less commonly, the epiglottis.
2. Aryepiglottoplasty is performed under general anesthesia using either insufflation or jet ventilation.
3. A Jako laryngoscope is advanced into the larynx exposing the region of the larynx that is collapsing on inhalation (Fig. 31–17**C**).
4. The redundant collapsing areas of the supraglottis (Fig. 31–17**D**) are resected with a laryngeal forceps and scissors, or with a $CO_2$ laser (Fig. 31–17**E**) to create an unobstructed supraglottis. Care is taken not to resect tissue in the posterior commissure, which could result in scarring and stenosis (Fig. 31–17**F**).
5. The child remains intubated overnight with an age-appropriate size endotracheal tube, is started on steroids, and is observed for airway obstruction in the intensive care unit. Extubation is performed on the first postoperative day and steroids are continued for 48 hours. Antibiotics are given for 10 days.

### Complications

1. Persistent laryngomalacia
2. Laryngeal edema causing airway obstruction
3. Stenosis

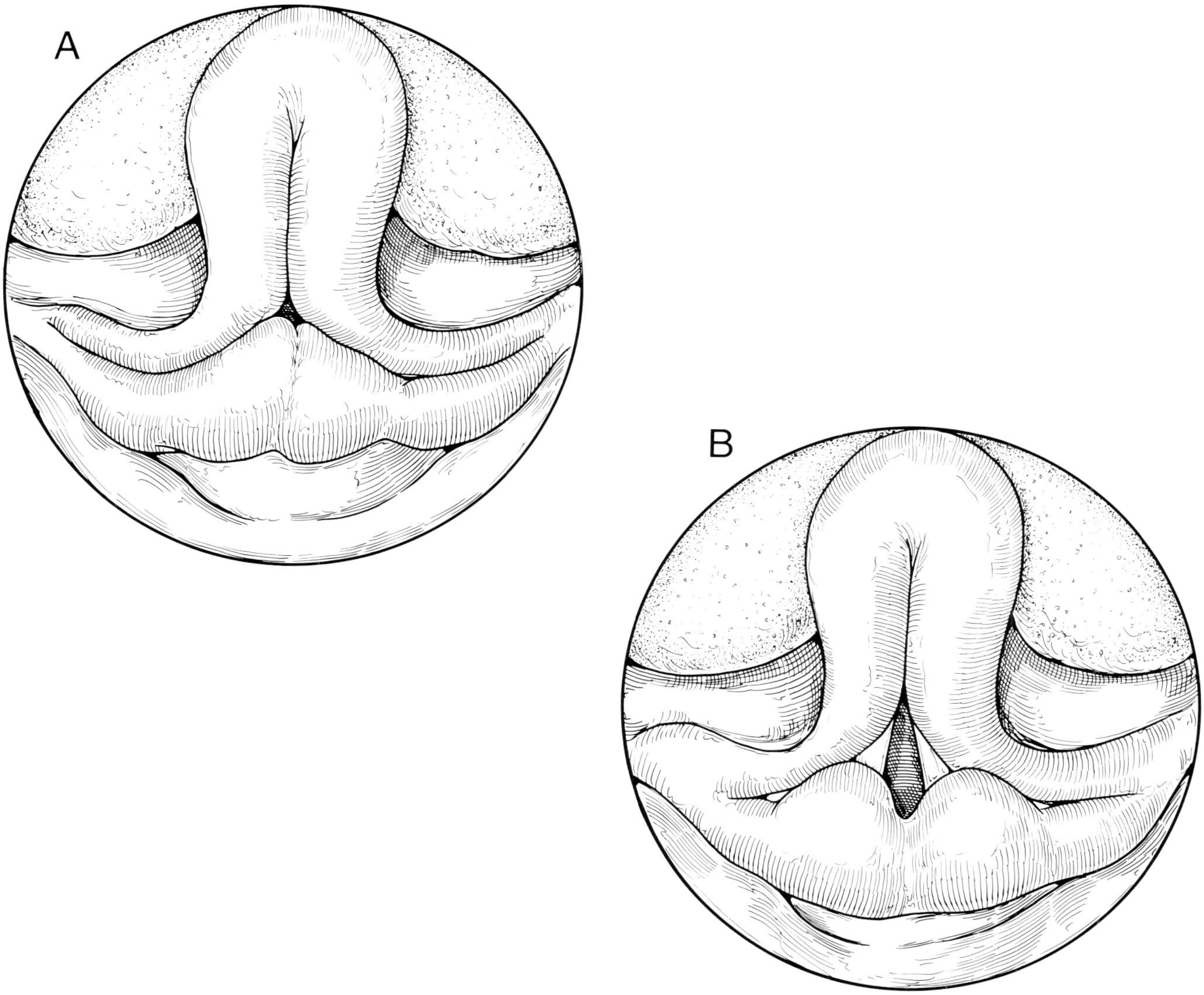


▸ **FIGURE 31-17**

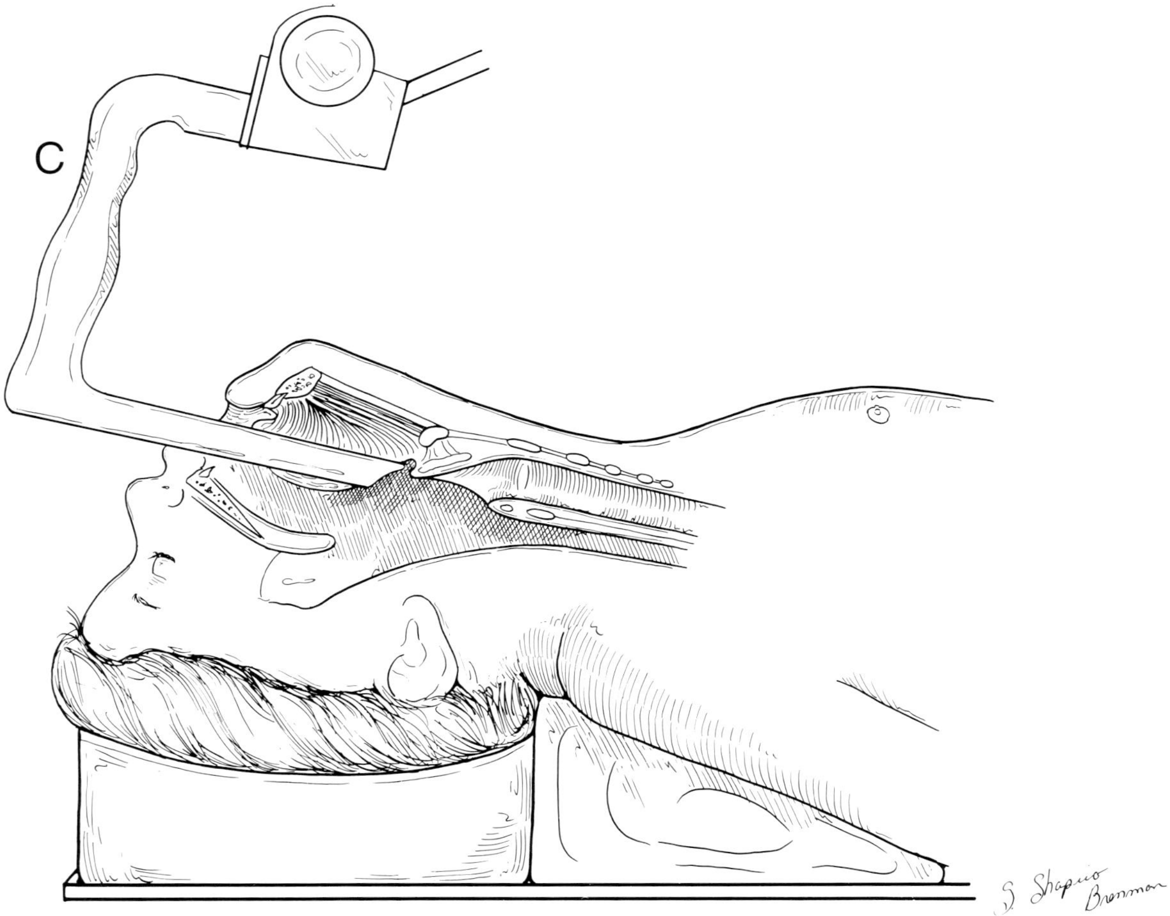


▶ **FIGURE 31-17**

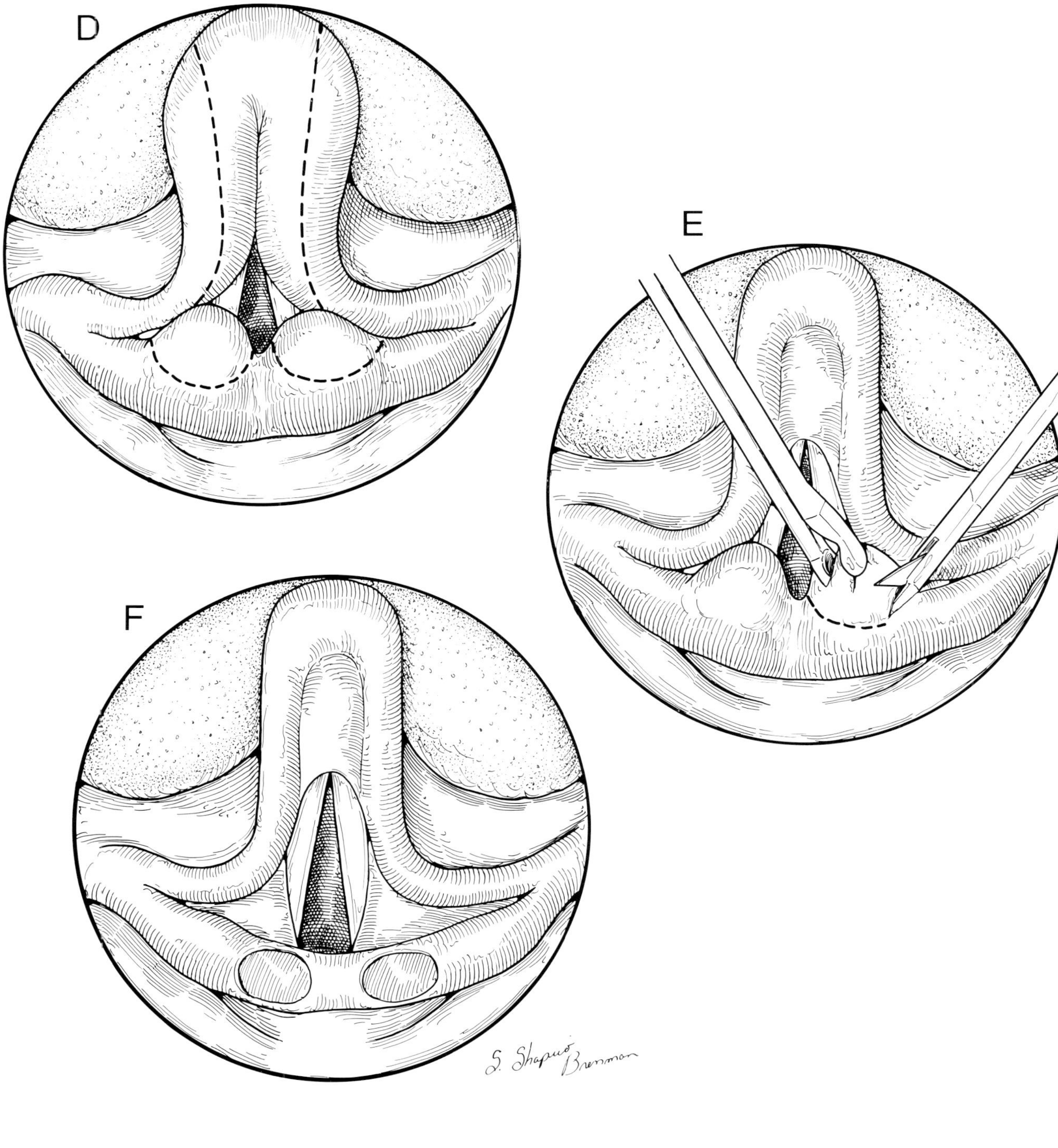


▶ **FIGURE 31-17**

# 32 ▶ Neck Mass

## ▶ 32-1 LYMPH NODE EXCISION

Cervical adenopathy is common in children and usually requires no intervention. However, in some instances, the nodes become large enough to cause suspicion of a malignancy. In those instances, excisional (if possible) biopsy of an enlarged node is indicated.

### Indications

The presence of a suspicious enlarged lymph node is the indication for excision of the mass.

### Preoperative Evaluation

A computed tomography (CT) or magnetic resonance imaging (MRI) scan is occasionally helpful if the lymph node is large or if there are numerous nodes over the cervical region. A chest x-ray is indicated if there is suspicion of a malignant process in the neck. If there is a strong suspicion of a malignancy, the oncologist should be notified and prepared to perform a lumbar puncture and/or bone marrow aspirate if a malignancy is confirmed or suspected on frozen section evaluation of the node.

### Operative Technique

1. An appropriate transverse skin crease overlying the lesion and approximately $1\frac{1}{2}$ cm below the margin of the mandible is selected. Care is taken to stay away from the course of the marginal mandibular nerve. One percent lidocaine with 1:100,000 epinephrine is injected to help in hemostasis.
2. An incision is made with a #15 scalpel through the skin and subcutaneous tissue (Fig. 32–1**A**).
3. The platysma muscle is incised using the cutting cautery to reduce bleeding (Fig. 32–1**B**).
4. Soft tissue overlying the node (or nodes) is gently dissected off using fine pickups and delicate scissors. A small gauze "peanut" may be helpful in this maneuver.
5. The node is gently grasped with fine forceps and dissected away from surrounding tissue with blunt and sharp dissection. Scissors are used to spread and then cut thin fibrous attachments. Every attempt is made to remove an intact node (Fig. 32–1**C**).
6. If a vascular pedicle is identified, this is clamped, cut, and tied with a 3-0 chromic suture (Fig. 32–1**D**).
7. If there is clinical suspicion of an infectious etiology for the node, a small piece is excised and sent for aerobic, fungal, and acid-fast cultures.
8. The node with its intact capsule is sent in a fresh state to the pathologist so that appropriate touch preps and stains may be performed.

9. A small rubber band drain is usually placed to prevent accumulation of fluid and/or blood in the dissected cavity. A safety pin or suture is attached to the distal end of the drain to prevent it being lost in the wound. The drain is removed within 24 hours.
10. The wound is closed in layers. The skin is closed with subcuticular sutures and Steri-strips are applied to keep the wound edges approximated (Fig. 32–1E).

## Complications

1. Hemorrhage from a major vessel
2. Marginal mandibular nerve injury

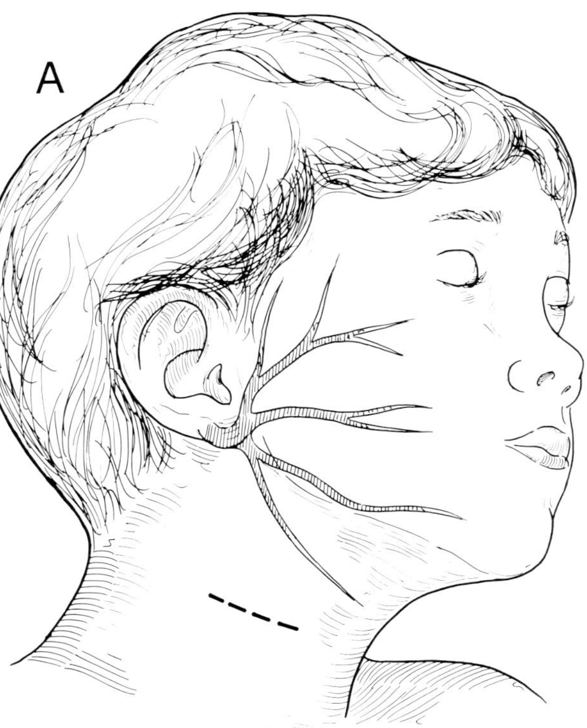


▶ **FIGURE 32-1**

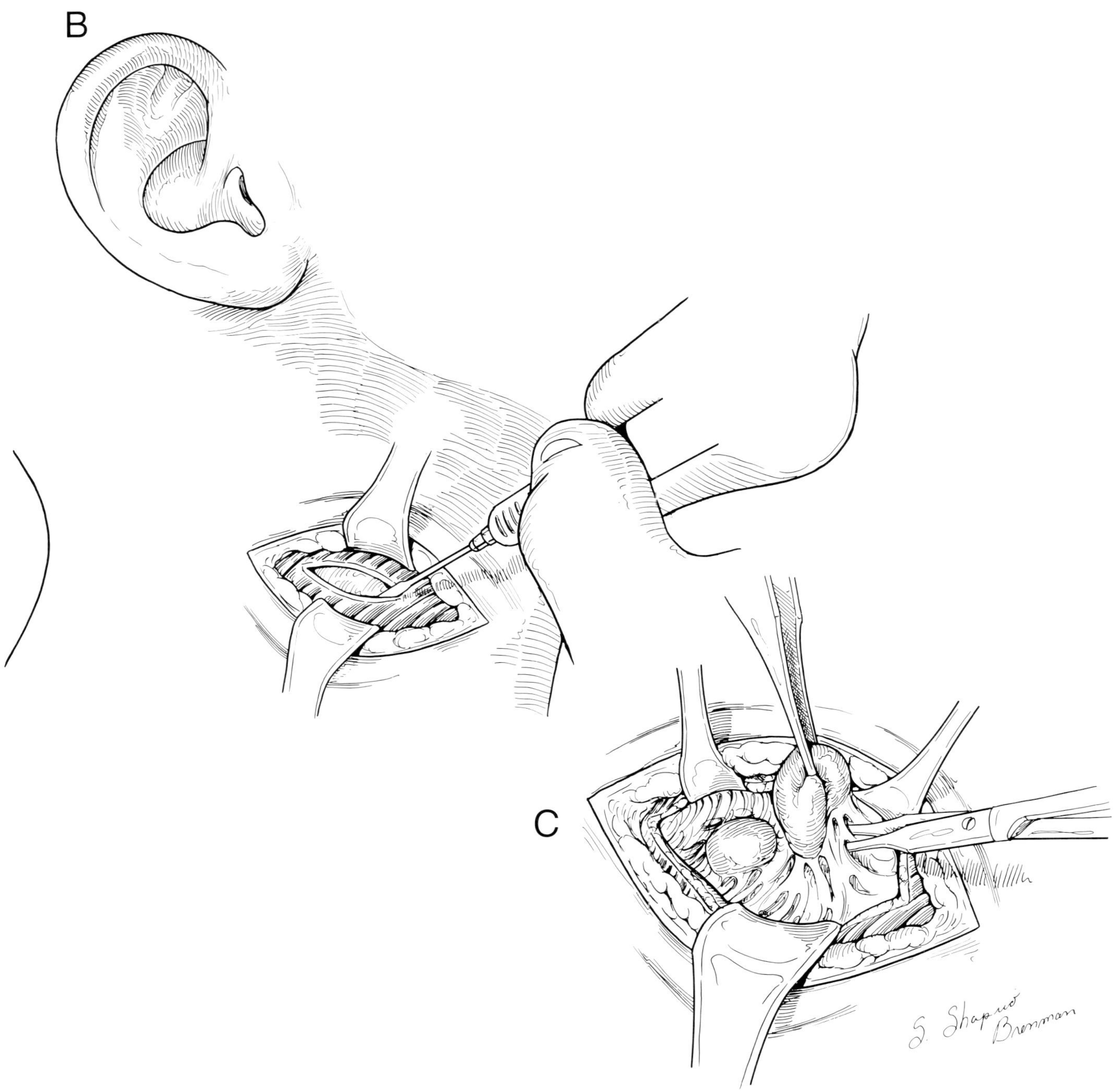


▶ **FIGURE 32-1**

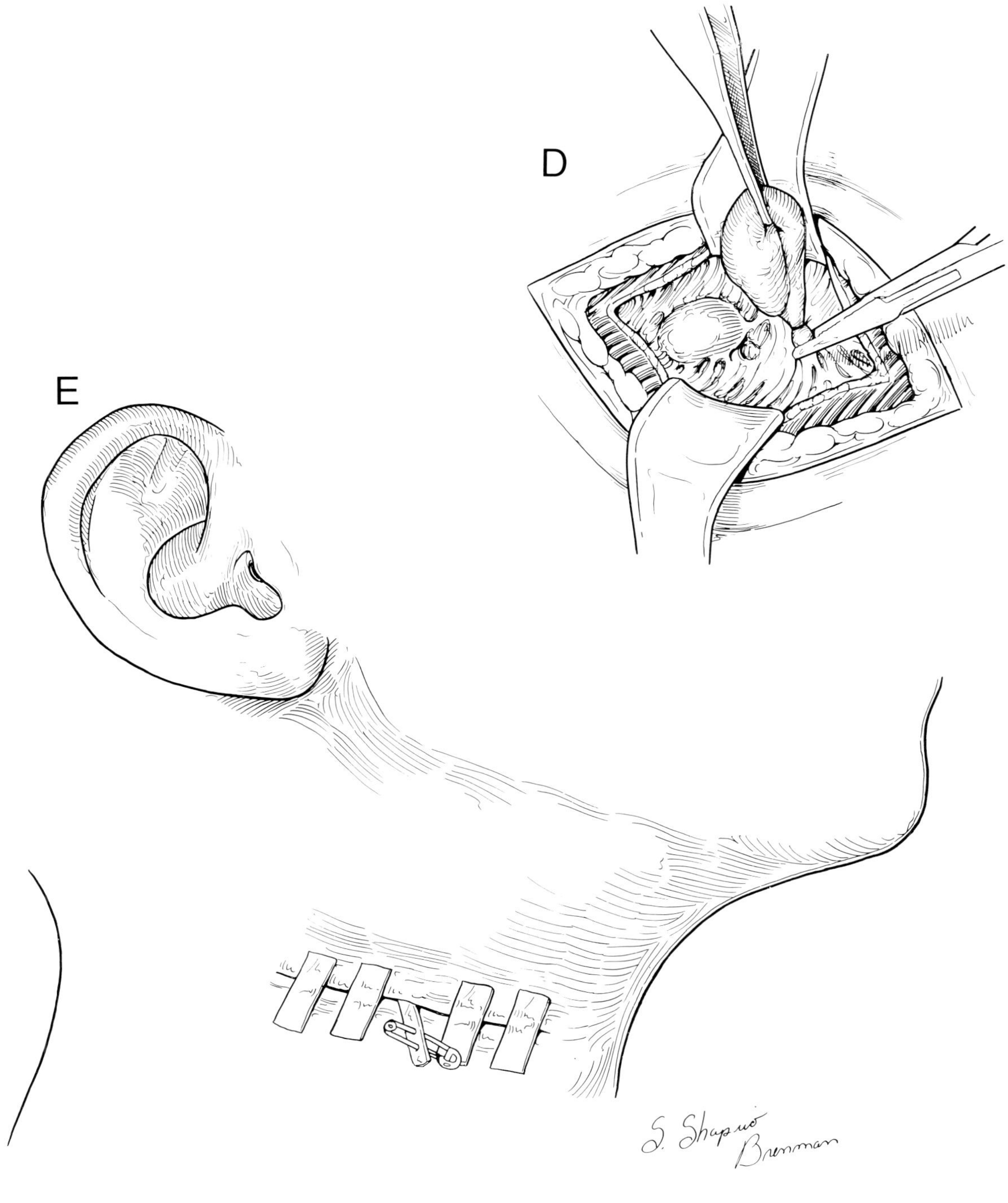


▶ **FIGURE 32-1**

## ▶ 32-2 EXCISION OF THYROGLOSSAL DUCT CYST

A cervical thyroglossal duct cyst may occur anywhere from the base of the tongue to the lower third of the neck. They usually lie close to the midline.

### Indications

Excision of a thyroglossal duct cyst is indicated before it becomes infected. Once infected, excision is associated with a higher rate of recurrence.

### Preoperative Evaluation

A thyroid ultrasound should be done prior to surgery to establish the presence of thyroid tissue in its normal location. If the thyroglossal duct cyst contains the child's only functioning thyroid tissue, thyroid replacement will be required after excision.

### Operative Technique

1. Excision of a thyroglossal duct cyst is performed under general anesthesia. One percent lidocaine with 1:100,000 epinephrine is injected to help with hemostasis.
2. The child is positioned supine on a shoulder roll with the neck extended (Fig. 32–2**A**).
3. A transverse incision is made through the skin, subcutaneous tissues and platysma muscle overlying the cyst (Fig. 32–2**B**).
4. Subplatysmal flaps are elevated with a scissors to a level above the hyoid bone and inferiorly to expose the cyst while being careful not to enter it. (Fig. 32–2**C**).
5. The cyst is dissected from its surrounding soft tissue attachments, including the thyrohyoid membrane (Fig. 32–3**D**).
6. If the tract enters the thyrohyoid membrane, it should be tied with suture, divided, and oversewn.
7. The cyst and its track usually extends to, and is attached to, the mid-portion of the hyoid bone.
8. The hyoid bone is exposed laterally by cutting the overlying soft tissue with a knife or Bovie at the junction of the lesser and greater cornua (Fig. 32–2**E**).
9. The hyoid bone is cut on each side at the lesser cornu with a bone cutter or heavy scissors (Fig. 32–2**F**).
10. The superior and inferior muscle attachments to the hyoid bone are released with a knife or Bovie (Fig. 32–2**G**).
11. If a tract is present above the hyoid, it must be removed to prevent recurrence.
12. The assistant surgeon breaks scrub to place the index finger of the left hand in the patient's vallecula, and the base of the tongue is depressed into the surgical field. The core of soft tissue and tract are removed by sharp dissection with a scissors up to the foramen cecum (Fig. 32–2**H**). Complete excision of the tract rarely requires entering the oropharynx. If the pharynx is

entered, one or two sutures of 3-0 chromic suture are usually all that is required to close the mucosal defect.

**13.** The wound is closed in layers with 3-0 chromic sutures to obliterate the dead space (Fig. 32–3**I**). A Penrose drain is placed in the wound and the skin may be closed with interrupted 5-0 nylon or subcuticular 4-0 Vicryl (Fig. 32–2**J**). A light gauze dressing is applied.

**14.** IV postoperative antibiotics should be administered until the drain is removed, usually 24 to 36 hours.

**15.** Oral antibiotics are used for 10 days.

## Complications

1. Seroma
2. Cyst recurrence

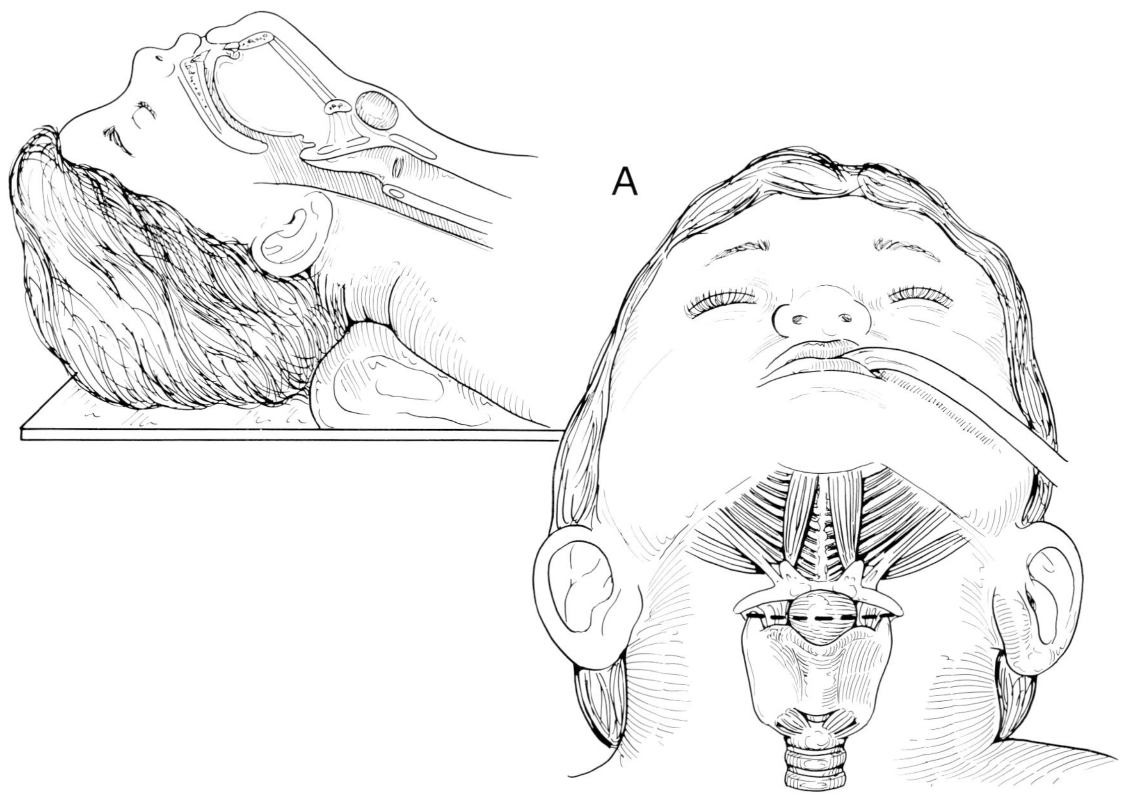


▶ **FIGURE 32-2**

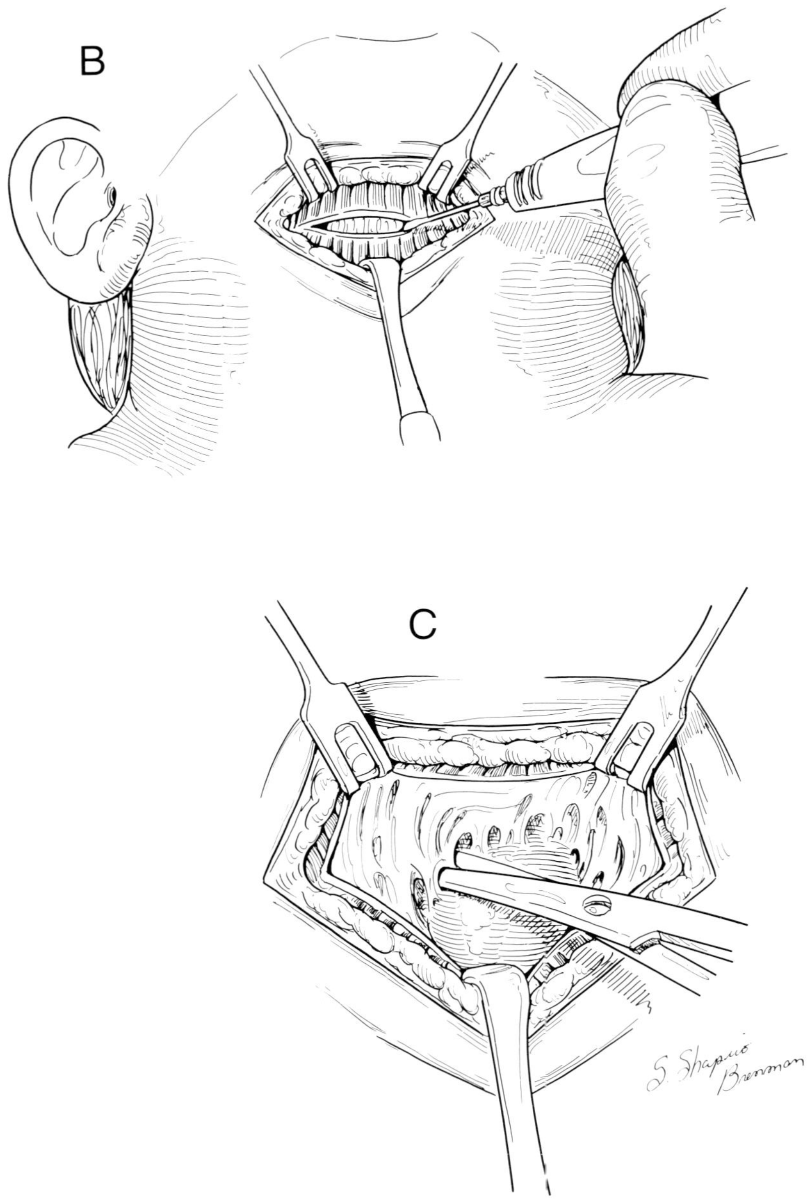


▶ **FIGURE 32-2**

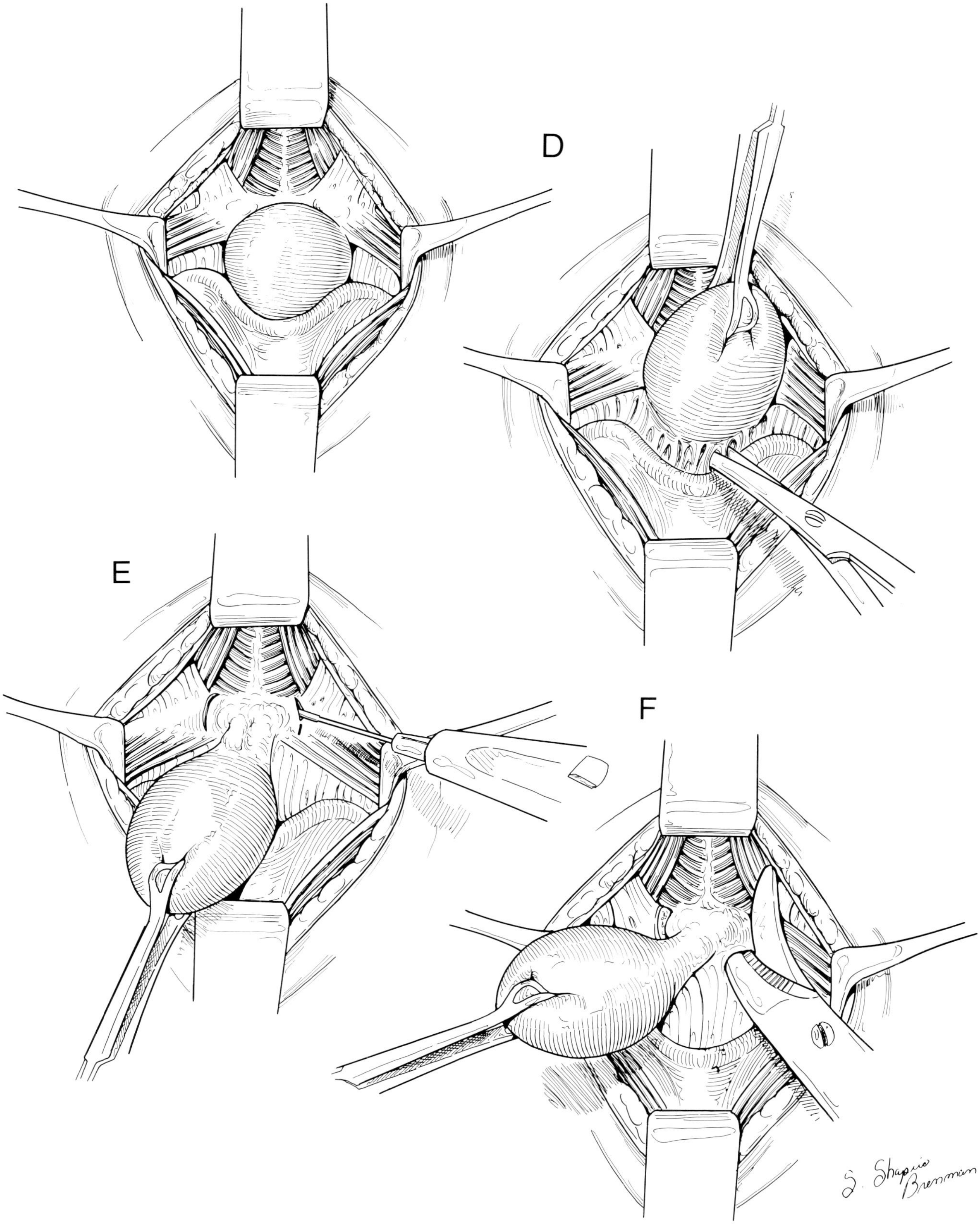


▶ **FIGURE 32-2**

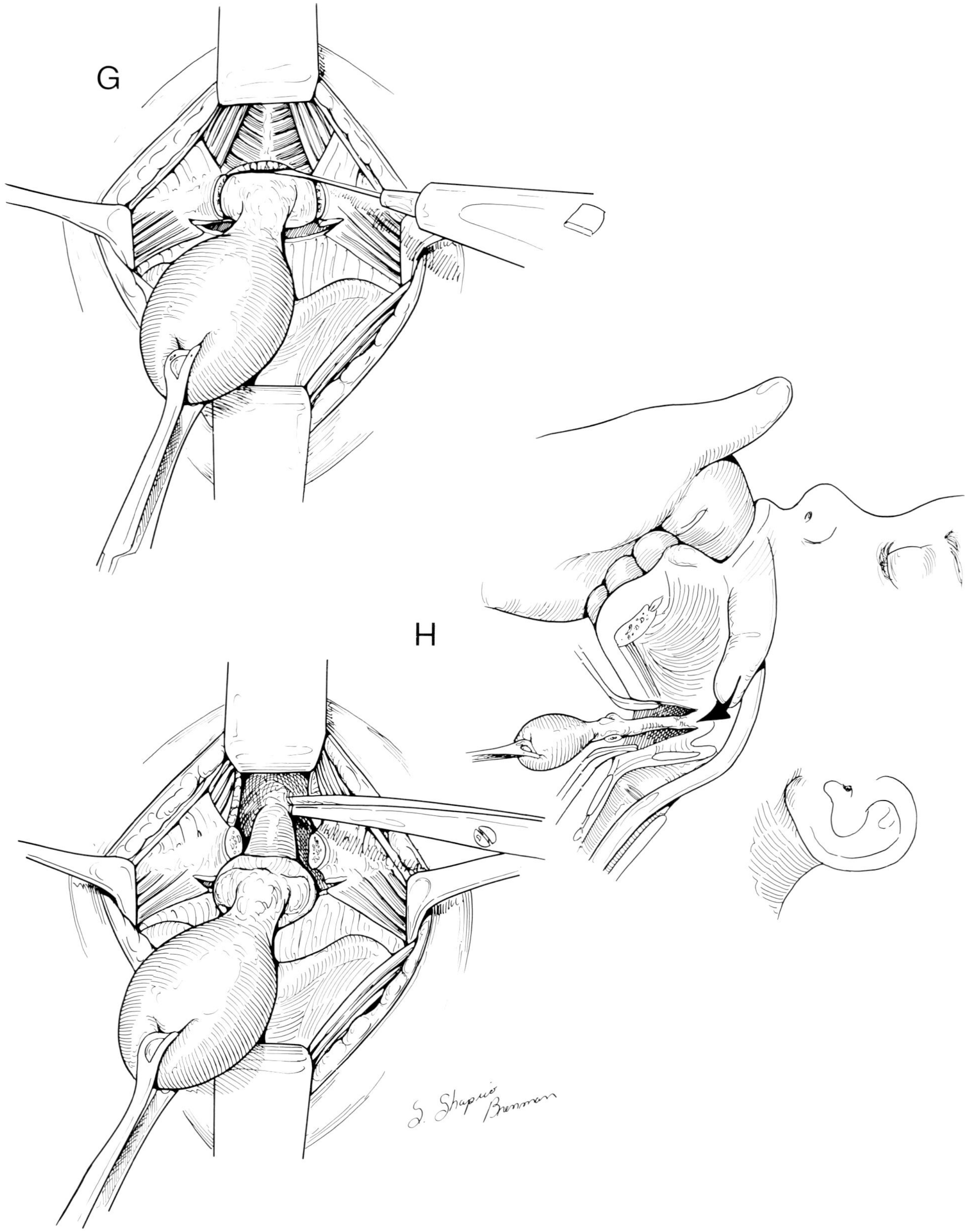


▶ **FIGURE 32-2**

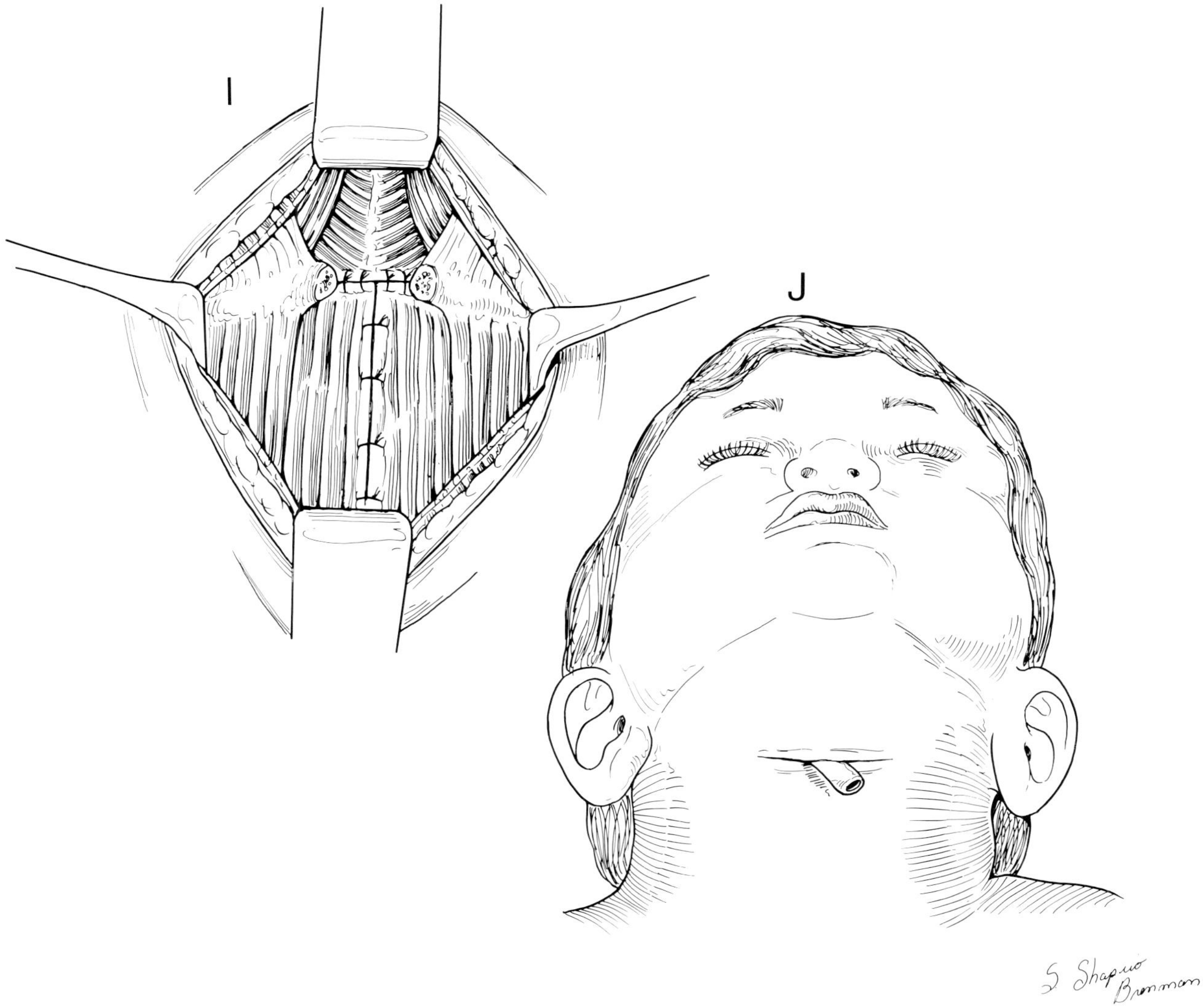


▶ **FIGURE 32-2**

## ▶ 32-3 EXCISION OF BRANCHIAL CLEFT CYST

Branchial cleft anomalies are remnants of the branchial arch apparatus that did not disappear during embryologic development. Cysts occur as a result of persistence of epithelial remnants between branchial arches. These lesions usually present as a soft swelling near the anterior border of the sternocleidomastoid muscle.

### Indications

The presence of a branchial cleft cyst is the indication for surgical excision both to confirm the diagnosis and to prevent infection of the cyst.

### Preoperative Evaluation

While clinical examination may suggest the diagnosis of branchial cleft cyst, radiographic studies such as ultrasound, computed tomography (CT) and magnetic resonance imaging (MRI) scans are helpful in confirming the diagnosis and determining the presence of an associated tract.

### Operative Technique

1. A transverse skin crease overlying the lesion and $1\frac{1}{2}$ cm below the margin of the mandible is selected. Care is taken to stay away from the course of the marginal mandibular nerve. One percent lidocaine with 1:100,000 epinephrine is injected to help with hemostasis.
2. The skin incision is made with a #15 blade through the skin and subcutaneous tissues (Fig. 32–3**A**).
3. The platysma muscle is divided with a cutting cautery (Fig. 32–3**B**).
4. The tissues overlying the cyst are gently dissected away with fine forceps and small scissors. A small gauze "peanut" may be helpful in this maneuver.
5. The cyst is gently grasped with a Babcock clamp. Surrounding tissue is dissected free from the cyst using small scissors to spread between the cyst capsule and surrounding tissue and then to cut through thin fibrous attachments (Fig. 32–3**C**).
6. If a pedicle or fibrous tract is identified, it is followed as far cephalic as possible before it is clamped, cut, and tied with a 3-0 chromic suture. It is not necessary to trace the tract all the way through the carotid bifurcation and into the pharynx (Fig. 32–3**D**).
7. A small rubber band drain is usually placed to prevent accumulation of fluid and/or blood in the dissected cavity. A safety pin or suture is attached to the distal end of the drain to prevent it being lost in the wound. The drain is removed within 24 hours.
8. The wound is closed in layers. The skin is closed with subcuticular sutures and Steri-strips are applied to keep the wound edges approximated (Fig. 32–3**E**).
9. Antibiotics are not employed unless the cyst was clinically infected or the contents were spilled during the dissection.

### Complications

1. Recurrence of the cyst from incomplete excision
2. Marginal mandibular nerve injury

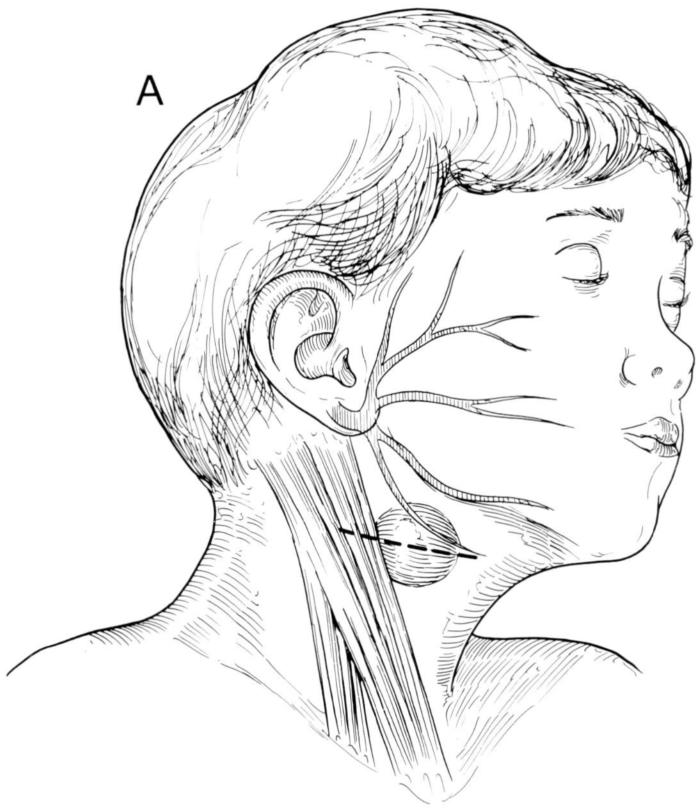


▶ **FIGURE 32-3**

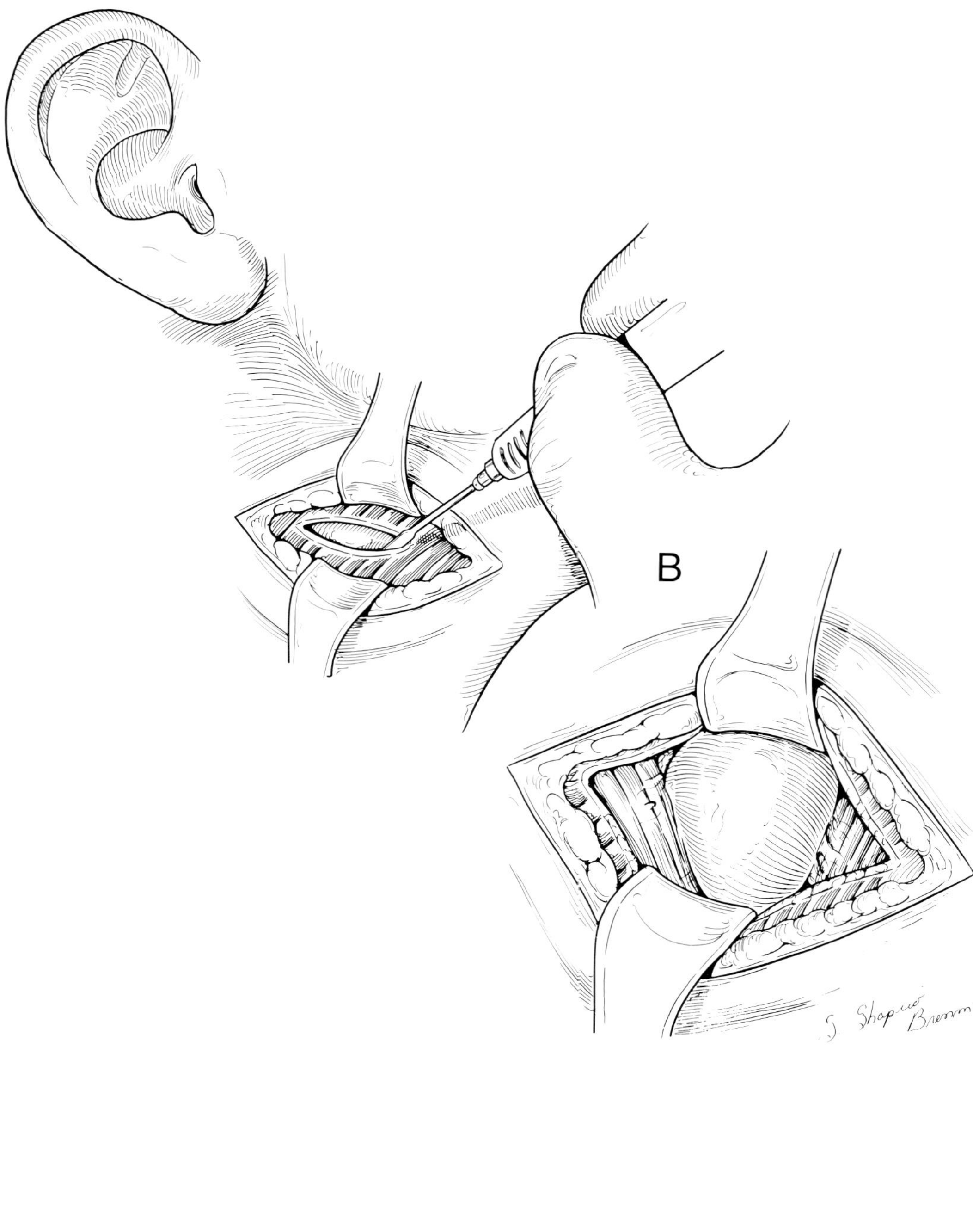


▶ **FIGURE 32-3**

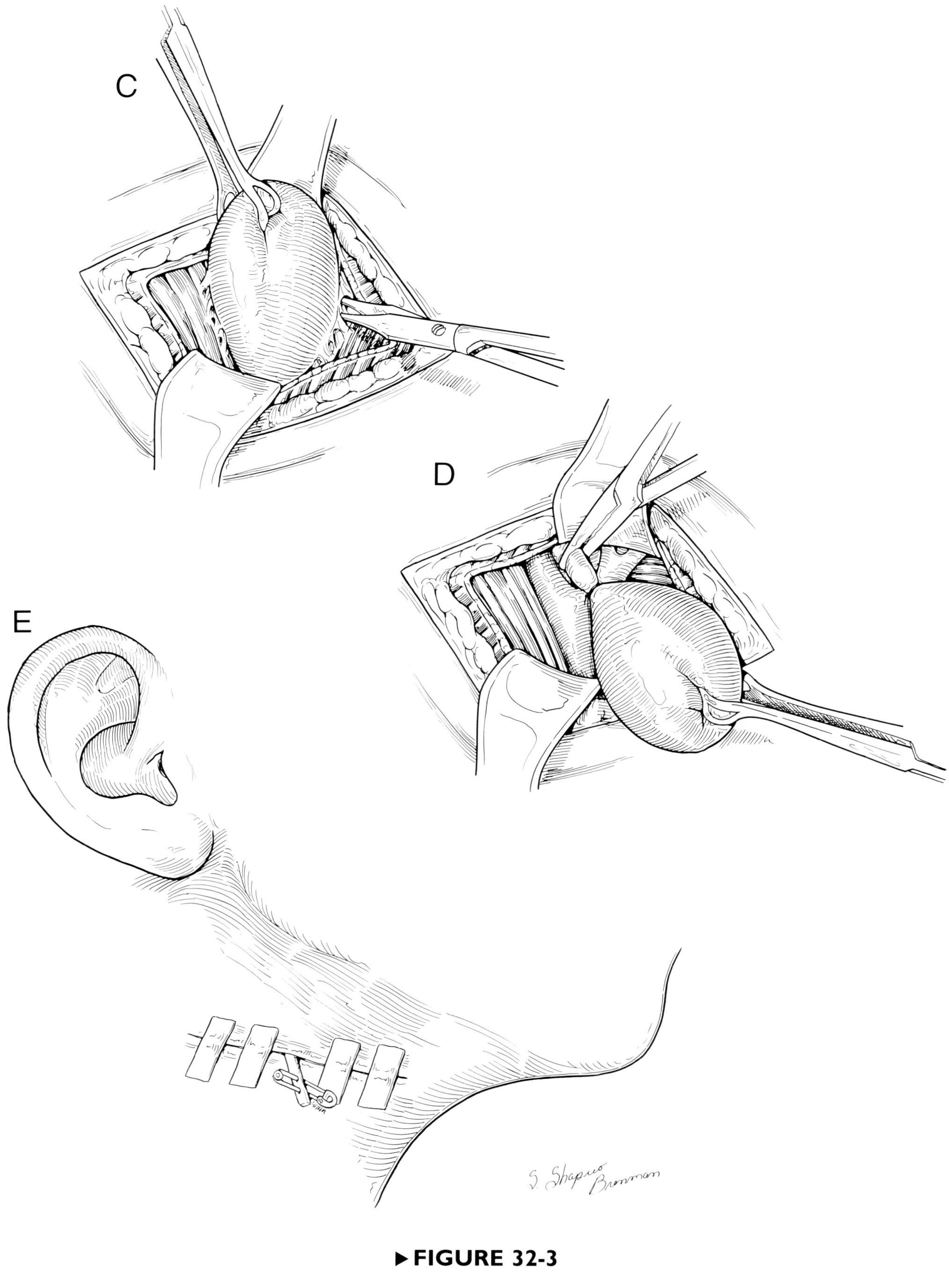


▶ **FIGURE 32-3**

## ▶ 32-4 EXCISION OF BRANCHIAL CLEFT SINUS/FISTULA

Branchial cleft sinuses/fistulas are epithelial remnants of the branchial arch system that maintain a connection to either the skin, mucous membrane of the oral cavity or pharynx, or both. An external sinus tract usually presents at the anterior border of the sternocleidomastoid muscle. Internal sinuses present at the tonsillar fossa or the pyriform sinus. First branchial cleft sinuses present as external openings near the angle of the mandible and course near the branches of the facial nerve to end in the external auditory canal or middle ear.

### Indications

The presence of a branchial cleft sinus/fistula is the indication for excision.

### Preoperative Evaluation

Computed tomography (CT) or magnetic resonance imaging (MRI) scan of the lesion may help to delineate the extent of the tract. It is not necessary to inject radio-opaque material into the fistula to visualize the tract. If a first branchial cleft sinus is suspected, an audiogram and a CT scan of the temporal bone is indicated preoperatively.

### Operative Technique

1. The area surrounding the external sinus (fistula) tract is injected with 1% lidocaine with 1:100,000 epinephrine.
2. A transverse elliptical incision is made encompassing the opening of the sinus tract (Fig. 32–4**A**).
3. Care is taken not to extend the superior limb of the incision too deeply where it may sever the tract.
4. Small blunt scissors are used to raise skin flaps superiorly and inferiorly (if necessary) staying superficial to the sinus tract (Fig. 32–4**B**).
5. The skin and distal end of the tract are grasped with an Allis clamp. Traction is maintained with the clamp as fibrous attachments to the tract are separated with the spreading of a small pair of blunt scissors and then cut (Fig. 32–4**C**).
6. The epithelial-lined sinus or fistula tract is followed superiorly as far as possible. Occasionally, a second, higher transverse incision ("stepladder") is needed to permit complete dissection of long sinus tracts.
7. The most proximal end of the tract is clamped, cut, and tied with a 3-0 silk suture (Fig. 32–4**D**).
8. If the fistula tract has an internal opening into the pharynx, this must be excised or ligated. In the case of a second branchial cleft fistula that drains into the tonsillar fossa, the involved tonsil is usually removed to allow complete excision of the fistula tract. Any defect in the wall of the pharynx (tonsillar fossa) must be closed with interrupted 3-0 chromic sutures.
9. If the fistula tract extends to the pyriform fossa (third branchial cleft), the opening must be ligated with a 3-0 chromic suture.
10. If the lesion is a first branchial cleft sinus, the lesion must be approached through a parotidectomy incision. A superficial parotidectomy (see section 35–2) is performed to identify and expose the trunk and branches of the fa-

cial nerve. Once this has been performed, the sinus tract can be dissected out to its termination in the external auditory canal or middle ear. If the sinus tract terminates in the external canal, the tract is transected at the entrance to the bony canal, and any epithelial remnants are removed with a curette. If the tract extends to the tympanic membrane or middle ear, a tympanoplasty (see section 3–2) may be necessary to allow complete removal of the lesion and reconstruction of the tympanic membrane.

11. A small rubber band drain is usually placed to prevent accumulation of fluid and/or blood in the dissected cavity. A safety pin is attached to the distal end of the drain to prevent it being lost in the wound. The drain is removed within 24 hours.
12. The wound is closed in layers. The skin incision (or incisions) is closed with subcuticular sutures and Steri-strips are applied to keep the wound edges approximated (Fig. 32–4E).
13. Antibiotics are not employed unless the tract was clinically infected or the contents were spilled during the dissection.

## Complications

1. Recurrence of the cyst from incomplete excision of the tract
2. Marginal mandibular nerve injury
3. Facial nerve injury (first branchial cleft cyst)
4. Tympanic membrane perforation (first branchial cleft cyst)

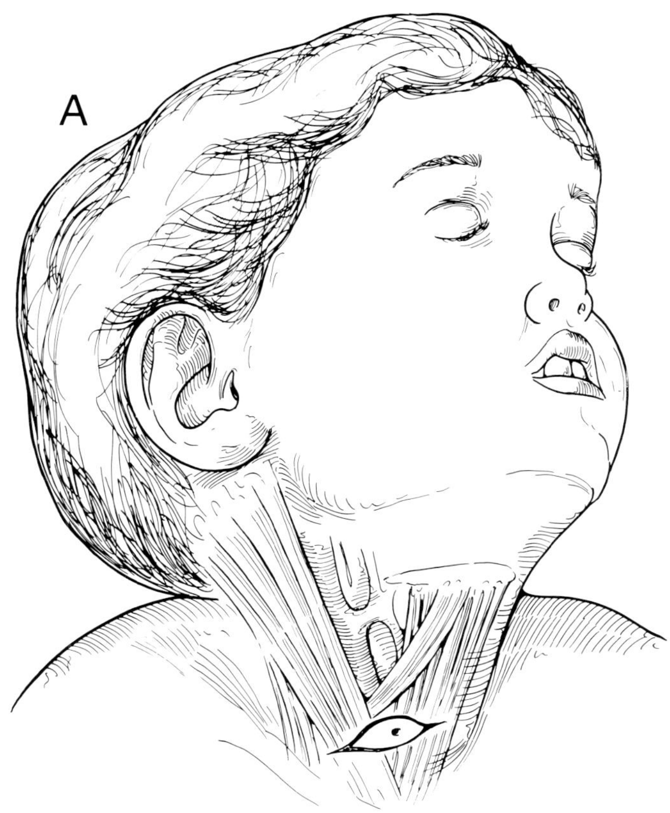


▶ **FIGURE 32-4**

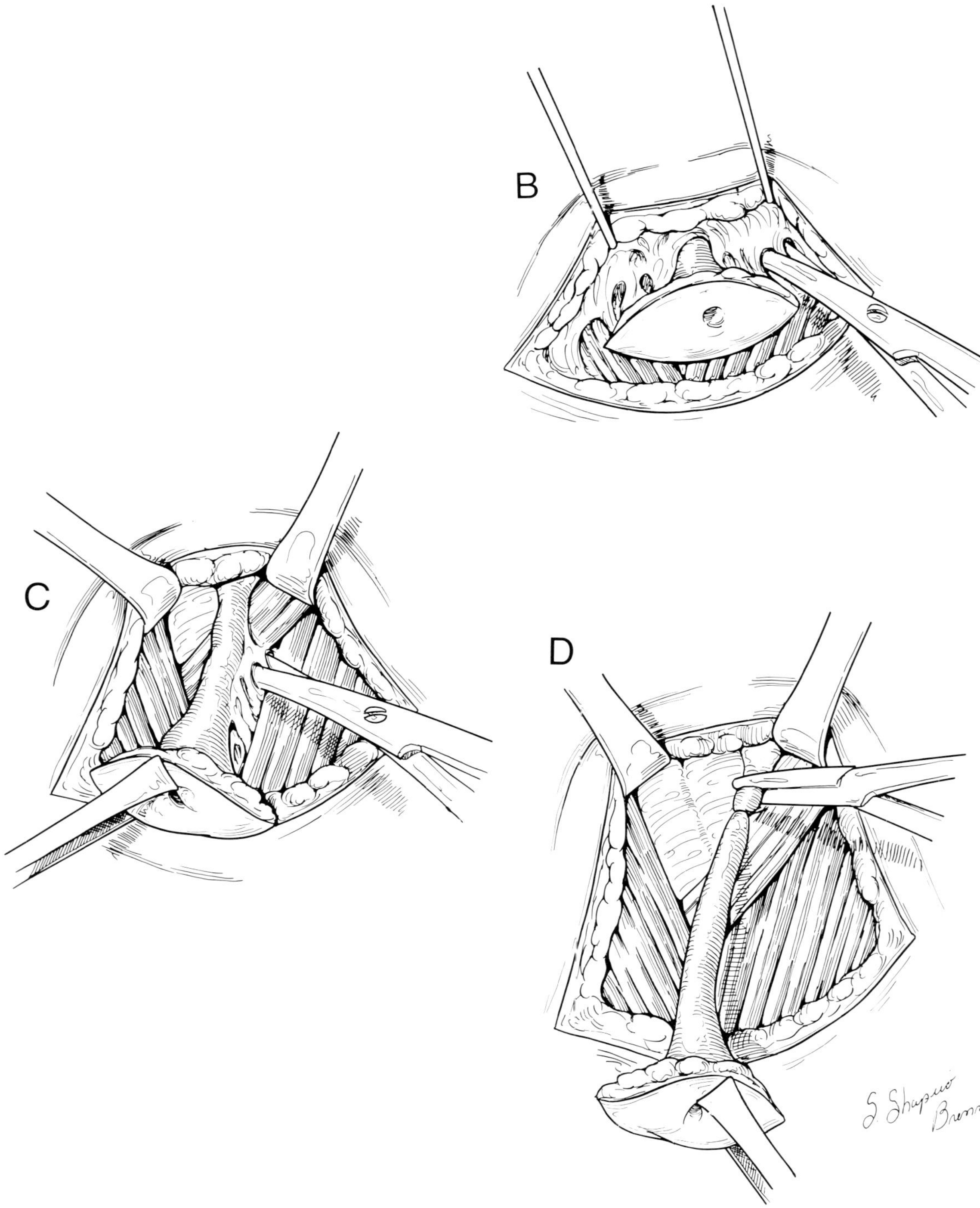


▶ **FIGURE 32-4**

E

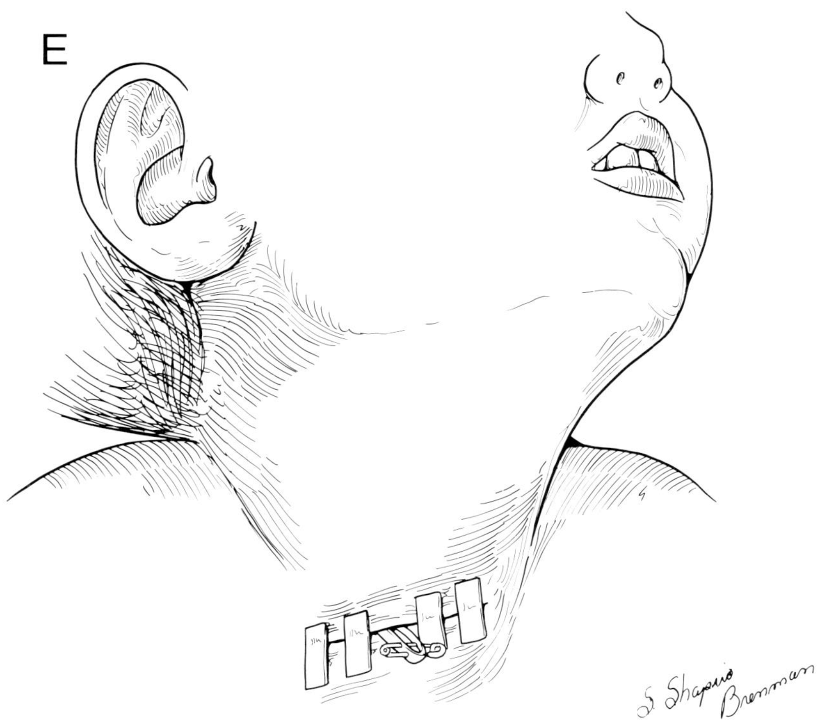

▶ **FIGURE 32-4**

## ▶ 32-5 DRAINAGE OF CERVICAL ADENITIS (ASPIRATION: INCISION AND DRAINAGE)

Inflammatory cervical adenitis is common in children and usually occurs concurrently with an upper respiratory infection. Rarely, a node breaks down to form a collection of purulent material.

### Indications

The indication for drainage of a cervical adenitis is the loculation of pus in a cervical node. Intravenous antibiotics should also be administered.

### Preoperative Evaluation

The preoperative evaluation of a cervical abscess includes a computed tomography (CT) or magnetic resonance imaging (MRI) scan to define the extent of the abscess.

### Operative Technique

1. Superficial cervical abscesses are aspirated without any anesthetic (Fig. 32–5A). Local anesthetics are usually not helpful in acutely inflamed tissue.
2. An 18 gauge needle is advanced into the abscess (Fig. 32–5B) and as much pus as possible is aspirated (Fig. 32–5C).
3. The needle should be moved to break septae and evacuate multiloculated pus (Fig. 32–5D).
4. Abscesses that do not respond to intravenous antibiotics and needle aspiration require incision and drainage under general anesthesia.
5. An incision is made into the abscess along the line of a skin crease (Fig. 32–5E).
6. Pus is evacuated from the abscess with a suction (Fig. 32–5F).
7. The septae in the abscess cavity are broken with a cotton tip applicator, finger, or clamp (Fig. 32–5G).
8. The abscess is packed with gauze to stop bleeding and allow it to drain (Fig. 32–5H).
9. No sutures are placed.
10. The packing is removed over 24 to 48 hours.
11. Antibiotics are administered based on culture findings (usually *Staphylococcus aureus*).

### Complications

1. Recurrence of abscess
2. Marginal mandibular nerve injury

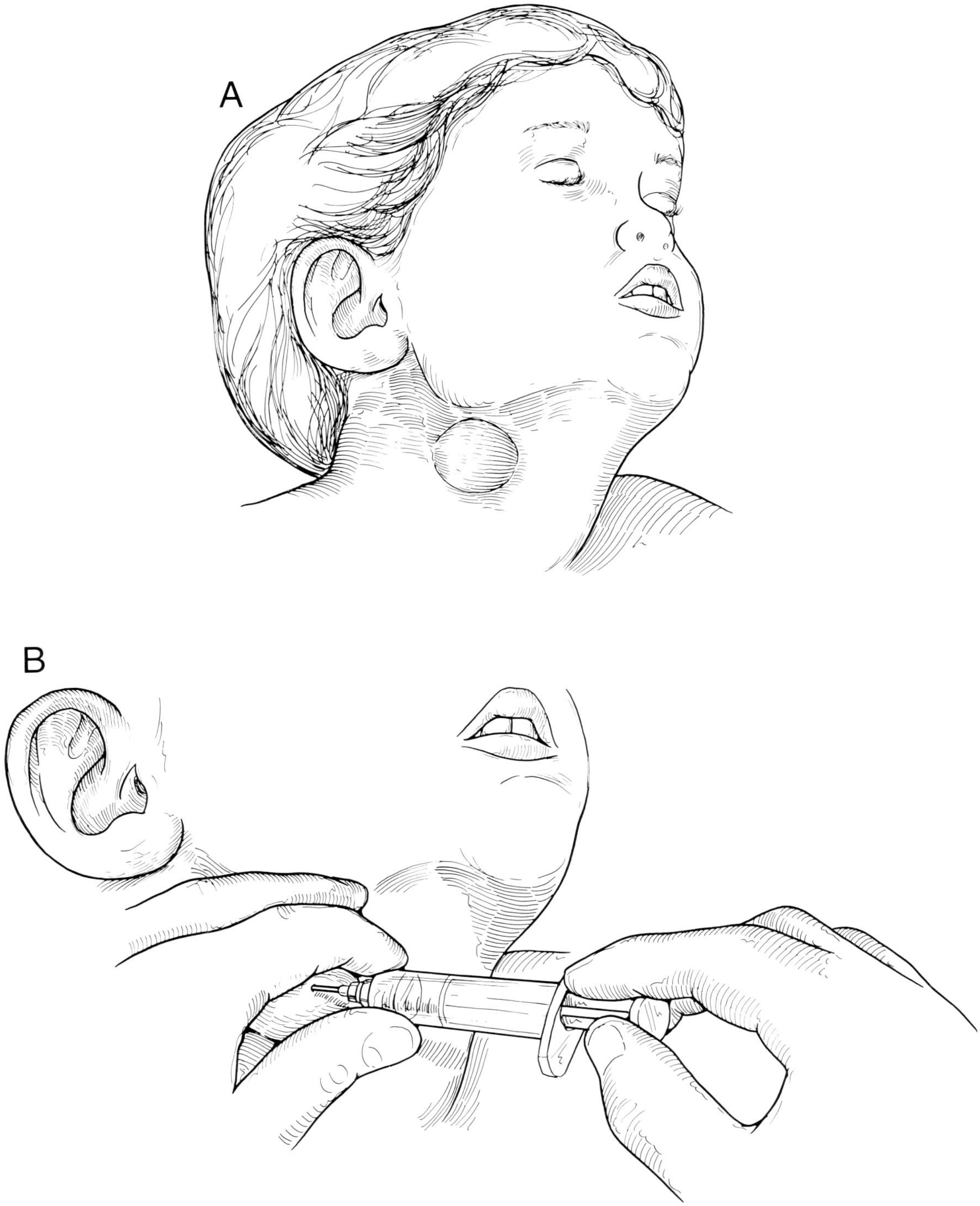


▶ **FIGURE 32-5**

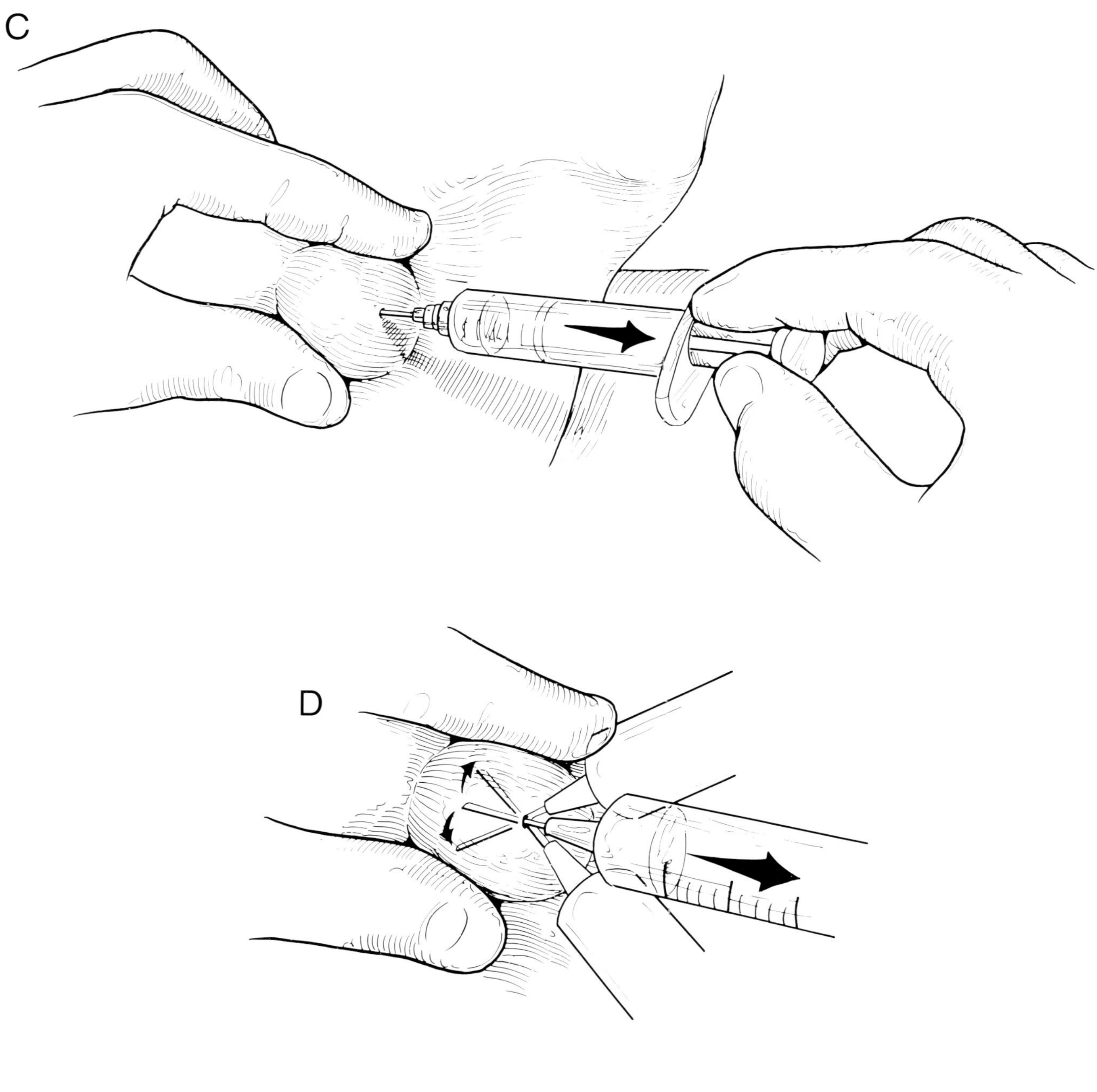


▶ **FIGURE 32-5**

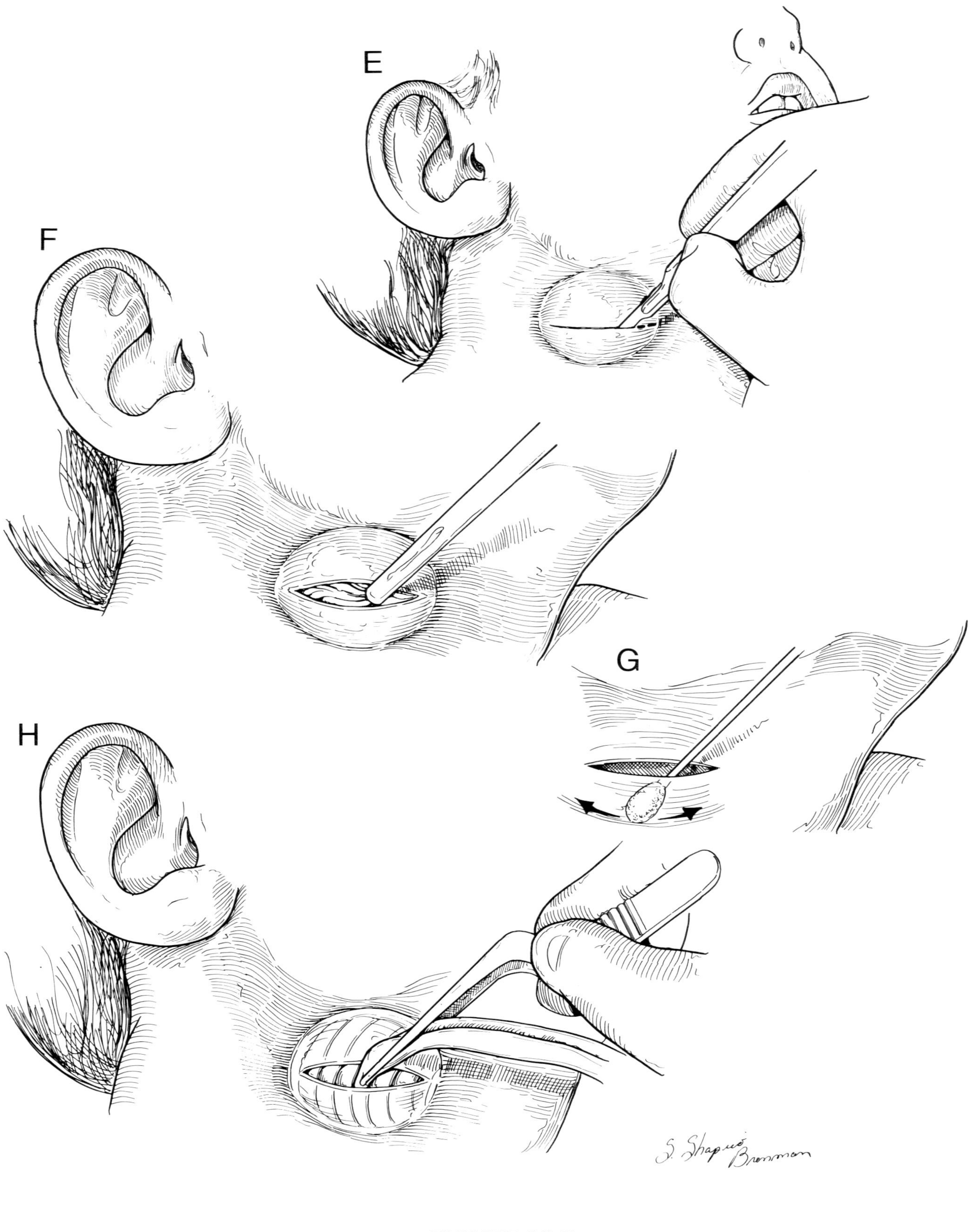


▸ **FIGURE 32-5**

## ▶ 32-6 CURETTAGE OF ATYPICAL MYCOBACTERIA

Atypical mycobacterial infection occurs uncommonly in children. It may involve any cervical lymph node, but most often presents at the lower border of the mandible in the posterior portion of the submandibular triangle. The overlying skin often has a deep red hue.

### Indications

These infections do not respond to antitubercular medications. Surgical excision is the treatment of choice. While either total excision or curettage can be utilized in the management of these lesions, curettage is equally effective and usually allows a more cosmetically acceptable result, especially in larger lesions.

### Preoperative Evaluation

Inspection and palpation of the involved mass is usually sufficient. A CT or MRI scan will define the extent of the deep nodes involved. The surgeon may elect to utilize intraoperative facial nerve monitoring during the surgical procedure.

### Operative Technique

1. Curettage of atypical mycobacteria cervical adenitis is performed under general anesthesia.,
2. An incision is made into the granulomatous abscess with a scalpel (Fig. 32–6**A**). The incision should be 2 cm below the edge of the mandible and in a skin crease. One percent lidocaine with 1:100,000 epinephrine may be injected subcutaneously at the site of the incision to aid in hemostasis.
3. The contents of the abscess are evacuated using a mastoid curette to clean out the granulomatous material (Fig. 32–6**B**).
4. Multiple nodes may be connected by granulomatous necrotic debris. These deeper nodes should be cleared out as well (Fig. 32–6**C**).
5. The skin incision is closed with interrupted 5-0 nylon suture. A rubber band drain is placed and removed in 24 to 36 hours (Fig. 32–6**D**).

### Complications

1. Recurrence of infection

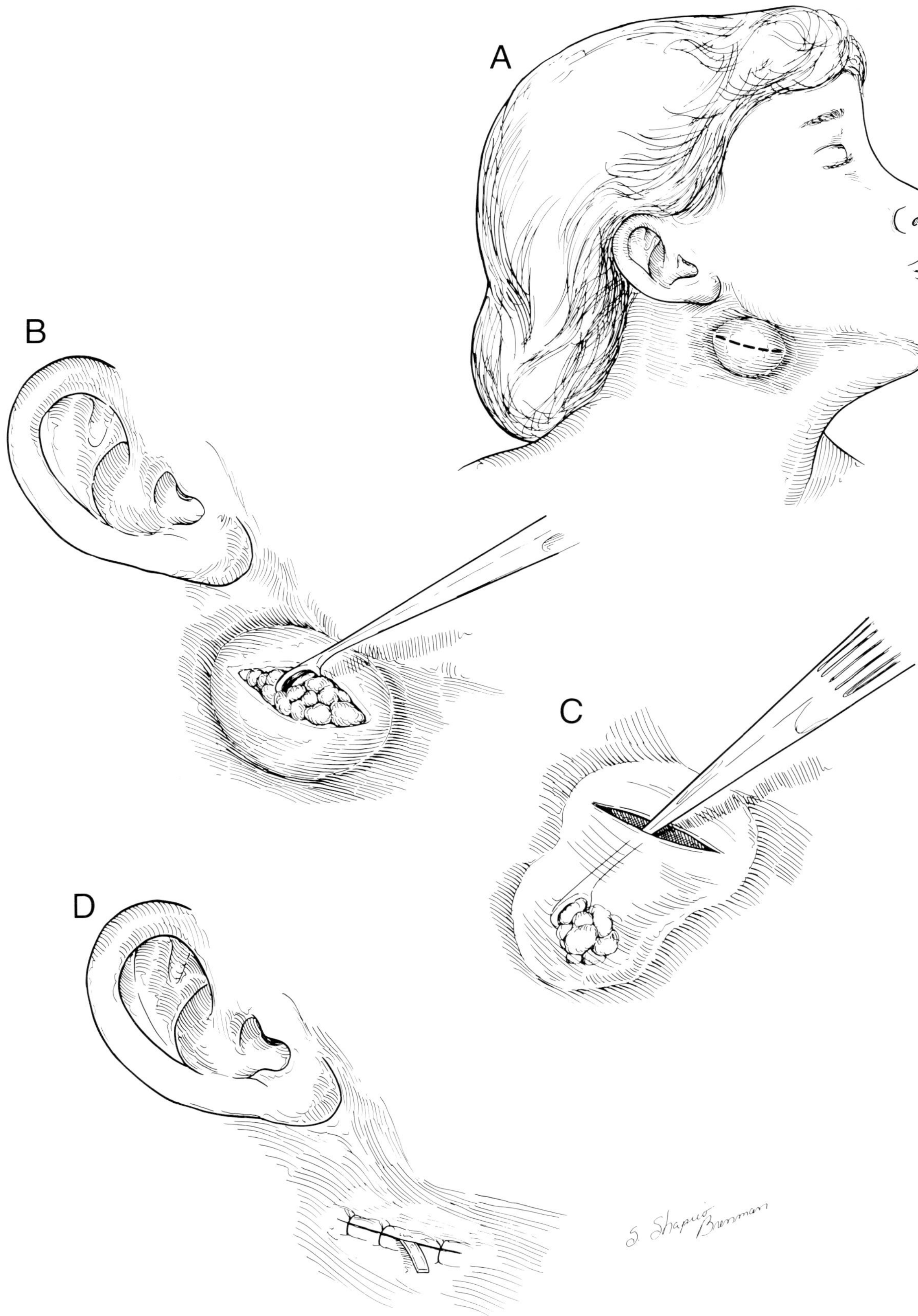


▶ **FIGURE 32-6**

## ▶ 32-7 THYROIDECTOMY

Thyroidectomy is an operation to excise one or both lobes of the thyroid gland. The most common indication for this procedure is the presence of a thyroid mass (suspicion of malignancy), which is rare in children.

### Indications

Thyroidectomy is indicated in the treatment of possible malignant disease in the thyroid gland.

### Preoperative Evaluation

Thyroid ultrasound and MRI are helpful to define disease in the thyroid gland and adjacent structures. Thyroid function tests and a chest radiograph should be performed pre-operatively.

### Operative Technique

1. Thyroidectomy is done under general anesthesia with the patient on a shoulder roll and the neck extended (see section 30–1).
2. A transverse incision is made in a skin crease in the lower neck after the area has been infiltrated with 1% lidocaine with 1:100,000 epinephrine to aid in hemostasis (Fig. 32–7**A**). The incision is carried through the subcutaneous tissue and the platysma muscle.
3. Inferior and superior sub-platysmal skin flaps are elevated with scissors exposing the strap muscles over the thyroid gland (Fig. 32–7**B**).
4. The strap muscles are separated in the midline and retracted laterally (Fig. 32–7**B**).
5. Using a clamp spreading in a vertical plane, the recurrent laryngeal nerve is identified in the tracheoesophageal groove near the inferior portion of the thyroid lobe (Fig. 32–7**C**).
6. Protecting the recurrent nerve, the thyroid veins and arteries are divided as the thyroid is dissected from its surrounding attachments with a clamp and scissors (Fig. 32–7**D**). If a parathyroid gland is identified, it should be preserved, if possible.
7. The thyroid lobe is reflected medially and the isthmus is cut with a Bovie (Fig. 32–7**E**).
8. The thyroid isthmus may be oversewn with chromic sutures to insure hemostasis.
9. If total thyroidectomy is required, the contralateral side is resected in a similar manner. In this instance, special care is taken to preserve at least one parathyroid gland.
10. The wound is closed with 4-0 Vicryl in the subcutaneous tissue and 4-0 interrupted subcuticular Vicryl in the skin (Fig. 30–7E).
11. A penrose drain is placed in the wound under the flap and removed in 24 to 36 hours.

### Complications

1. Recurrent laryngeal nerve injury
2. Hypoparathyroidism

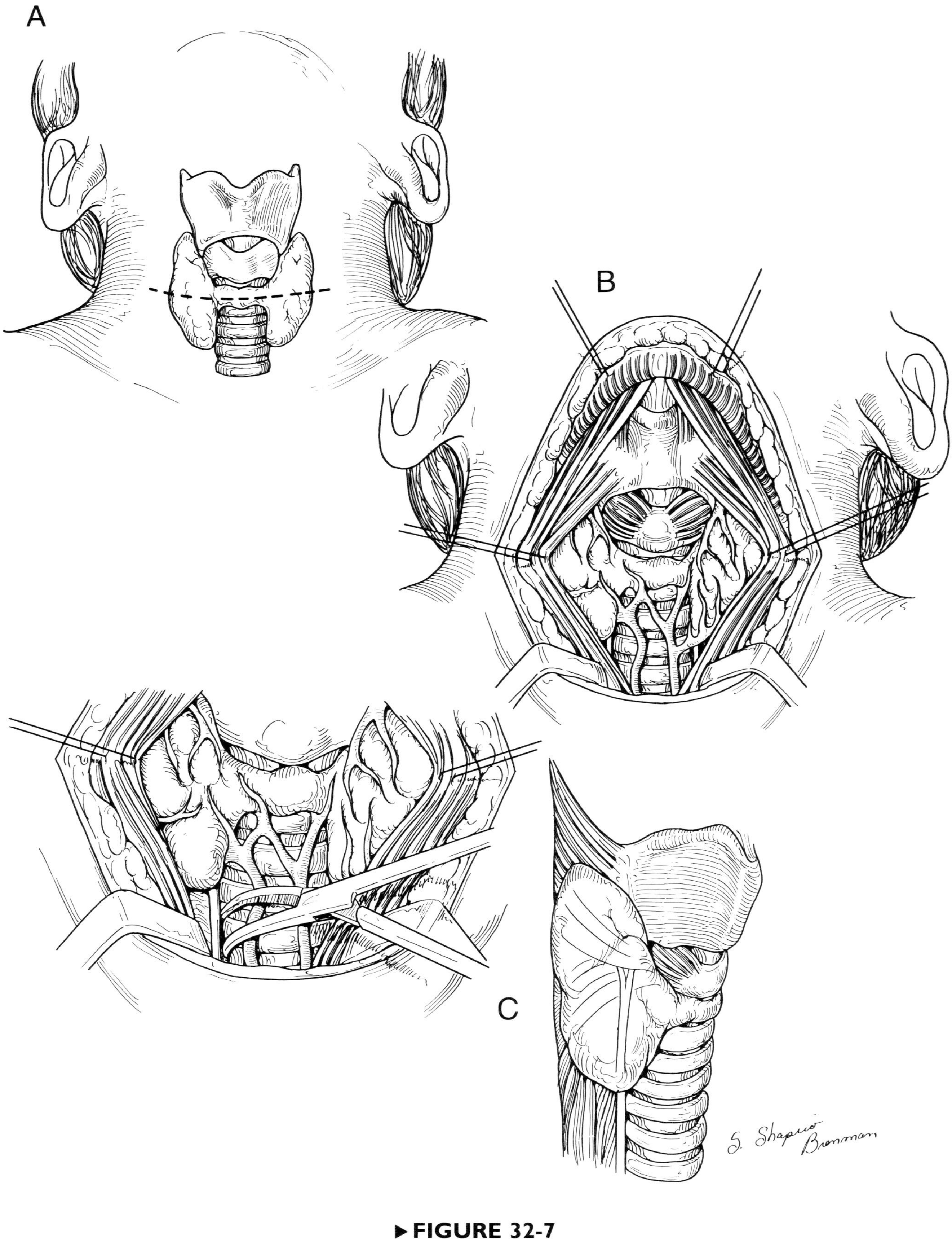


▶ **FIGURE 32-7**

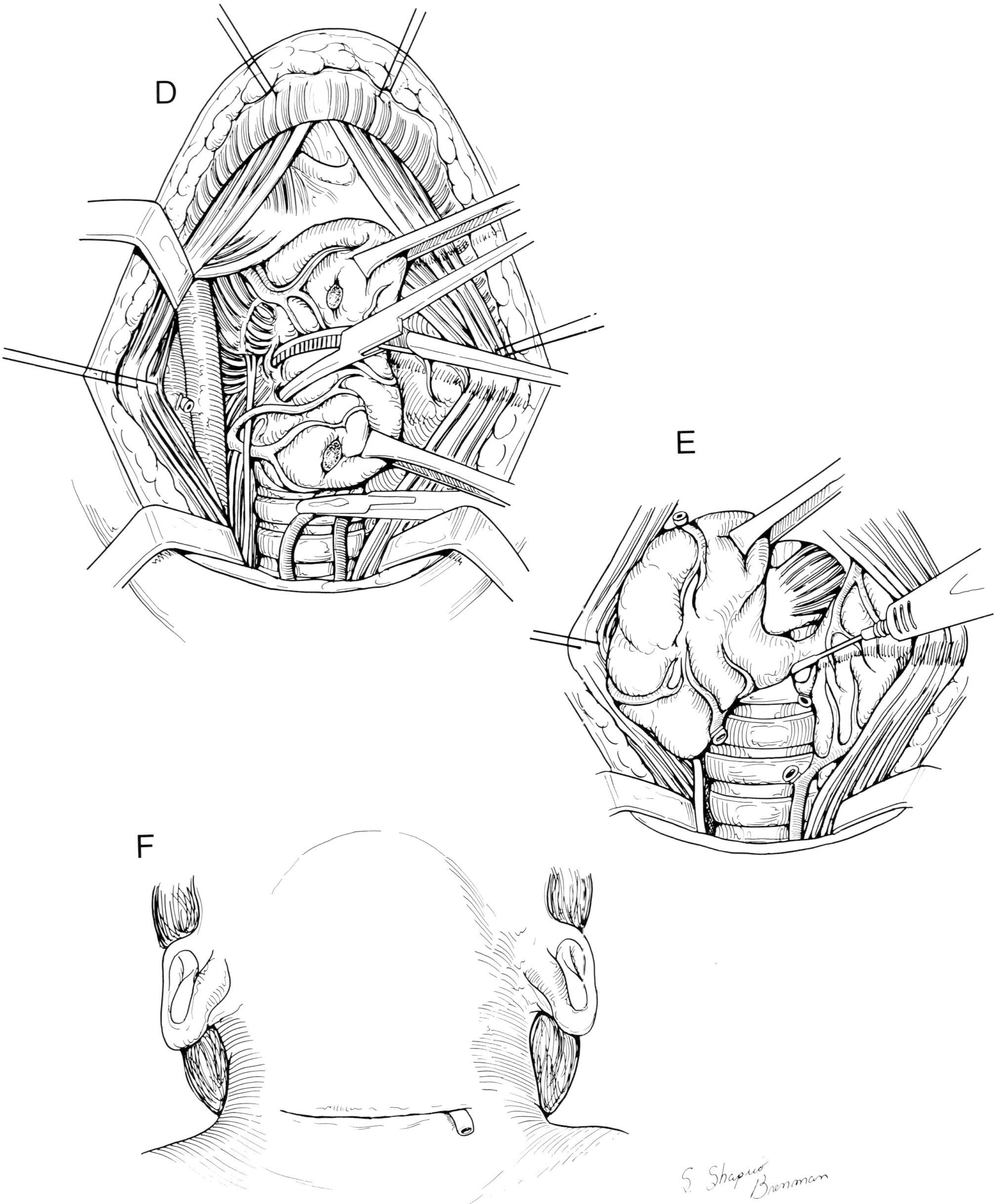


▶ **FIGURE 32-7**

# PART VI

# The Salivary Gland

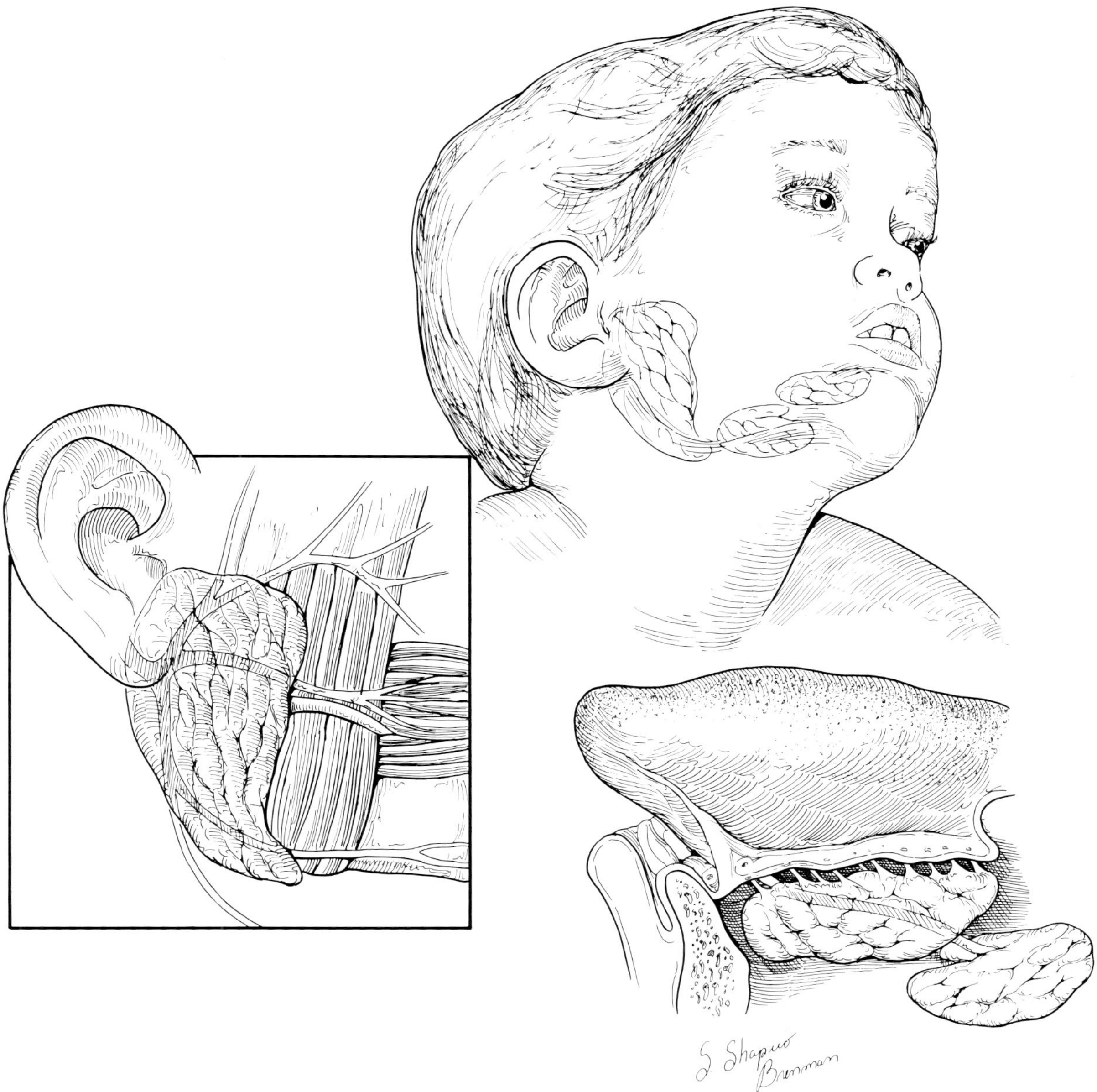

# 33 ▸ Salivary Duct Surgery

## ▸ 33 - 1 PAROTID DUCT LIGATION

Parotid duct ligation reduces salivary production and causes atrophy of the gland.

### Indications

Parotid duct ligation is performed in neuromuscularly impaired children to help control drooling. The indications for the operation are based on the history and observance of drooling that is a problem both for the child and for his caregiver. It is usually performed bilaterally and simultaneously with bilateral submandibular gland excision. Submandibular gland excision is described in section 34–1.

### Preoperative Evaluation

Preoperative radiographic studies are not helpful.

### Operative Technique

1. Parotid duct ligation is performed utilizing general nasotracheal anesthesia. This provides good oral exposure.
2. A lacrimal probe is inserted into the parotid duct to stabilize the papilla (Fig. 33–1**A**). One percent lidocaine with 1:100,000 epinephrine is injected into the mucosa surrounding the papilla.
3. An elliptical incision is made around the papilla (Fig. 33–1**B**).
4. The papilla is grasped with a clamp and traction is placed on the duct while dissecting the duct free from surrounding tissue with a scissors (Fig. 33–1**C**).
5. The duct is ligated twice with 3-0 silk suture and the papillary mucosa is excised by transecting the distal portion of the duct (Fig. 33–1**D**).
6. The duct is allowed to retract into the soft tissue of the cheek (Fig. 33–1**E**) and the oral mucosa is sutured with 3-0 chromic suture (Fig. 33–1**F**).

### Complications

1. Temporary painful parotid swelling

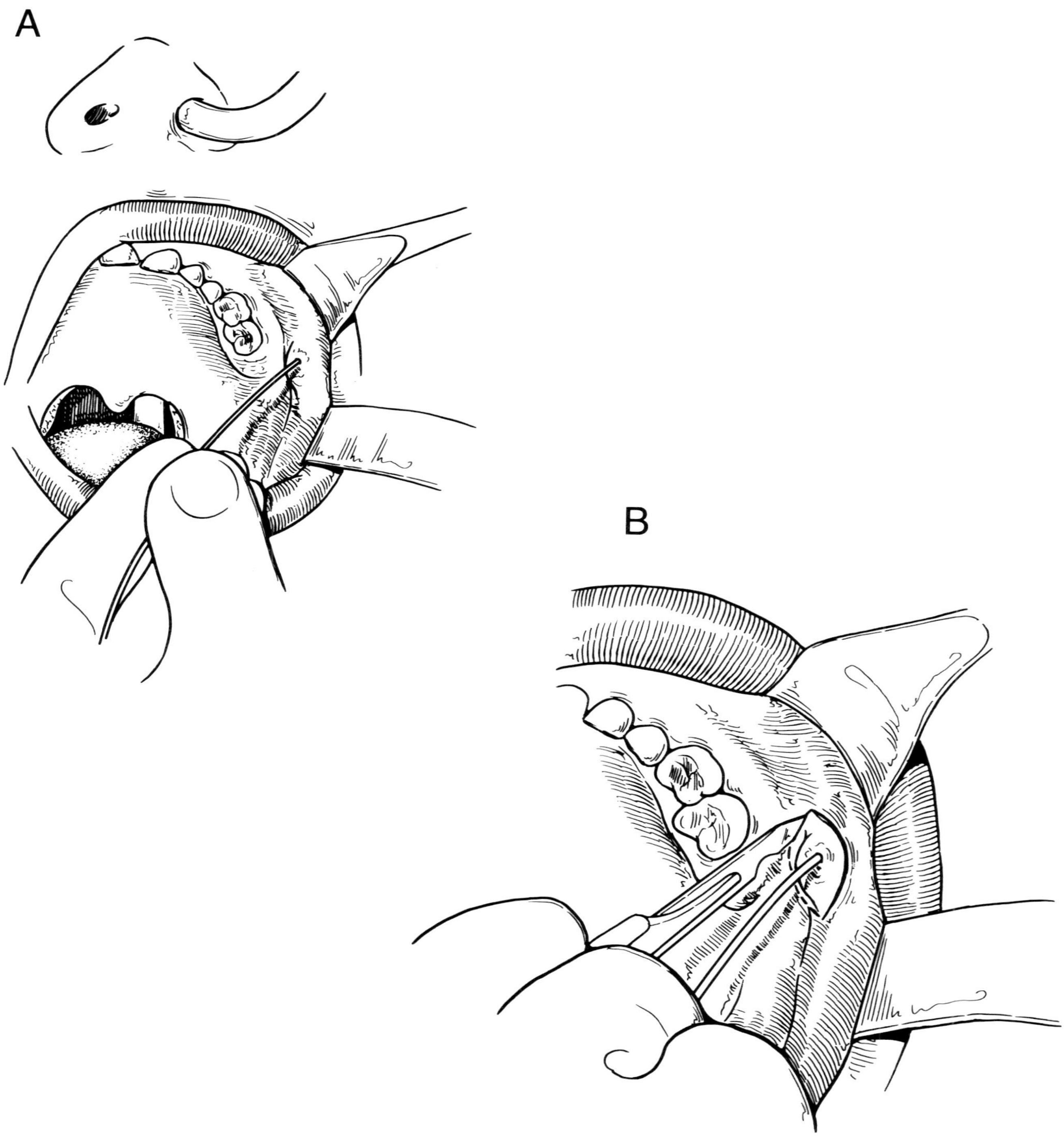


▶ **FIGURE 33-1**

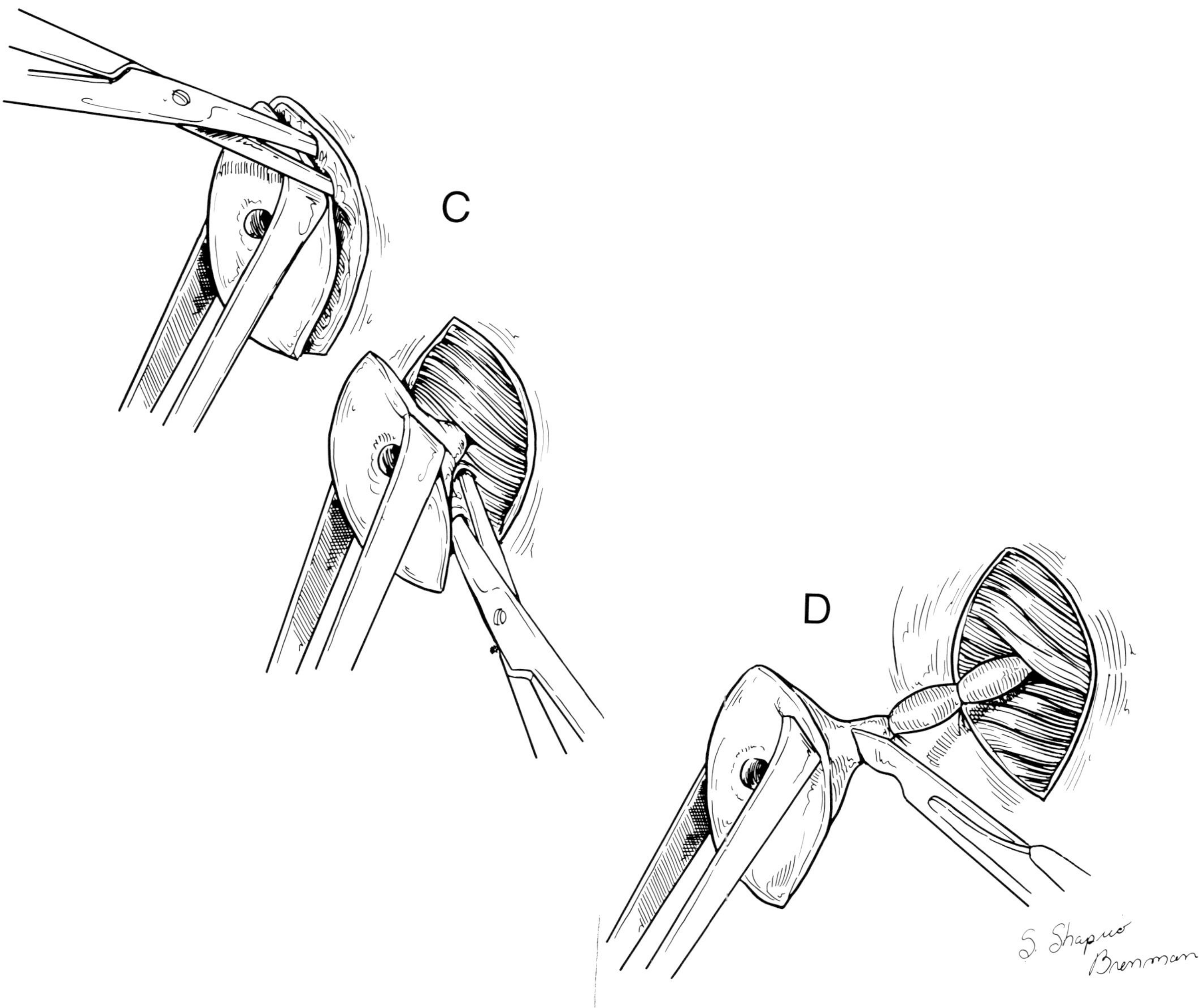


▶ **FIGURE 33-1**

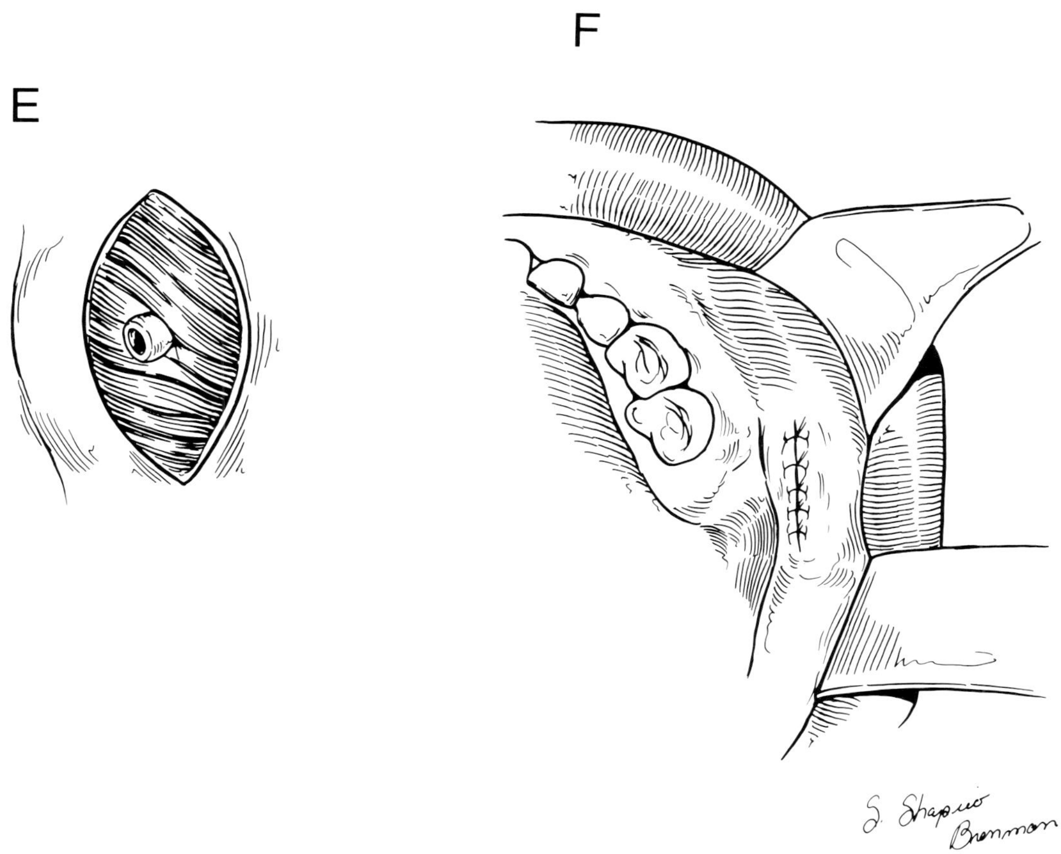


▶ **FIGURE 33-1**

## ▶ 33-2 REMOVAL OF DISTAL SALIVARY DUCT STONES (SUBMANDIBULAR AND PAROTID)

Salivary duct stones usually present with acute painful swelling of the involved gland. Some degree of bacterial infection from chronic stasis is often present.

### Indications

Removal of salivary duct stones is indicated in cases of chronic or intermittent salivary gland swelling secondary to a ductal stone.

### Preoperative Evaluation

Inspection of the duct in the oral cavity may reveal a turbid discharge. The stone usually can be palpated by passing the index finger along the course of the duct intraorally.

Standard radiographic films are rarely helpful because salivary duct stones are usually not calcified. Sialography or magnetic resonance imaging (MRI) may be useful to demonstrate the position of the stone.

### Operative Technique

1. Stones near the papilla of the submandibular gland are removed utilizing general anesthesia and nasotracheal intubation to provide optimal intraoral exposure.
2. The duct is dilated with lacrimal probes (Fig. 33–2**A**).
3. The duct is cut by placing one blade of a sharp-pointed scissors in the dilated duct and closing the blades to open the duct in a slit-like manner (Fig. 33–2**B**, **C**).
4. The stone is expressed from the duct or removed with a curette (Fig. 33–2**D**).
5. The ductal incision is not closed. Salivary flow will keep this new larger orifice open.
6. Stones near the orifice of the parotid duct are treated in the same fashion.

### Complications

1. Stricture of the duct

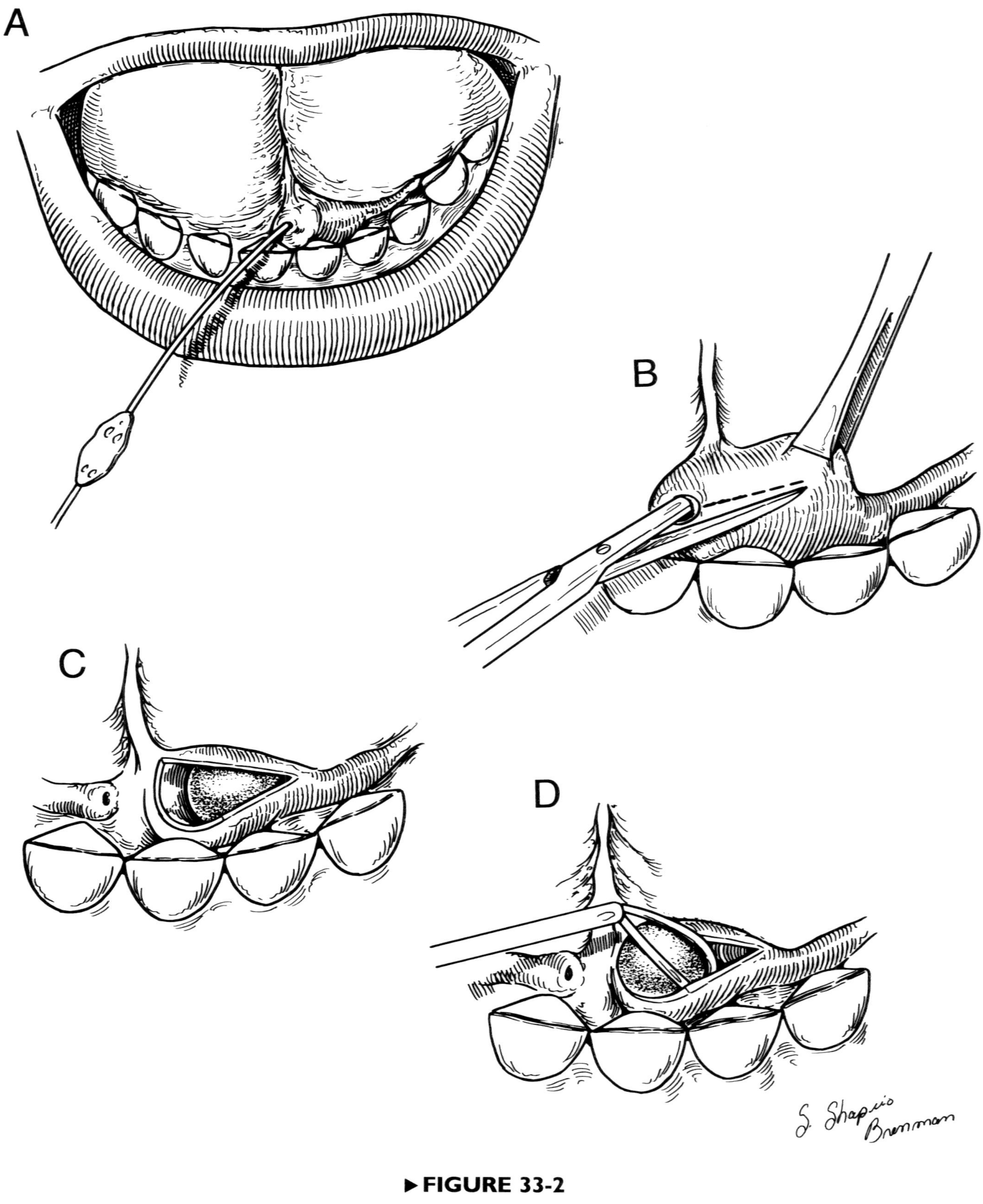


▶ **FIGURE 33-2**

## ▶ 33-3 REMOVAL OF SUBMANDIBULAR DUCT STONES (PROXIMAL)

Salivary duct stones usually present with acute painful swelling of the involved gland. Some degree of bacterial infection from chronic stasis is often present.

### Indications

The presence of a salivary duct stone causing swelling and/or infection of the involved gland is the indication for surgical removal.

### Preoperative Evaluation

Inspection of the duct in the oral cavity may reveal a turbid discharge. The stone usually can be palpated by passing the index finger along the course of the duct intraorally.

Standard radiographic studies are rarely helpful because salivary duct stones are usually not calcified. Sialography or magnetic resonance imaging (MRI) may be useful to demonstrate the position of the stone.

### Operative Technique

1. Submandibular duct stones are removed utilizing general anesthesia and nasotracheal intubation for maximum exposure.
2. With a lacrimal probe in the duct and a finger in the floor of the mouth, the stone is located by palpation (Fig. 33–3**A**).
3. A silk suture is passed around the duct proximal to the stone to prevent the stone from slipping back into the gland (Fig. 33–3**B**).
4. The portion of the duct containing the stone is opened with a knife and the stone is removed (Fig. 33–3**B**,**C**).
5. The mucosal incision is closed loosely with 4-0 interrupted chromic sutures. It is not necessary to suture the duct since the obstruction has been relieved and attempts at closure of the duct can cause stenosis (Fig. 33–3**D**).

Submandibular duct stones that are deep within the proximal portion of the ductal system should be removed by resection of the involved gland (see section 34–1, Submandibular Gland Excision).

### Complications

1. Stricture of the submandibular duct

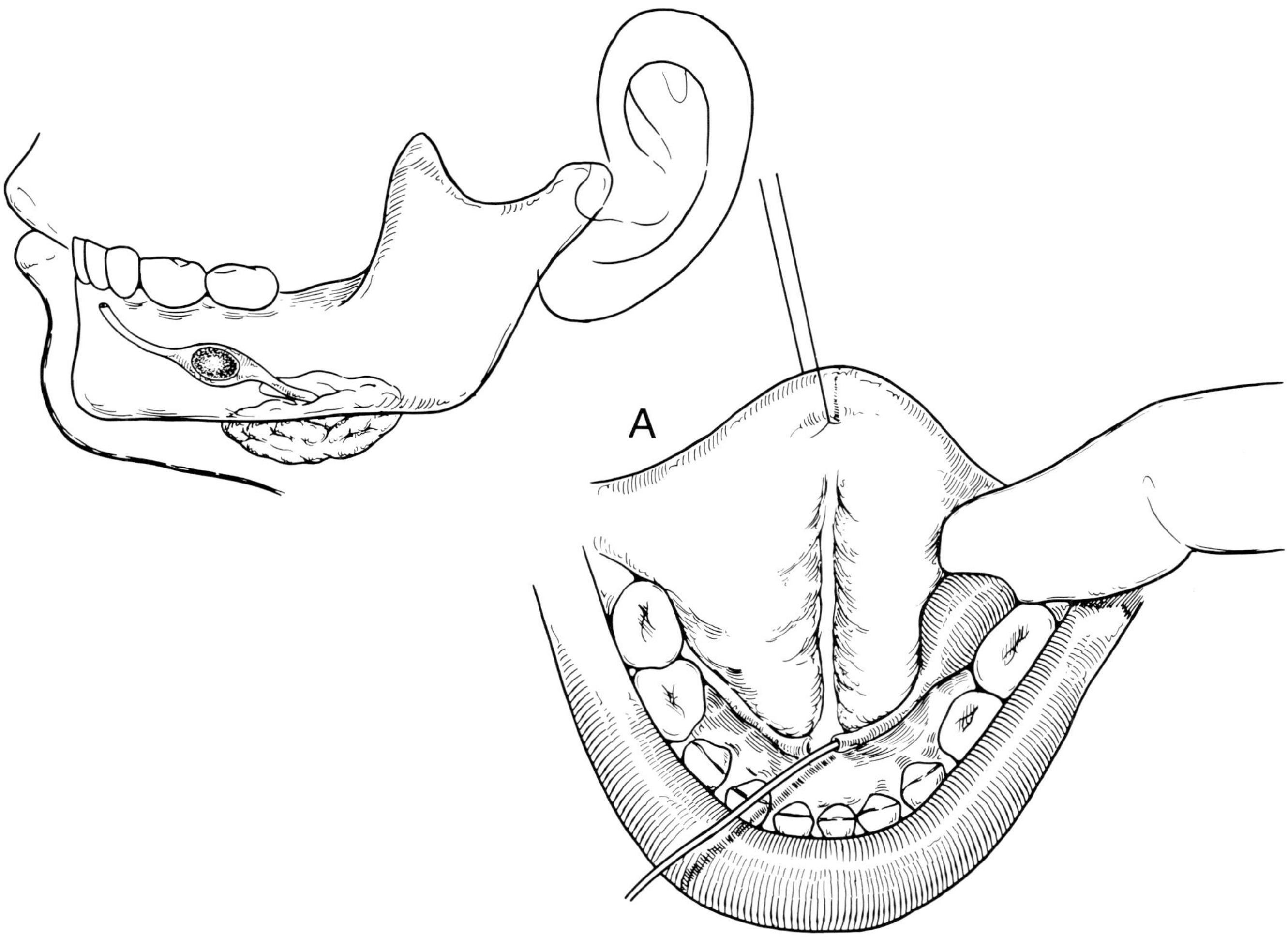


▶ **FIGURE 33-3**

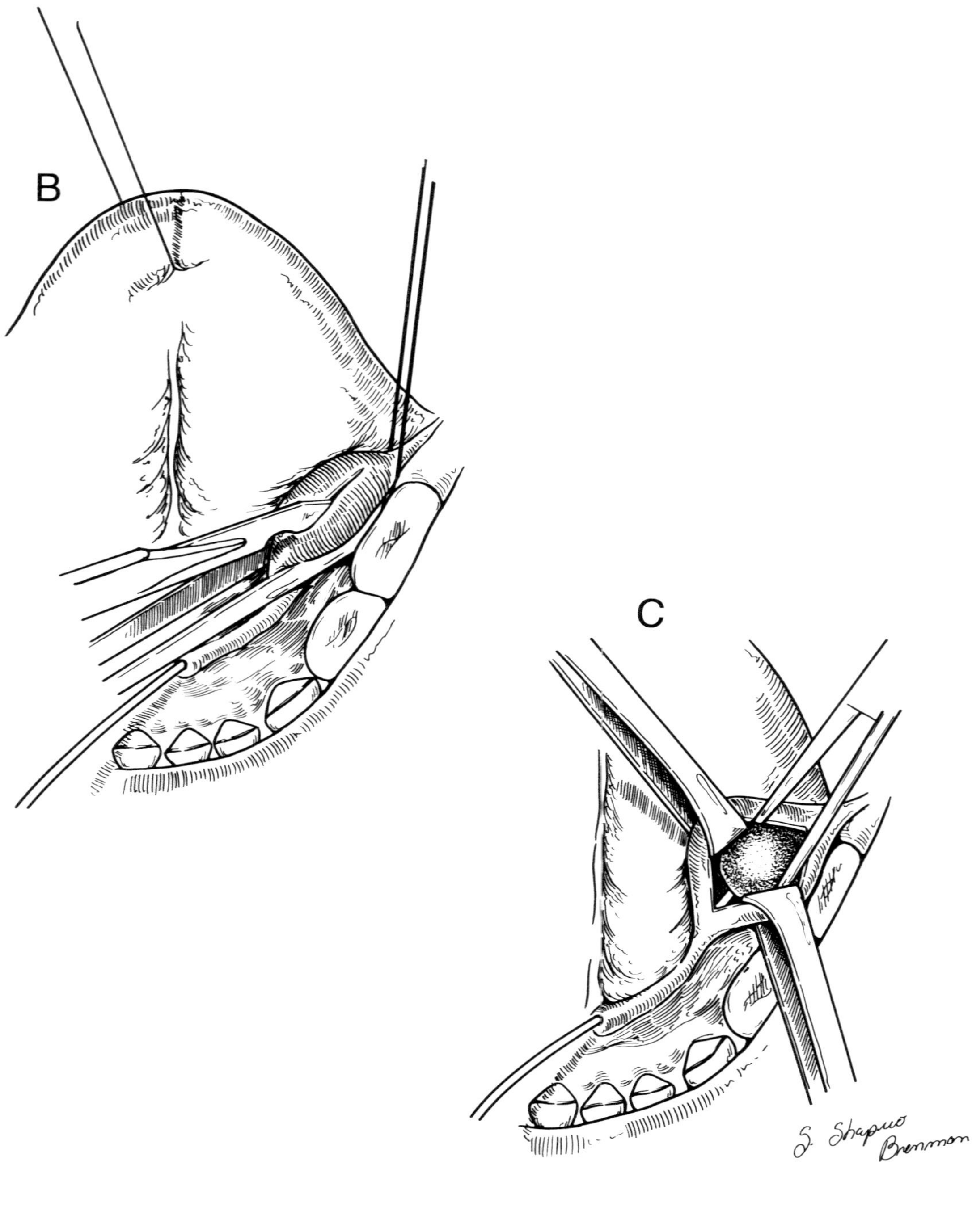


▶ **FIGURE 33-3**

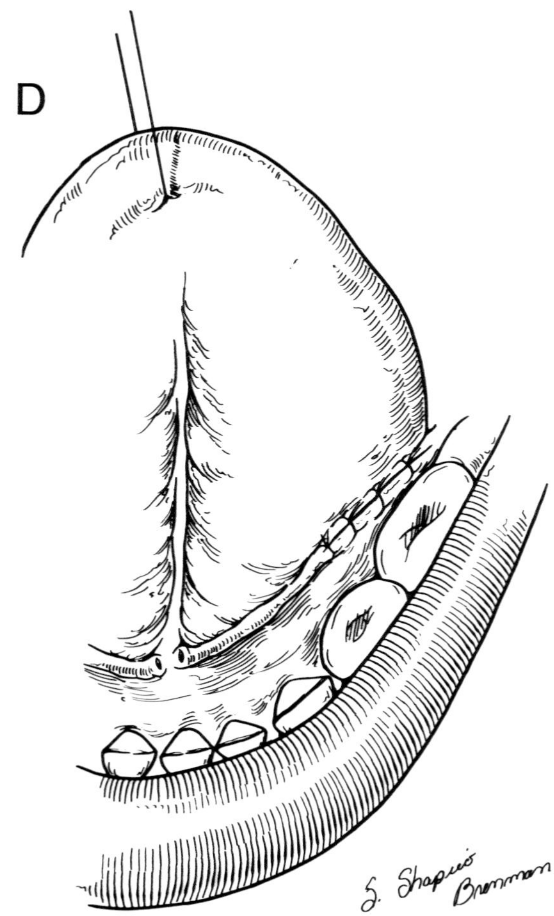


▶ **FIGURE 33-3**

## ▶ 33-4 REMOVAL OF PAROTID DUCT STONES (PROXIMAL)

Salivary duct stones usually present with acute painful swelling of the involved gland. Some degree of bacterial infection from chronic stasis is usually present.

### Indications

The presence of a salivary duct stone causing swelling and/or infection of the involved gland is the indication for surgical removal.

### Preoperative Evaluation

Inspection of the duct in the oral cavity may reveal a turbid discharge. The stone can usually be palpated by passing the index finger along the course of the duct intraorally.

Standard radiographic studies are rarely helpful because salivary duct stones are usually not calcified. Sialography or magnetic resonance imaging (MRI) may be useful to demonstrate the position of the stone.

### Operative Technique

1. Parotid stones are removed utilizing general anesthesia and nasotracheal intubation for maximum exposure.
2. The parotid duct is cannulated with a polyethylene tube or lacrimal probe until the stone is palpated (Fig. 33–4A).
3. A suture is placed in the mucosa medial to the papilla to be used for traction (Fig. 33–4B).
4. A vertical incision is made along the lateral border of the papilla (Fig. 33–4B).
5. The course of the duct is followed by sharp and blunt dissection until the stone is reached (Fig. 33–4C).
6. The portion of the duct containing the stone is incised with a knife and the stone is removed (Fig. 33–4D, E).
7. The duct and mucosal incision are closed with 5-0 interrupted chromic suture (Fig. 33–4F). Parotid stones that are deep within the proximal portion of the ductal system should be removed by resection of the involved gland (see section 34–2, Parotidectomy).

### Complications

1. Stricture of the parotid duct

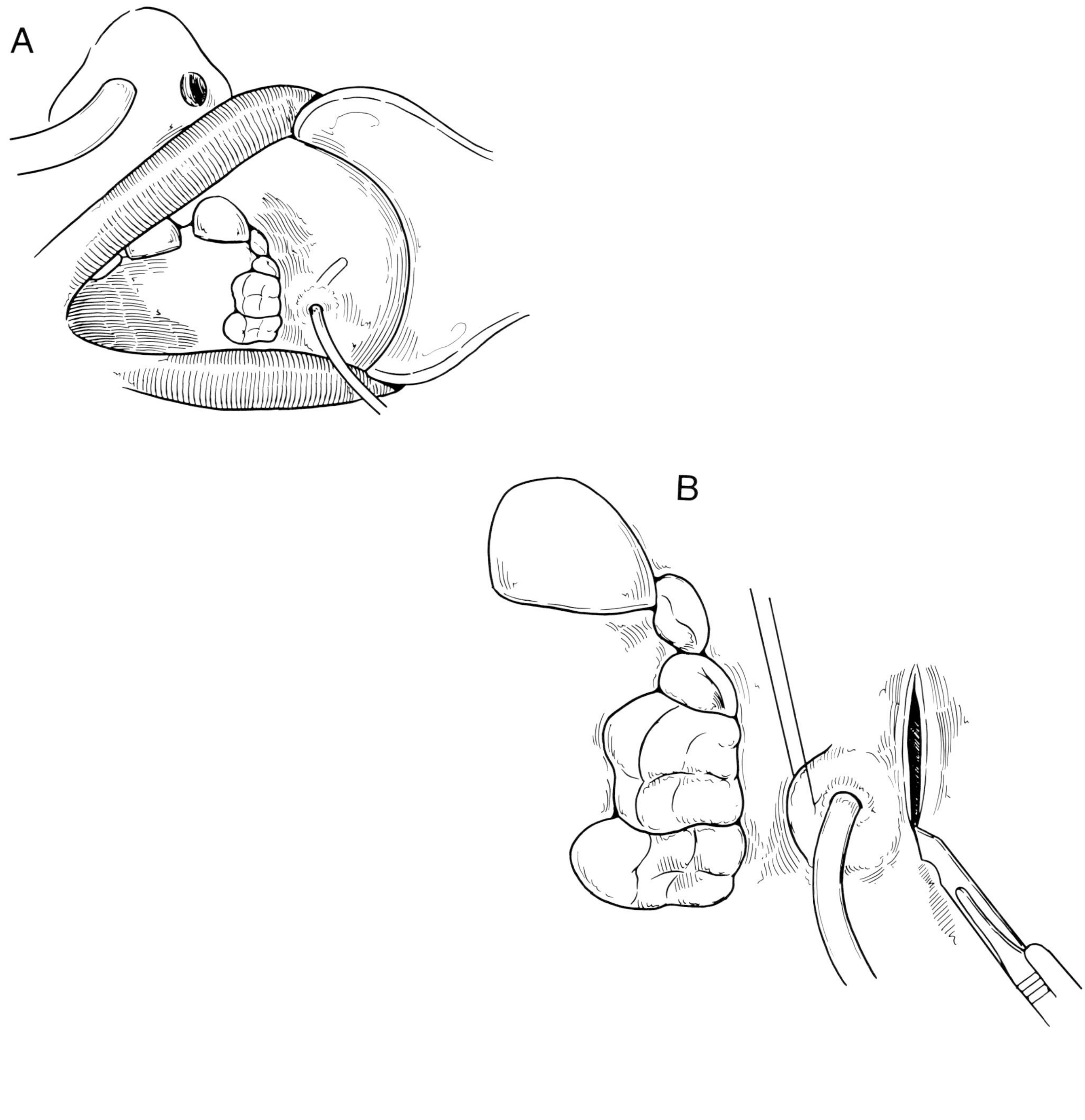


▶ **FIGURE 33-4**

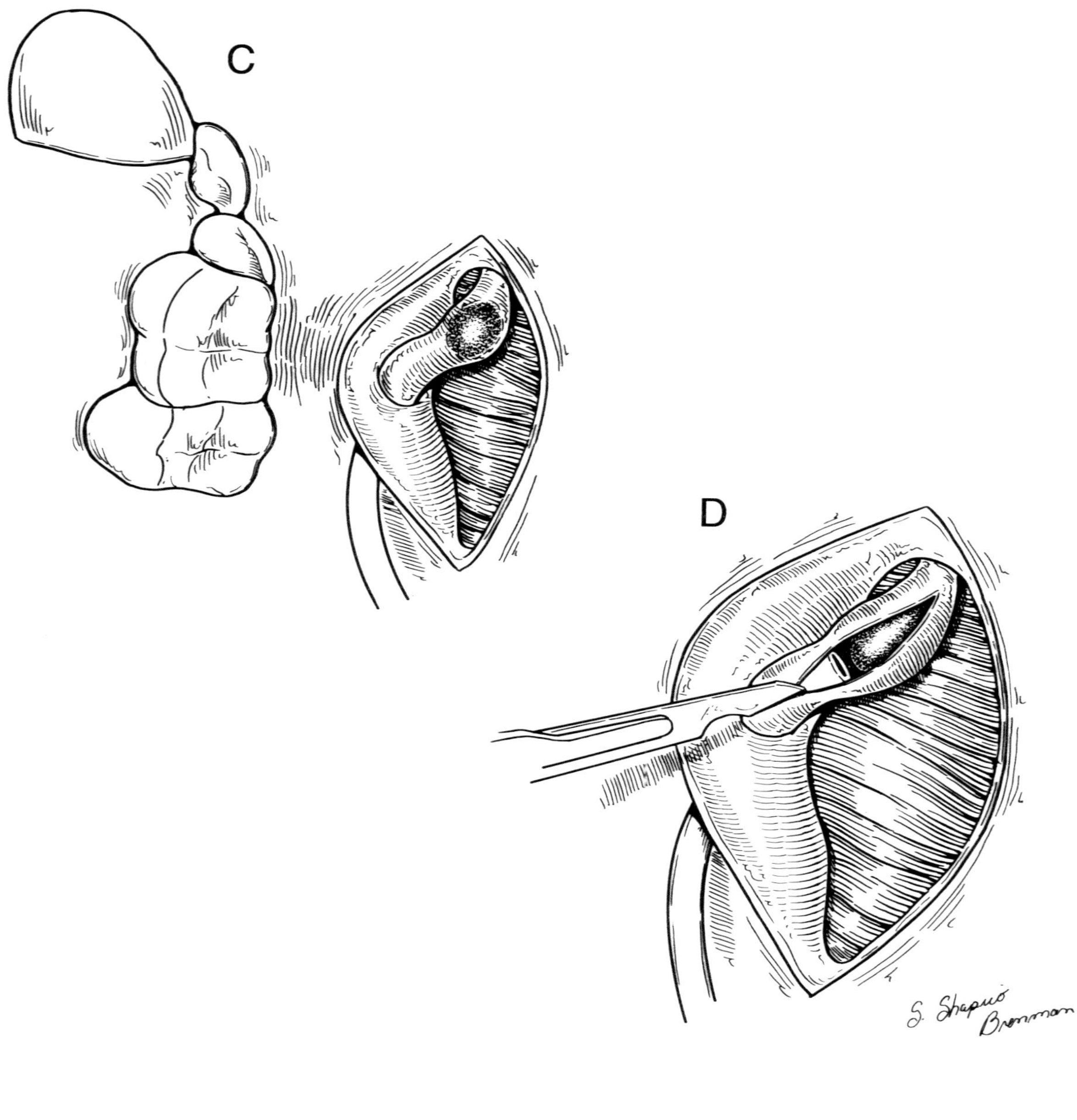


▶ **FIGURE 33-4**

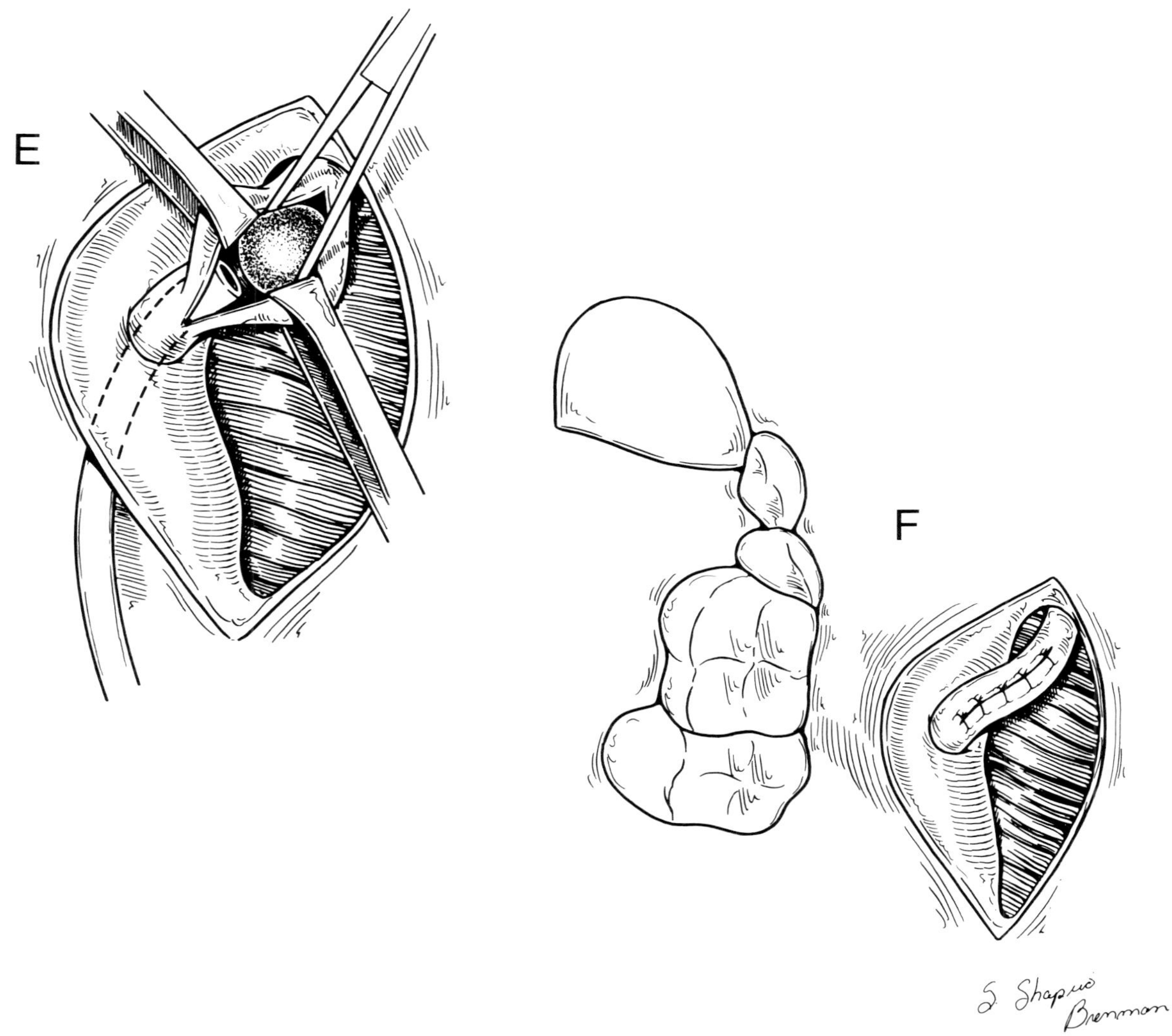


▶ **FIGURE 33-4**

## ▶ 33-5 PAROTID DUCT REPAIR

The parotid duct is vulnerable to injury whenever there is soft tissue trauma to the face (Fig. 33–5A).

### Indications

Repair of the parotid duct is indicated when there is salivary flow out of a cheek wound. Deep wounds involving the masseter muscle should be explored for injury to the parotid duct.

### Preoperative Evaluation

Facial nerve integrity should be assessed preoperatively. A sialogram may be helpful to demonstrate the cut duct and salivary leak.

### Operative Technique

1. Wound exploration and ductal reanastomosis is best accomplished utilizing general anesthesia administered through a nasotracheal tube.
2. A polyethylene tube is passed into the distal duct through the papilla. The catheter exits the cut distal portion of the duct in the wound (Fig. 33–5B).
3. The proximal portion is then found and both ends are cut cleanly on an angle to increase the circumference of the anastomosis (Fig. 33–5C).
4. The proximal cut end is held with a 6-0 nylon suture and the polyethylene tube is passed into that portion of the duct (Fig. 33–5D).
5. The ends of the duct are then sutured with 6-0 or 7-0 interrupted Vicryl suture over the tube (Fig. 33–5E).
6. The polyethylene tube is secured by passing a 4-0 nylon or silk suture through the tube and suturing it to the adjacent oral mucosa. The end of the tube is cut to allow 5 mm to extend intraorally (Fig. 33–5F).
7. The facial wound is then closed using conventional plastic surgical techniques. Postoperative antibiotics and wound drainage are utilized.
8. The polyethylene tube is removed after 3 weeks.

### Complications

1. Sialocutaneous fistula
2. Stricture of parotid duct

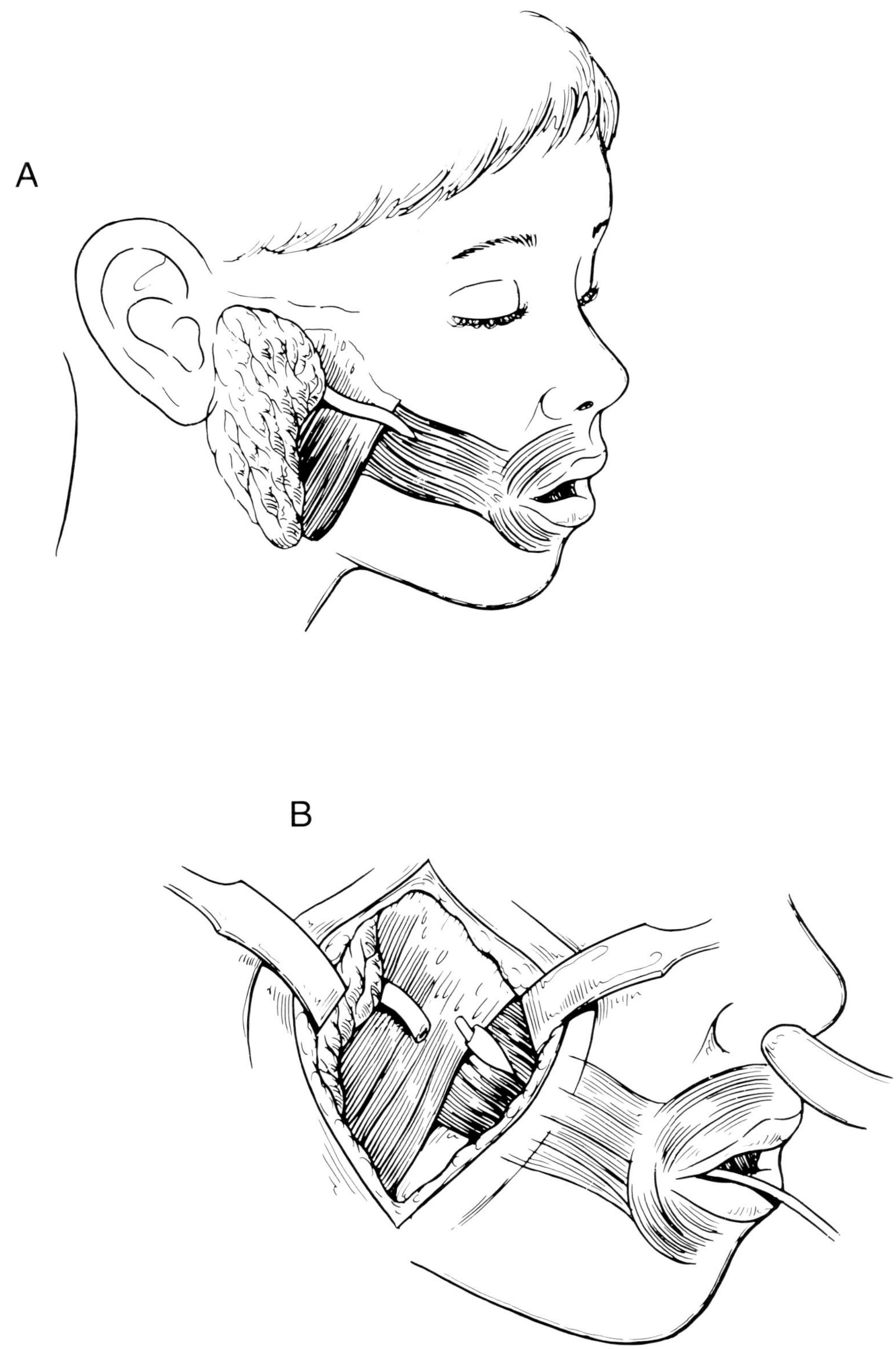


▶ **FIGURE 33-5**

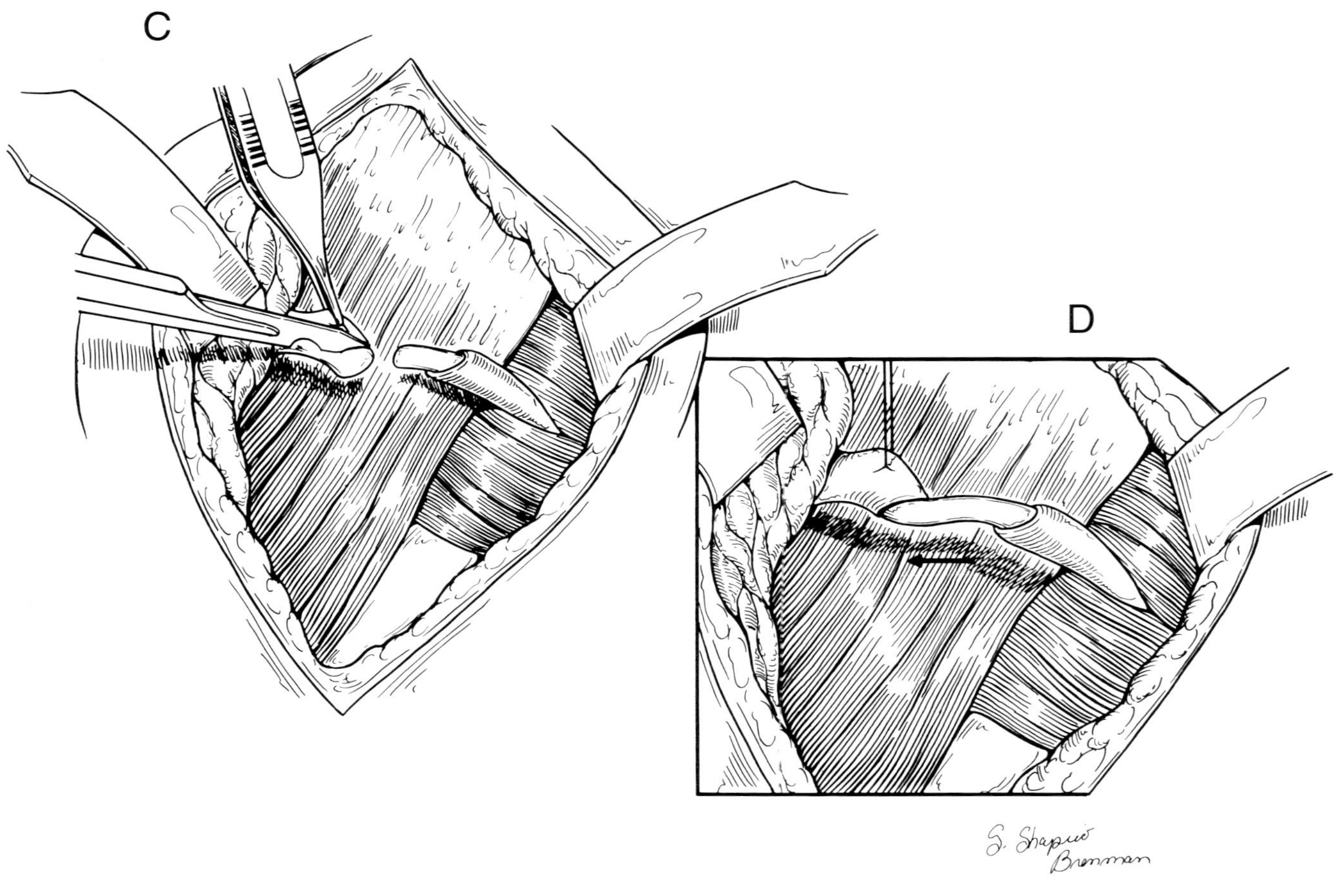


▶ **FIGURE 33-5**

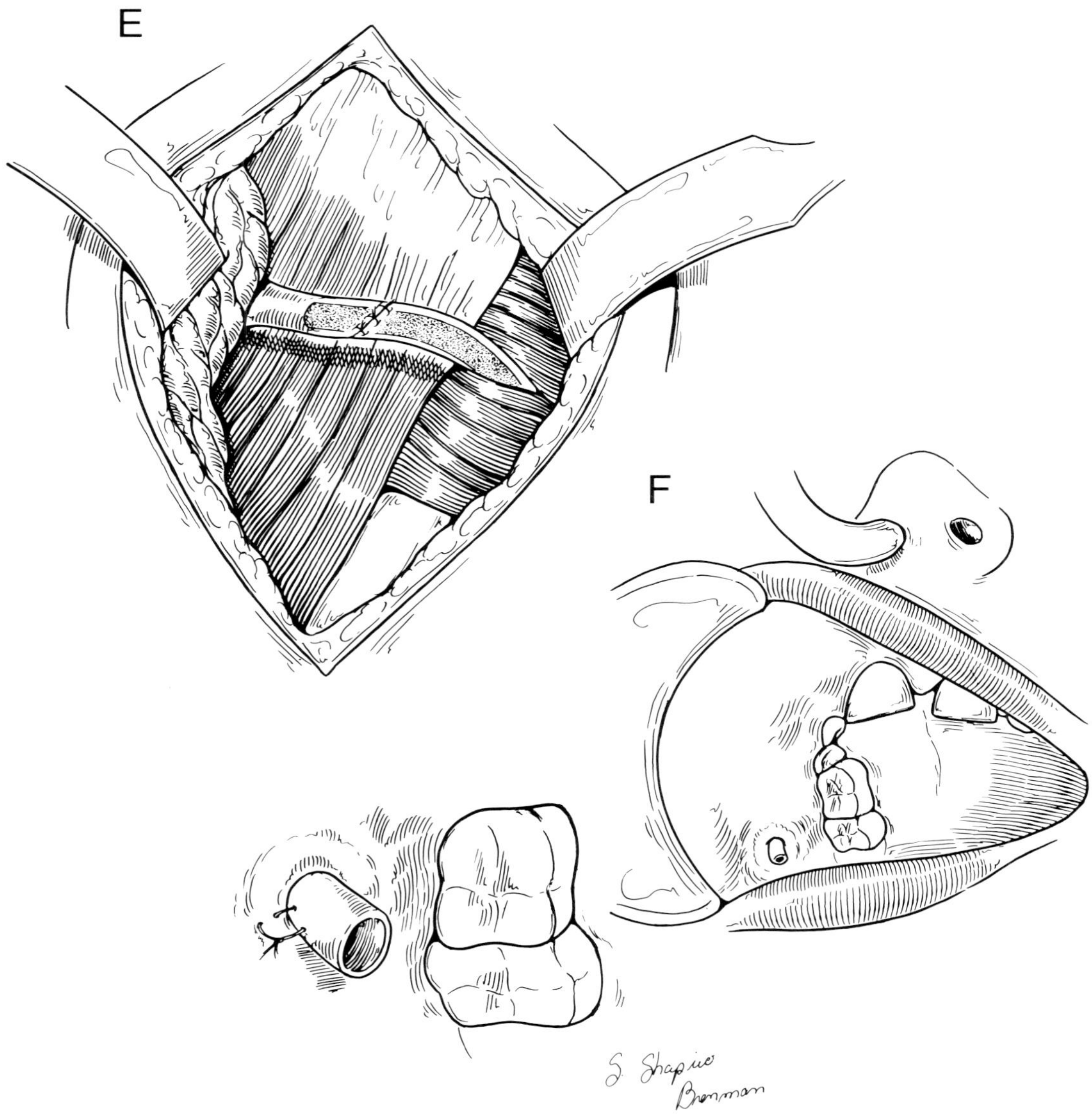


▶ **FIGURE 33-5**

# ▶ 33-6 SUBMANDIBULAR DUCT REPOSITION

Submandibular duct repositioning is one of the techniques used to decrease drooling. By repositioning the ducts into the posterior oral cavity, saliva is directed to the posterior oropharynx.

## Indications

Parotid duct ligation is performed in neuromuscularly impaired children to help control drooling. The indications for the operation are based on the history and observance of drooling that is a problem both for the child and for his caregiver. It is usually performed bilaterally and simultaneously with bilateral parotid duct ligation. Alternately, the submandibular glands may be removed completely (see section 34–1).

## Operative Technique

1. Submandibular duct reposition is performed under general anesthesia administered through a nasotracheal tube.
2. The papillae of the submandibular ducts are released and separated by incising around the ducts with a knife (Fig. 33–6**A**).
3. With traction on the duct by using an atraumatic clamp or sutures, the duct is dissected from surrounding tissue attachments with a scissors (Fig. 33–6**B**).
4. A tunnel is made with a clamp to the posterior floor of the mouth. The mucosa of the mouth is cut with a knife down to the clamp (Fig. 33–6**C**).
5. The duct is delivered through the tunnel and the papilla is sewn in place with 3-0 chromic suture (Fig. 33–6**D**).
6. The surgical defect in the anterior floor of the mouth is closed with 3-0 chromic suture.

## Complications

1. Submandibular duct stricture
2. Continued drooling

**▶ FIGURE 33-6**

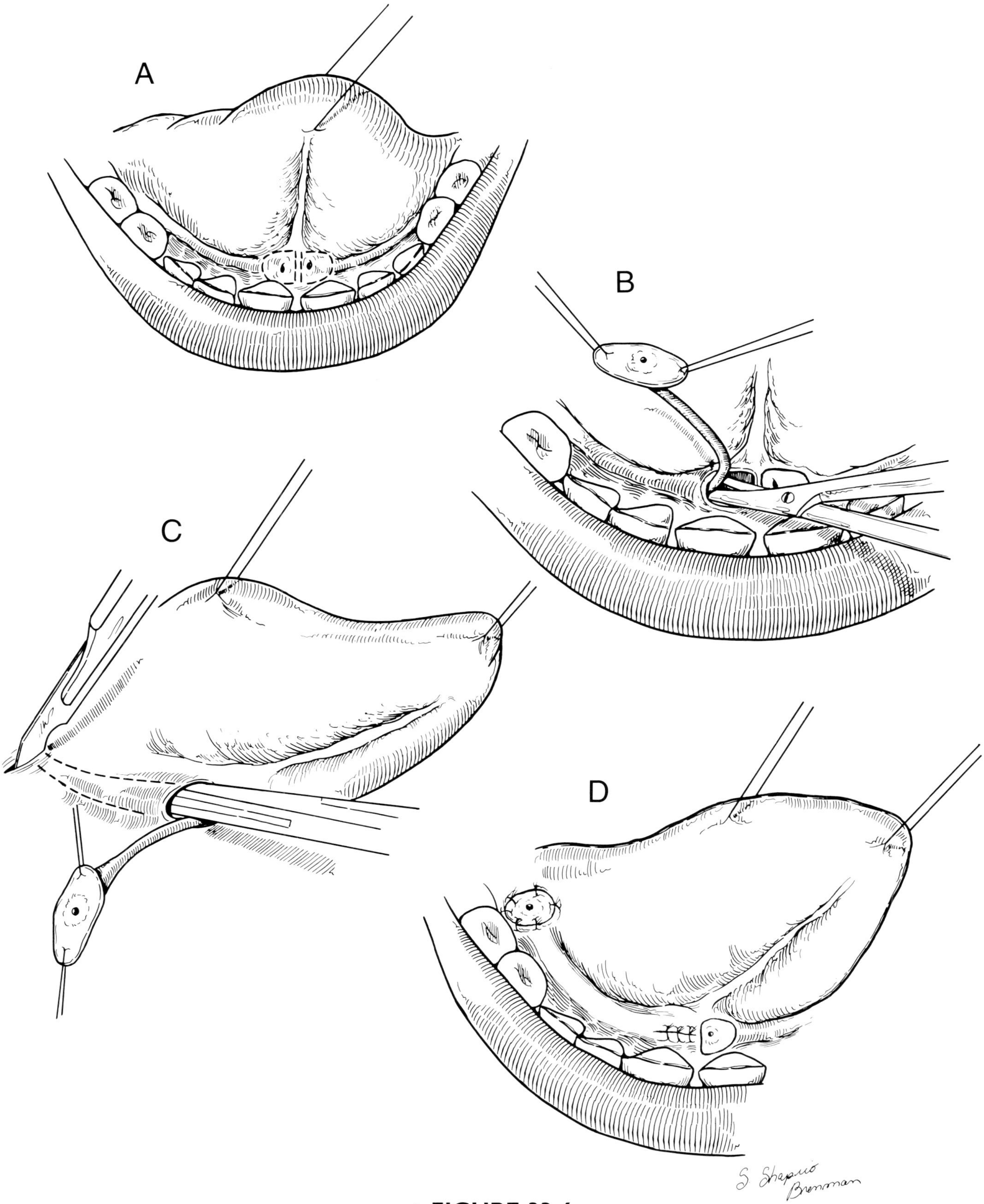


▶ **FIGURE 33-6**

## ▶ 33-7 REPAIR OF PAPILLARY SALIVARY DUCT STRICTURE (PAROTID AND SUBMANDIBULAR)

Papillary salivary duct strictures occur as a result of chronic inflammation or intraoral trauma. These usually respond well to surgical correction.

Strictures may also occur in the proximal portion of the duct distant from the papilla. These strictures may respond to interval dilatation with a lacrimal probe.

### Indications

A papillary stricture that is causing recurrent swelling, pain or infection of the associated gland is the indication for operative intervention.

### Preoperative Evaluation

Sialography may be helpful to define the location and severity of the stricture. However, the stricture may preclude cannulation of the duct that is necessary for sialography.

### Operative Technique

1. Papillary ductal stricture is corrected utilizing general anesthesia administered through a nasotracheal tube.
2. The papilla is identified and the orifice is dilated with lacrimal dilators (Fig. 33–7**A**).
3. One blade of an iris scissors is inserted into the duct and the scissors are closed to create a slit posteriorly (Fig. 33–7**B**, **C**).
4. The edges of the duct are sutured to the edges of the mucosa with 5-0 Vicryl suture, creating a wider opening into the oral cavity (Fig. 33–7**D**).

### Complications

1. Restricture of the duct

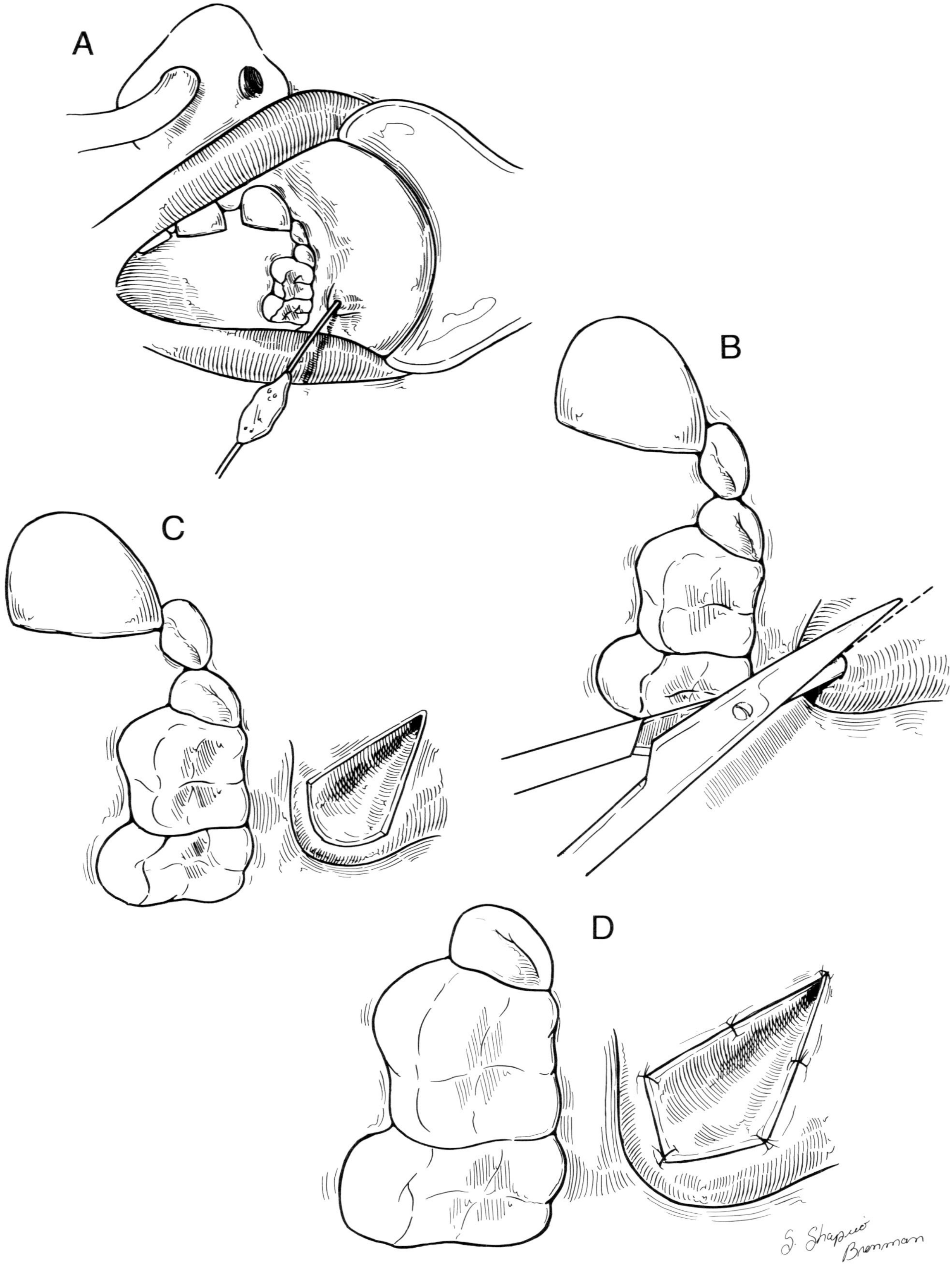


▶ **FIGURE 33-7**

# 34 ▶ Salivary Gland Excision

## ▶ 34-1 SUBMANDIBULAR GLAND EXCISION

### Indications

Submandibular gland excision is indicated in the treatment or chronic salivary gland infections, salivary gland stones, suspicion of neoplasm, and as an adjunct to surgical treatment for drooling.

### Preoperative Evaluation

Palpation of the submandibular gland is usually sufficient to detect a mass. Sialography defines chronic inflammatory disease, stones, or strictures. Computed tomography (CT) or magnetic resonance imaging (MRI) is a more appropriate study to evaluate masses in the submandibular area. The surgeon may elect to utilize intraoperative facial nerve monitoring.

### Operative Technique

1. Submandibular gland excision is performed utilizing general endotracheal anesthesia.
2. The patient is positioned on a shoulder roll. The head is hyperextended and turned to the opposite side. This brings the submandibular gland into position (Fig. 34–1**A**).
3. One percent lidocaine with 1:100,000 epinephrine is injected in a skin crease near the lower border of the gland for hemostasis. This should be approximately 2 to 3 cm below the edge of the mandible to avoid the marginal mandibular branch of the facial nerve (Fig. 34–1**B**).
4. The platysma muscle is divided with a knife and minimal flaps are developed superiorly and inferiorly exposing the cervical fascia overlying the gland (Fig. 34–1**C**).
5. The cervical fascia is incised and the gland exposed (Fig. 34–1**D**). By staying deep to this fascia, injury to the marginal mandibular nerve, which lies between the platysma and the fascia of the gland, is avoided.
6. The facial artery and vein over the posterior aspect of the gland are divided (Fig. 34–1**E**) and elevated superiorly, further protecting the marginal mandibular nerve.
7. The submandibular gland is then mobilized by blunt and sharp dissection out of the digastric sling and off the hyoglossus muscle. The hypoglossal nerve deep to the gland is preserved and vessels are divided releasing the gland (Fig. 34–1**F**).
8. The mylohyoid muscle is then retracted anteriorly as the submandibular gland is retracted posteriorly (Fig. 34–1**G**). This stretches and exposes the duct, which should be double ligated with 3-0 silk and divided.
9. The gland is then retracted posterior-inferiorly and the submandibular ganglion and accompanying vein are transected with a knife, allowing the lin-

gual nerve to retract up under the mandible and releasing the entire gland for removal (Fig. 34–1**H**).

**10.** The wound is closed in layers (platysma, subcutaneous tissue, and subcuticular chromic) and a small Penrose drain is placed in the wound (Fig. 34-1**I**). The drain is removed in 12 to 24 hours.

## Complications

1. Marginal mandibular nerve weakness
2. Hypoglossal nerve weakness

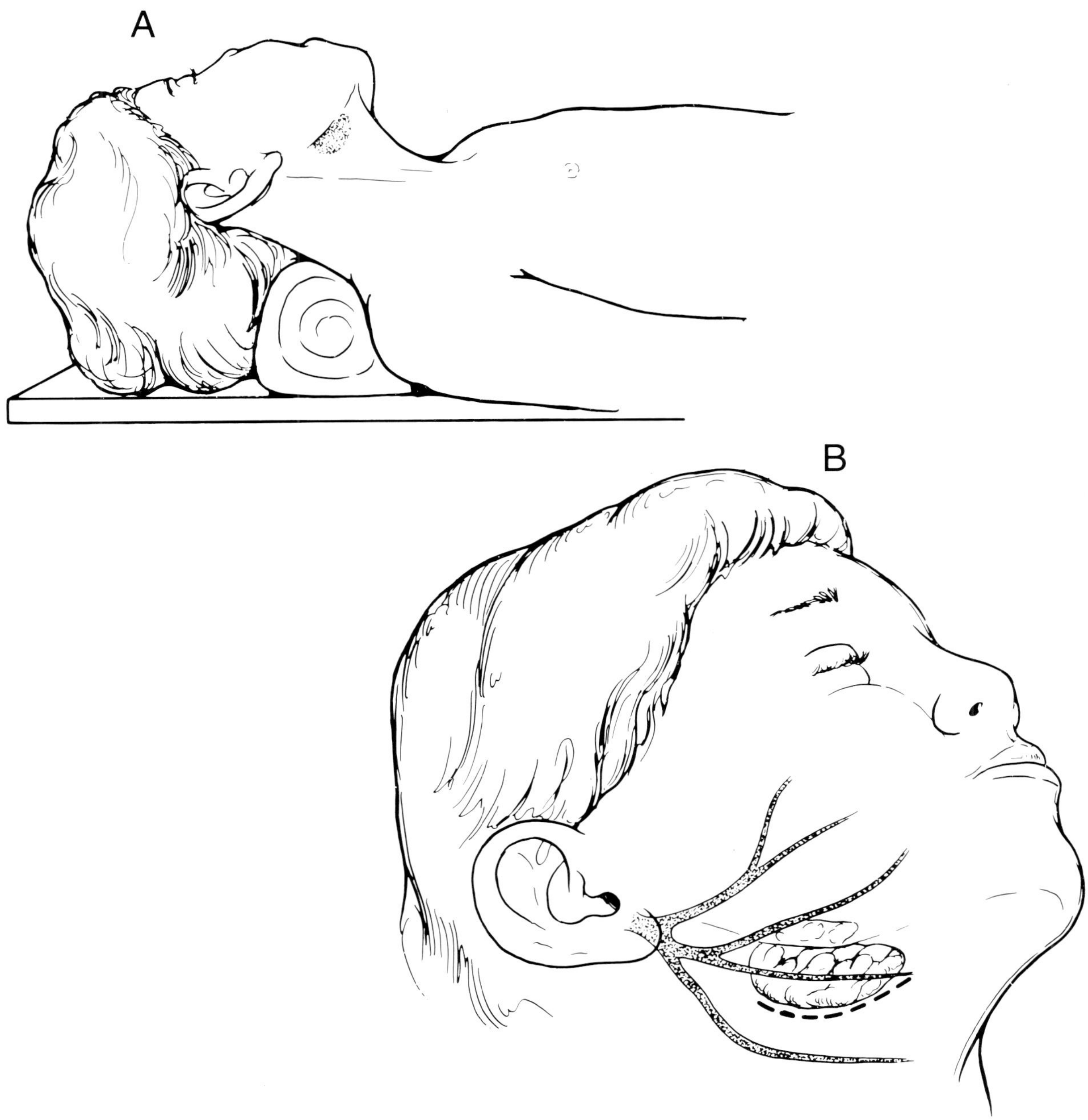


▶ **FIGURE 34-1**

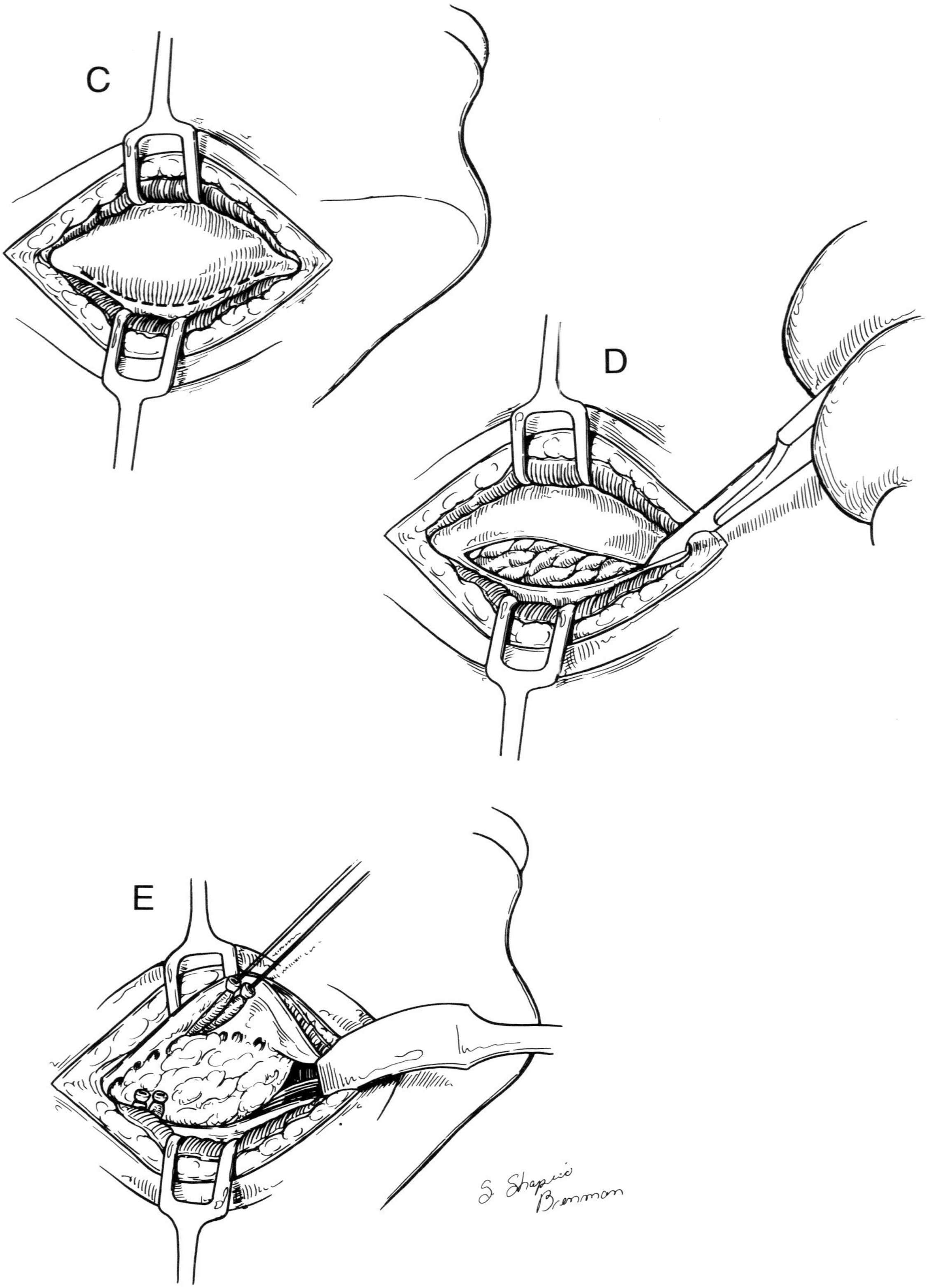


▶ **FIGURE 34-1**

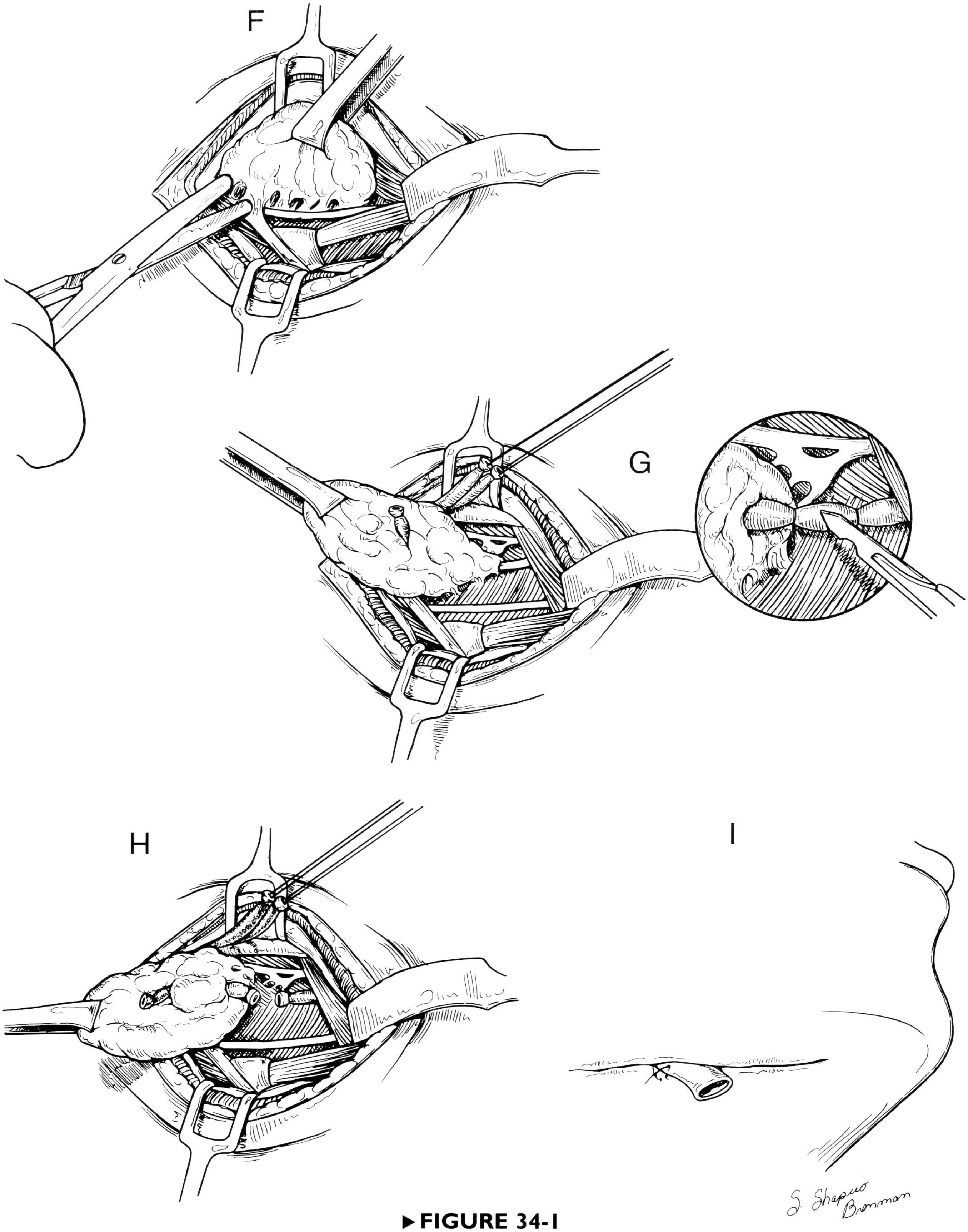


▶ **FIGURE 34-1**

## ▶ 34-2 PAROTIDECTOMY

Parotidectomy is most commonly performed in children to excise a mass (suspected neoplasm) in the parotid gland. Rarely, parotidectomy may be required to treat chronic inflammatory disease or stones.

### Indications

A mass in the parotid gland or chronic and recurrent parotiditis are indications for parotidectomy.

### Preoperative Evaluation

Sialography, computed tomography (CT) or magnetic resonance imaging (MRI) may help define a mass in the parotid gland, but these studies do not have histologic specificity. A suspected neoplasm must be removed for treatment and histologic diagnosis. The surgeon may elect to utilize intraoperative facial nerve monitoring.

### Operative Technique

1. Parotidectomy is performed utilizing general endotracheal anesthesia without using any long-acting paralyzing agents. This permits intraoperative facial nerve monitoring and stimulation.
2. The patient is positioned on a shoulder roll with the neck slightly hyperextended and the head turned to the opposite side (Fig. 34–2**A**).
3. An incision is made starting in the preauricular line in front of the tragus. This is curved around the ear lobe, over the mastoid process, and continued onto the neck sufficiently below the mandible to avoid the mandibular branch of the facial nerve (Fig. 34–2**B**, **C**).
4. The skin flap overlying the parotid gland is elevated with a scissors anteriorly in the plane of subcutaneous fat (Fig. 34–2**D**). The ear lobule is retracted posteriorly with a 2-0 silk suture. This exposes the parotid gland fascia over the tumor (Fig. 34–2**E**).
5. The superficial fascia between the parotid gland and the sternocleidomastoid muscle is cut with a scissors (Fig. 34–2**F**).
6. Dissection along the anterior and inferior surface of the cartilaginous external auditory canal is carried out with a clamp spreading in the direction of the nerve (Fig. 34–2**G**).
7. As the parotid gland is retracted forward, the facial nerve is stretched across the line of dissection and can be found in the groove between the mastoid tip and the bony canal (Fig. 34–2**G**). The facial nerve in the child is more superficial than in an adult and the usually described bony and cartilaginous landmarks for finding the nerve in adults rarely apply in the child (Fig. 34–2**H**).
8. As the parotid gland is reflected forward, the facial nerve can often be detected with a gentle fingertip as it enters the gland from the stylomastoid foramen.
9. Sufficient care and time should be taken to find the trunk of the nerve before any further dissection of the parotid gland is carried out.
10. Once the glistening white facial nerve trunk is found, its presence should be confirmed by testing with a facial nerve stimulator (Fig. 34–2**I**).

**11.** Dissection is then carried out by using a clamp over the nerve. While elevating and opening the clamp to lift the parotid tissue from the facial nerve, the parotid tissue is cut with a knife or scissors. The nerve is kept in view at all times (Fig. 34–2**J**).

**12.** Once the nerve trunk, bifurcation, and branches beyond the mass are dissected free, the parotid tissue between the areas over the nerve is released by either blunt or sharp dissection (Fig. 34–2**K**).

**13.** The mass is then removed with a cuff of normal parotid gland.

**14.** If the parotid duct is exposed, it should be ligated to prevent leak of saliva (Fig. 34–2**L**).

**15.** No attempt is made to remove all remaining parotid tissue such as that in the region of the zygomatic temporal branch or tail of the parotid unless it is involved in the disease process.

**16.** When a mass or diseased tissue is present in the deep lobe of the parotid gland, this tissue is removed by sharp dissection from the masseter muscle as the branches of the facial nerve are gently retracted out of the way (Fig. 34–2**L**).

**17.** The branches or main trunk of the facial nerve are again tested to confirm integrity, and the wound is closed with 3-0 chromic in the subcutaneous tissue and 4-0 interrupted subcuticular chromic in the skin (Fig. 34–2**M**).

**18.** A small, Penrose drain is placed in the wound and brought out inferiorly for drainage (Fig. 34–2**N**). No suction is applied. Suction drains work well to prevent hematoma formation but often create a noticeable depression in the region of the excised gland. The drain is removed in 24 to 36 hours.

## Complications

1. Facial nerve injury
2. Gustatory sweating (Frey's syndrome)
3. Salivary fistula

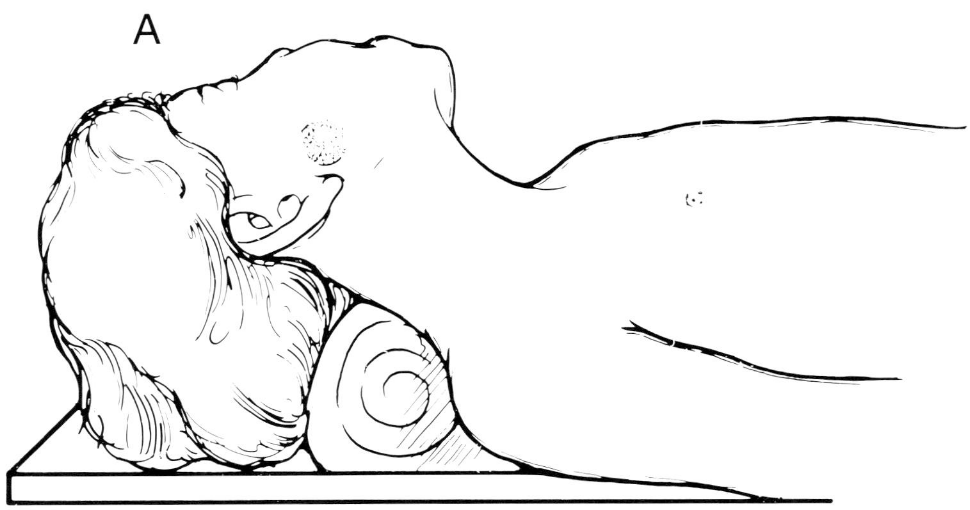


▶ **FIGURE 34-2**

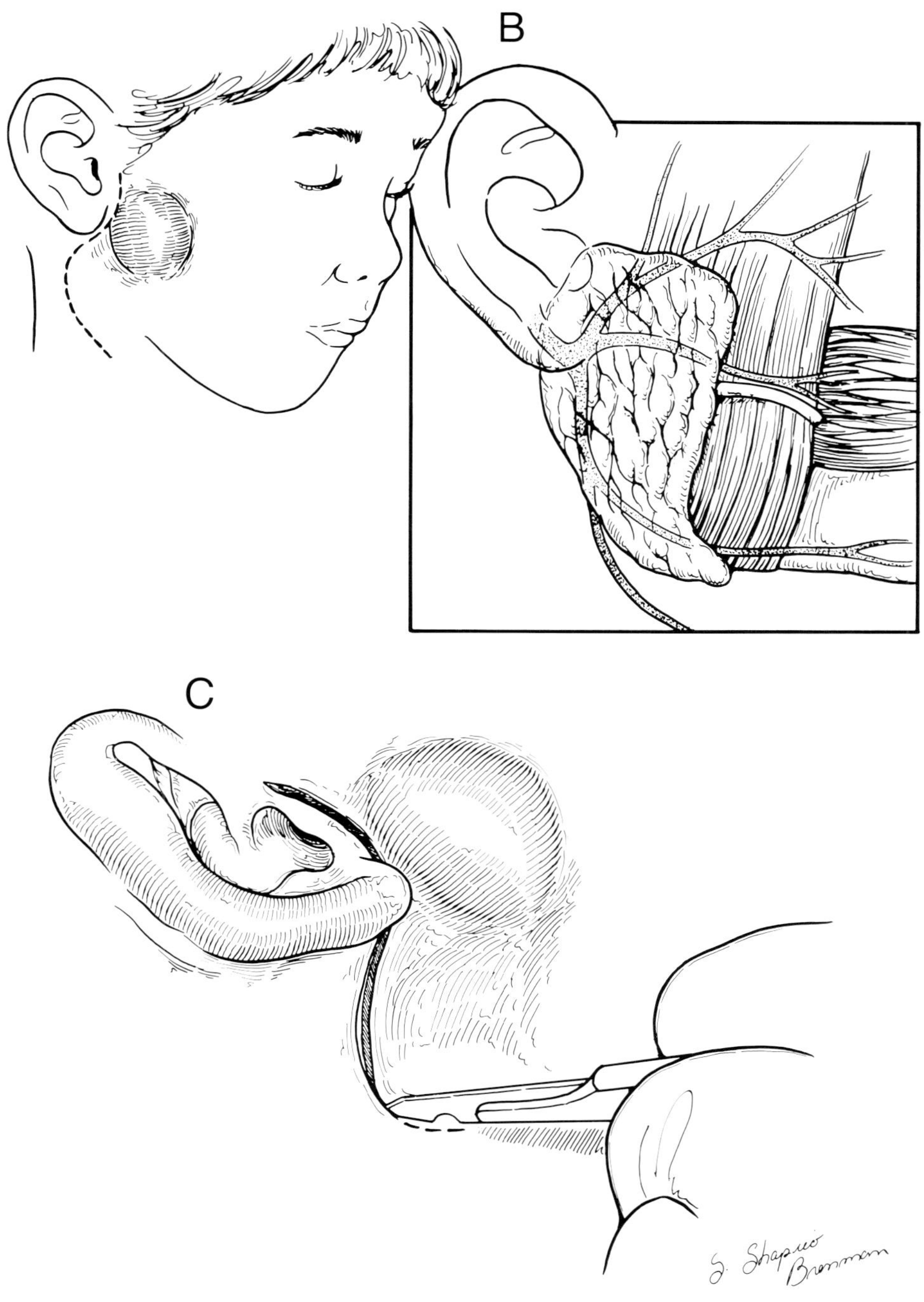


▶ **FIGURE 34-2**

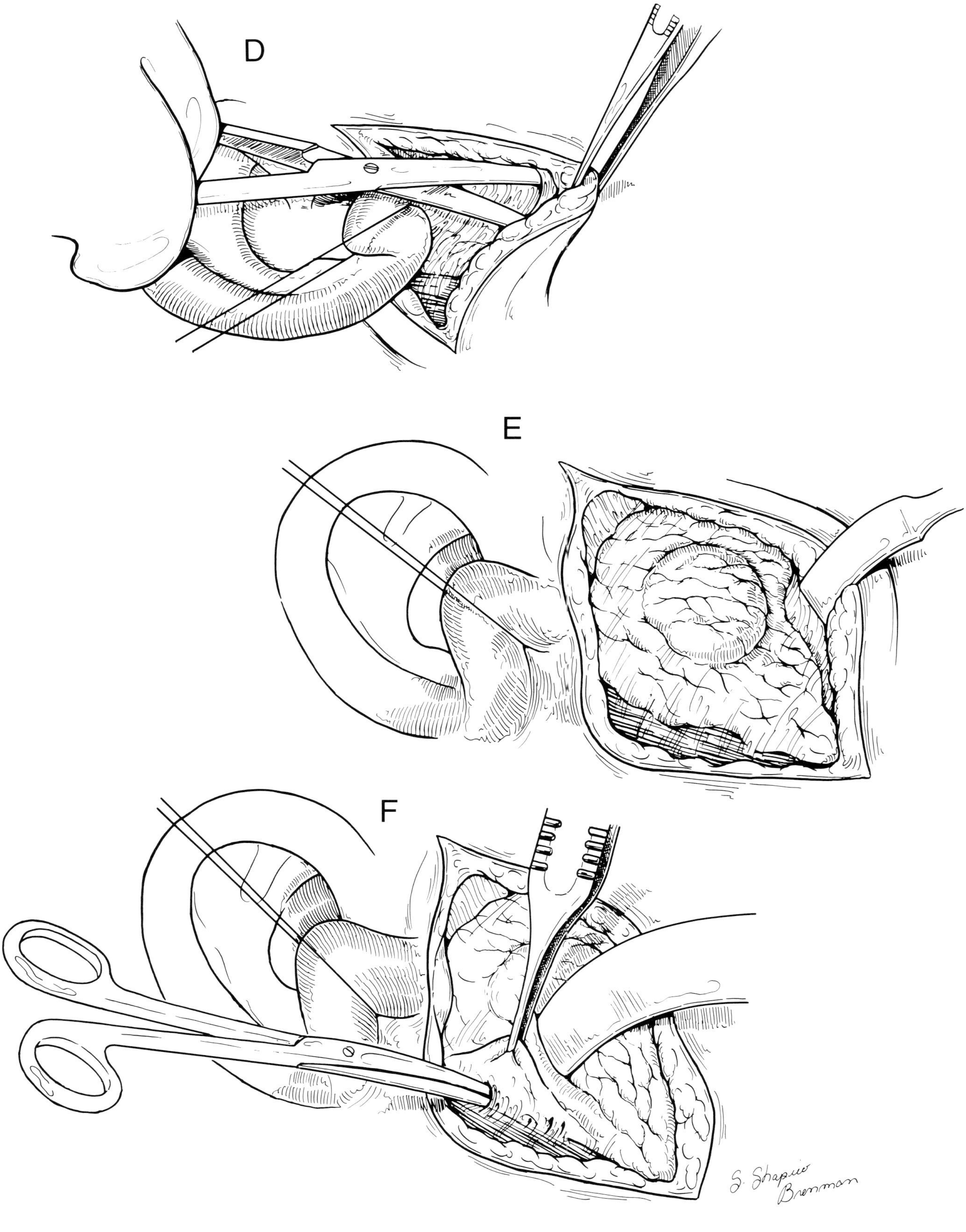


▶ **FIGURE 34-2**

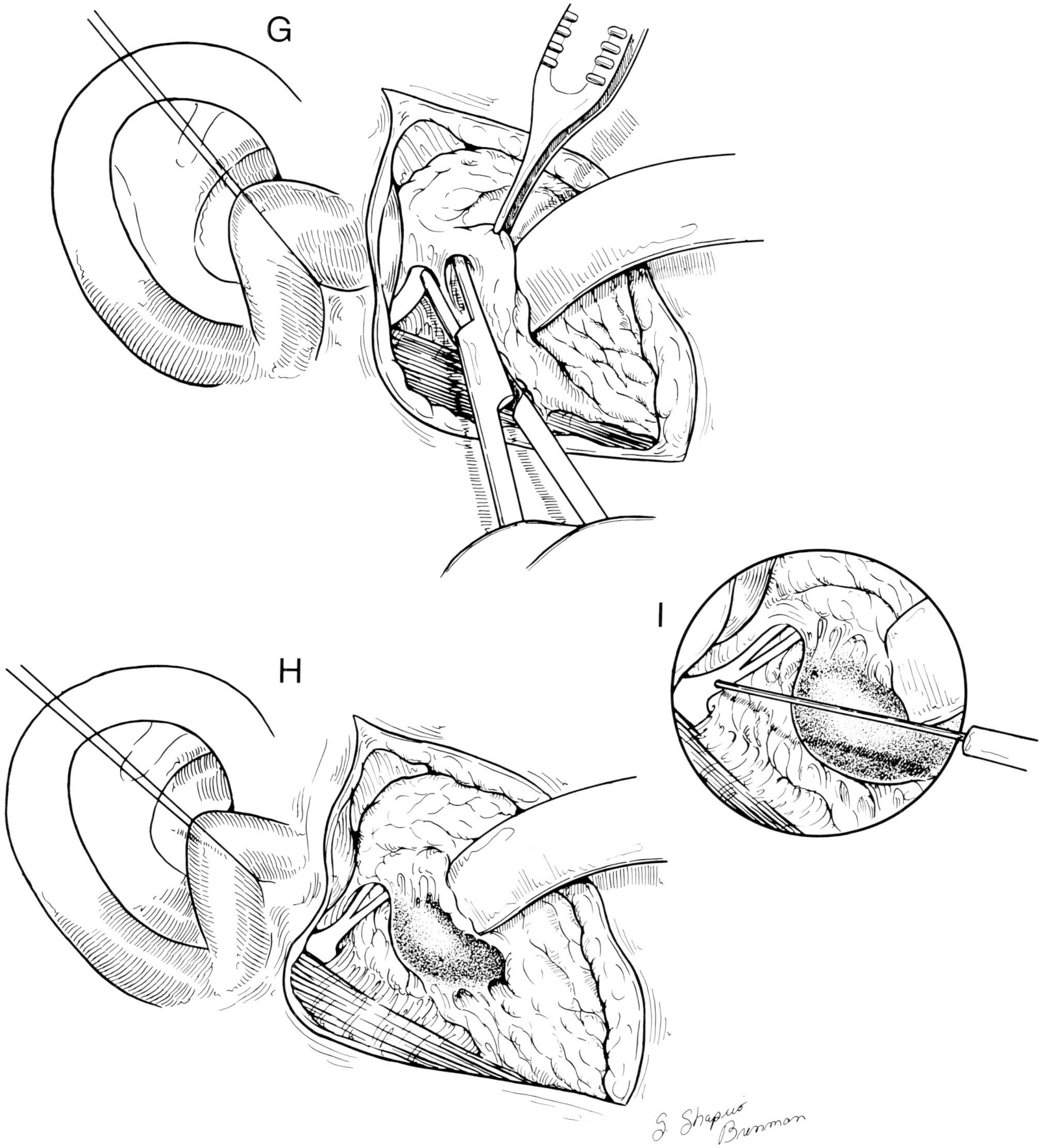


▶ **FIGURE 34-2**

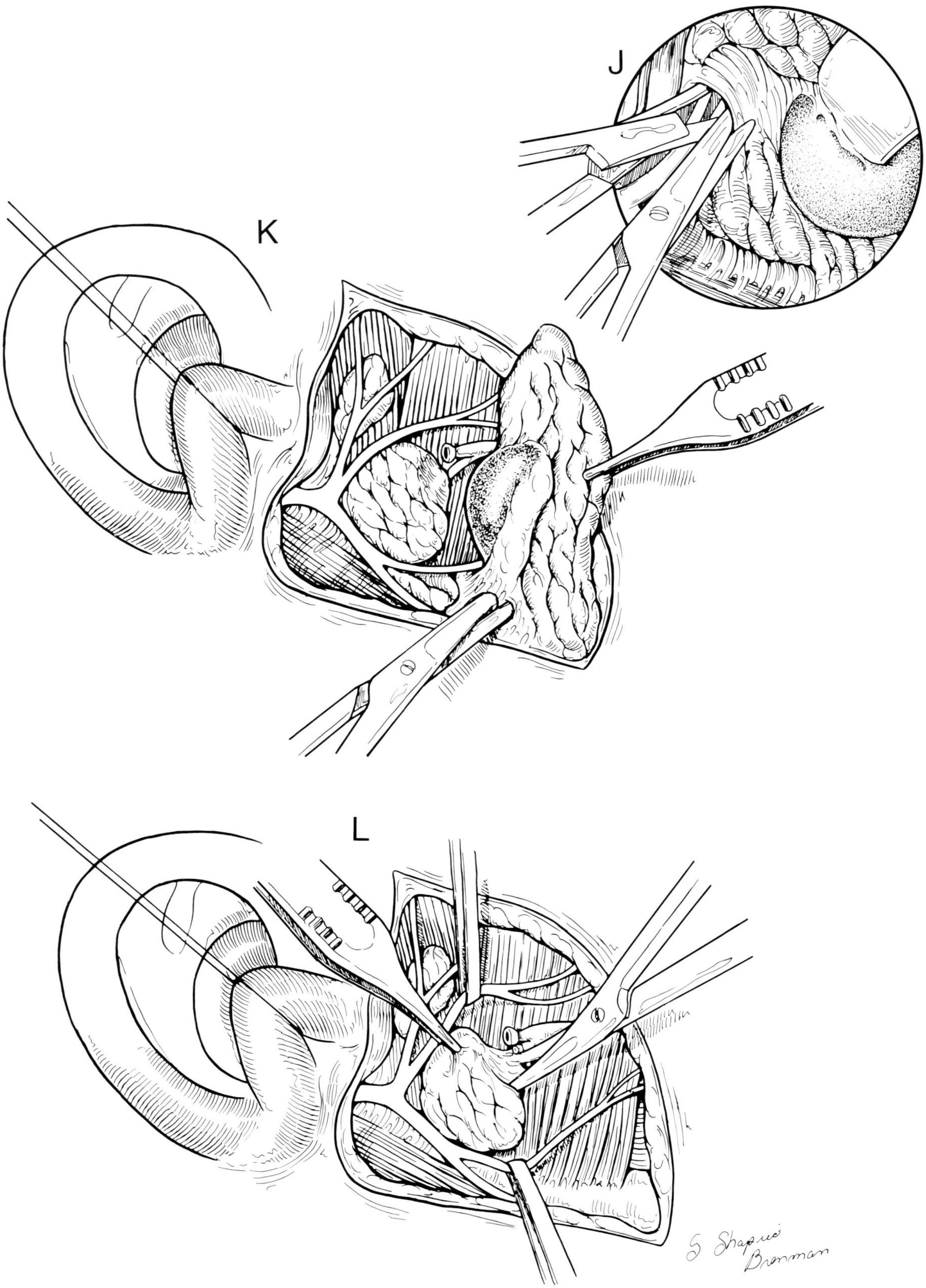


▶ **FIGURE 34-2**

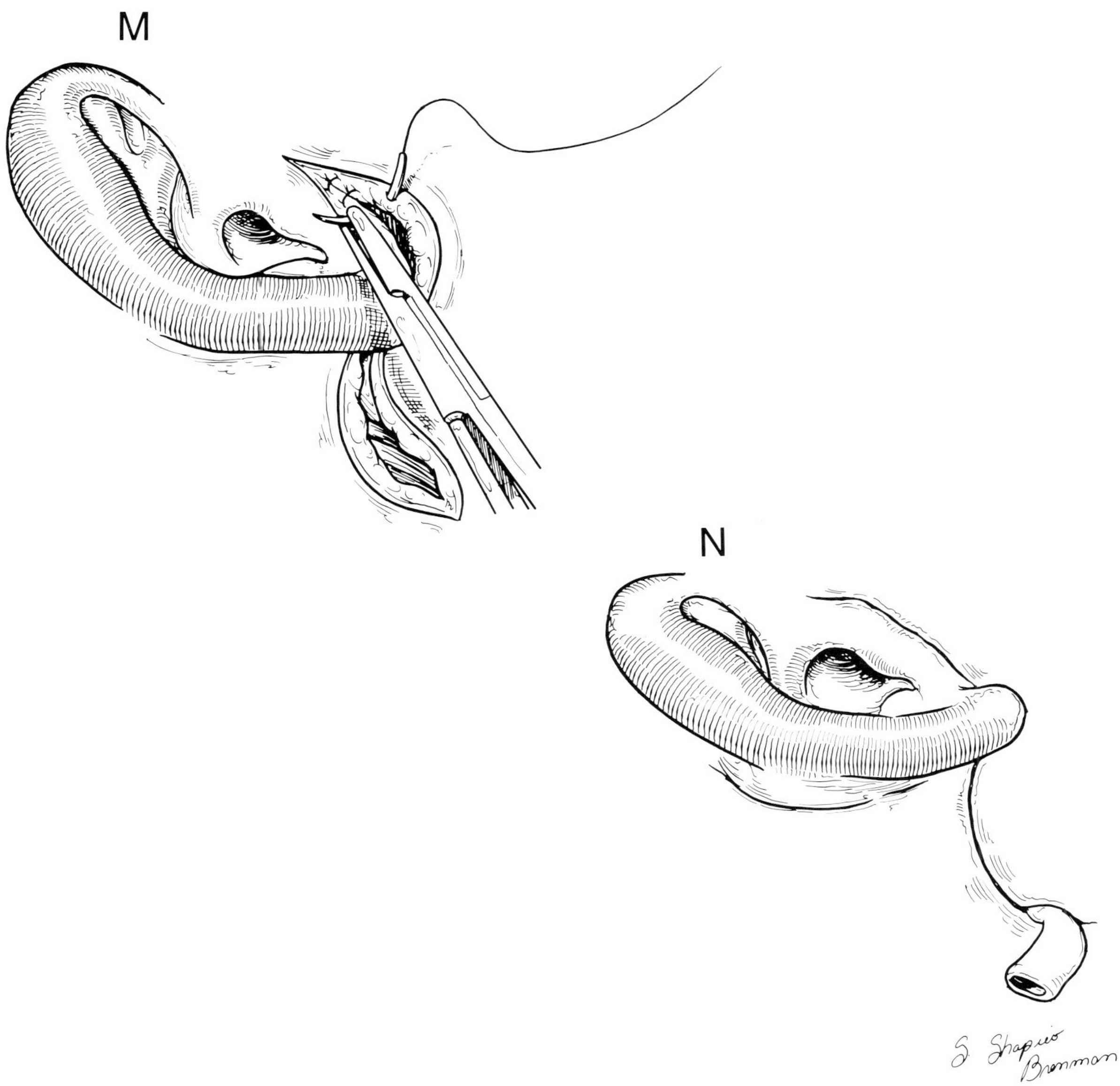


▶ **FIGURE 34-2**

# 35 ▸ Surgery of Salivary Mucocele

## ▸ 35-1 MUCOCELE (RANULA)

Ranulas and mucoceles develop from blocked minor (such as sublingual) salivary gland ducts. They usually present as a bluish, soft, fluctuant mass under the tongue (Fig. 35–1**A**).

### Indications

The presence of a ranula is the indication for surgical treatment.

### Preoperative Evaluation

Computed tomography (CT) or magnetic resonance imaging (MRI) may be helpful to define the ranula, especially if it extends deep to the mylohyoid muscle. One usually relies on history and clinical examination alone.

### Marsupialization—Operative Technique

1. Marsupialization is performed utilizing general nasotracheal anesthesia for maximum exposure.
2. An incision is made into the lumen of the cyst along the floor of the mouth avoiding the submandibular duct (Fig. 35–1**A**). The mucoid contents of the cyst can be evacuated with a suction (Fig. 35–1**B**).
3. The redundant portions of the oral mucosa and cyst wall are excised, widely opening the cyst (Fig. 35–1**C**).
4. The mucosal edges of the floor of the mouth are sutured to the remaining cyst wall with 3-0 or 4-0 chromic suture (Fig. 35–1**D**).

### Complications

1. Recurrence of the ranula
2. Trauma to the submandibular duct

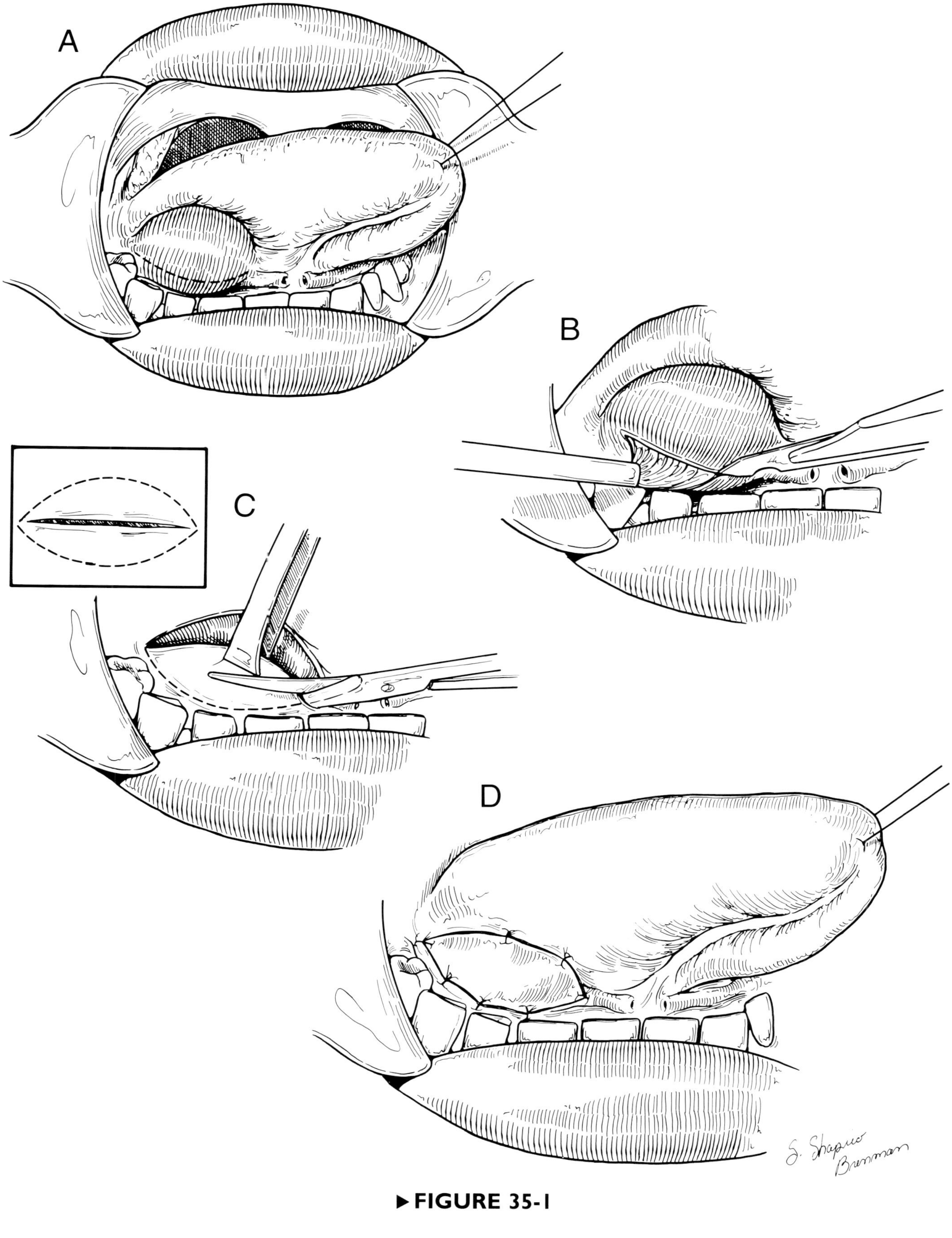


▶ **FIGURE 35-1**

## ▶ 35-2 RANULA EXCISION (INTRAORAL)

Ranula is a cystic dilation of a sublingual salivary gland.

### Indications

An enlarging or painful ranula should be removed.

### Preoperative Evaluation

If a ranula is suspected to have an extension deep to the mylohyoid muscle, computed tomography (CT) or magnetic resonance imaging (MRI) scan may be helpful to define its extent. Ranulas extending deep to the mylohyoid muscle should be removed through an external approach as described for submandibular gland excision (see section 34-1).

### Operative Technique

1. General anesthesia administered by nasotracheal tube is best for maximum exposure of the floor of the mouth.
2. The submandibular duct is cannulated with a polyethylene tube to aid in identification and protection of the duct during the dissection. The papilla may be dilated with lacrimal probes to permit the cannula to enter the duct (Fig. 35–2**A**).
3. A linear incision is made over the cyst along the course of the duct staying away from the duct itself (Fig. 35–2**A**).
4. Mucosal flaps are elevated superiorly and inferiorly by sharp and blunt dissection exposing the borders of the cyst (Fig. 35–2**B**).
5. The cyst is removed with attached salivary gland tissue by careful blunt and sharp dissection along the floor of the cyst (Fig. 35–2**C**) protecting the submandibular duct and lingual nerve, which lies on the floor of the mouth (Fig. 35–2**D**).
6. The mucosal incision is closed loosely with 3-0 chromic suture (Fig. 35–2**E**).

### Complications

1. Submandibular duct stricture
2. Lingual nerve injury

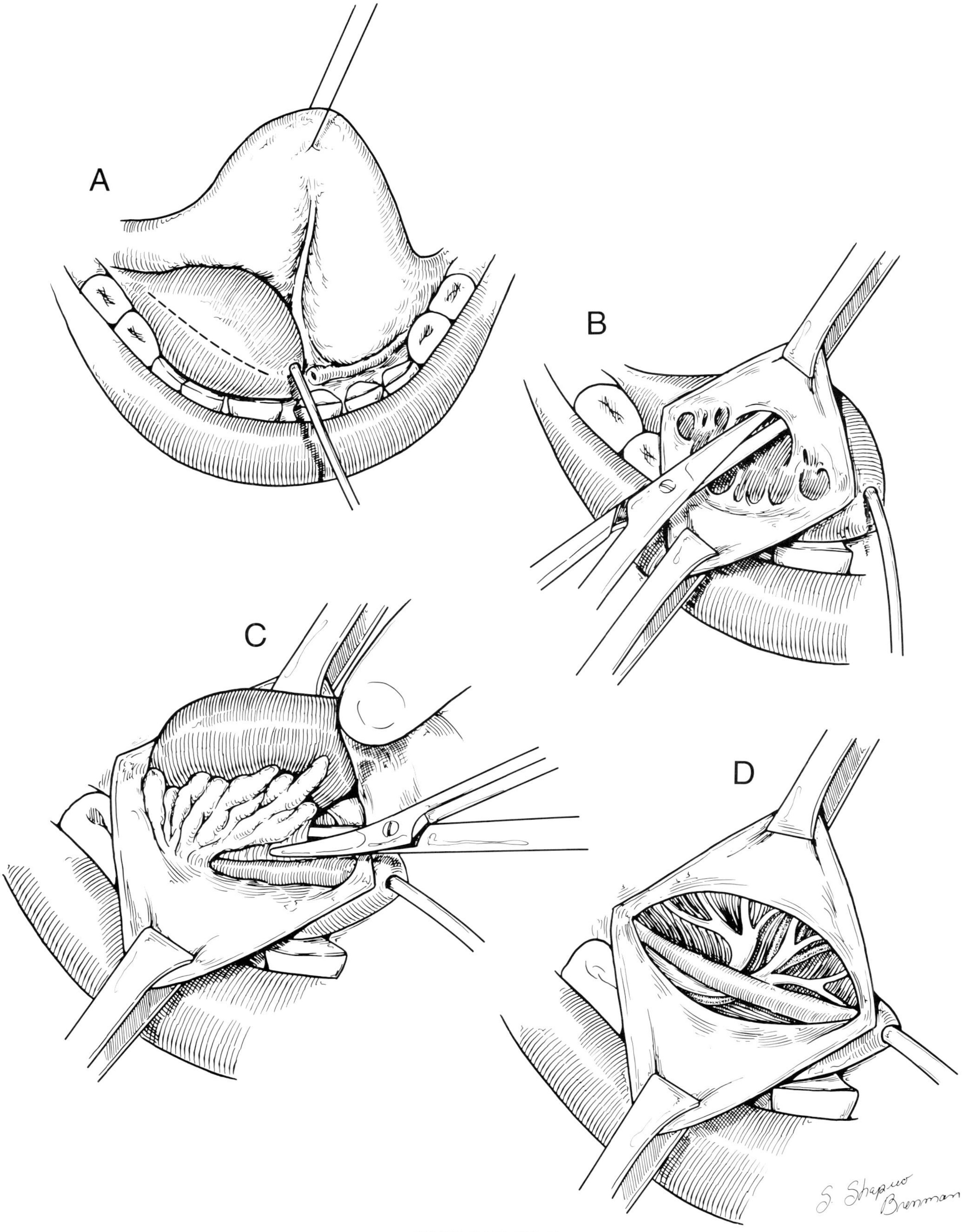


▶ **FIGURE 35-2**

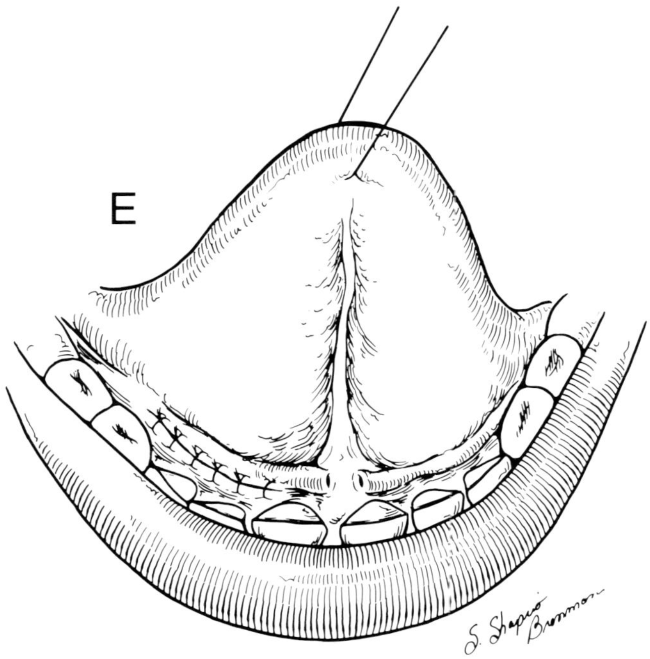


▶ **FIGURE 35-2**

# PART VII

# Endoscopy

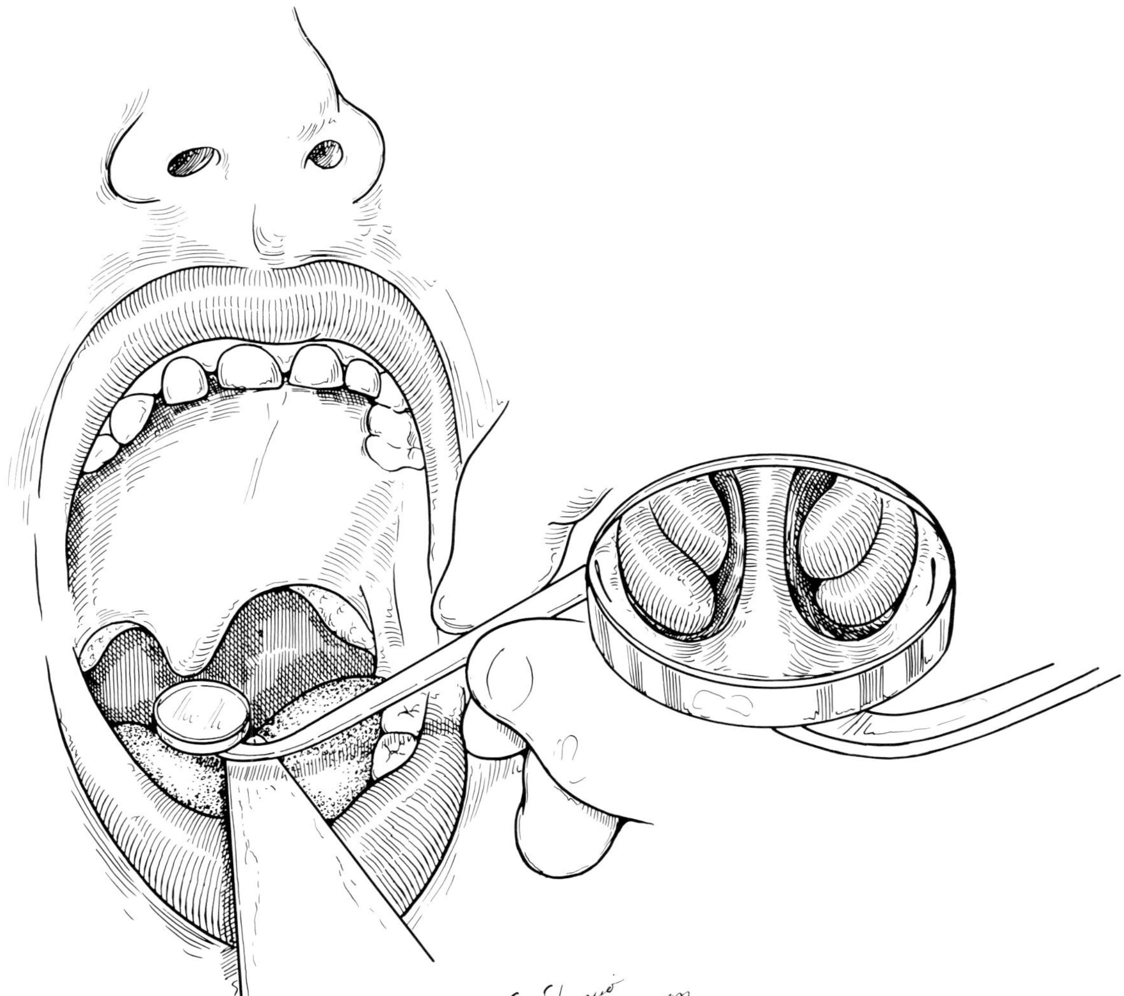

# 36 ▶ Endoscopy

Examination of the internal cavities of the head and neck has become a very common practice in the pediatric otolaryngologic examination. In no other area of pediatric otolaryngology have there been such advances in techniques and methods as in pediatric endoscopy. Fiberoptic instruments (both flexible and rigid) and improvements in pediatric anesthesia have combined to permit endoscopy in any child in almost any condition. These procedures are useful in providing information to help direct further evaluation and treatment. In many instances, the endoscopic examination may spare the child more invasive procedures.

## ▶ 36-1 RHINOSCOPY

Rhinoscopy is part of the standard otolaryngologic examination of the child.

### Indications

Epistaxis, foreign body, or anterior nasal mass require rhinoscopy.

### Preoperative Evaluation

Usually no preoperative preparation is required. However, a plain radiograph may be helpful in identifying a radiopaque foreign body.

### Operative Technique

1. No anesthetic or vasoconstricting substance is necessary for limited anterior rhinoscopy.
2. The child is in the upright position seated in a chair or in the parent's lap.
3. The child's mobile nasal tip is gently elevated with the examiner's thumb as a directed light source is shone into the nasal cavity. In this way, the anterior nasal septum, nasal vestibule, the inferior and, occasionally, the middle turbinate can be examined easily (Fig. 36–1**A**).
4. If redundant or collapsible tissue or nasal hairs prevent adequate visualization, a standard nasal speculum can be inserted gently into the nasal vestibule and the internal structures visualized.
5. Care must be taken to stabilize the instrument with the examiner's forefinger on the patient's nasal tip so that the instrument will follow any movements of the child's head (Fig. 36–1**B**). An otoscope with a large speculum may be substituted for the nasal speculum.
6. If examination of the more posterior aspect of the nasal cavity is needed, posterior rhinoscopy can be performed utilizing a straight telescope. Topical anesthesia and vasoconstriction is obtained using cotton pledgets soaked in 4% cocaine (alternately, any combination of a topical vasoconstrictor and local anesthetic may be used). The telescope can then be advanced into the nasal cavity to inspect the deeper aspects of the turbinates and the nasal septum

(Fig. 36–1C). Rigid telescopes are available in different viewing angles so that the entire nasal cavity can be examined.

7. A flexible telescope may be inserted and angulated in different directions to view the entire nasal cavity (Fig. 36–1D).

## Complications

1. Mucosal abrasions
2. Epistaxis

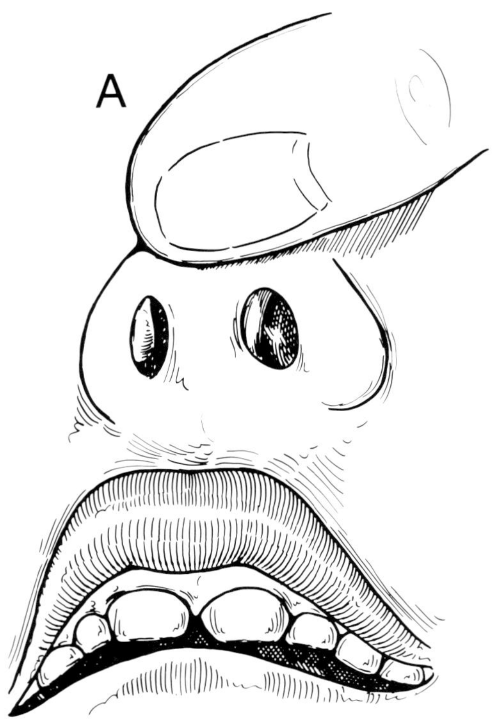


▶ **FIGURE 36-1**

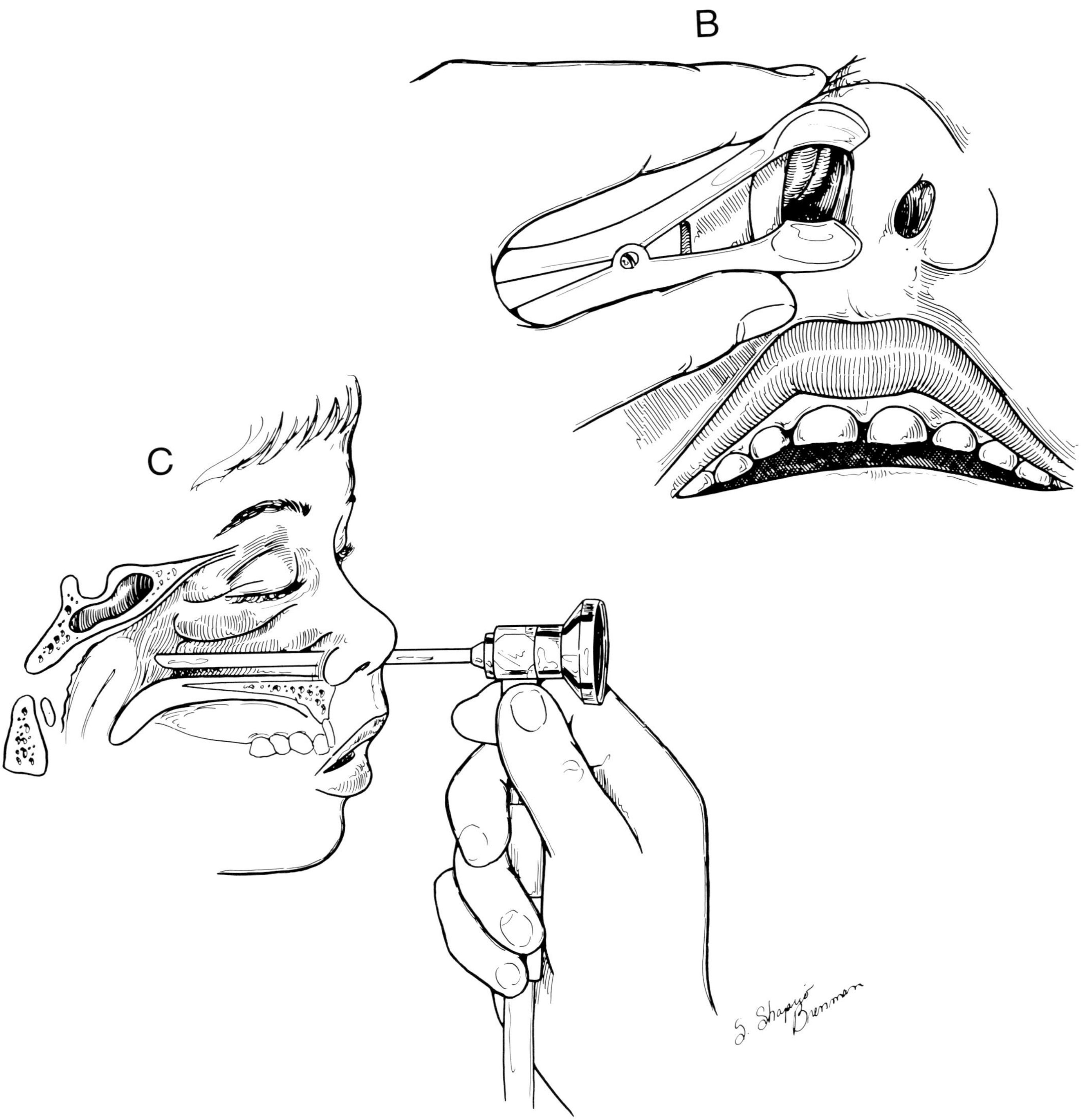


▶ **FIGURE 36-1**

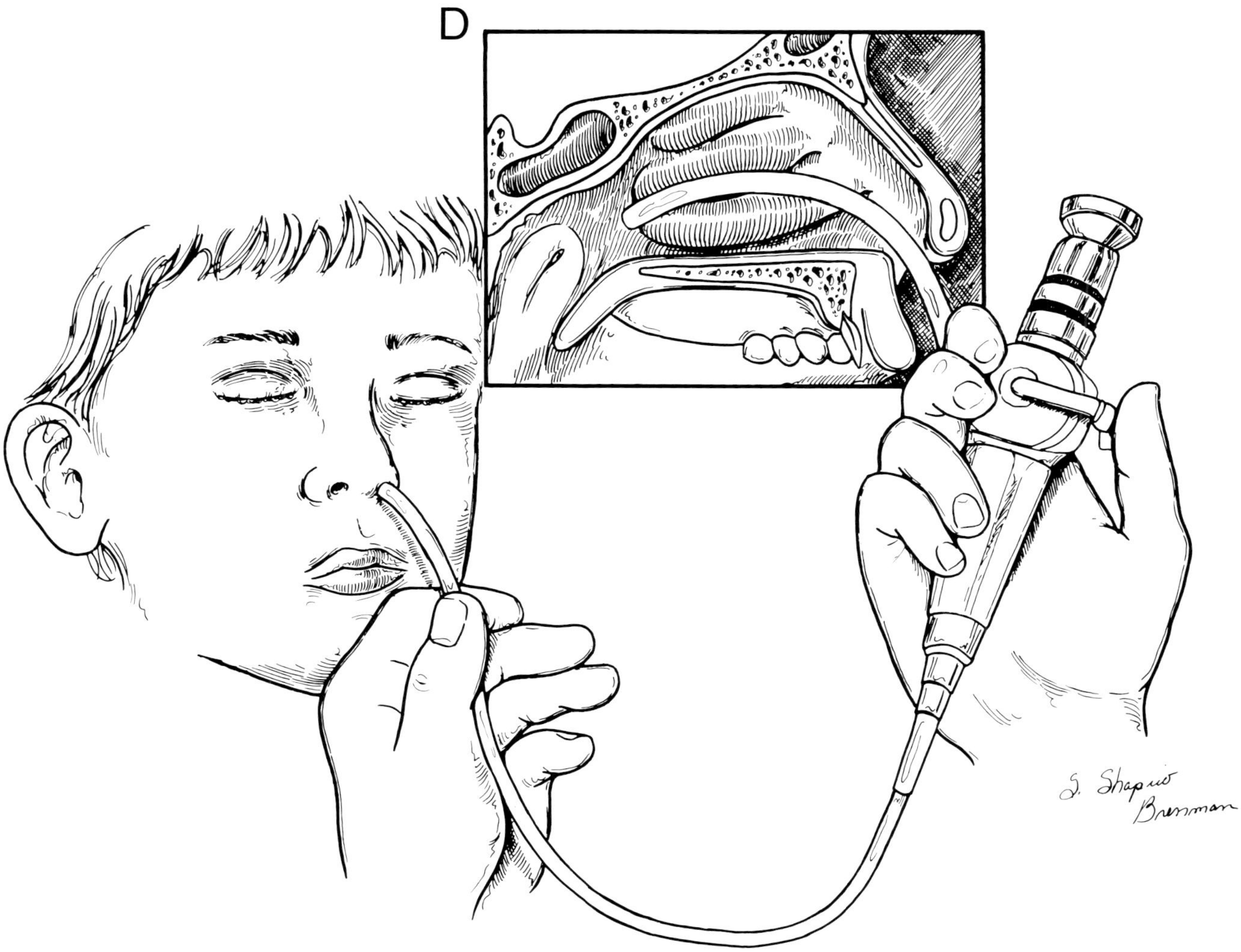


▶ **FIGURE 36-1**

# 37 ▸ Sinoscopy

## ▸ 37-1 SINOSCOPY

Sinoscopy is a technique that is used to examine the maxillary sinus through a patent nasal-antral window or enlarged maxillary sinus ostia after sinus surgery. While the procedure can also be performed through a puncture of the anterior wall of the maxillary sinus, the developing maxillary tooth buds in the child make this a less-desirable approach.

### Indications

Presence of maxillary sinus disease in a child with a patent nasal-antral window or enlarged natural maxillary ostia.

### Operative Technique

Sinoscopy may be performed under general anesthesia or under topical anesthesia in the office.

1. The child is in the upright position seated in a chair or in the parent's lap.
2. Topical anesthesia and vasoconstriction is obtained using cotton pledgets soaked in 4% cocaine (alternately, any combination of a topical vasoconstrictor and local anesthetic may be used).
3. The telescope is then gently inserted into the nasal cavity and angulated laterally to enter the previously created nasal-antral window or enlarged natural ostia. Rigid telescopes of varying viewing angles are utilized to examine the entire maxillary sinus cavity (Fig. 37–1**A**).

### Complications

1. Mucosal abrasions
2. Epistaxis

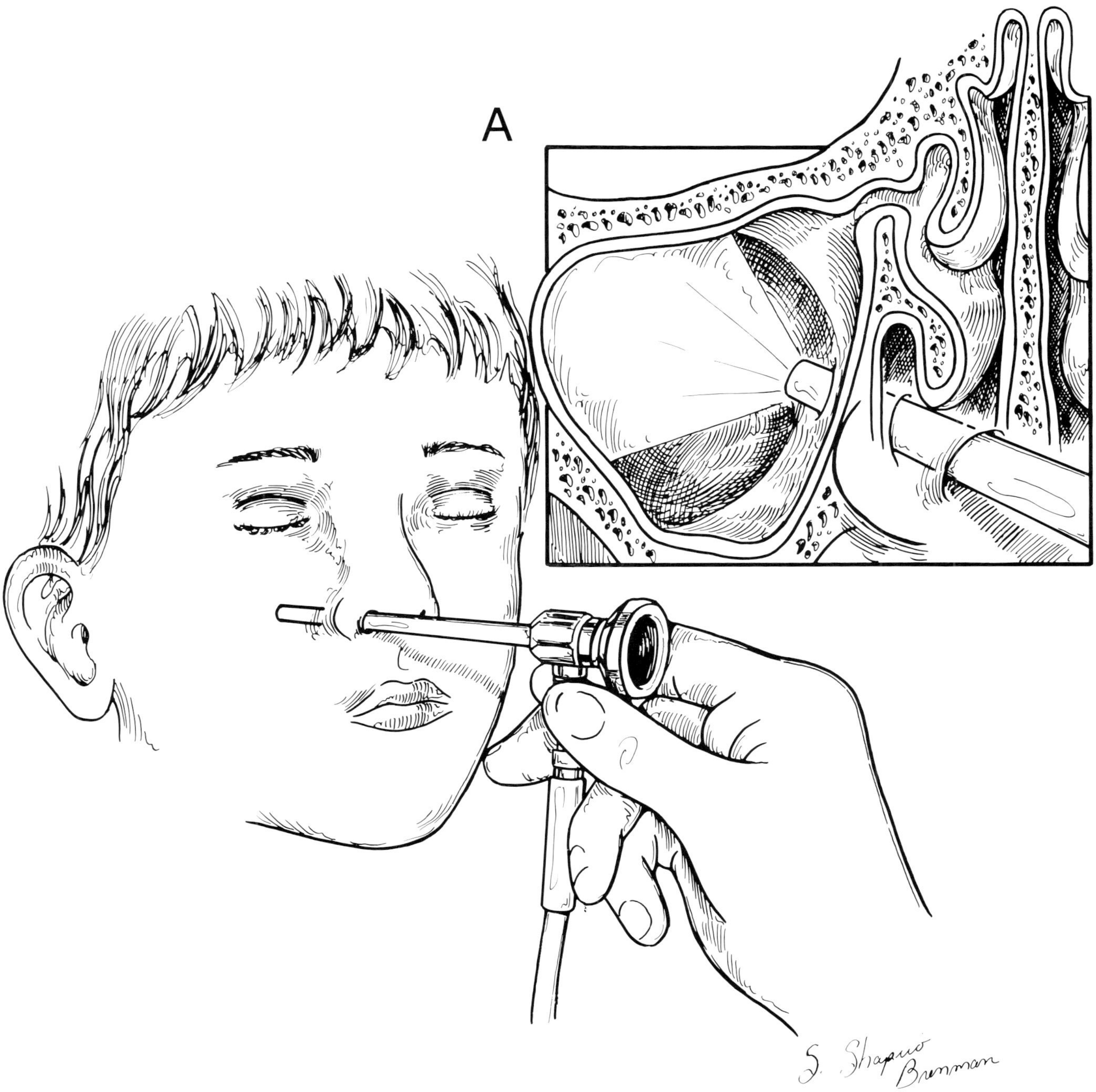


▶ **FIGURE 37-1**

# 38 ▶ Nasopharyngoscopy

Nasopharyngoscopy is a very important technique in evaluating palatal function, eustachian tube anatomy and physiology, adenoid size and the presence of any nasopharyngeal lesion. Several techniques are available to the otolaryngologist in the evaluation of this area.

### Indications

Nasopharyngoscopy is indicated when visualization of the nasopharynx is desired to assess enlarged adenoids, a nasopharyngeal mass or velopharyngeal insufficiency.

## ▶ 38 - 1 MIRROR NASOPHARYNGOSCOPY

This technique rarely requires topical anesthesia and provides excellent visualization of the entire nasopharynx. However, it is not useful in assessing dynamic motion of the palate or eustachian tube.

### Operative Technique

1. The child is in the upright position seated in a chair or on the parent's lap.
2. The neck is flexed and the head extended in the "sniffer's position."
3. The examiner faces the child and wears a headlight or head mirror with a focused light source beside the child's head.
4. The child is asked to open his mouth but not to protrude his tongue.
5. A tongue blade is used to depress the central portion of the tongue, taking care not to touch the more sensitive posterior aspects of the tongue.
6. A warmed or defogged nasopharyngeal mirror is gently inserted into the pharynx, behind the uvula, and angulated upward so that the examiner can view the entire nasopharynx (Fig. 38–1**A**). The warmed mirror should be touched to the examiner's hand prior to inserting it into the patient's mouth to prevent burning the oral mucosa.
7. The child is asked to breathe through his nose or to "pant like a puppy" in order to allow the palate to relax and allow visualization of the nasopharynx.

### Complications

None

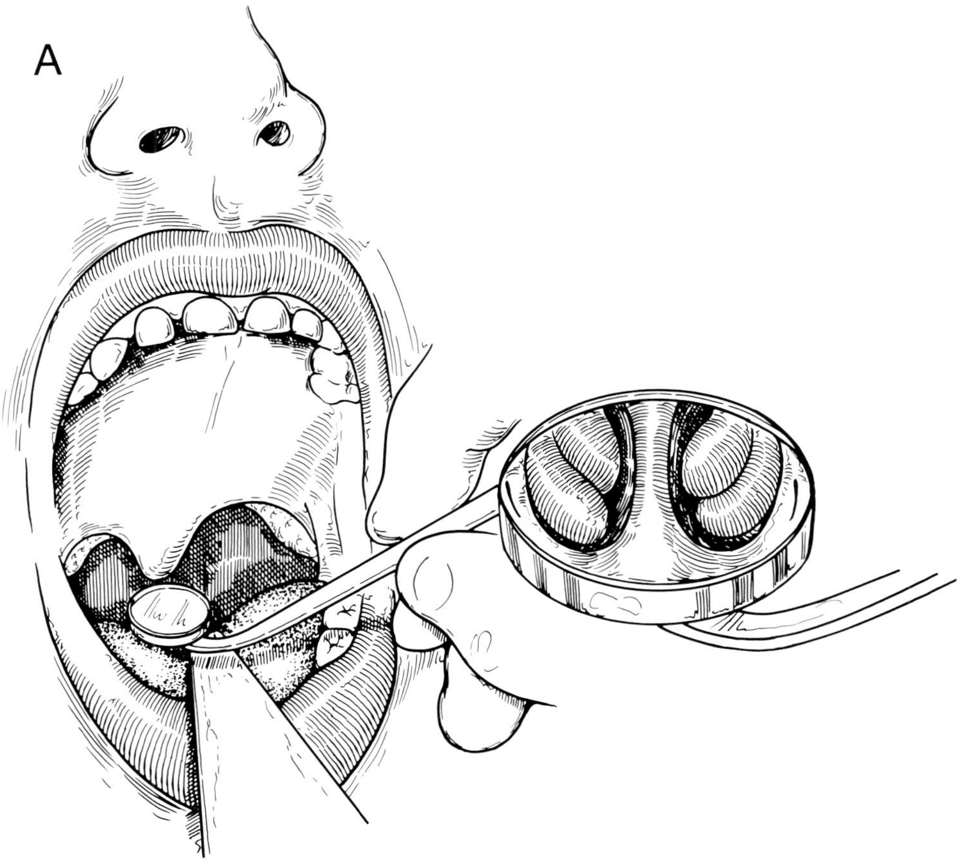


▶ **FIGURE 38-1**

## ▶ 38 - 2 RIGID NASOPHARYNGOSCOPY

This examination has the advantage of allowing excellent telescopic visualization of the entire nasopharynx. However, it fails to provide information regarding palatal movement.

### Operative Technique

1. The preparation for this technique is the same as described above for the mirror examination.
2. A defogged telescopic rod with a 90° viewing angle is inserted in the mouth over a tongue blade that depresses the central position of the tongue (Fig. 38–2**B**).
3. Care is taken not to touch the base of the tongue or posterior pharynx.
4. The child is asked to breathe through his nose or to "pant like a puppy" in order to allow the palate to relax and allow visualization of the nasopharynx.

### Complications

1. Mucosal abrasions
2. Epistaxis

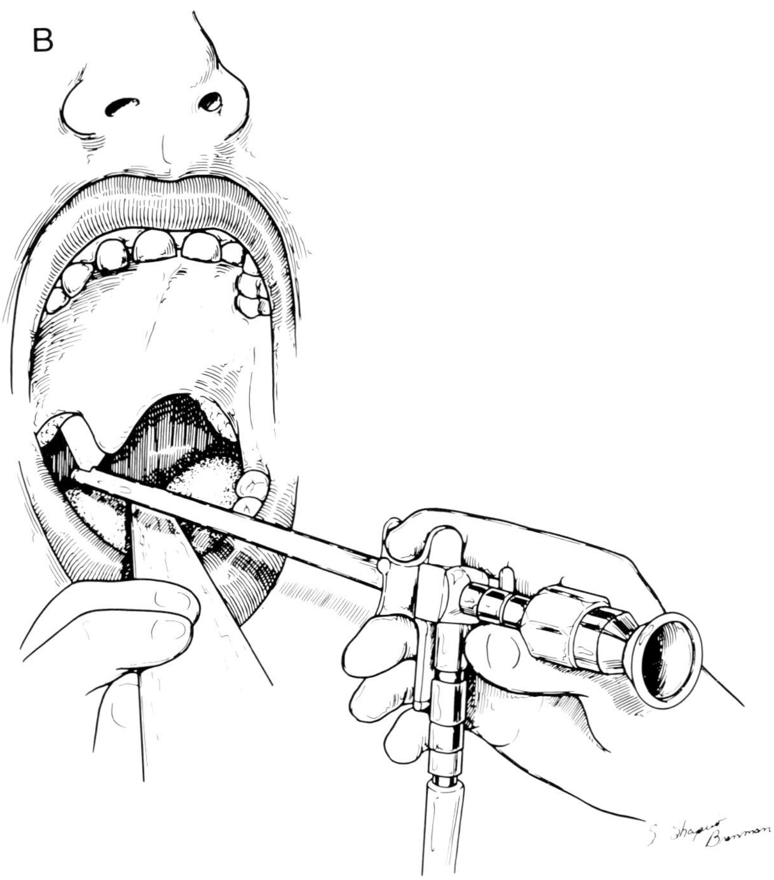


▶ **FIGURE 38-2**

## ▶ 38-3 FLEXIBLE NASOPHARYNGOSCOPY

This technique has the disadvantage of usually requiring topical anesthesia, yet it provides the most information regarding palatal movement and eustachian tube dynamics. It also allows for normal phonation and articulation without objects in the mouth.

### Operative Technique

1. The child's position is the same as described above.
2. Topical anesthesia and vasoconstriction of the nasal mucosa is obtained using cotton pledgets soaked in 4% cocaine (alternately, any combination of a topical vasoconstrictor and local anesthetic may be used). In some older, more cooperative patients, the newer, thinner instruments may be used without local anesthesia.
3. The flexible nasopharyngoscope is gently inserted along the floor of the nose or in the middle meatus area until the posterior aspect of the hard palate is identified (Fig. 38–3C).
4. The telescope is deflected downward so that the adenoid pad can be identified and palatal closure monitored during phonation. Eustachian tube dynamics can also be observed.

### Complications

1. Mucosal abrasions
2. Epistaxis

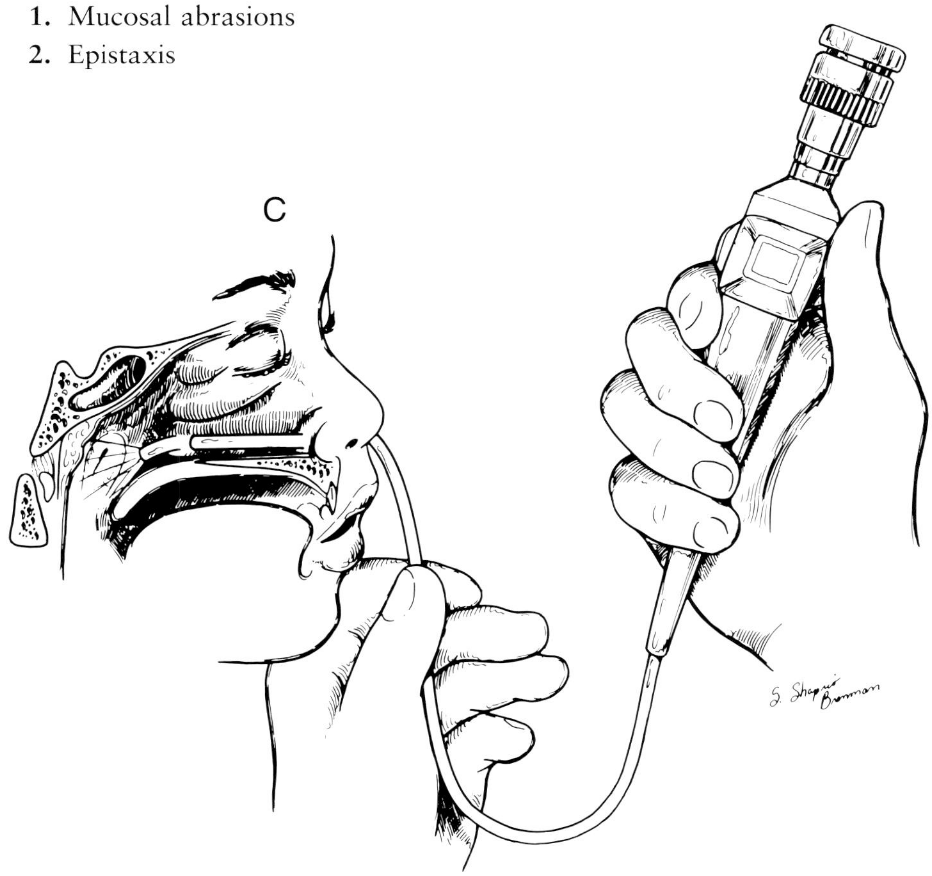


▶ **FIGURE 38-3**

# 39 ▶ Indirect Laryngoscopy

Indirect laryngoscopy is an office procedure that is often a part of the complete otolaryngologic examination of the child. It should precede any direct laryngoscopy under anesthesia. Several techniques are available to perform this examination.

## ▶ 39-1 MIRROR INDIRECT LARYNGOSCOPY

### Operative Technique

1. The child is positioned in the upright position seated in a chair or on his parent's lap.
2. The child's head is extended and the neck flexed in the classic "sniffer's position."
3. The examiner is facing the child using a headlight or head mirror with a focused light source beside the child's head.
4. The child is asked to open his mouth and protrude his tongue. The anterior portion of the tongue is grasped with a gauze sponge.
5. A warmed or defogged laryngeal mirror is gently inserted into the oral cavity and elevates the uvula and distal soft palate (Fig. 39–1**A**). The warmed mirror should be touched to the examiner's hand prior to inserting it into the patient's mouth to prevent burning the oral mucosa.
6. The instrument is angulated until the examiner is able to obtain excellent visualization of the laryngeal and hypopharyngeal structures.
7. The child is asked to say "ee" so that active vocal cord adduction can be observed.
8. If the child begins to gag with the instrument in place, he is asked to "pant like a puppy." This tends to relax the palate and allows completion of the examination.

### Complications

None

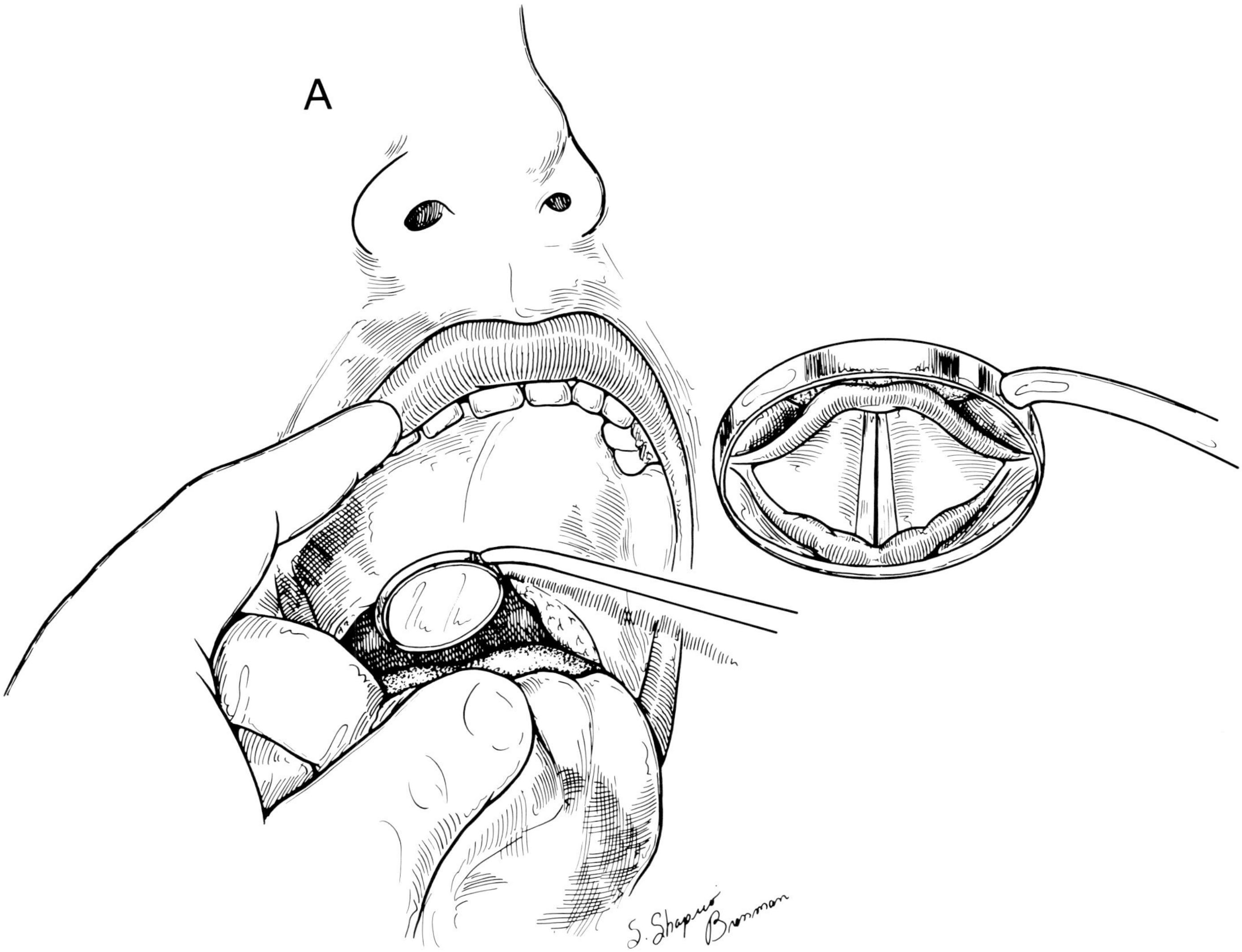


▶ **FIGURE 39-1**

## ▶ 39-2 RIGID TELESCOPIC DIRECT LARYNGOSCOPY

### Operative Technique

1. This technique utilizes the same preparation as mentioned above.
2. The anterior tongue is grasped with a gauze sponge.
3. A defogged telescopic rod with a 90° viewing angle is inserted over the surface of the tongue, taking care not to touch the posterior tongue or posterior pharyngeal wall (Fig. 39–2**A**).
4. Visualization of the laryngeal and hypopharyngeal structures is obtained in the same manner as described for the mirror (Fig. 39–2**B**).
5. If the child begins to gag with the instrument in place, he is asked to "pant like a puppy." This tends to relax the palate and allows completion of the examination.

### Complications

None

B

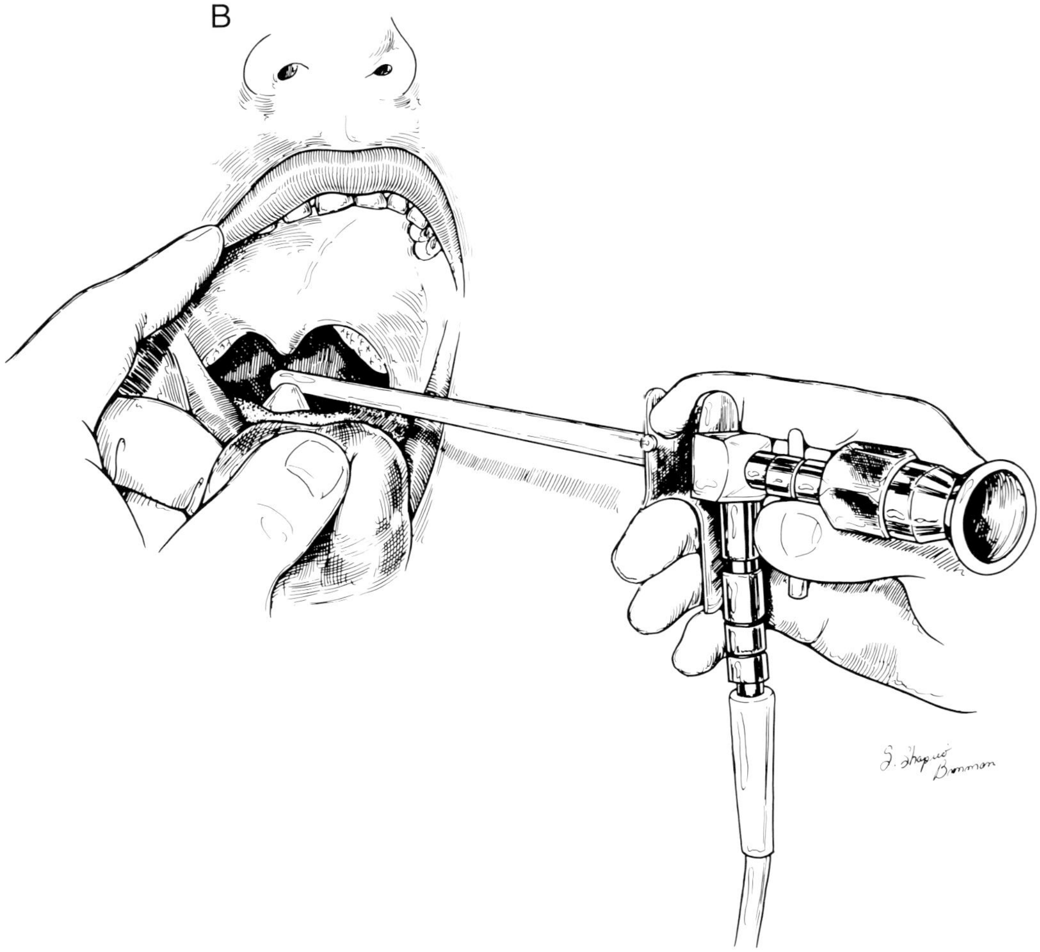

**▶ FIGURE 39-2**

## ▶ 39-3 FLEXIBLE DIRECT LARYNGOSCOPY

Because the tongue is not held by the examiner, the phonated sounds are more normal and the range of sounds is greater than that allowed by the mirror or rigid telescope techniques.

### Operative Technique

1. This technique is an extension of the flexible nasopharyngoscopy described previously (see section 38–3).
2. The flexible nasopharyngoscope is advanced further into the oropharynx, passing the soft palate and approaching the epiglottis (Fig. 39–3**C**). Care is taken not to touch any of the laryngeal structures which could cause laryngospasm.
3. The child is asked to say "ee" and the laryngeal dynamics are observed.

### Complications

1. Mucosal abrasions
2. Epistaxis
3. Laryngospasm

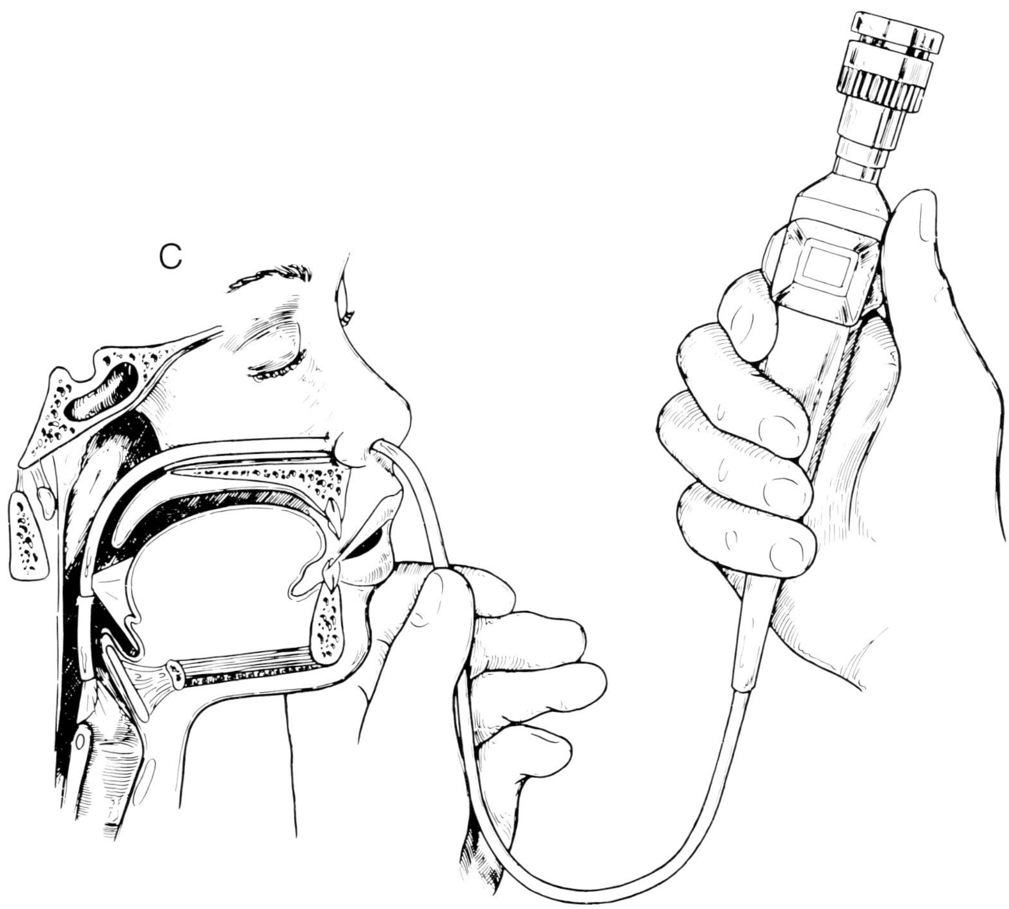


▶ **FIGURE 39-3**

# 40 ▶ Direct Laryngoscopy (General Anesthesia)

## ▶ 40 - 1 FLEXIBLE DIRECT LARYNGOSCOPY (GENERAL ANESTHESIA)

Flexible direct laryngoscopy allows for complete evaluation of the larynx and for manipulation and instrumentation of the larynx, if indicated.

### Indications

Stridor, laryngeal masses, foreign body, unexplained hoarseness, and history of chronic aspiration all require direct laryngoscopy.

### Preoperative Evaluation

Direct laryngoscopy should be preceded by indirect laryngoscopy and/or lateral neck radiography of the larynx.

### Flexible Technique

This technique, under a general anesthesia, allows for the best examination of the laryngeal structures and dynamics under spontaneous respiration. It is the procedure of choice to evaluate vocal cord mobility, laryngomalacia, and to assess the laryngeal airway in cases of suspected laryngeal foreign body. We utilize a 3.5-mm Olympus bronchoscope (with suction channel) for this procedure because it provides excellent visualization of the larynx, permits suctioning of secretions, and can be used to continue the examination into the trachea and bronchi if necessary.

While this technique has the advantage of allowing the best visualization for laryngeal structure, mobility, and physiology, it does not allow for immediate airway management, intervention, or protection.

### Operative Technique

1. The child is supine on the operating room table.
2. General anesthesia is induced utilizing a mask with an inhalation agent. Transparent masks are used so the face can be seen during this whole procedure.
3. Intravenous lines are placed to allow for drug administration as necessary.
4. Oxymetazoline is placed in both nostrils to decongest the nasal mucosa.
5. A shoulder roll is placed under the child's shoulders to provide maximum extension of the head on the neck.
6. The anesthesiologist's hand is able to maintain an open airway by elevating the mandible and supporting the submental and supralaryngeal soft tissues.
7. An oropharyngeal airway may be inserted, if necessary, to maintain an open airway.

8. A special adapter (Swivel-Flex Elbow-Life Design Systems, Carrollton, TX) (Fig. 40–1**A**) is placed at the junction of the mask and the anesthetic tubing to allow entrance of the endoscope without losing the ability to ventilate.
9. The endoscope is gently advanced through the adapter and into the mask area.
10. The endoscope is directed into the nasal cavity. Usually, it is necessary to remove the mask for a second or two to manually place the endoscope in the nasal cavity (Fig. 40–1**B**). Once this has been accomplished, the mask is replaced on the face and adequate ventilation is resumed.
11. The child is ventilating spontaneously during this entire procedure.
12. The endoscope is advanced through the nasal cavity and into the nasopharynx. The tip of the endoscope is deflected inferiorly past the soft palate and adenoid area until the oropharynx and larynx are identified. The endoscope is advanced to the level of the epiglottis (Fig. 40–1**C**).
13. Care is taken not to touch the epiglottis in order to prevent laryngospasm. If the level of anesthesia is too light, this can also cause laryngeal closure. Intravenous lidocaine is often given before this point in the procedure to help in reducing the incidence of laryngospasm.
14. If the level of anesthesia is too deep, spontaneous ventilation ceases, and no vocal cord mobility can be identified. In this case, the anesthesia level is lightened so that spontaneous ventilation resumes and vocal cord movement can be observed. In this way, vocal cord paralysis, paresis, and laryngomalacia can be observed and even documented by video recorder.
15. Care must be taken by the anesthesiologist to avoid applying high continuous positive airway pressure (CPAP), as this may make detection of laryngomalacia difficult.
16. If the child has a tracheostomy tube in place, and the anesthesia is induced through the tracheostomy tube, the same procedure as described above can be performed to assess laryngeal function. However, since there is no traction to the mandible or submandibular structures by the anesthesiologist, there may be some collapse of the tongue and epiglottis into the oropharyngeal airway. This can be overcome by opening the mouth and grasping the tongue with a gauze sponge. Gentle traction upward is applied to bring the larynx into view in the hypopharyngeal area (Fig. 40–1**D**).

## Complications

1. Mucosal abrasions
2. Epistaxis
3. Laryngospasm
4. Glottic edema

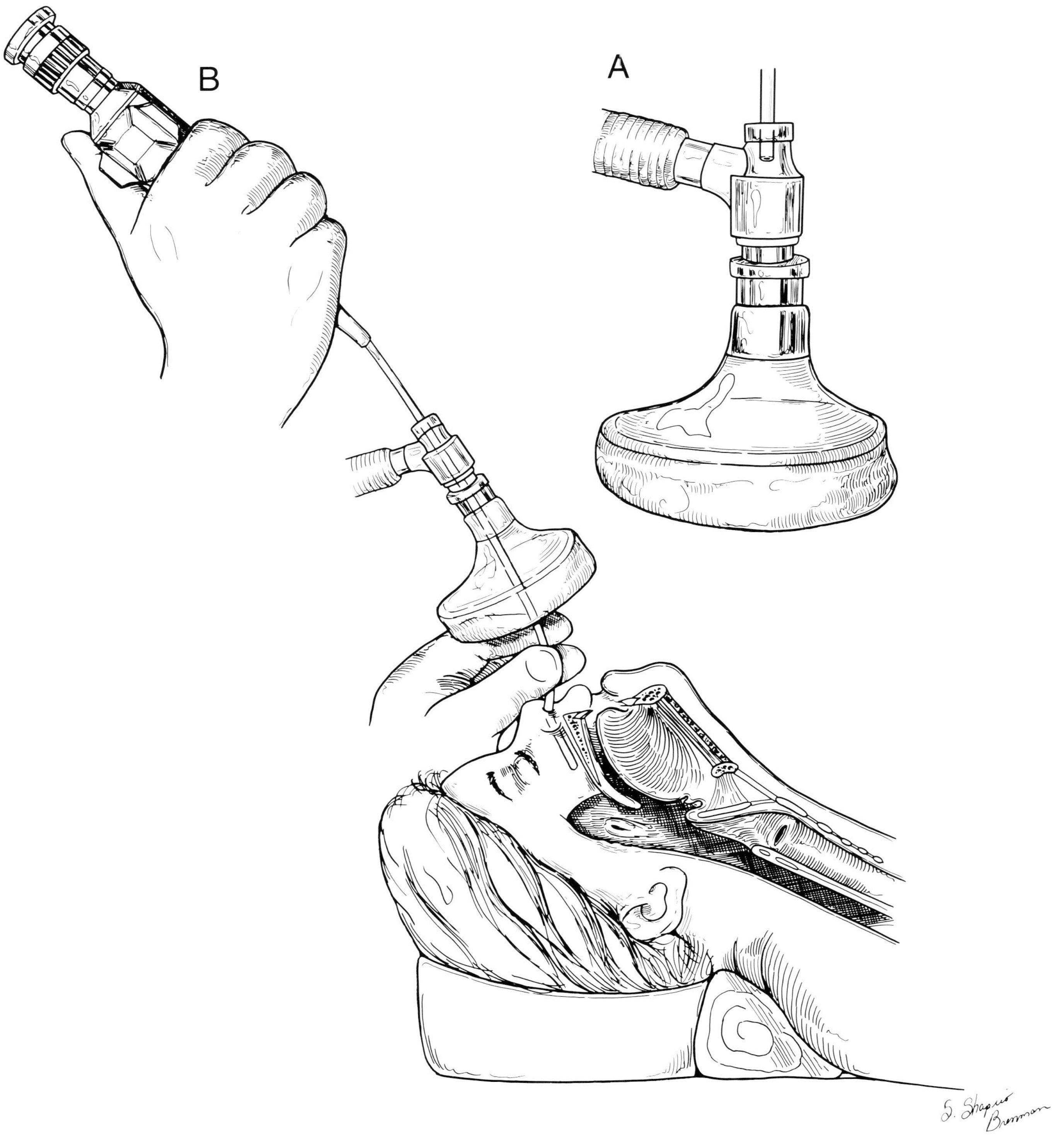


▶ **FIGURE 40-1**

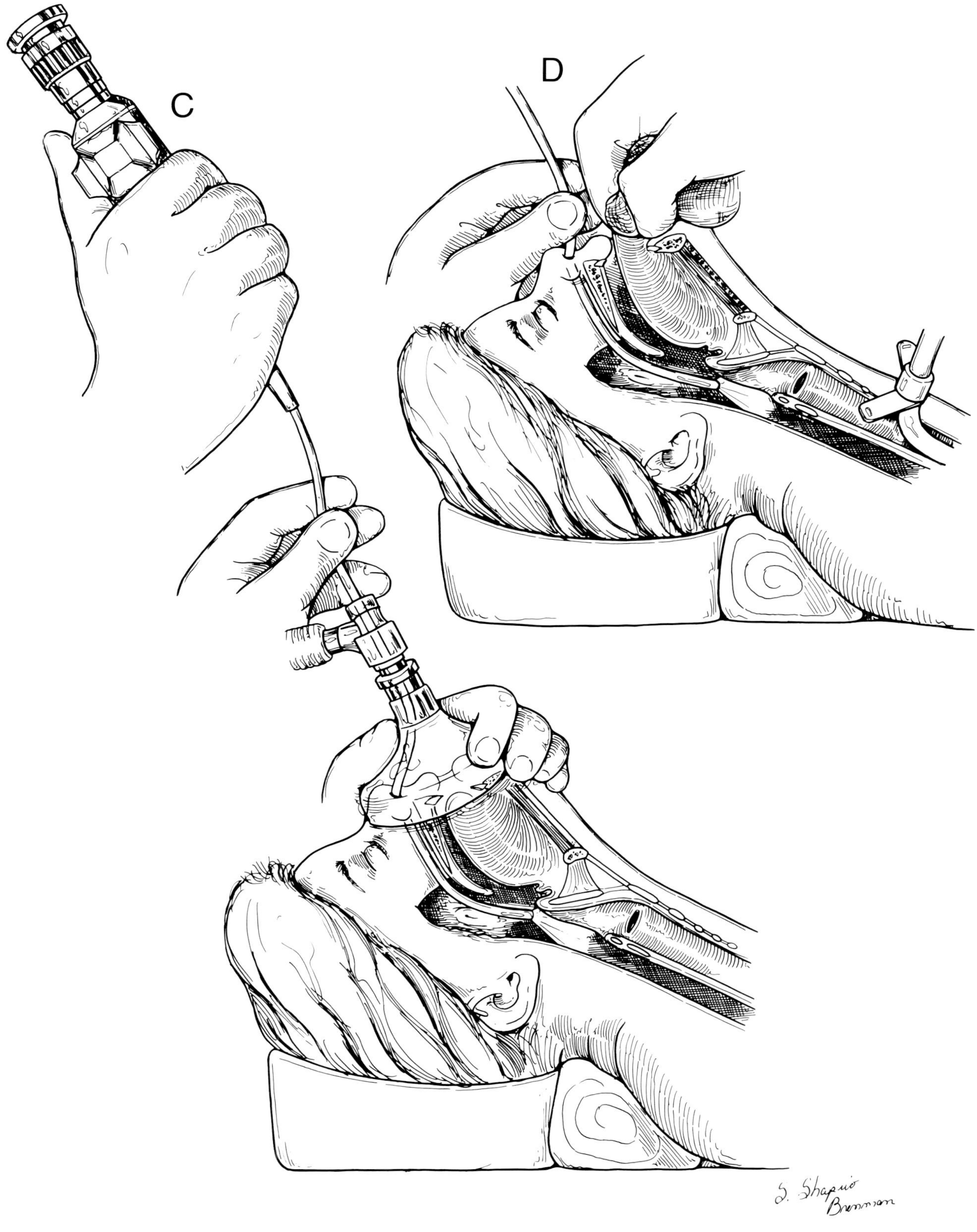


▶ **FIGURE 40-1**

## ▶ 40-2 RIGID DIRECT LARYNGOSCOPY (GENERAL ANESTHESIA)

This is the classic technique for examination of the larynx that allows for instrumentation and intervention as indicated. However, it does not allow for as good an evaluation of the dynamics of the larynx as the flexible technique described above.

The size and type of laryngoscope depends on the age of the child and the indication for the laryngoscopy. The anterior commissure (Holinger) laryngoscopes are utilized if examination of the endolarynx is desired. The Jackson slide or open laryngoscopes are indicated if instrumentation of the larynx (e.g., removal of foreign body, intubation, introducing a bronchoscope) is needed. The sizes of the laryngoscopes and their use in children are indicated below:

| Size of laryngoscope (diameter) | Approximate age of child |
|---|---|
| 9 mm | newborn to 2 years |
| 12 mm | 2 years to 8 years |
| 16–17 mm | 8 years to adolescent |

Note: These are approximate guidelines and requirements may vary depending upon the actual size of the child.

### Operative Technique

1. The patient is supine on the operating table. Anesthesia is induced utilizing a mask with an inhalation agent.
2. The table is then turned 90° to the anesthesiologist so that the examiner is at the head of the bed.
3. A shoulder roll is placed under the child's shoulders so that there can be maximum extension of the head on the neck (Fig. 40–2**A**).
4. The anesthetic level is deepened until the child is apneic. At that time, the anesthesia mask is removed and the examiner begins the laryngoscopy.
5. A small moist gauze sponge is placed on the upper gum or teeth to protect this area.
6. The mouth is opened widely using the examiner's first finger and thumb of the right hand.
7. The laryngoscope (held in the left hand) is then inserted at the right side of the mouth. The tongue is gently swept to the left. This technique allows for easier insertion of the laryngoscope and avoids the often protruding incisors (Fig. 40–2**B**).
8. Secretions are cleared from the end of the laryngoscope utilizing long suction instruments.
9. The tip of the epiglottis is visualized.
10. The observer's end of the scope is moved to the midline to provide an undistorted view of the larynx.
11. If possible, the laryngoscope is placed in the vallecula and the tongue gently elevated (Fig. 40–2**C**). This brings the epiglottis and the laryngeal structures into direct view in the open end of the laryngoscope (Fig. 40–2**D**). If the epiglottis obscures the view of the larynx, the tip of the laryngoscope is elevated to improve visualization.

**12.** As the anesthesia level is lightened, spontaneous ventilation is observed. Vocal cord mobility and laryngomalacia can be identified. Since this technique involves direct contact with the base of tongue and laryngeal structures, intravenous lidocaine and/or topical lidocaine spray may be useful to reduce the incidence of laryngospasm. As the child's level of anesthesia lightens, there may be excessive swallowing and muscular movement in the field, which prevent adequate visualization. If this occurs, the laryngoscope is removed and the anesthesiologist's mask replaced. The child is ventilated and the anesthesia level deepened to allow for a second or subsequent look at the larynx.

**13.** If placement of the tip of the laryngoscope in the vallecula does not provide a view of the larynx, the instrument may be placed under the epiglottis (Fig. 40–2E) and advanced up to the false cords for better visualization of the larynx (Fig. 40–2F). However, this technique carries the increased risk of laryngospasm and may cause distortion of the larynx by compressing the epiglottis.

**14.** Constant attention is paid to elevating the tongue anteriorly with the tip of the laryngoscope and not to pry or lever on the upper teeth in the attempt to view the larynx.

**15.** If the anterior commissure laryngoscope is inadequate to observe the larynx or instrumentation of the larynx is anticipated, the operating or Jackson slide laryngoscope is utilized. This instrument allows for easier instrumentation of the larynx and for passage of the bronchoscope, if necessary.

## Complications

1. Laryngospasm
2. Glottic edema
3. Dental trauma

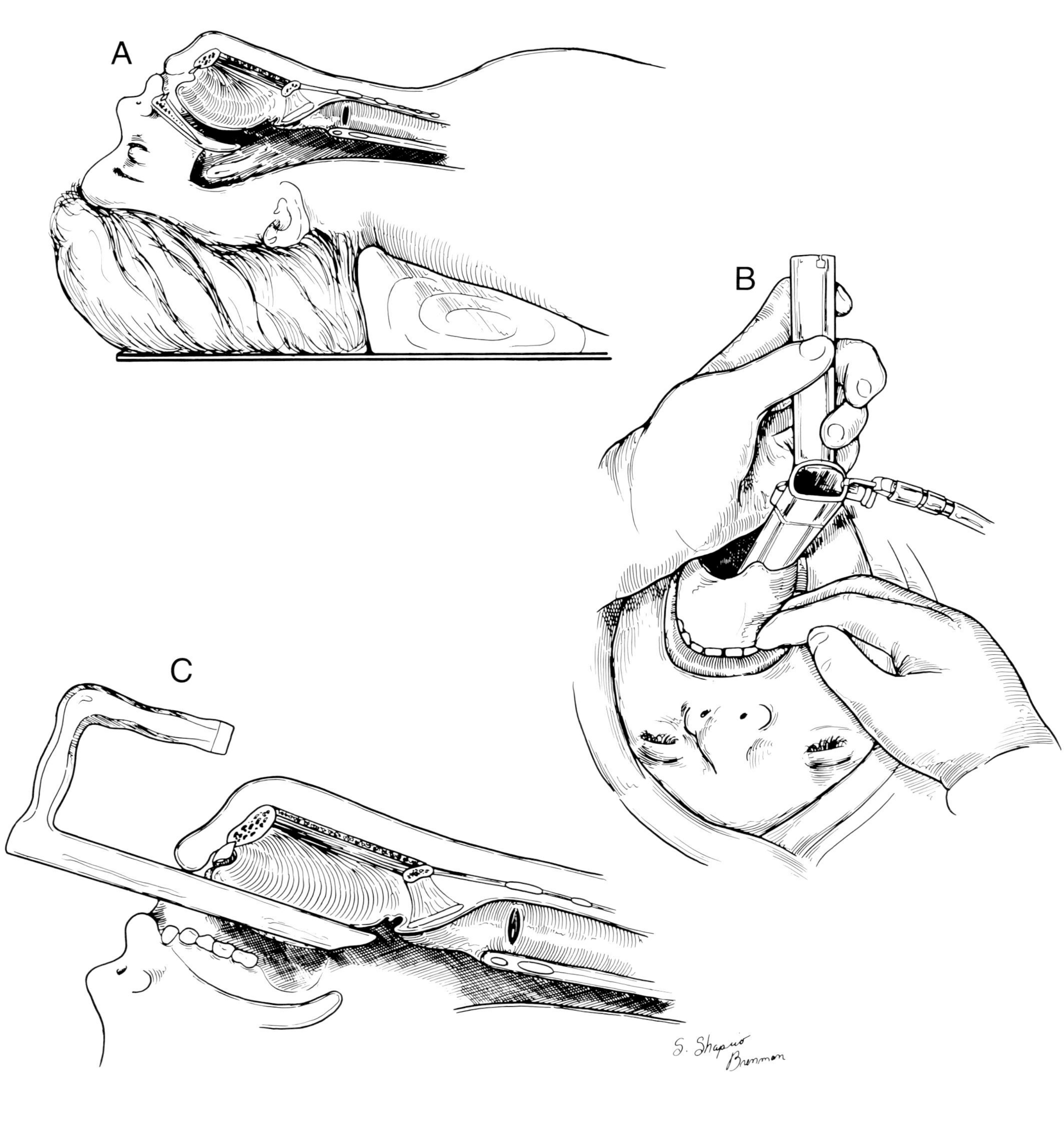


▶ **FIGURE 40-2**

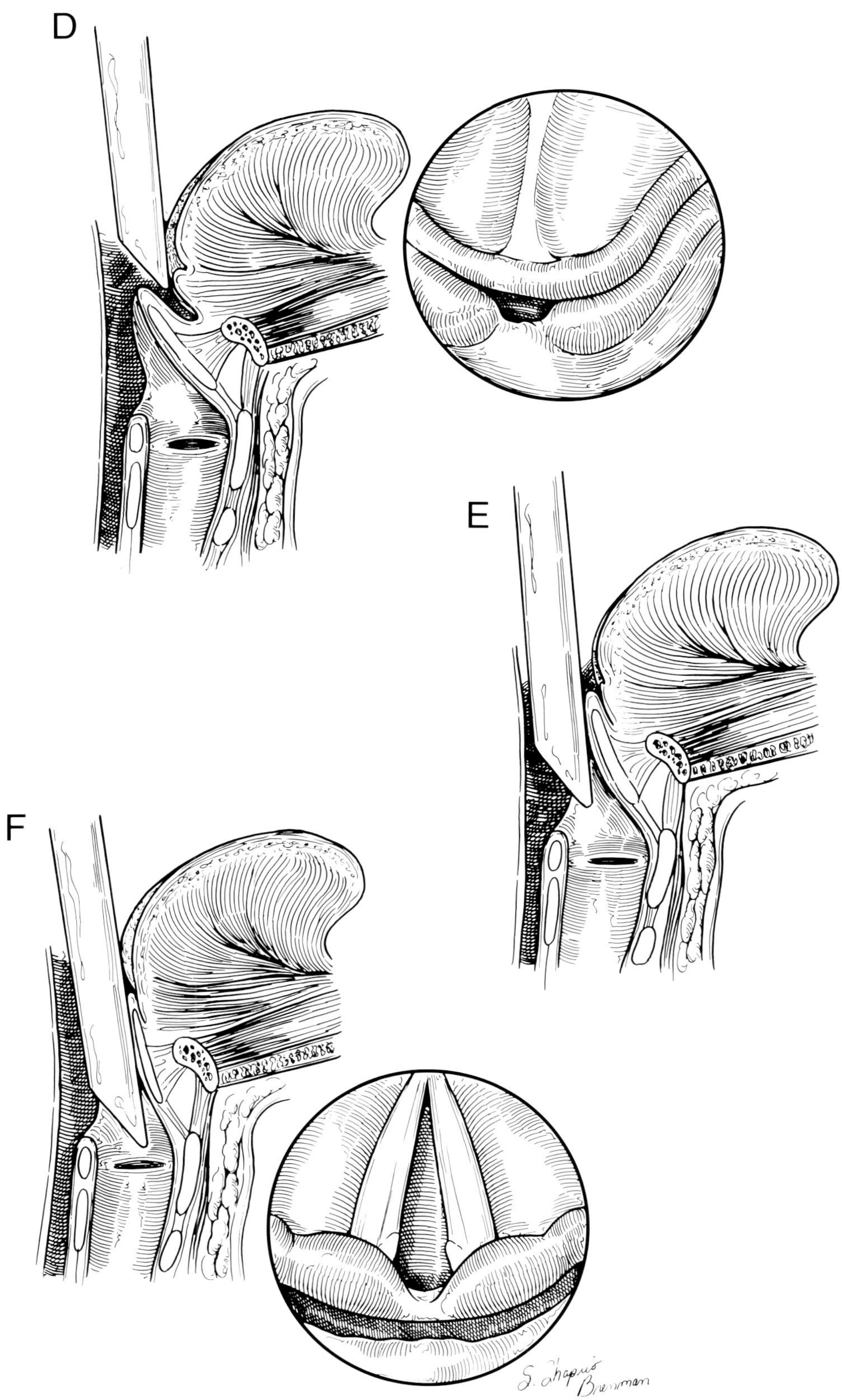


▶ **FIGURE 40-2**

# 41 ▶ Intubation

## ▶ 41-1 INTUBATION

Endotracheal intubation in children with mandibular hypoplasia (Pierre Robin sequence, Treacher-Collins syndrome) as well as other craniofacial anomalies has provided a challenge to otolaryngologists and anesthesiologists alike. In addition to the small mandible, several other features of these patients contribute to the difficult intubation: macroglossia, glossoptosis, trismus related to temporomandibular joint (TMJ) abnormalities, and prominent maxillary or mandibular incisors. Most of the traditional techniques that have been described for intubation in problem cases are difficult or impossible to use in infants and young children with mandibular hypoplasia or craniofacial anomalies. We have developed a modification of the standard direct laryngoscopic procedure, utilizing the anterior commissure laryngoscope and an optical stylet in the task of exposing and intubating the larynx of a child with mandibular hypoplasia. This procedure may be used in older children with craniofacial malformations by using appropriately sized instruments.

### Indications

A child with mandibular hypoplasia or other craniofacial anomaly in which standard intubation techniques are unlikely to be successful.

### Preoperative Evaluation

Patency of the nasal airway, size of tongue, TMJ mobility, and presence of prominent teeth must be determined preoperatively.

### Operative Technique

1. Infants in the first few weeks of life are usually not anesthetized prior to laryngoscopy and intubation. Awake intubation with continuous administration of oxygen is preferred.
2. In older patients, anesthesia is induced using 100% oxygen with halothane, and spontaneous ventilation is preserved.
3. Muscle relaxants are best avoided in patients with difficult airway problems.
4. We have chosen to use a 9 cm (pediatric) Holinger anterior commissure laryngoscope for this procedure rather than the various anesthesia laryngoscopes or the Jackson standard laryngoscope. Its straight enclosed barrel design prevents the tongue from obscuring the view of the larynx as so often occurs with the other more open instruments. In addition, its narrow profile throughout its entire length permits easier access to the laryngeal inlet and allows the barrel of the laryngoscope to slip more completely laterally into the oral commissure. Suctioning of excess secretions can be performed easily through this instrument using a straight laryngoscopic suction. Other techniques that utilize curved laryngoscopic blades, blind intubation, or flexible fiberoptic laryngoscopes do not allow such complete and easy clearing of pharyngeal secretions.

5. The dicta of Jackson regarding the position of the patient are still of prime importance. The patient is supine with the head elevated above the shoulders. The neck is flexed forward and the head extended at the atlanto-occipital joint to bring the axes of the mouth, pharynx, and larynx into alignment.
6. The laryngoscope is introduced into the mouth and advanced along the right side of the anterior two-thirds of the tongue (Fig. 41–1**A**, position a).
7. Instead of shifting the whole laryngoscope toward the midline in the traditional manner (Fig. 41–1**A**, position b), only the laryngoscope tip is directed toward the midline, while the proximal end is shifted far laterally into the oral commissure. This allows 20–30° additional anterior angulation of the blade (Fig. 41–1**B**, position a). This anterior angulation is not possible with the laryngoscope in the standard midline position because of the bulky tongue, hypoplastic mandible, and the prominent maxilla or maxillary teeth common in these children (Fig. 41–1**B**, position b).
8. With the instrument approaching the larynx from the right side, the epiglottis is visualized and elevated with the tip of the laryngoscope.
9. Visualization of the larynx within the lumen of the laryngoscope may be facilitated by external pressure over the cricoid area in the posterior and lateral (toward the laryngoscope) direction.
10. With the larynx visualized, placement of an endotracheal tube requires a special sequence of maneuvers.
    - **a.** The 15 mm adapter is removed from a tube of appropriate size and a water-soluble lubricant is placed on the outside of the tube to facilitate movement of the tube within the barrel of the laryngoscope.
    - **b.** The tube is placed in the lumen of the laryngoscope and passed beyond the vocal cords.
    - **c.** This step may be aided by the use of an optical stylet (2.7 mm diameter telescope, 27018A Karl Storz Endoscopy-America, Inc.) placed inside the endotracheal tube (Fig. 41–1**C**). (If a stylet is used, it should also be coated with a water-soluble lubricant to promote easy insertion into and removal from the endotracheal tube.)
    - **d.** The proximal end of the endotracheal tube is grasped and stabilized in its position with a laryngeal alligator forceps as the laryngoscope is withdrawn (Fig. 41–1**D**).
    - **e.** The 15 mm adapter is reinserted into the endotracheal tube and ventilation is commenced in the usual manner (Fig. 41–1E).
    - **f.** Placement of the endotracheal tube in the trachea is confirmed by auscultation for bilateral air entry and observation of bilateral chest movement.

## Complications

1. Laryngospasm
2. Glottic edema
3. Dental trauma

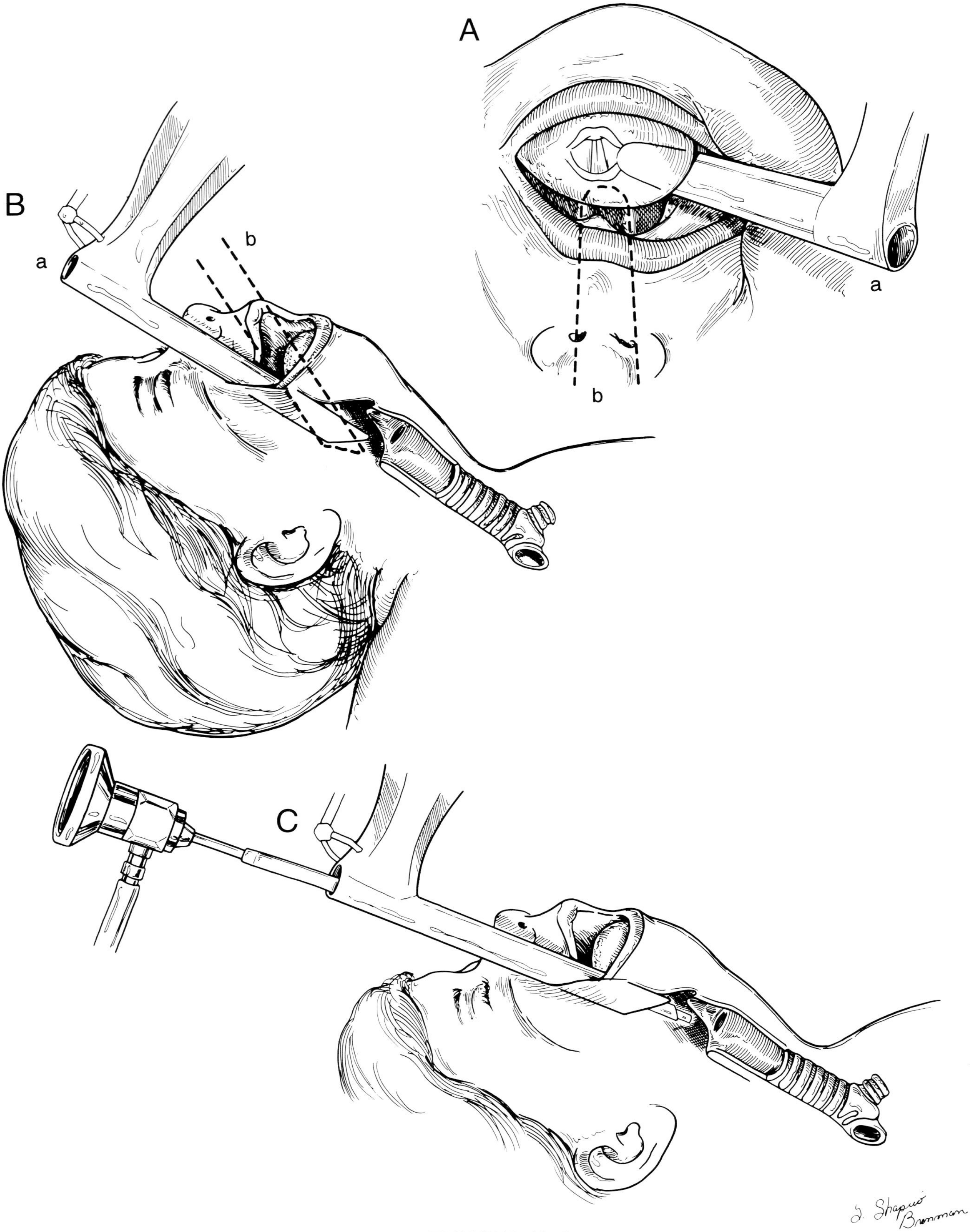


▶ **FIGURE 41-1**

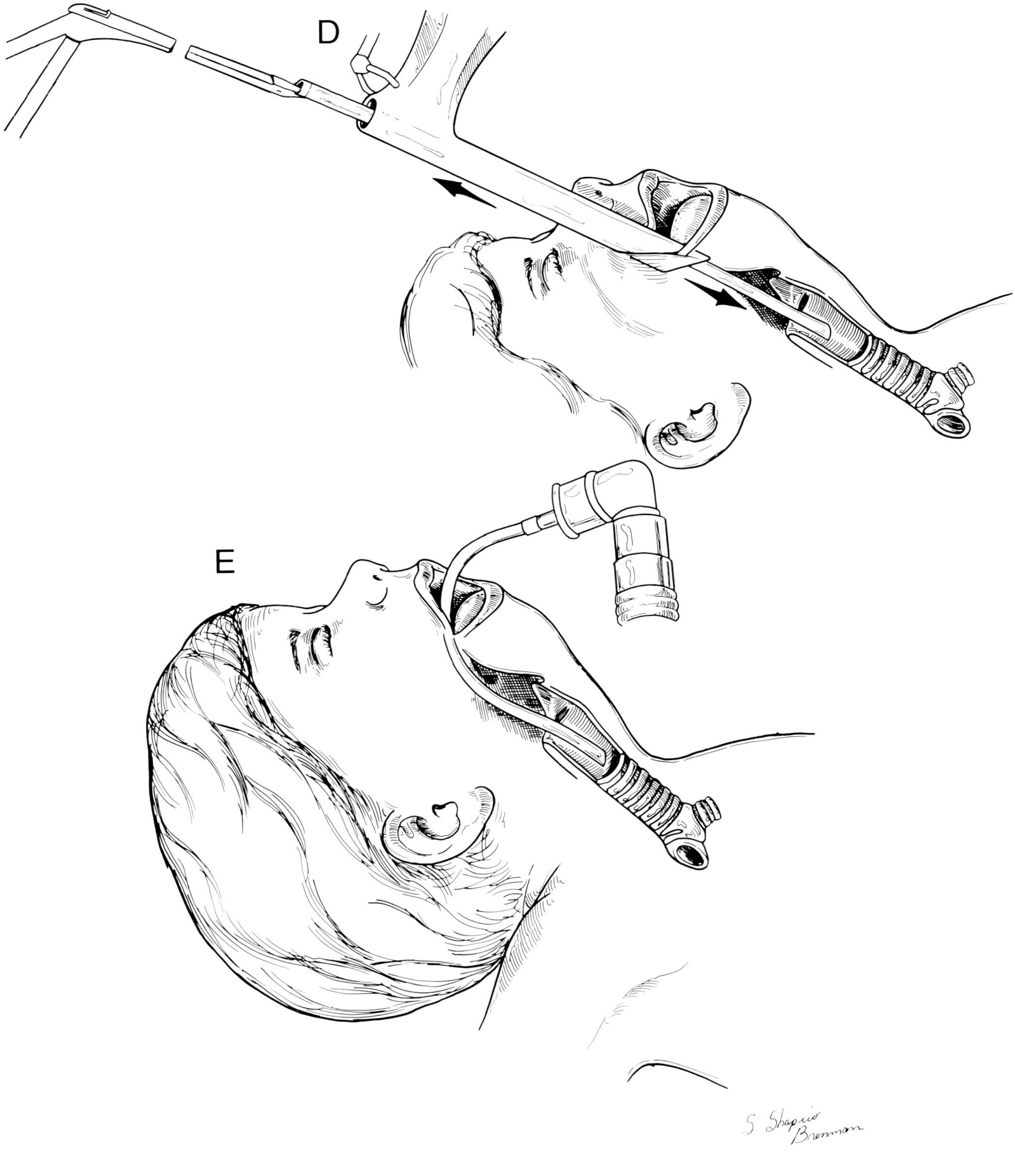


▶ **FIGURE 41-1**

# 42 ▶ Microlarynogoscopy

## ▶ 42-1 Microlaryngoscopy

In the event of laryngeal pathology that requires microscopic manipulation and removal (laryngeal papilloma, vocal cord nodules, vocal cord web, etc.), it is necessary to place a laryngoscope and stabilize its position to allow for the instrumentation. This frees both of the surgeon's hands to accomplish the surgery.

### Operative Technique

1. The child is supine on the operating room table.
2. The anesthesiologist intubates the larynx with a small foil-wrapped red rubber or metal tube (Fig. 42–1**A**) (if laser use is anticipated) taped to the left side of the mouth.
3. A roll is placed beneath the shoulders to allow for complete extension of the head on the neck.
4. The table is placed in reverse Trendelenburg position to allow for comfortable viewing of the larynx through the operating microscope.
5. The laryngoscope is introduced as described previously.
6. When the larynx is adequately visualized, the observer's end of a self-retaining laryngoscope (Jako, Dedo, etc.) can be brought over to the midline so that minimal distortion of tissues is noted.
7. The laryngoscope is inserted deeply enough to view the entire anterior laryngeal structures (Fig. 42–1**B**).
8. The suspension apparatus is attached to the laryngoscope and then suspended from a Mayo stand or attached to the operating room table. Suspending the laryngoscope from a table attached to the bed allows for movement of the entire table without disturbing the position of the laryngoscope.
9. The operating microscope is brought into place and the larynx is visualized utilizing a 400 mm lens (Fig. 42–1**C**). Instrumentation of the larynx can proceed with micro instruments and/or laser as indicated.
10. If a $CO_2$ laser is used, the patient's face must be covered with moist towels and the eyes with moist eye pads. No part of the patient's face can be exposed. Operating room personnel must wear protective eyewear.
11. If examination of the posterior commissure area is required and this area is obscured by the endotracheal tube, the tube is removed and ventilation is continued using a Venturi Jet ventilation device. The Venturi device is placed through one of the light carrier channels of the laryngoscope and positioned above the laryngeal inlet. When adequately positioned, chest wall movement can be seen after each "jet" of air, and the laryngoscopy may continue without any obstruction in the larynx (Fig. 42–1**D**).
12. A rigid suction instrument placed through one of the light carrier channels can aid in continuous smoke evacuation during laser procedures. This is

possible because illumination for this procedure is provided by the operating microscope.

**13.** At the termination of the procedure, the patient may be re-intubated to recover from the anesthesia. This can be accomplished in one of two methods:

   **a.** The laryngoscope can be removed and the patient intubated in a normal manner.

   **b.** The child can be re-intubated with the laryngoscope still in place.

      **1.** The appropriate endotracheal tube (without the anesthesia adapter) is placed through the laryngoscope and into the laryngeal lumen (Fig. 42–1E).

      **2.** The observer's end of the tube is grasped with an alligator forceps and gently advanced as the laryngoscope is withdrawn (Fig. 42–1F).

      **3.** The endotracheal tube is grasped at the level of the lips as it becomes visible as the laryngoscope is withdrawn.

      **4.** The laryngeal forceps are removed.

      **5.** The endotracheal tube adapter is placed on the end of the tube and adequate ventilation is resumed (Fig. 42–1G).

## Complications

1. Laryngospasm
2. Glottic edema
3. Dental trauma

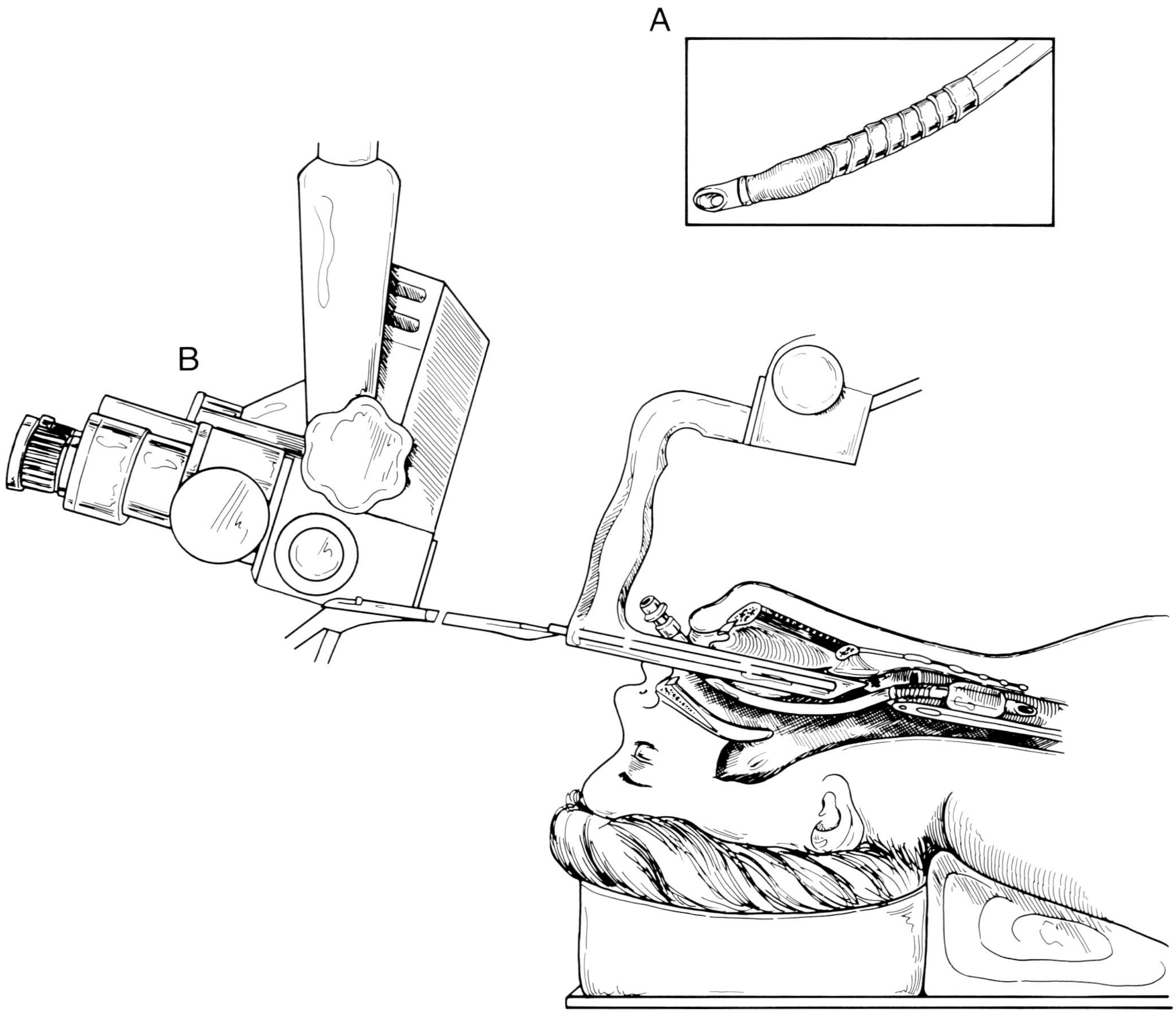


▶ **FIGURE 42-1**

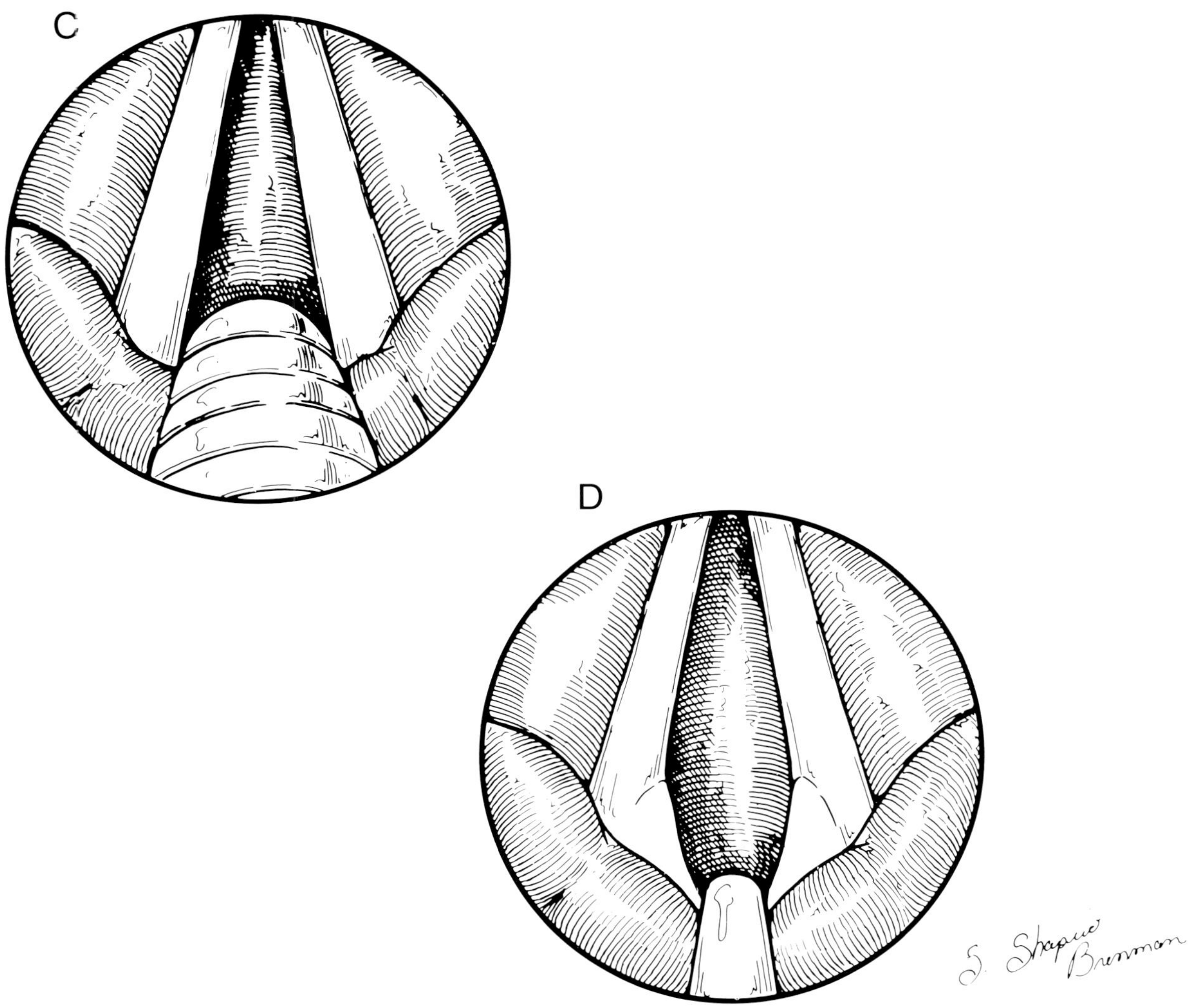


▶ **FIGURE 42-1**

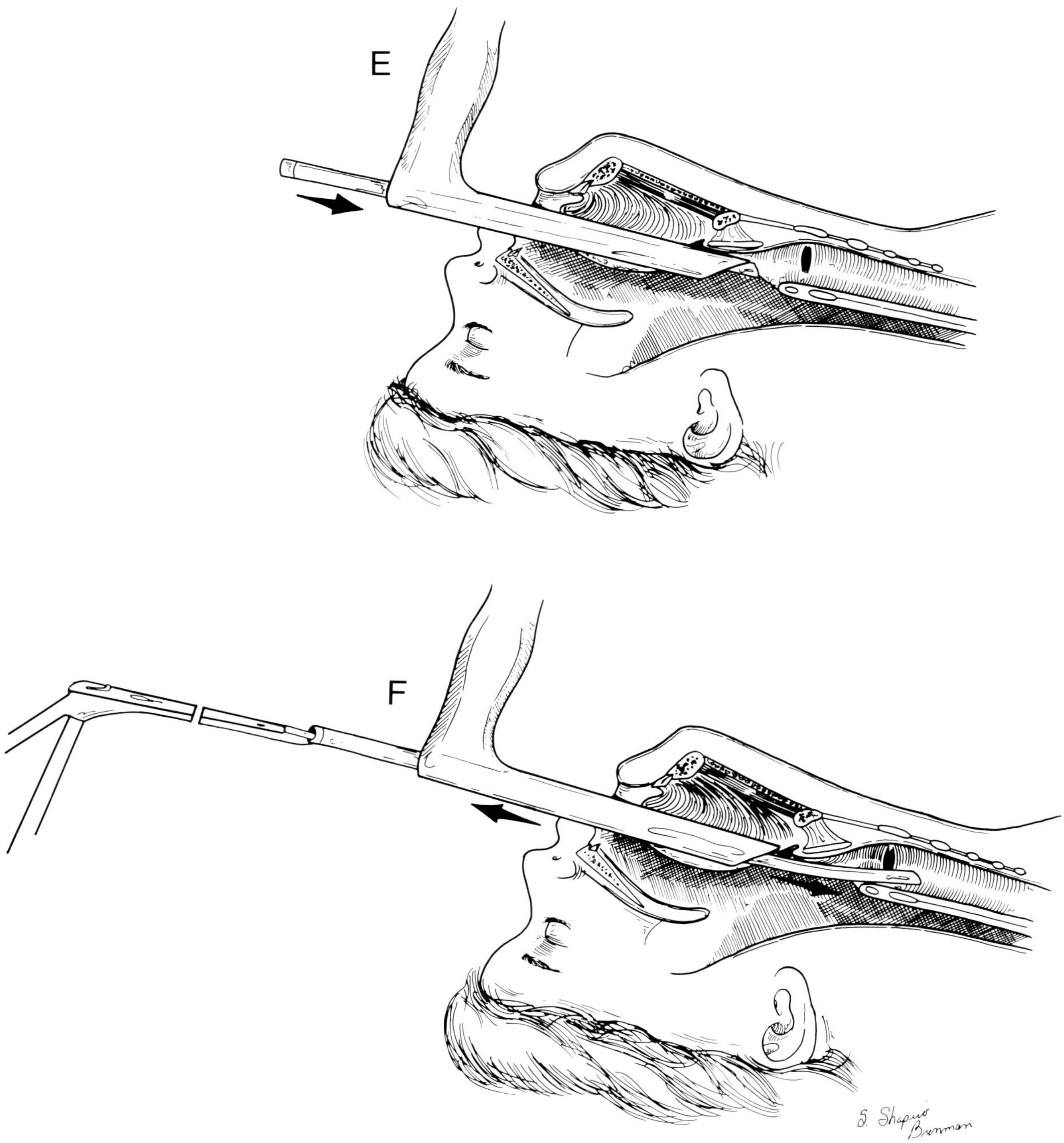


▶ **FIGURE 42-1**

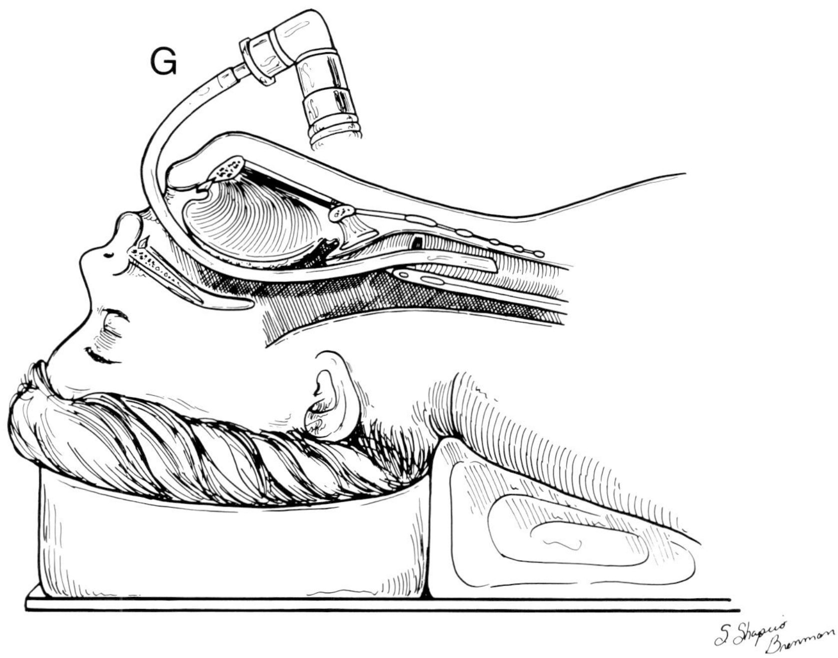


▶ **FIGURE 42-1**

# 43 ▶ Bronchoscopy

Bronchoscopy is the visual examination of the tracheobronchial tree. Both flexible and rigid instruments are available for this procedure. Rigid bronchoscopy permits instrumentation of the airway and allows for continued ventilation. Flexible bronchoscopy, while giving better visualization of the more distal bronchi, does not allow for easy foreign body removal and cannot be used to maintain an airway unless it is passed through or alongside an endotracheal tube. However, the laryngeal lumen requirement for this arrangement precludes its use in small children. Direct laryngoscopy (either flexible or rigid) always precedes bronchoscopy.

## ▶ INDICATIONS

Foreign body, lesions in the trachea or bronchi, or mucus plugging of the bronchi are indications for bronchoscopy.

## ▶ PREOPERATIVE EVALUATION

Anteroposterior and lateral chest radiographs are necessary in the preoperative evaluation in the child undergoing bronchoscopy. Computed tomography (CT) may prove helpful in localizing the disease process. Indirect laryngoscopy is useful in the preparation for the endoscopic examination.

## ▶ 43 - 1 FLEXIBLE BRONCHOSCOPY

Flexible bronchoscopy is the procedure best suited to viewing respiratory dynamics of the trachea and bronchi and details of the distal airway.

### Operative Technique

1. Flexible bronchoscopy occurs after successful flexible direct laryngoscopy has been performed.
2. As preparation is made to pass the bronchoscope through the vocal cords, the child is paralyzed or the anesthesia level is deepened sufficiently to prevent laryngospasm.
3. The bronchoscope is advanced into the subglottic space and then into the trachea and bronchi (Fig. 43–1A).
4. Usually the anesthesiologist can maintain an adequate fit with the mask and adequate ventilation can be maintained. However, if the bronchoscope is too snug in the subglottic or laryngeal area, ventilation may be limited. In this case, the bronchoscope must be withdrawn periodically to the level of the laryngeal inlet so that adequate ventilation can be maintained.
5. The bronchoscope is advanced so that the right and left bronchi are inspected in an orderly manner.

**6.** The bronchoscope is withdrawn and ventilation maintained by the anesthesiologist utilizing a mask or endotracheal tube, depending upon the situation.

## Complications

1. Laryngospasm
2. Glottic edema
3. Dental trauma

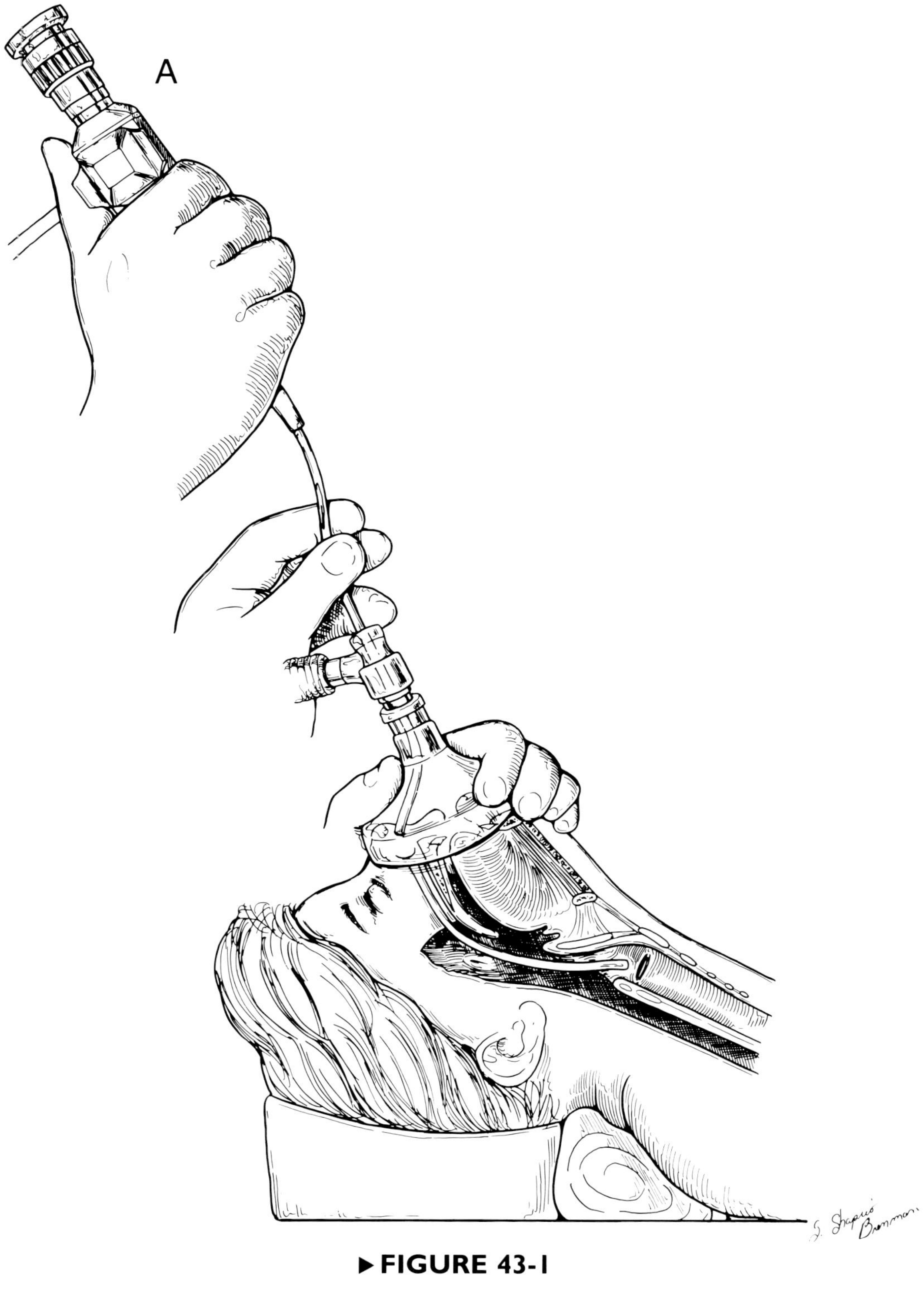


▶ **FIGURE 43-1**

## ▶ 43 - 2 RIGID BRONCHOSCOPY

### Indications

Rigid bronchoscopy is the technique of choice when management and/or manipulation of the airway is required.

### Operative Technique

1. Direct laryngoscopy has already been performed utilizing the slide or open blade operating laryngoscope.
2. The laryngoscope is placed in the vallecula, holding up the posterior tongue so that the epligottis and laryngeal inlet fall in the view of the scope. However, in some instances, it may be necessary to place the tip of the laryngoscope under the epiglottis to visualize the laryngeal inlet.
3. The bronchoscope is inserted with the examiner's right hand and advanced down the shaft of the laryngoscope until the laryngeal lumen is identified (Fig. 43–2**A**).
4. The bevel of the bronchoscope is kept in the anteroposterior direction so that it can be insinuated between the vocal cords (Fig. 43–2**B**). Occasionally, it is necessary to gently twist the bronchoscope to push the vocal cords apart to allow passage of the instrument.
5. As the instrument is passed below the subglottic space, the laryngoscope is removed and the anesthesiologist connects his tubing to the end of the bronchoscope. Adequate ventilation is ascertained by auscultating both lung fields to determine proper placement of the bronchoscope.
6. The bronchoscope is then advanced to the area of the carina to visualize both mainstream orifices (Fig. 43–2**C**). The head is rotated to the right so that the left bronchus and its branches can be examined. The scope is withdrawn to the carina and the head is turned to the left so that the right bronchus and orifices can be examined in a similar manner.
7. At the termination of the procedure, the bronchoscope is withdrawn. The endotracheal tube is replaced by the anesthesiologist or the otolaryngologist so that the child may be awakened with an endotracheal tube in place.

### Complications

1. Laryngospasm
2. Glottic edema
3. Dental trauma

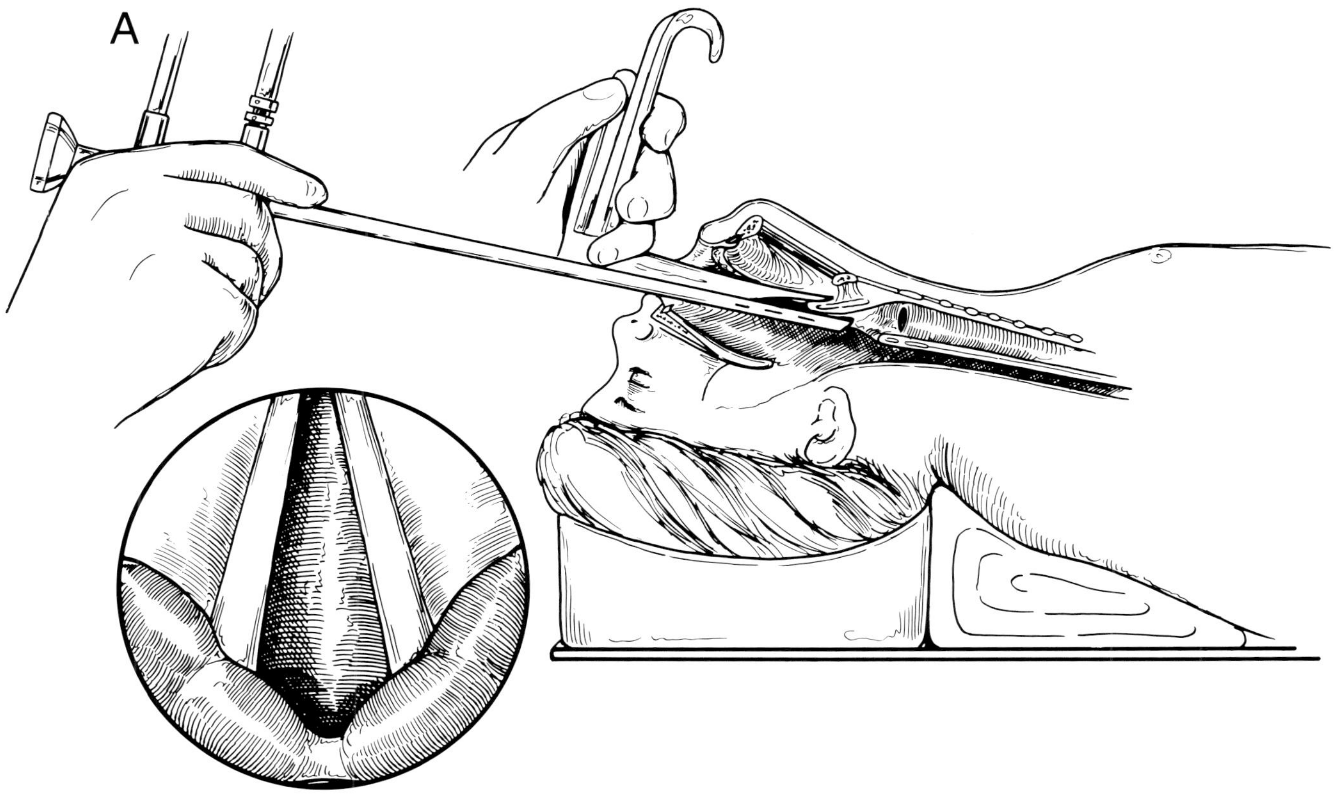


▶ **FIGURE 43-2**

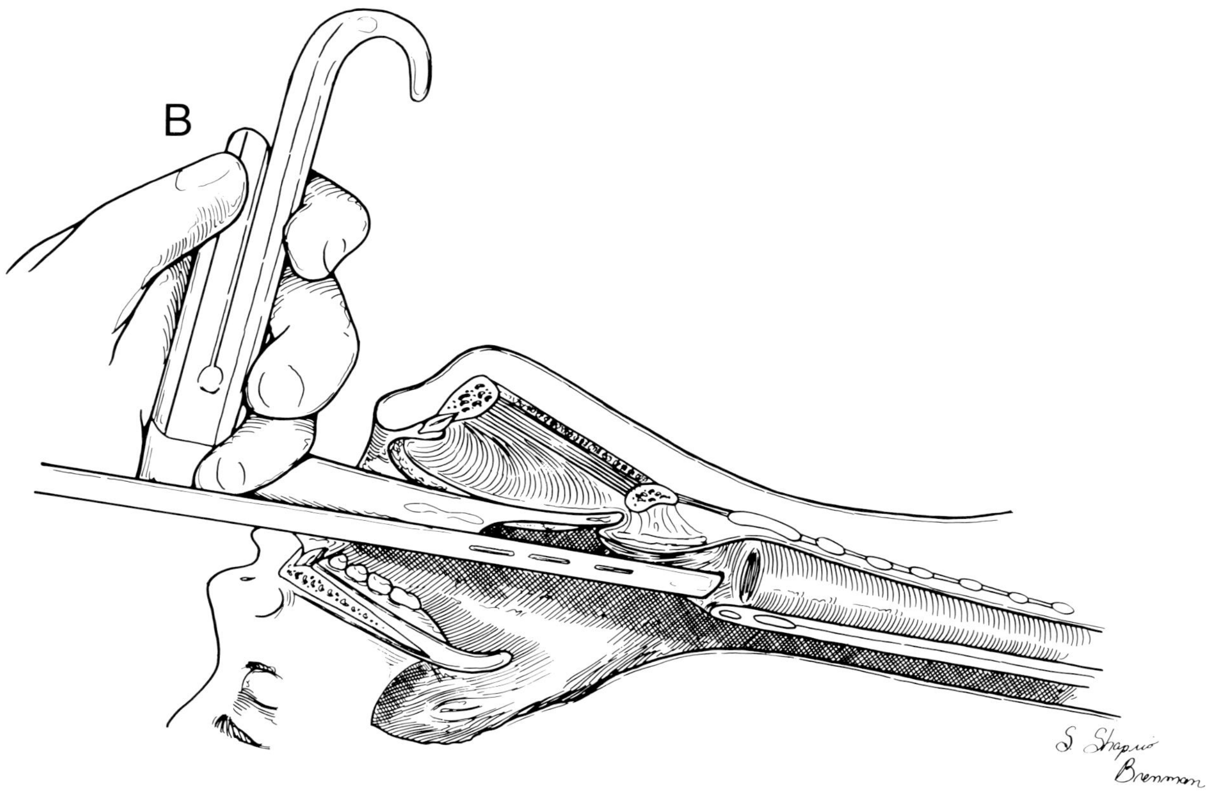


▶ **FIGURE 43-2**

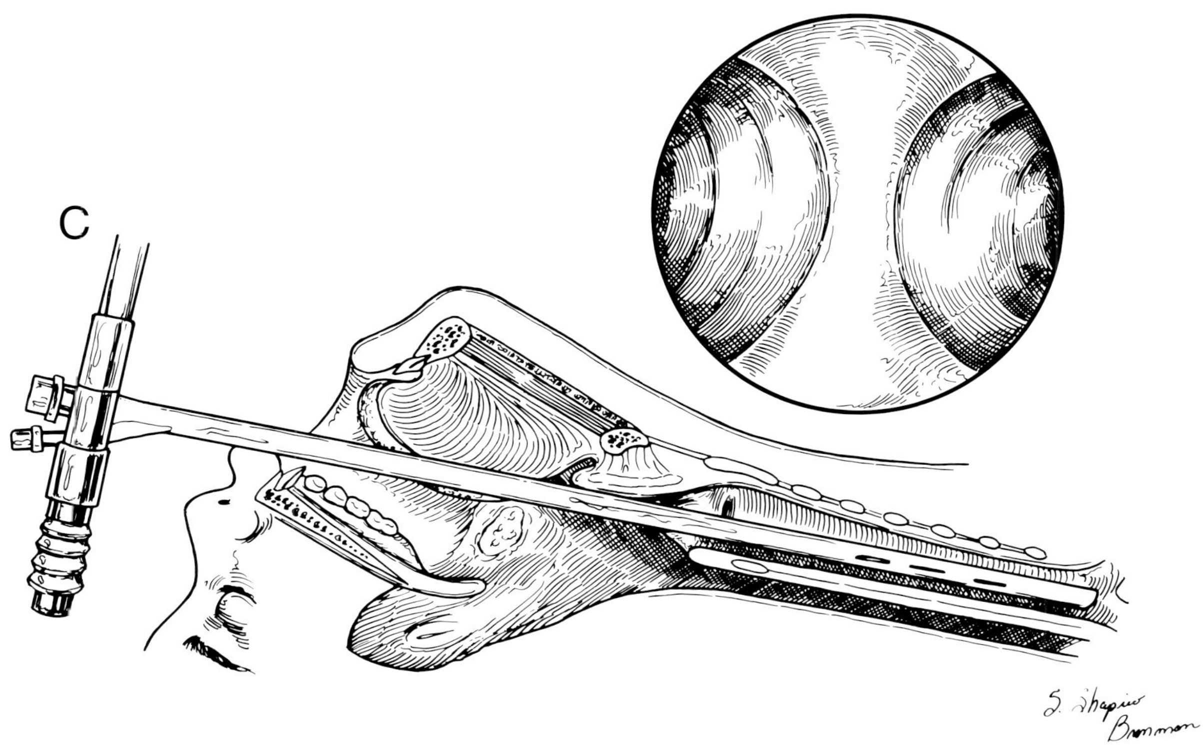


▶ **FIGURE 43-2**

# 44 ▶ Esophagoscopy

Esophagoscopy is the visual examination of the esophagus. Both flexible and rigid instruments are available for this procedure.

## ▶ INDICATIONS

The presence or suspected presence of esophageal pathology (burn, stricture, fistula) or foreign body is the indication for esophagoscopy.

## ▶ PREOPERATIVE EVALUATION

Radiographic evaluation with plain film and/or contrast study is usually performed prior to esophagoscopy.

## ▶ 44-1 FLEXIBLE ESOPHAGOSCOPY

Flexible esophagoscopy has the advantage of being relatively atraumatic, but is unsuited for foreign body removal, dilatation, or other instrumentation of the esophagus. However, excellent examination of the mucosa can be obtained using this technique.

### Operative Technique

1. The child is supine and under adequate endotracheal anesthesia.
2. The esophagoscope is inserted into the mouth and advanced to the area of the esophageal inlet (Fig. 44–1**A**).
3. The flexible instrument is advanced through the esophagus (Fig. 44–1**B**) as the lumen is continually in view until the rugal folds are identified (Fig. 44–1**C**).
4. The esophagus is examined again as the instrument is withdrawn.

### Complications

1. Esophageal perforation

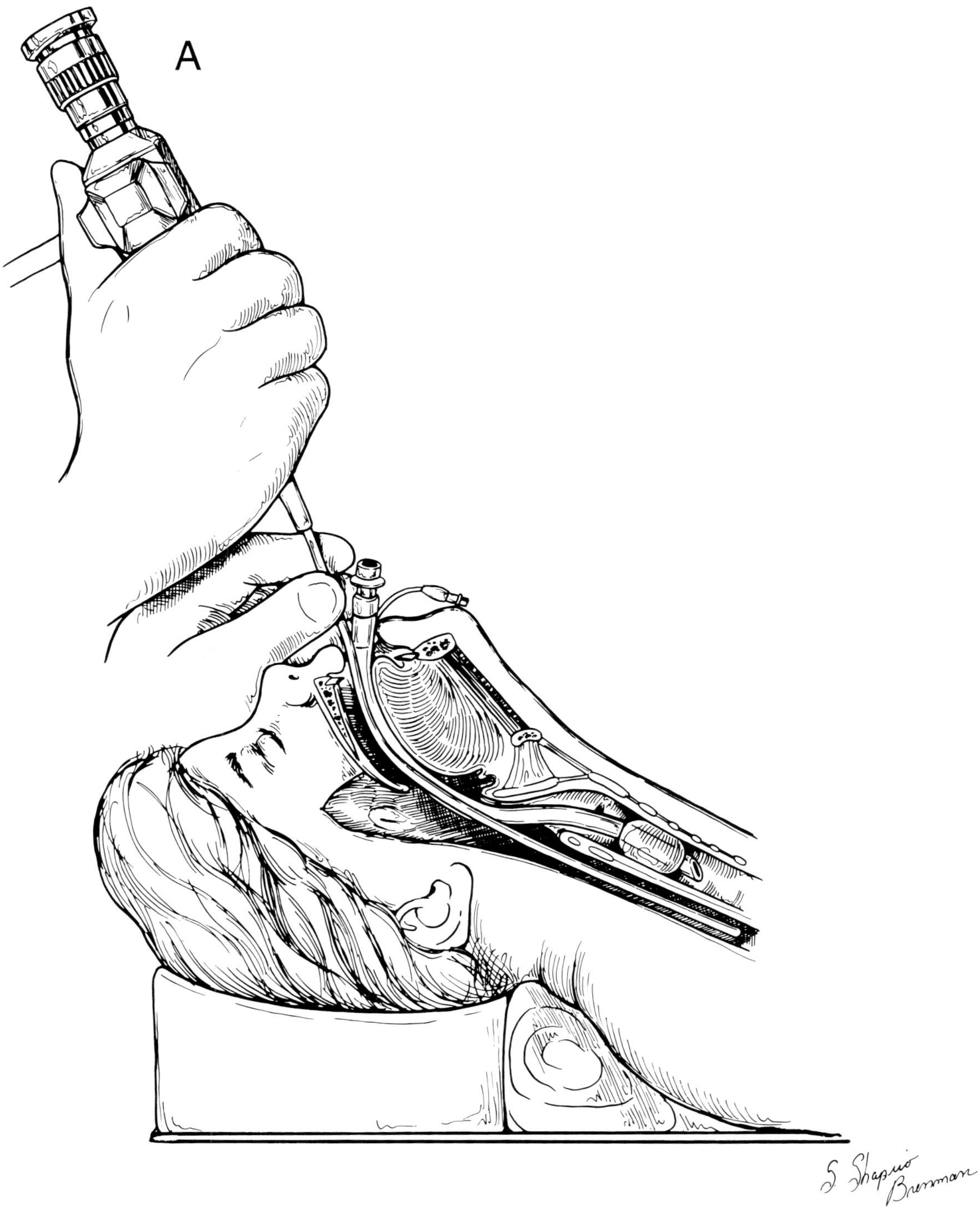


▶ **FIGURE 44-1**

B

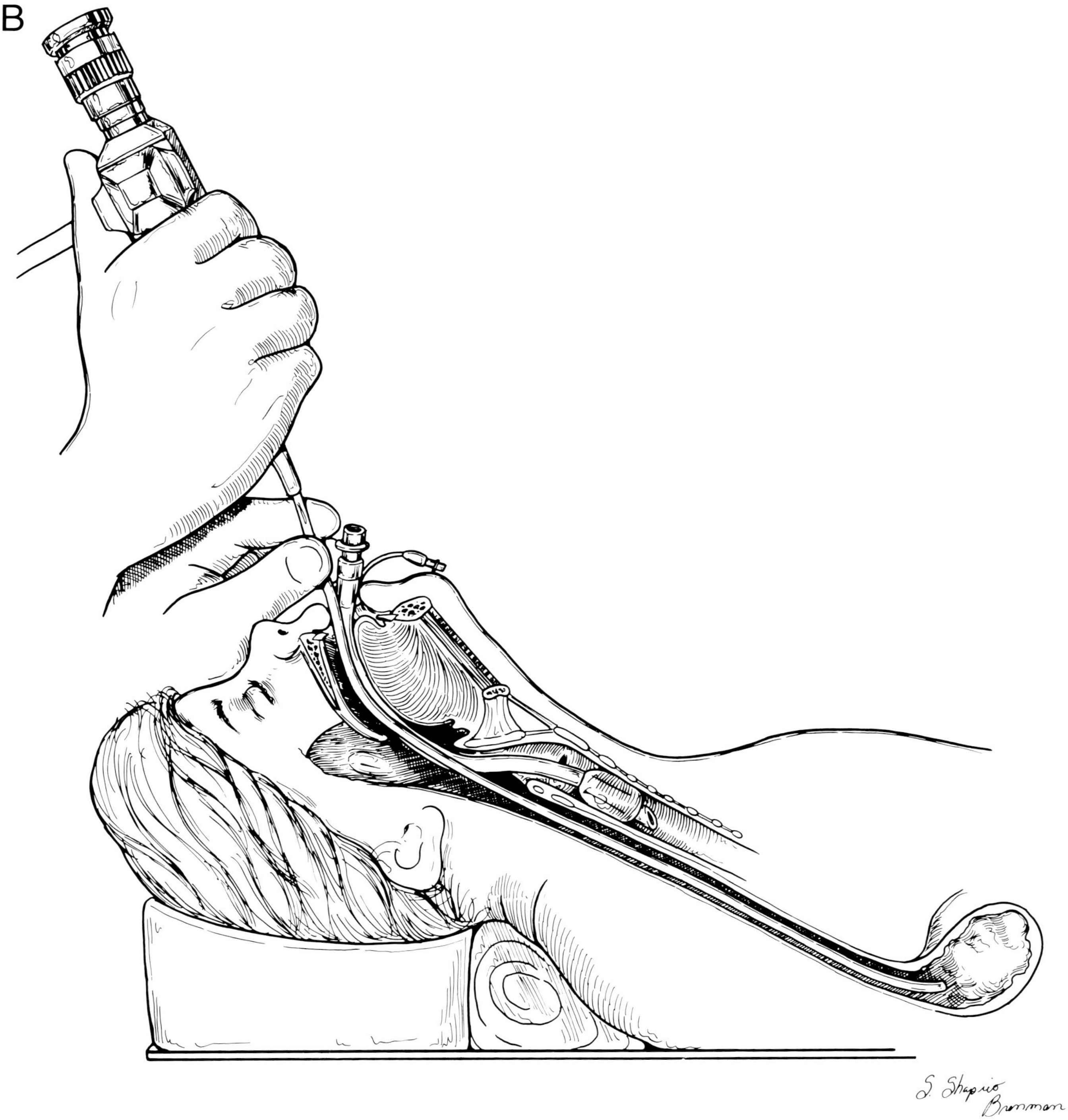

▶ **FIGURE 44-1**

C

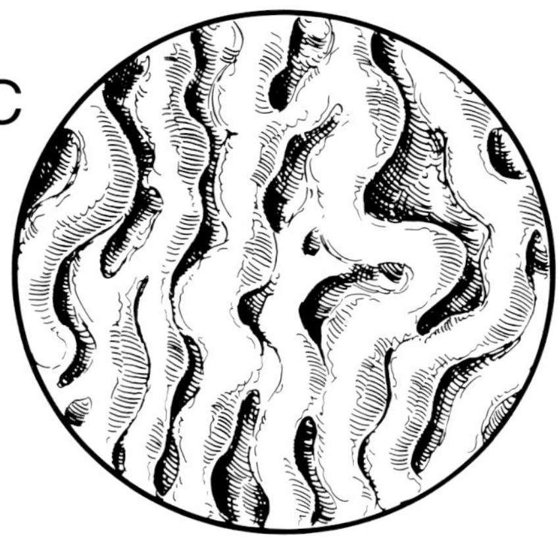

▶ **FIGURE 44-1**

## ▶ 44-2 RIGID ESOPHAGOSCOPY

Rigid esophagoscopy is the procedure of choice in almost all cases because it allows for precise and gentle instrumentation of the esophagus.

### Operative Technique

1. The child is supine and under adequate endotracheal anesthesia with the tube taped to the left side.
2. The slide or open blade operating laryngoscope is utilized as described in the section on laryngoscopy to visualize the laryngeal structures.
3. The postcricoid area is identified and the esophagoscope is inserted (with the right hand) (Fig. 44–2A) to the level of the cricopharyngeus (Fig. 44–2B).
4. The laryngoscope is removed and the esophagoscope is gently advanced using both hands.
5. The surgeon's left hand rests on the child's mouth to guide the esophagoscope.
6. The esophagoscope is only advanced when an adequate lumen is identified.
7. Secretions are cleared from the esophagoscope utilizing long suction instruments.
8. Telescopic examination of the mucosa can be utilized, as necessary (Fig. 44–2C).
9. The esophagoscope is gently advanced to the area of the gastroesophageal junction (Fig. 44–2D).
10. The termination of the procedure is indicated by the appearance of gastric rugal folds in the distal end of the scope.
11. The esophagus is examined again as the instrument is withdrawn.

### Complications

1. Dental trauma
2. Esophageal perforation

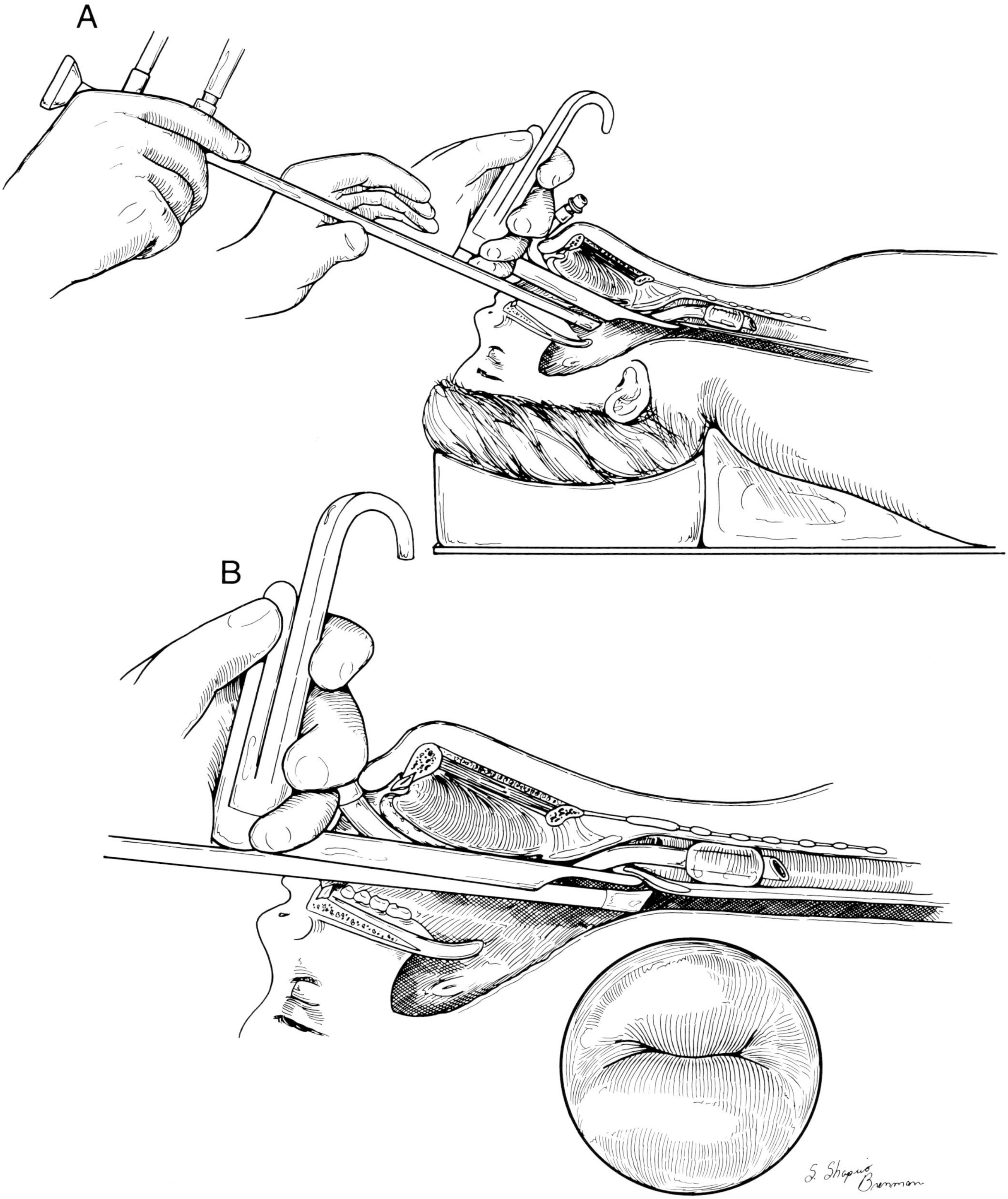


▸ **FIGURE 44-2**

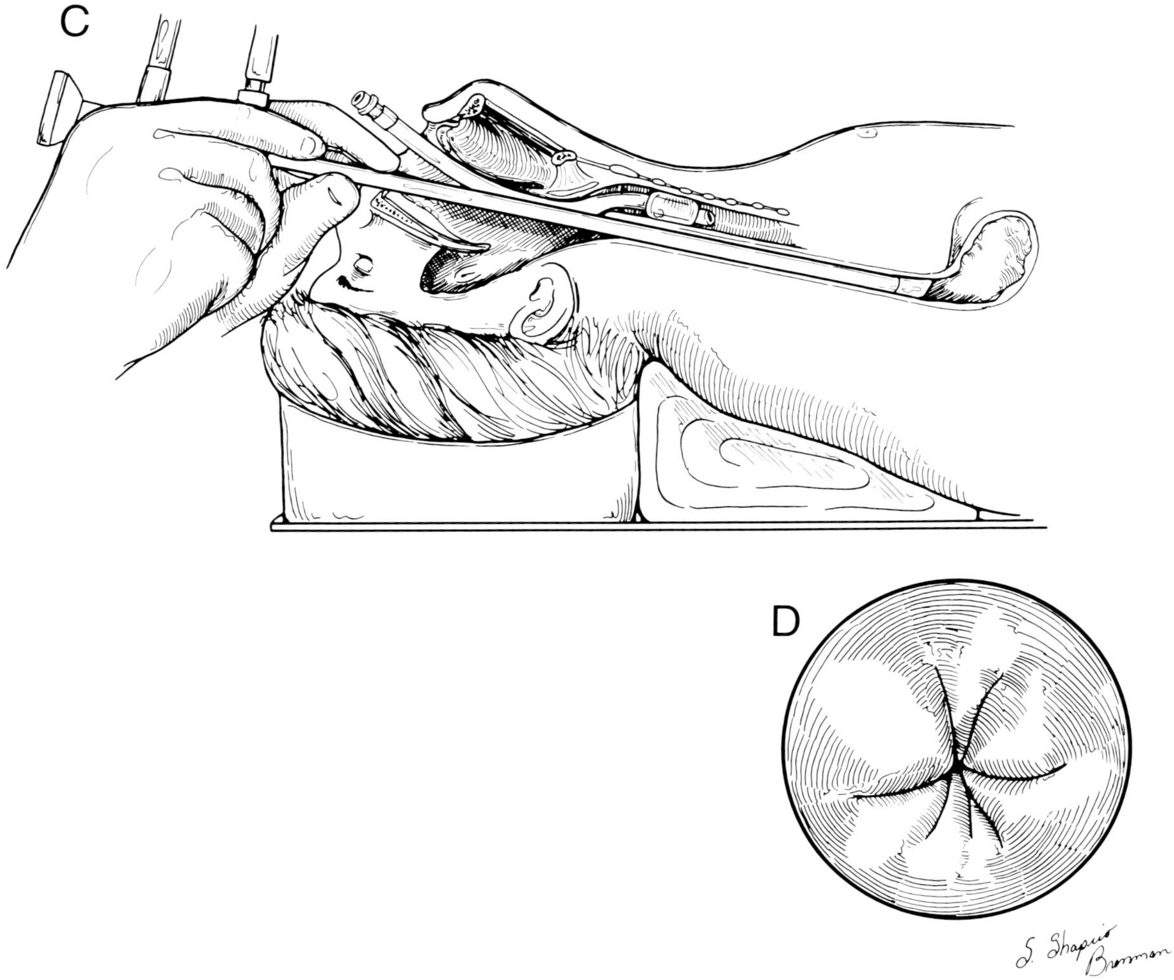


▶ **FIGURE 44-2**

# PART VIII

# Facial Trauma

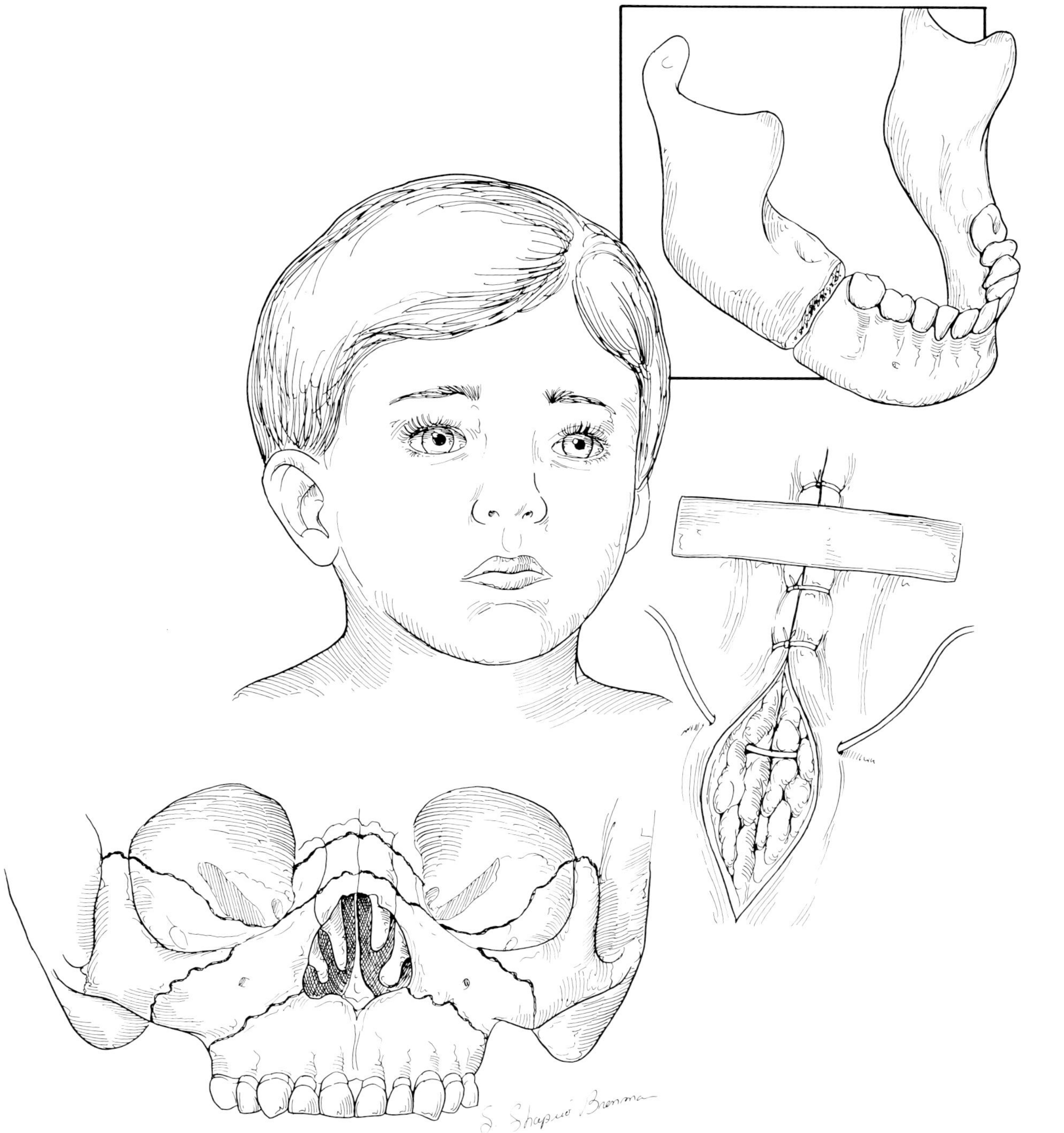

# 45 ▶ Facial Lacerations

Facial lacerations are common in children as a result of their frequent falls and accidents. The majority of these injuries are superficial and require minimal care. However, some of these lacerations have deeper and/or associated injuries that must be detected and treated.

## ▶ 45 - 1 REPAIR OF LACERATIONS

### Indications

A facial laceration through the dermis that is too large to approximate with Steri-strips should be sutured.

### Preoperative Evaluation

The presence of any associated injury must be determined. Facial x-rays are indicated if fractures are suspected.

### Operative Technique

1. Small lacerations may be sutured using local anesthesia, but larger, complex lacerations of the head and neck are best closed utilizing general anesthesia.
2. Lacerations should be cleaned of any foreign debris.
3. Subcutaneous absorbable sutures (4-0 or 5-0 chromic) are useful to help close the deep lacerations, but should be kept to a minimum to reduce tissue reaction in the wound. It is helpful to start in the middle of the laceration to aid in lining up the edges correctly.
4. The skin is closed with interrupted buried subcuticular absorbable sutures when possible (Fig. 45–1**A**,**B**,**C**).
5. Care is taken to take a larger "bite" of the dermis and subcutaneous tissue than the epidermis in order to evert the wound and bury the knot (Fig. 45–1**D**).
6. Steri-strips are then applied to reduce skin tension (Fig. 45–1**C**, **E**).
7. If an interrupted subcutaneous closure is not possible, an interrupted closure with 6-0 mild chromic (which usually do not need to be removed) or nylon can be used, again being careful to evert the wound edges (Fig. 45–1**E**, **F**).
8. Steri-strips can be applied across the closure to reduce wound tension, if desired. (Fig. 45–1**E**).
9. Facial sutures are removed at 3 to 4 days to prevent stitch marks. Neck sutures are removed in 4 to 6 days.

### Complications

1. Widened scar
2. Uneven skin edges

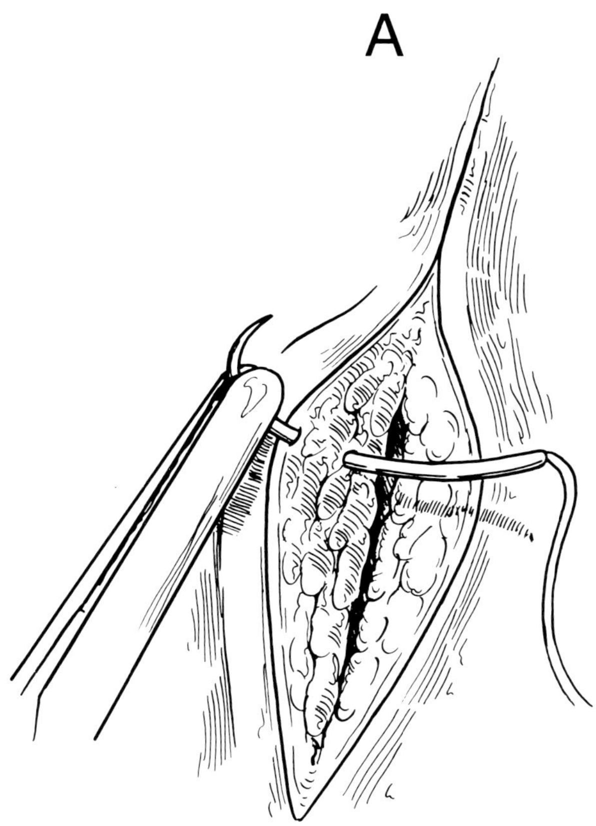


▶ **FIGURE 45-1**

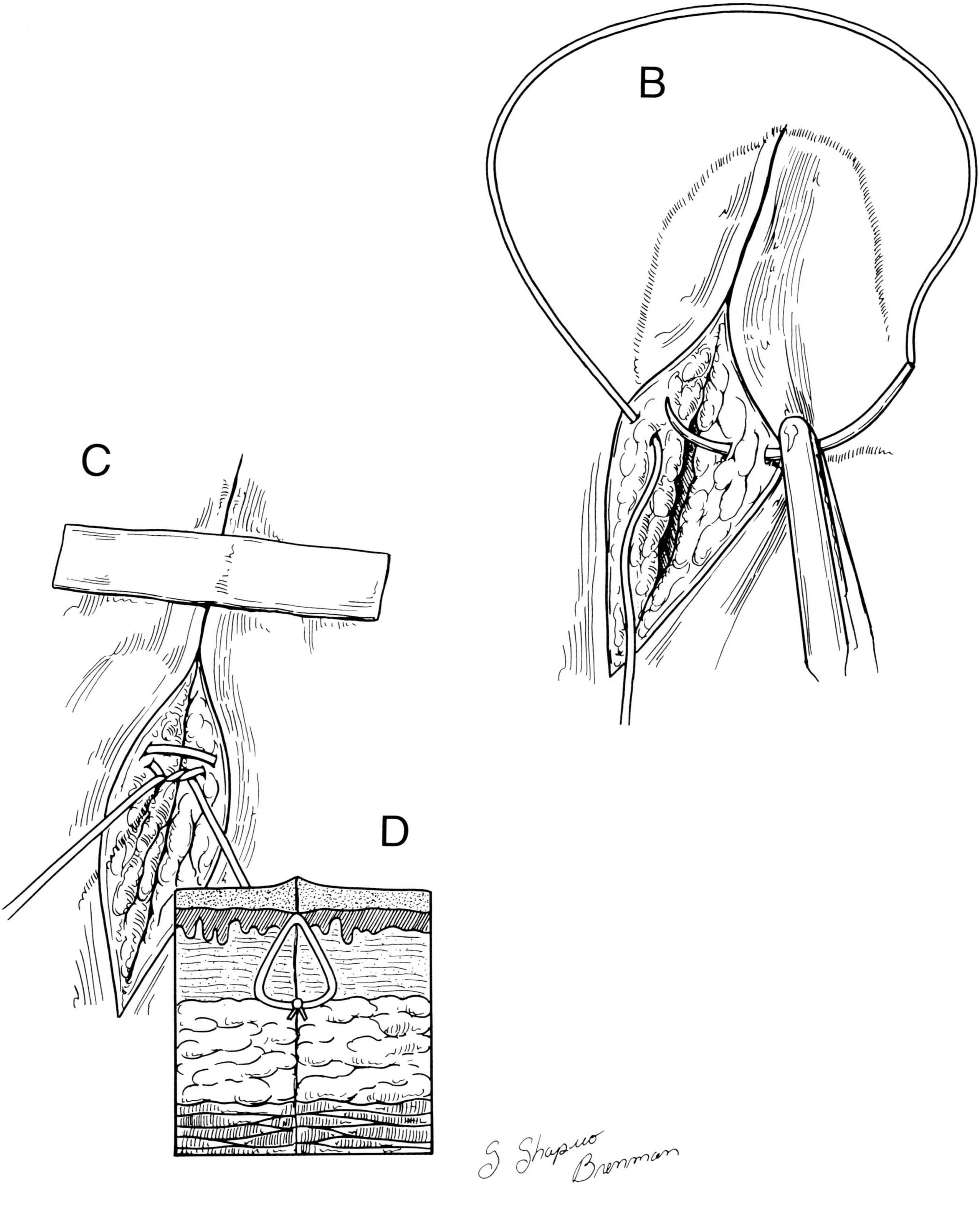


▶ **FIGURE 45-1**

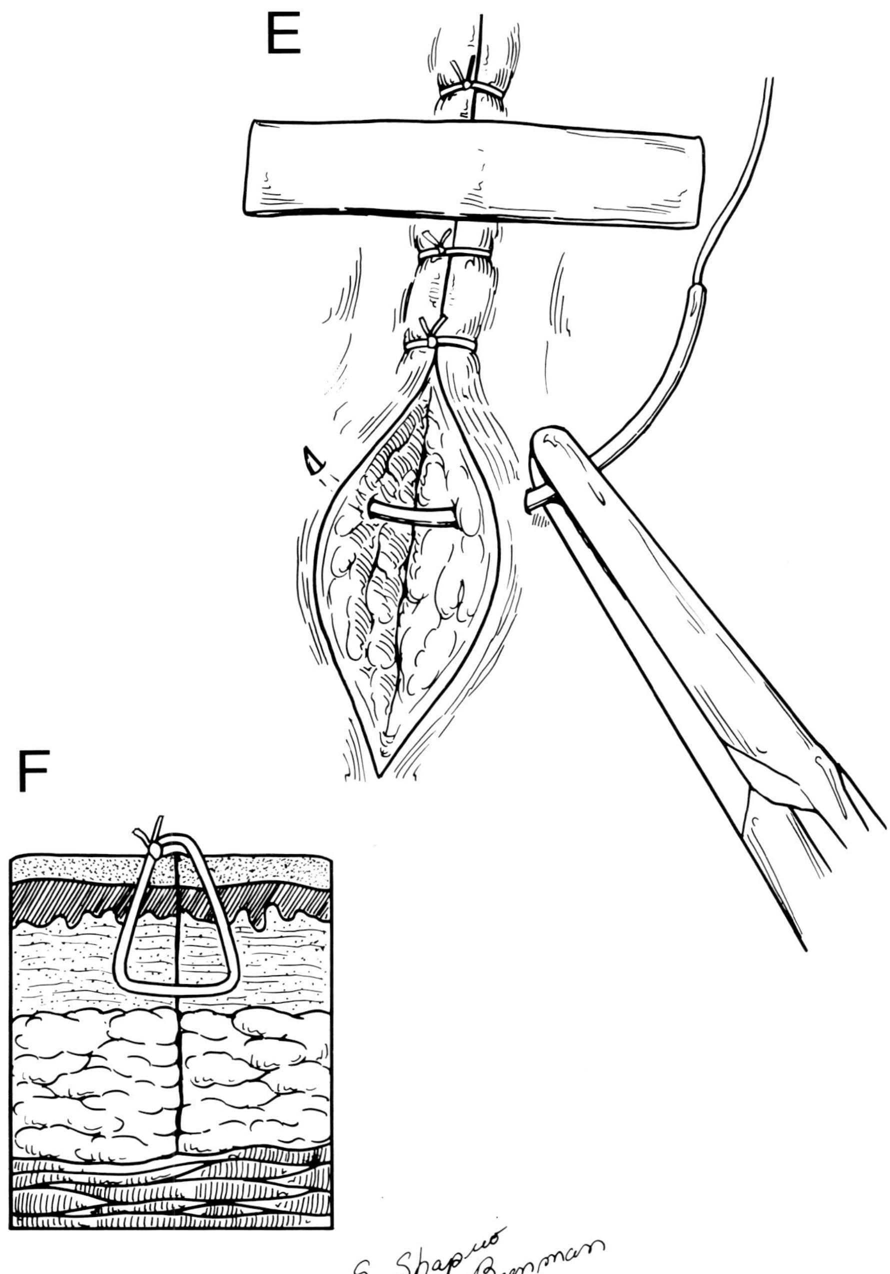


▶ **FIGURE 45-1**

# 46 ▸ Nasal Fractures

Nasal fractures may occur at any age, but are uncommon in early childhood. They account for the largest group of facial fractures because of the nose's prominent position on the face.

## ▸ 46-1 TREATMENT OF NASAL FRACTURES

### Indications

Reduction of nasal fractures is indicated if there is significant cosmetic or functional deformity.

### Preoperative Evaluation

A complete examination of the nose and surrounding structures is necessary. Associated injuries to the orbit must be identified and treated. Inspection of the nose will usually reveal the nasal deformity. Palpation of the nose may detect bone irregularities (stepoffs) on the nasal bones. However, if 30 to 60 minutes have passed, the edema over the bony structures may obscure the deformity.

If the patient is seen several hours after the injury and edema is present, the patient should be reexamined 5 to 7 days later to determine the presence of any nasal deformity after the acute edema has resolved.

Septal hematomas should be detected and treated immediately (see section 11–1, Evacuation of Septal Hematoma and Abscess).

Nasal bone radiographs are occasionally helpful in identifying a fracture site, but only the clinical examination can determine if the cosmetic deformity present is sufficient to justify intervention (Fig. 46–1**A**).

Nasal fracture reduction is best carried out 4 to 7 days following the injury. This allows tissue edema from the injury to subside and permits a more precise reduction.

### Operative Technique

1. Nasal reduction in children is best accomplished under general anesthesia.
2. The nose is packed with 4% cocaine hydrochloride using neurosurgical pledgets for decongestion and hemostasis (alternately, any combination of a topical vasoconstrictor and local anesthetic may be used).
3. A flat, blunt instrument (such as a Boies nasal fracture elevator) is placed in the nose, and the depressed nasal bone is mobilized anterolaterally (Fig. 46–1B).
4. If the opposite nasal bone is displaced laterally, it is reduced to its normal position manually.
5. The fractured fragments are then gently replaced in their normal position by manual palpation (Fig. 46–1C).
6. Care is taken to make sure that the septum is in its normal midline position.
7. Gelfoam or oxycel (Surgicel) is then placed in the nose to support the fracture fragments, if necessary. This is rarely needed in young children.

8. An external nasal splint of plaster or a prefabricated material is placed to prevent reinjury while the nose heals (Fig. 46–1D). This is removed after 1 week.

## Complications

1. Cosmetic deformity secondary to inadequate reduction
2. Epistaxis

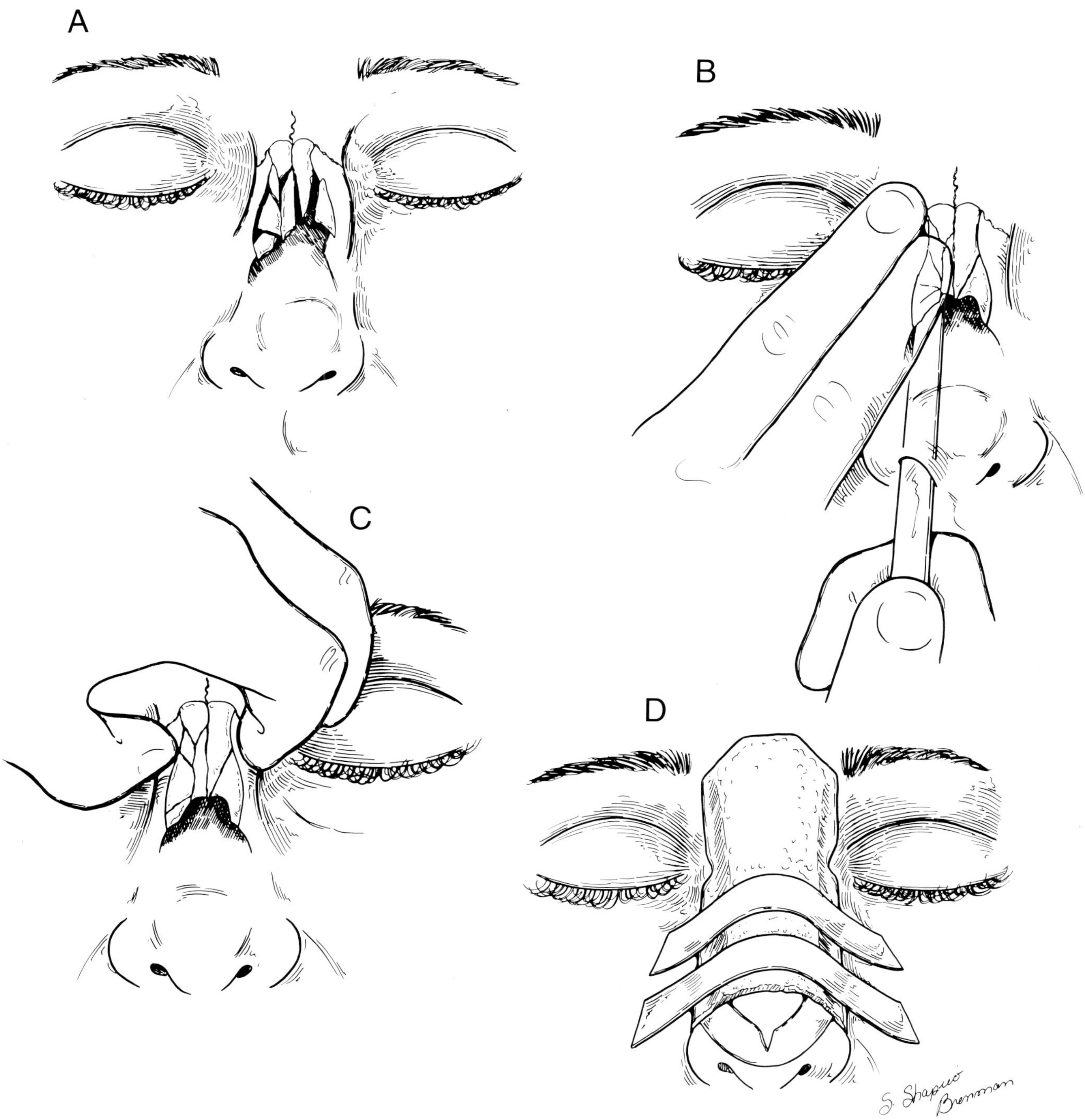


▶ **FIGURE 46-1**

# 47 ▸ Zygomatic Arch Fractures

Zygomatic arch fractures occur from direct trauma to the side of the face. The arch is most often fractured in two or three places; the fragments are usually depressed, causing a visible flat deformity of the cheek.

## ▸ 47-1 TREATMENT OF ZYGOMATIC ARCH FRACTURES

### Indications

If a zygomatic fracture results in a cosmetic deformity or trismus, operative intervention is required.

### Preoperative Evaluation

While plain radiographs of the face can demonstrate the fracture, computed tomography (CT) provides the best evaluation of the fracture and any associated injuries.

### Operative Technique

1. Zygomatic arch fractures are elevated in children utilizing general nasotracheal anesthesia.
2. A small incision is made in the buccal mucosa lateral to the maxilla (Fig. 47–1A). One percent lidocaine with 1:100,000 epinephrine is injected at the incision site to aid in hemostasis.
3. An elevator or bar is inserted under the zygoma. Using the maxilla as a fulcrum, the fracture is elevated into place (Fig. 47–1B).
4. No splint is needed and two or three chromic sutures are sufficient for closure of the intraoral incision (Fig. 47–1C).

### Complications

1. Insufficient reduction

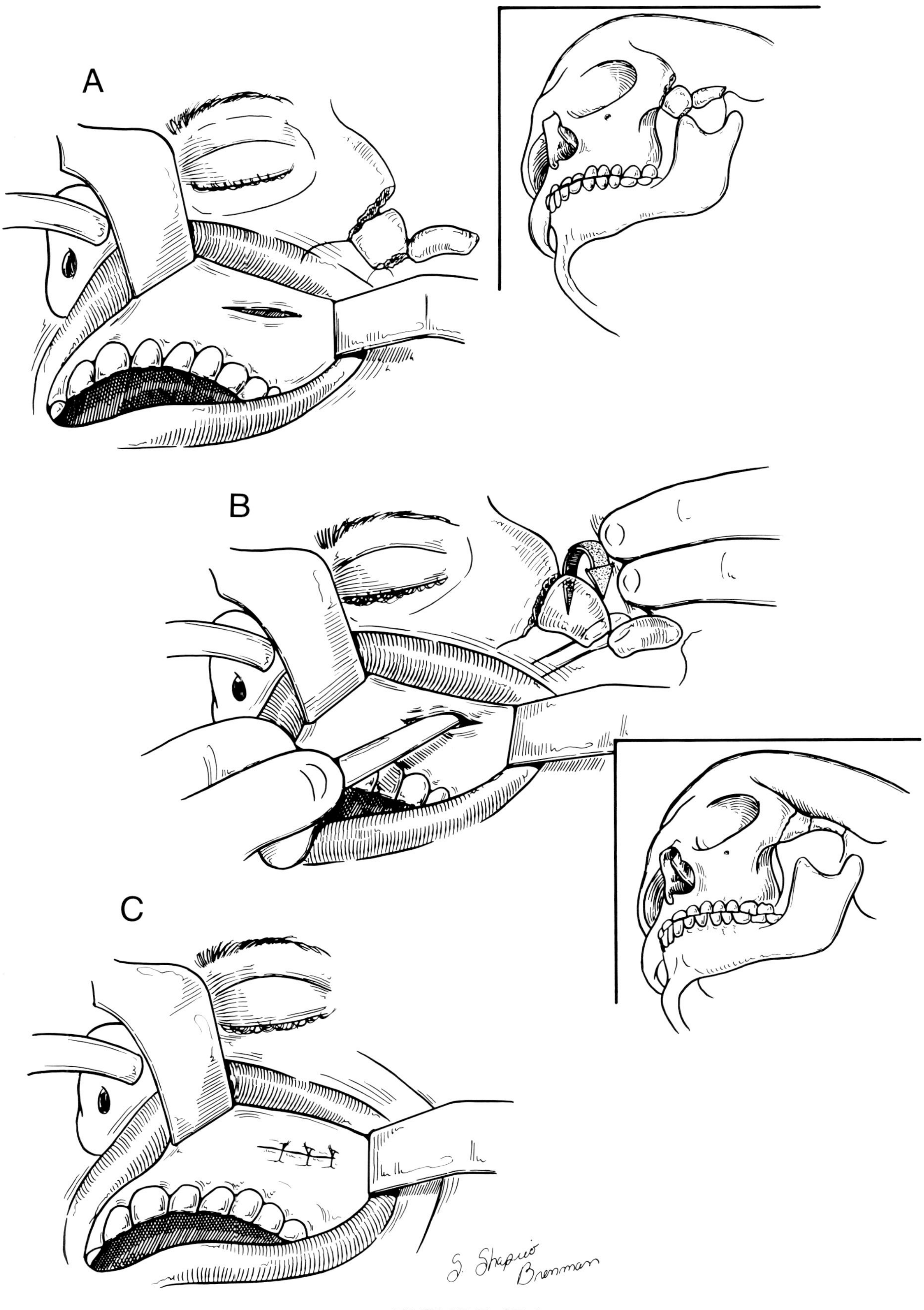


▶FIGURE 47-1

# 48 ▸ Malar Fractures

Malar fractures usually occur as a result of direct trauma to the malar eminence (cheekbone). The malar bone fractures at its frontal, temporal, and maxillary attachments. The resulting fracture is often depressed and rotated (Fig. 48–1**A**).

## ▸ 48 - 1 TREATMENT OF MALAR FRACTURES

### Indications

A depressed malar fracture with cosmetic deformity requires surgical intervention.

### Preoperative Evaluation

Fracture stepoffs can often be palpated along the inferior orbital rim and at the zygomatic frontal attachment. Infraorbital hypesthesia may be present from injury to the infraorbital nerve. CT of the facial bones is best to demonstrate the fracture and any associated injuries. Ophthalmologic evaluation should be obtained prior to surgical intervention. Fracture reduction should be carried out when the patient's general condition is stable and the edema has subsided (usually 4 days).

### Operative Technique

**1.** Malar fractures are best reduced in children utilizing general anesthesia.

**2.** Incisions are made over the zygomatic-frontal area and in a skin crease below the lower lid lashes through the skin, subcutaneous tissue, and periosteum (Fig. 48–1**A**). No hair is shaved for the incisions. One percent lidocaine with 1:100,000 epinephrine is injected at the incision site to aid in hemostasis.

**3.** The periosteum is elevated for a small distance to expose the fracture fragments (Fig. 48–1**B**).

**4.** The malar eminence is reduced and rotated into position by lifting the bone with an elevator inserted behind the zygoma from the frontal incision (Fig. 48–1**C**). The orbital floor is checked for fractures (see section 49–1, Treatment of Orbital Floor Fractures).

**5.** Holes are drilled on either side of the frontal and maxillary fractures and the fragments are wired in place with 26 stainless steel wire (Fig. 48–1**D, E, F, G**).

**6.** Alternately, the fractures may be secured with minicompression plates (Fig. 48–1**H**).

**7.** The incisions are closed with 3-0 interrupted chromic in the subcutaneous tissues and 4-0 interrupted subcuticular chromic.

**8.** No dressings or splints are necessary.

### Complications

1. Insufficient reduction
2. Osteomyelitis
3. Enophthalmos

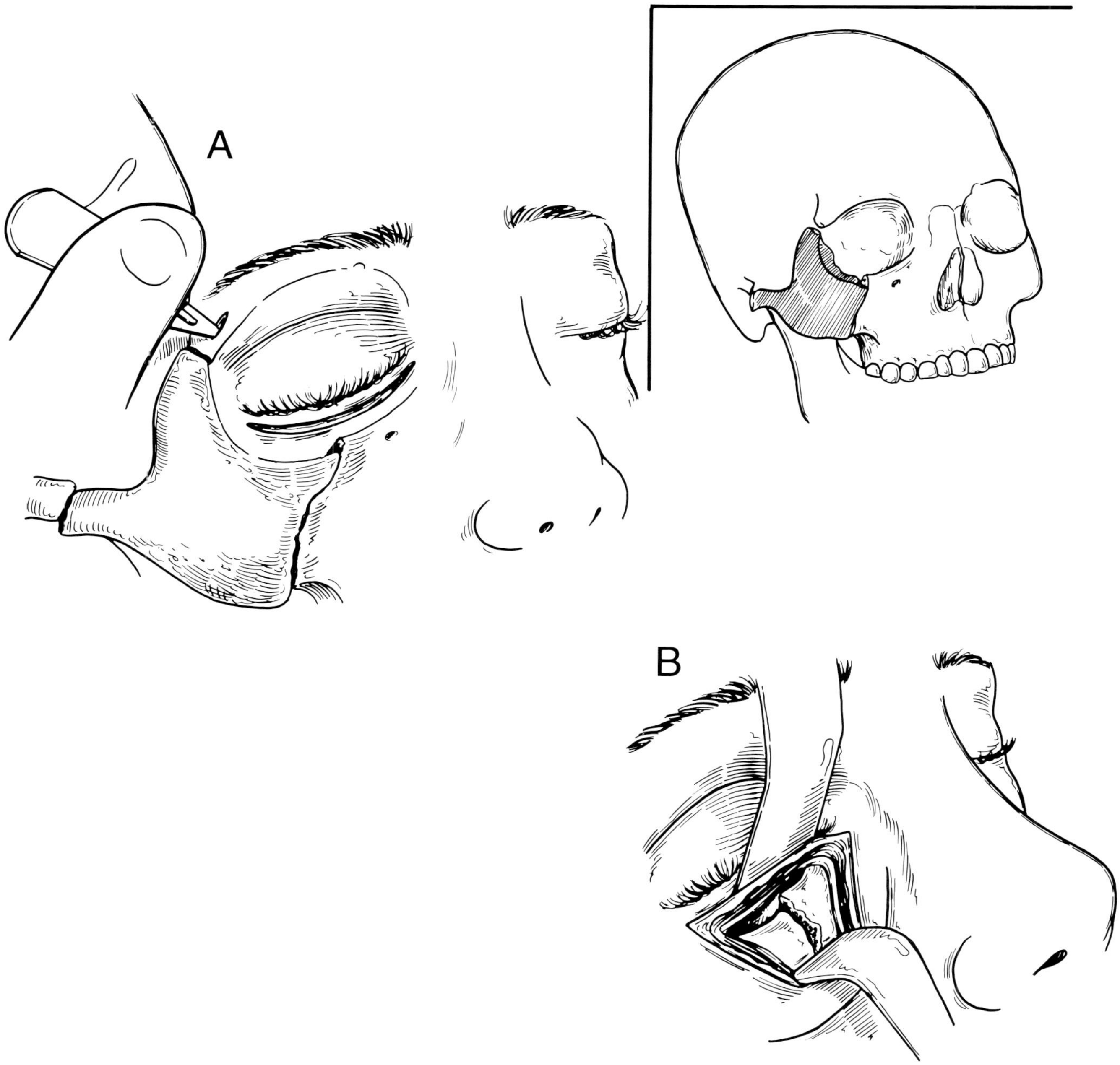


▶ **FIGURE 48-1**

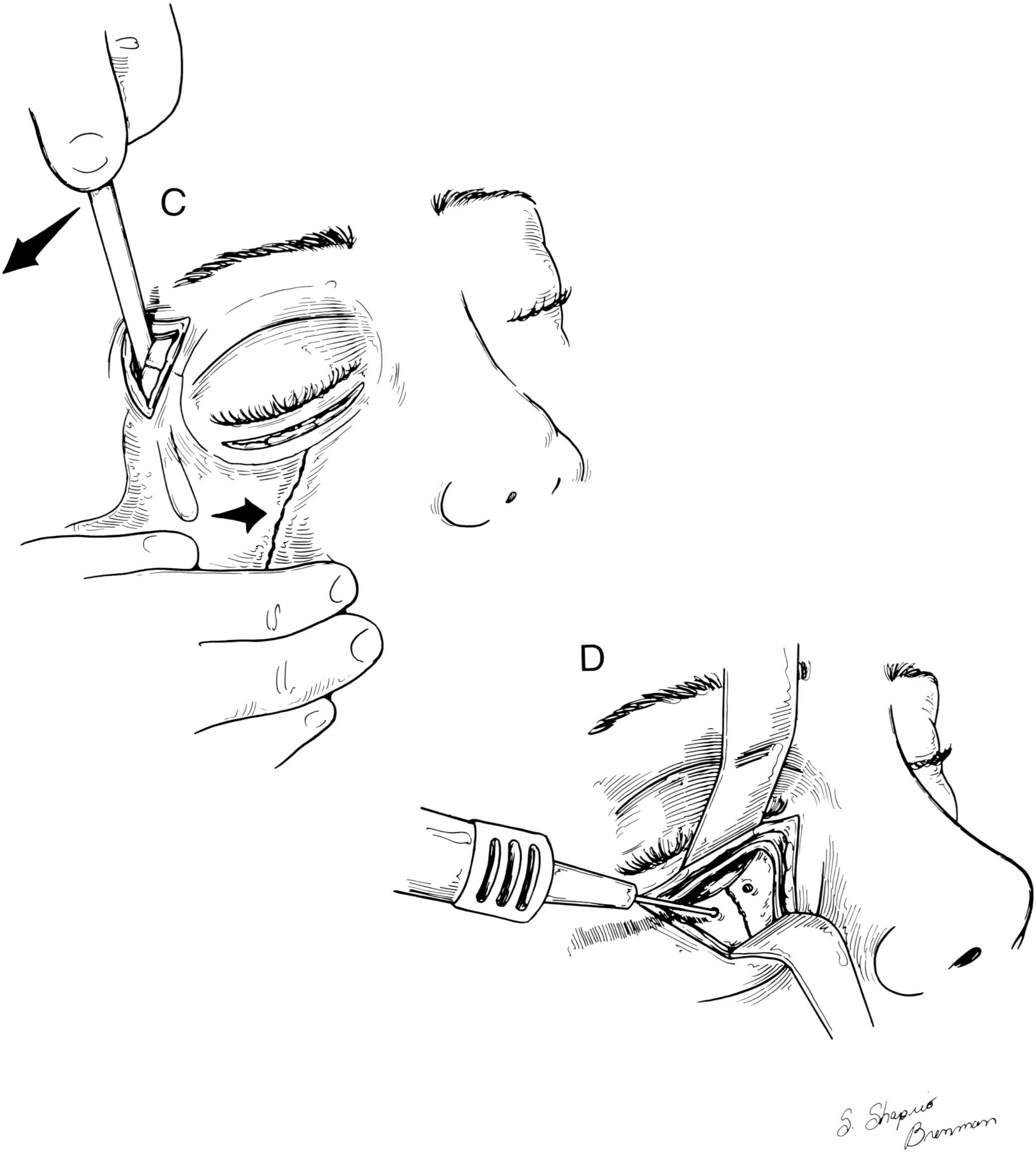


▶**FIGURE 48-1**

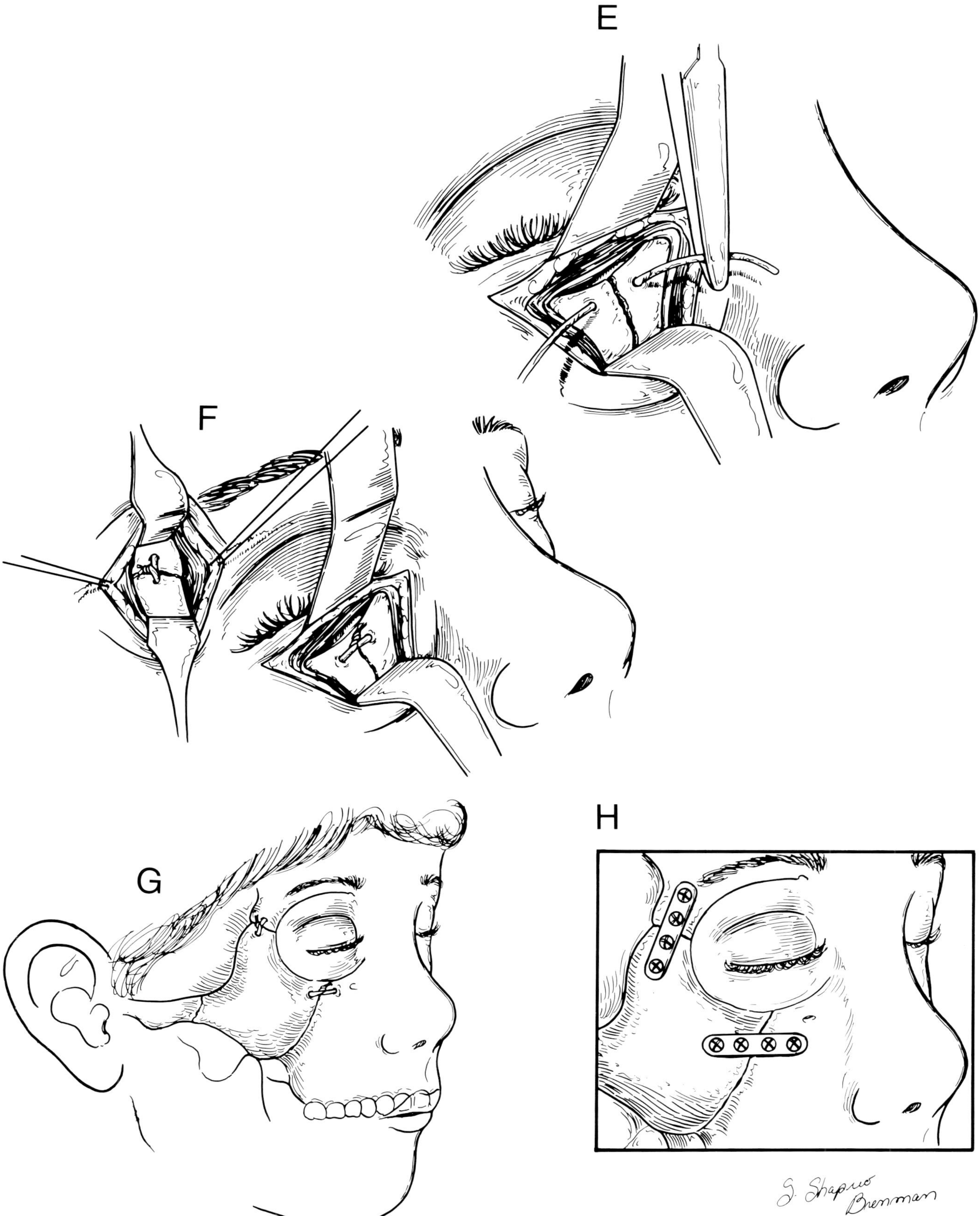


▶**FIGURE 48-1**

# 49 ▶ Orbital Fractures

Direct trauma to the eye may transmit force to the floor of the orbit causing multiple fractures in the floor while the orbital rim remains intact. Herniation of fat and muscle through the bony defect may cause a restriction of upward gaze and resultant diplopia. Presence of an orbital floor fracture with enophthalmos and/or restriction of ocular mobility is an indication for surgical exploration.

## ▶ 49 - 1 TREATMENT OF ORBITAL FLOOR FRACTURES

### Preoperative Evaluation

A careful examination of the eye to rule out ocular injury (e.g., hyphema) is essential.

Plain radiographs may demonstrate the herniated orbital contents extending through the fracture into the maxillary sinus. However computed tomography (CT) provides the best definition of the fracture.

Reduction of the fracture should be carried out after edema has substantially resolved, usually about 4 days following the injury.

### Operative Technique

1. Orbital floor fractures are best reduced utilizing general anesthesia.
2. A tarsonaphy suture of 6-0 nylon is placed to protect the cornea (Fig. 49–1**A**, **B**). An incision is made through the skin of the lower eyelid in a skin crease just below the lash line (Fig. 49–1**A**). One percent lidocaine with 1:100,000 epinephrine is injected at the incision site to aid in hemostasis.
3. The skin flap is elevated to the inferior orbital rim with a fine scissors (Fig. 49–1**B**).
4. The periosteum is incised along the orbital rim and elevated posteriorly, exposing the fracture (Fig. 49–1**C**).
5. Orbital fat and muscle entrapped in the fracture are released with an elevator (Fig. 4–1**D**).
6. The depressed fracture fragments are lifted with an elevator (Fig. 49–1**E**).
7. A sheet of Gelfilm is inserted along the orbital floor to protect the fractures and prevent reherniation of orbital contents (Fig. 49–1**F**, **G**).
8. The incision is closed with 4-0 interrupted chromic in the periosteum and subcutaneous tissue. The skin is closed with 5-0 interrupted subcuticular chromic (Fig. 49–1**G**).

### Complications

1. Persistent diplopia
2. Persistent enophthalmos

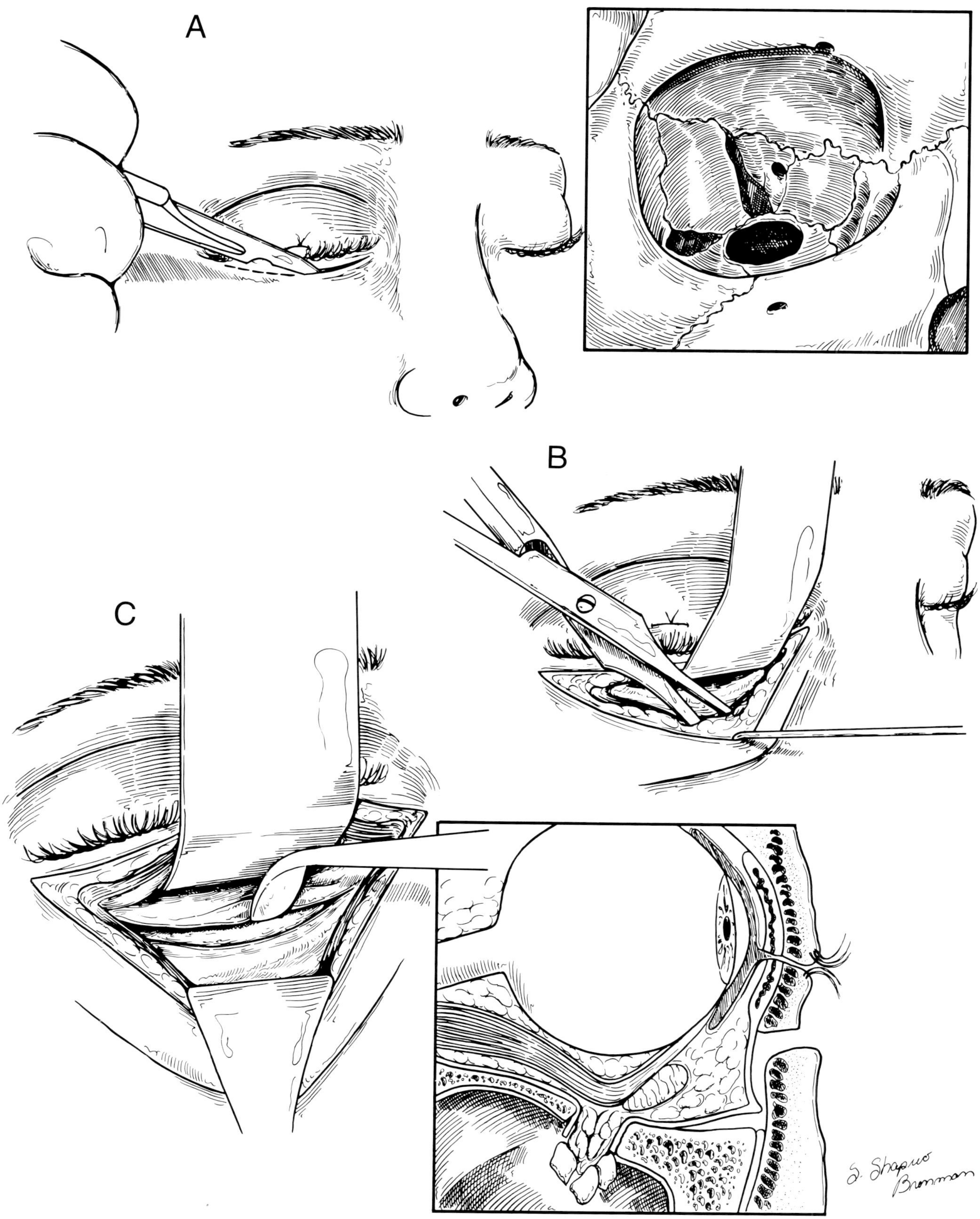


▶ **FIGURE 49-1**

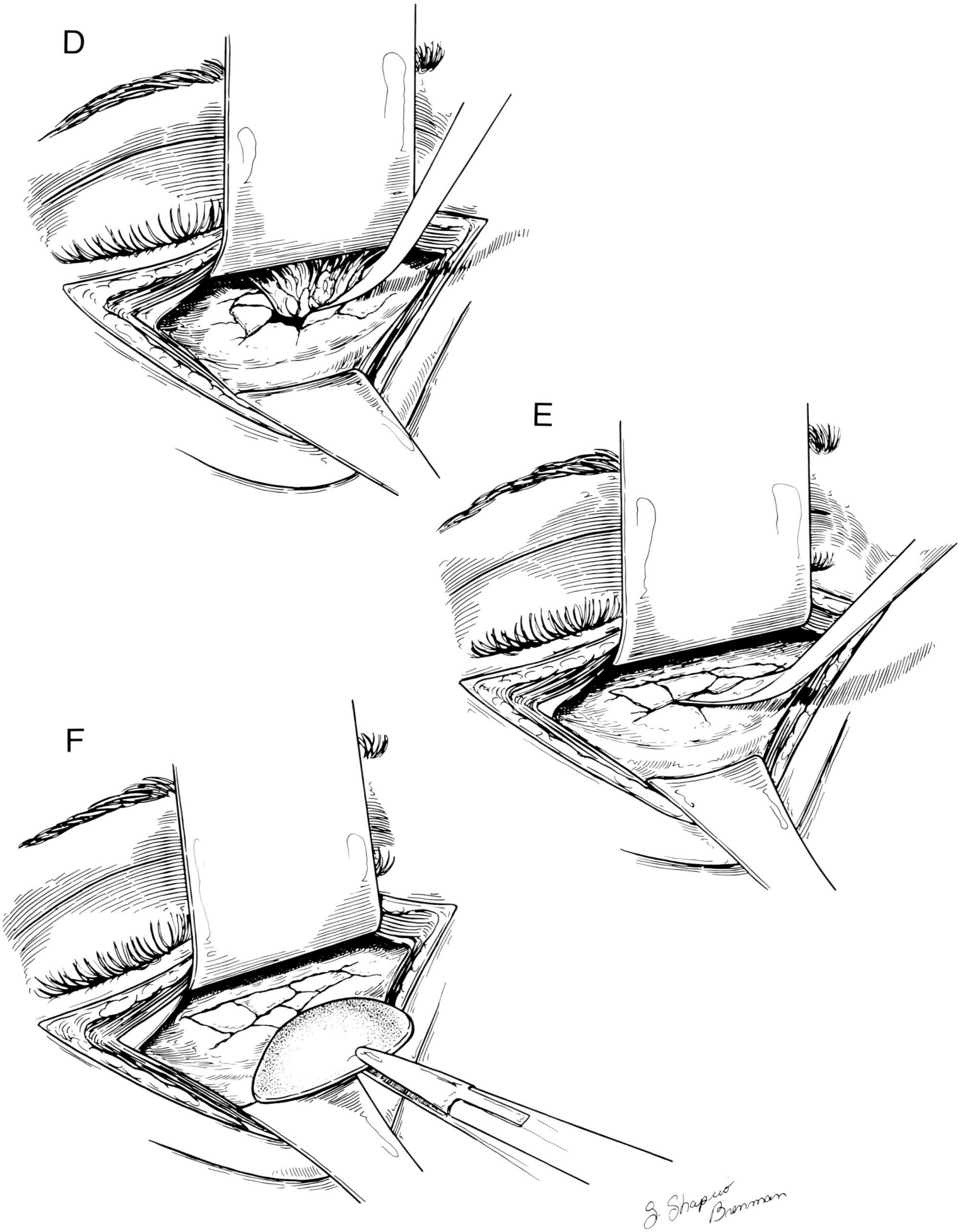


▶ **FIGURE 49-1**

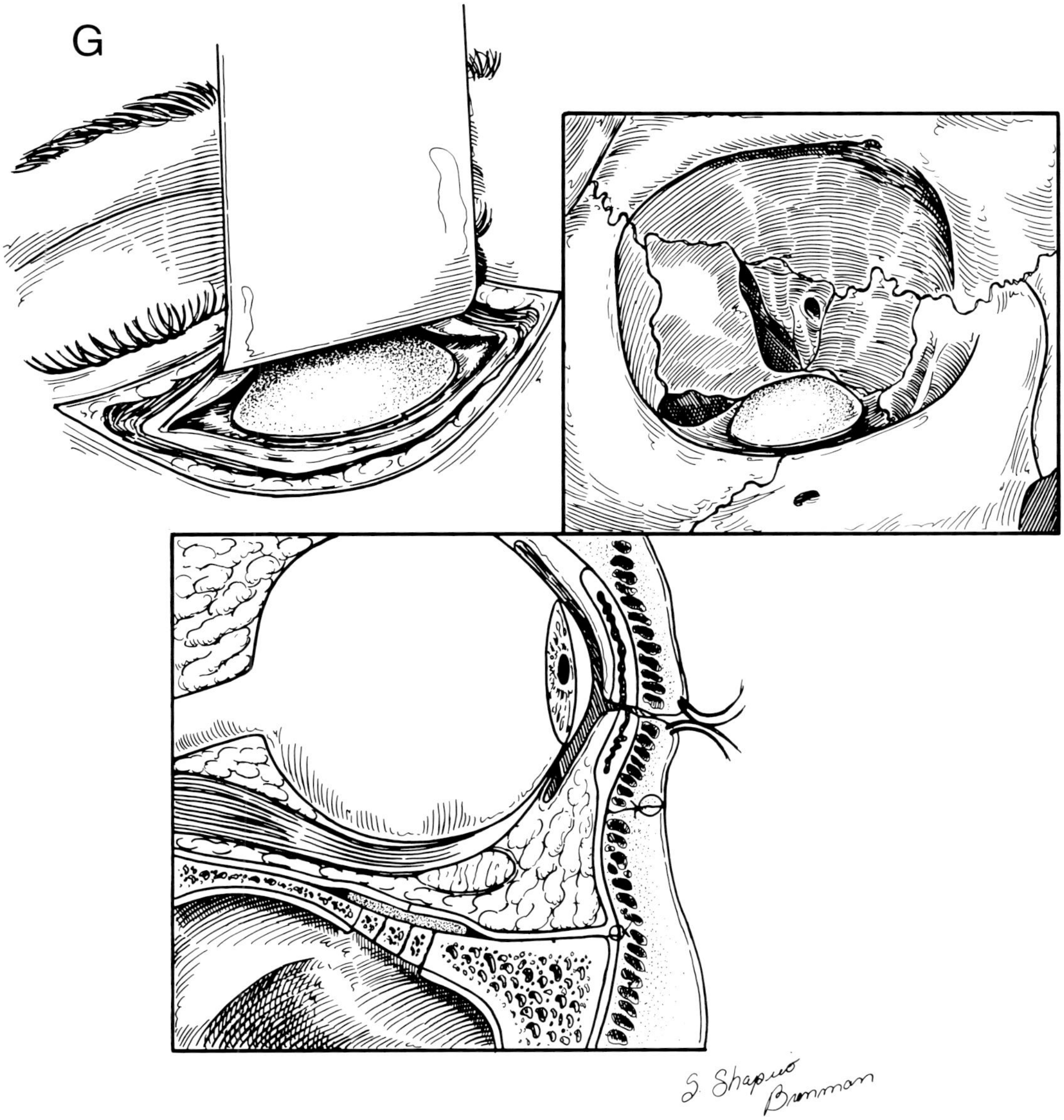


▶ **FIGURE 49-1**

# 50 ▶ Midface Fractures

Midface fractures are rare in children because this portion of the child's face occupies a relatively small portion of the head. Also, the poorly developed paranasal sinuses result in crush or greenstick injuries rather than complete fractures.

## ▶ 50 - 1 TREATMENT OF MIDFACE FRACTURES

### Indications

A mobile/depressed midface requires surgical treatment.

### Preoperative Evaluation

Computed tomography (CT) of the facial bones is the best study to define the fractures. Because the injuries are usually the result of severe trauma, associated injuries must be suspected. The airway may also be compromised. The injury is categorized by the location of the fracture: Le Fort I, II, III (Fig. 50–1**A**,**B**). Location of the fracture is important to determine the stable site on the facial skeleton that is to be used for fixation and immobilization. The principles of management include restoration of appearance and normal occlusion and fixation by wire suspension.

### Operative Technique

1. Midfacial fractures are best reduced utilizing general anesthesia.
2. The posteriorly displaced maxilla is reduced by grasping the maxilla with a forceps and pulling forward as the maxilla is rocked in a superior-inferior direction (Fig. 50–1**C**).
3. The maxilla is fixed in place with a wire. A trocar is first passed medial to the zygoma and into the oral cavity. The wire is passed through the trocar into the oral cavity and grasped with a clamp (Fig. 50–1**D**).
4. The trocar is then withdrawn from the skin and the wire. It is passed lateral to the zygoma back into the oral cavity (Fig. 50–1**E**). The upper end of the wire is fed into the trocar and the trocar removed through the mouth (Fig. 50–1**F**). The ends of the wire are "sawed" back and forth until the wire forms a snug sling against the zygoma (Fig. 50–1**G**).
5. To suspend the wire from the frontal process, the wire is passed into the oral cavity after it is put through a drill hole in the frontal bone above the fracture (Fig. 50–1**G**).
6. The suspension wire is twisted to create a sling, and a second wire is passed around the sling and placed on the teeth. It is then twisted to fix the maxilla in place (Fig. 50–1**G**).
7. The attachment of the suspension wire to the teeth can be accomplished utilizing an arch bar, bonded hooks, wire loops, or a dental plate. Assistance from a dentist or orthodontist can be very helpful in this step.
8. Intermaxillary fixation (IMF) is accomplished utilizing ivy loops or bonded hooks on the mandibular teeth (see Fig. 51–1**C**, section 51–1, Treatment of Mandible Fractures).

9. The IMF is released 3 weeks after the reduction to prevent temporomandibular joint ankylosis. The maxillary suspension wires are removed at 6 weeks.

10. Fractures may also be secured with minicompression plates when possible (Fig. 50–1H).

## Complications

1. Malunion
2. Osteomyelitis
3. Malocclusion

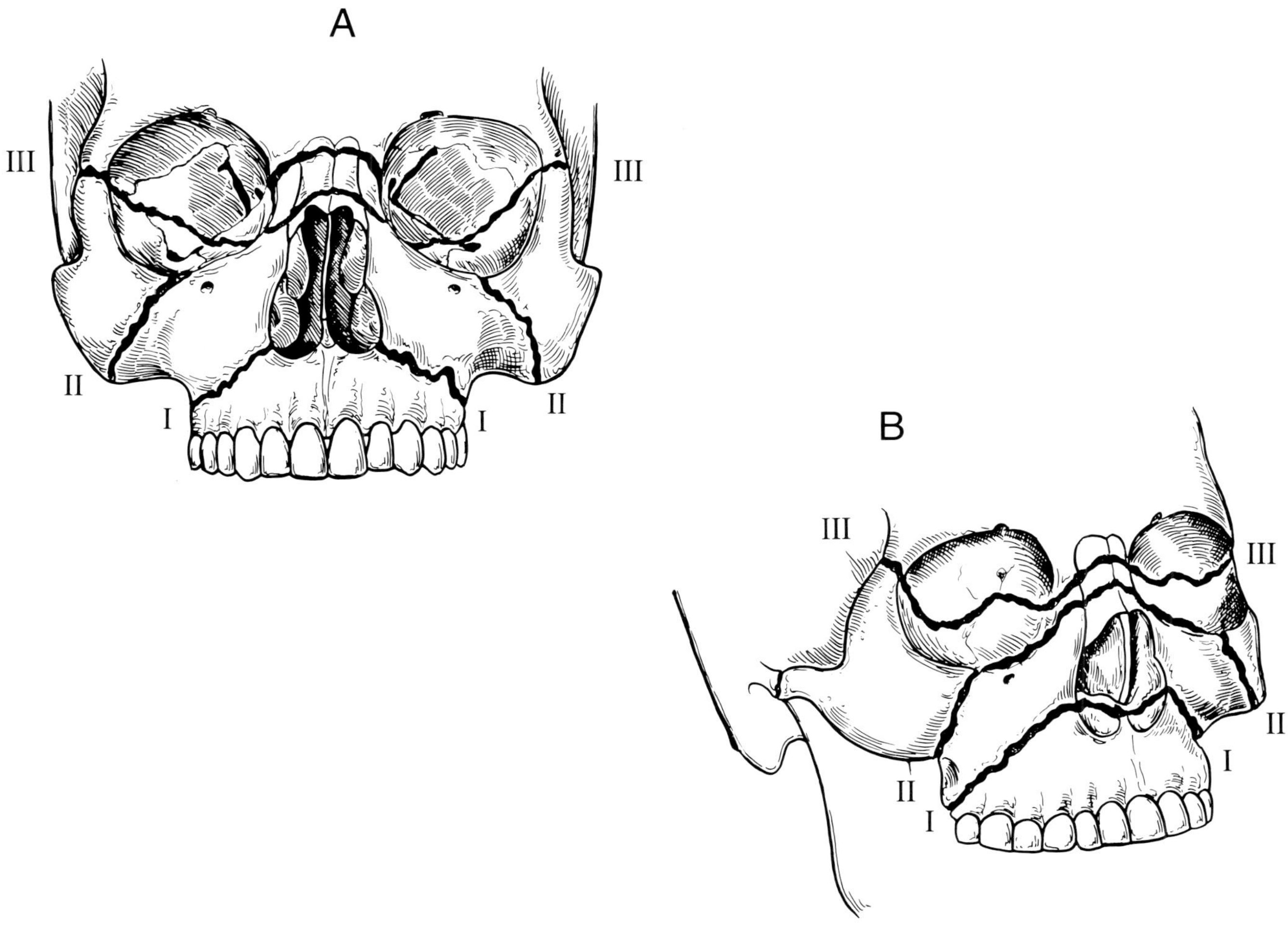


▶ **FIGURE 50-1**

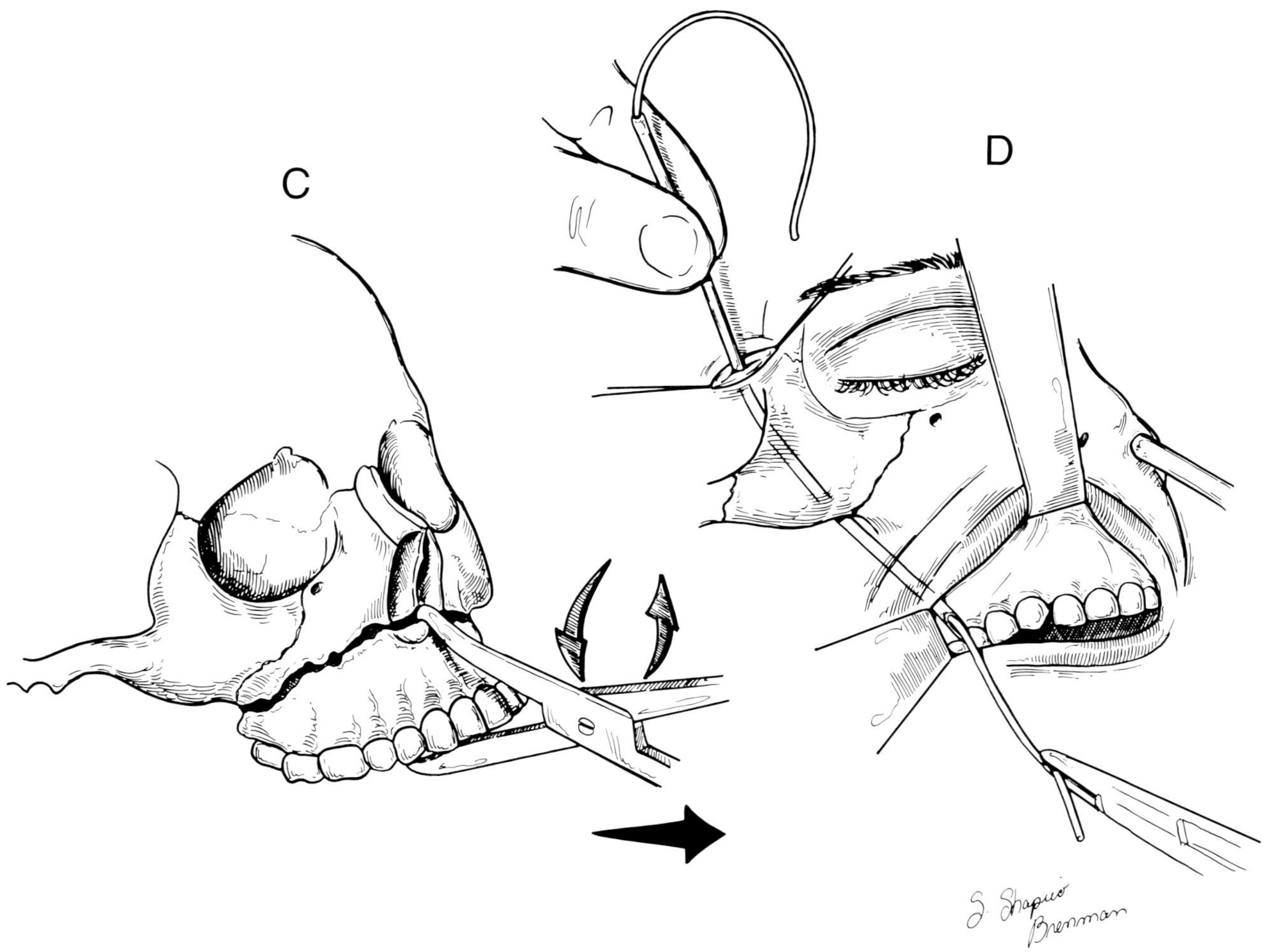


▸ **FIGURE 50-1**

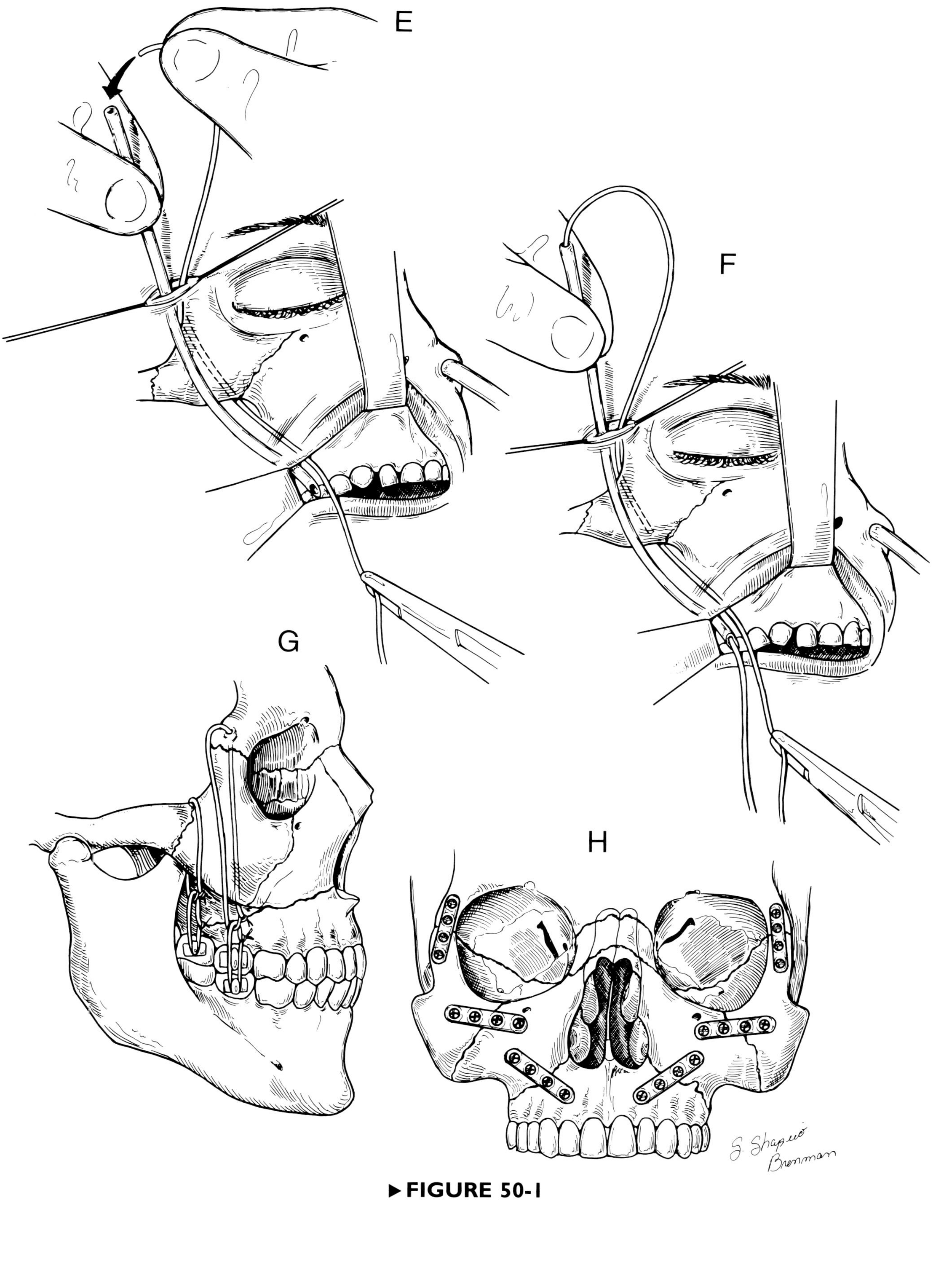


▶ **FIGURE 50-1**

# 51 ▶ Mandibular Fractures

Mandibular fractures are uncommon in children. They usually occur as a result of severe trauma and are often associated with other injuries.

## ▶ 51-1 TREATMENT OF MANDIBULAR FRACTURES

### Indications

All fractures of the mandible require some treatment.

### Preoperative Evaluation

Some degree of malocculsion and trismus usually accompany mandibular fractures. Radiographs should be obtained to document the suspected fractures and to search for the frequent second fracture. Panoramic dental films are useful to determine dental fractures. Most mandibular fractures do not require immediate reduction. They should be managed as soon as the patient's general condition has stabilized and when facial edema has resolved (usually 2 to 5 days).

### Operative Technique

1. Uncomplicated subcondylar fractures in children do not require reduction if occlusion is reasonably good (Fig. 51–1**A**). Soft diet should be used for approximately 4 to 6 weeks until the child can eat without pain. An immobilization dressing (Barton bandage) may help to reduce discomfort by restricting jaw motion (Fig. 51–1**B**).
2. Mandible arch fractures in children are best reduced and immobilized utilizing general anesthesia.
3. If a single fracture is present and the fragments are not displaced, simple immobilization for 1 to 3 weeks will allow the fracture to heal.
4. When teeth are present, Ivy loops fashioned from 26-gauge stainless steel wire are utilized to immobilize the mandible and may be used to reduce the fracture as well. Because of the narrow neck on primary dentition, the wire loops may become loose or may gradually pull the tooth from its socket.
5. A 26-gauge stainless steel wire is bent around a suction approximately 2 to 3 mm in diameter (Fig. 51–1**C**).
6. The wire is grasped with a clamp or needle holder and twisted clockwise, creating a loop (Fig. 51–1**D**).
7. The trailing wires are then passed between two teeth (molars or premolars) at the gum line. One end is passed back around one tooth and the second end is passed back around the other tooth (Fig. 51–1**E**).
8. The ends of the wires are tightened by twisting clockwise with a needle holder (Fig. 51–1**F**).
9. The twisted ends of the wire are bent toward the gingiva to prevent buccal lacerations (Fig. 51–1**G**).

10. The loops on the mandible and maxilla are then wired together to create intermaxillary fixation (IMF), which immobilizes the mandible (Fig. 51–1H).
11. When secondary teeth are available for reduction and fixation, arch bars may be used (Fig. 51–1I).
12. A 26-gauge wire is passed around each of the premolars and molars. The wires are twisted and tightened with a needle holder to hold the arch bars in place on the maxillary or mandibular teeth (Fig. 51–1I).
13. The arch bars are secured together with rubber bands or wire to immobilize the mandible (Fig. 51–1I).
14. Severely displaced fractures require open reduction and fixation with wires or minicompression plates.
15. An incision is made below the lower edge of the mandible, taking care to avoid the marginal mandibular division of the facial nerve (Fig. 51–1J). One percent lidocaine with 1:100,000 epinephrine is injected at the incision site to aid in hemostasis.
16. The platysma muscle is divided with a knife (Fig. 51–1K).
17. The inferior edge of the mandible is exposed by cutting through masseter muscle or periosteum as needed (Fig. 51–1L).
18. The periosteum is reflected with an elevator and a hole is drilled in the mandible on each side of the fracture. The fragments are reduced with forceps (Fig. 51–1M). The hole must be in a solid portion of bone and close enough to the lower border of the mandible to avoid injury to the tooth buds (Fig. 51–1M).
19. The wire is then passed in a figure-eight configuration and tightened by twisting with a needle holder in a clockwise direction (Fig. 51–1N).
20. Alternately, the fracture may be stabilized utilizing minicompression plates (Fig. 51–1O).
21. The wound is closed in layers with absorbable subcutaneous and subcuticular sutures. The wound is drained with a small Penrose drain if needed.
22. The mandible is immobilized against the maxilla by loops or arch bars as previously described.
23. Postoperative antibiotics are given for 10 days. The drain is removed in 24 to 36 hours.
24. IMF should be removed in approximately 3 weeks to avoid ankylosis of the condyle.

## Complications

1. Malunion/nonunion
2. Osteomyelitis
3. Infected wires or plates
4. Loosened teeth
5. Reduced range of motion of TMJ

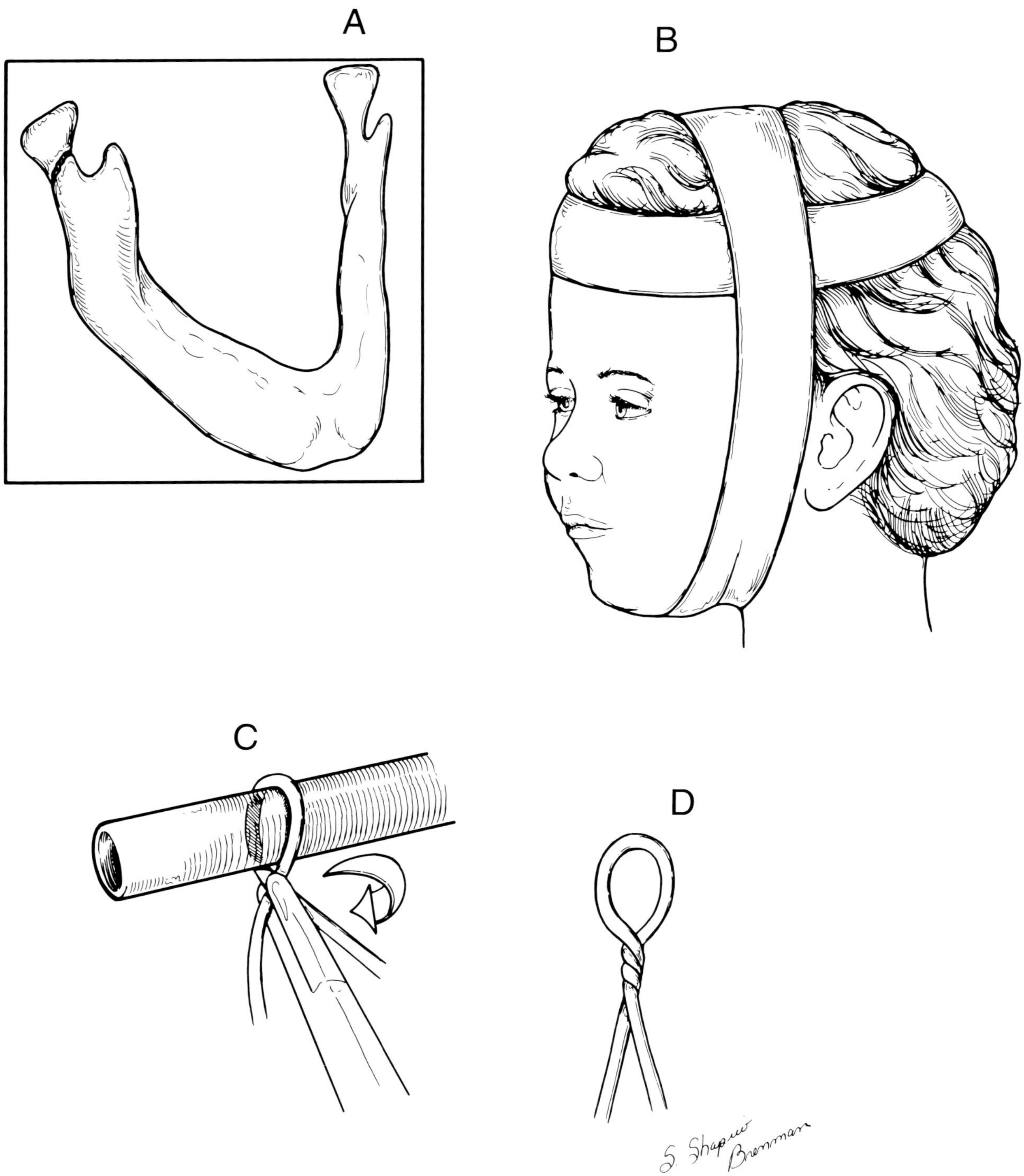


**▶ FIGURE 51-1**

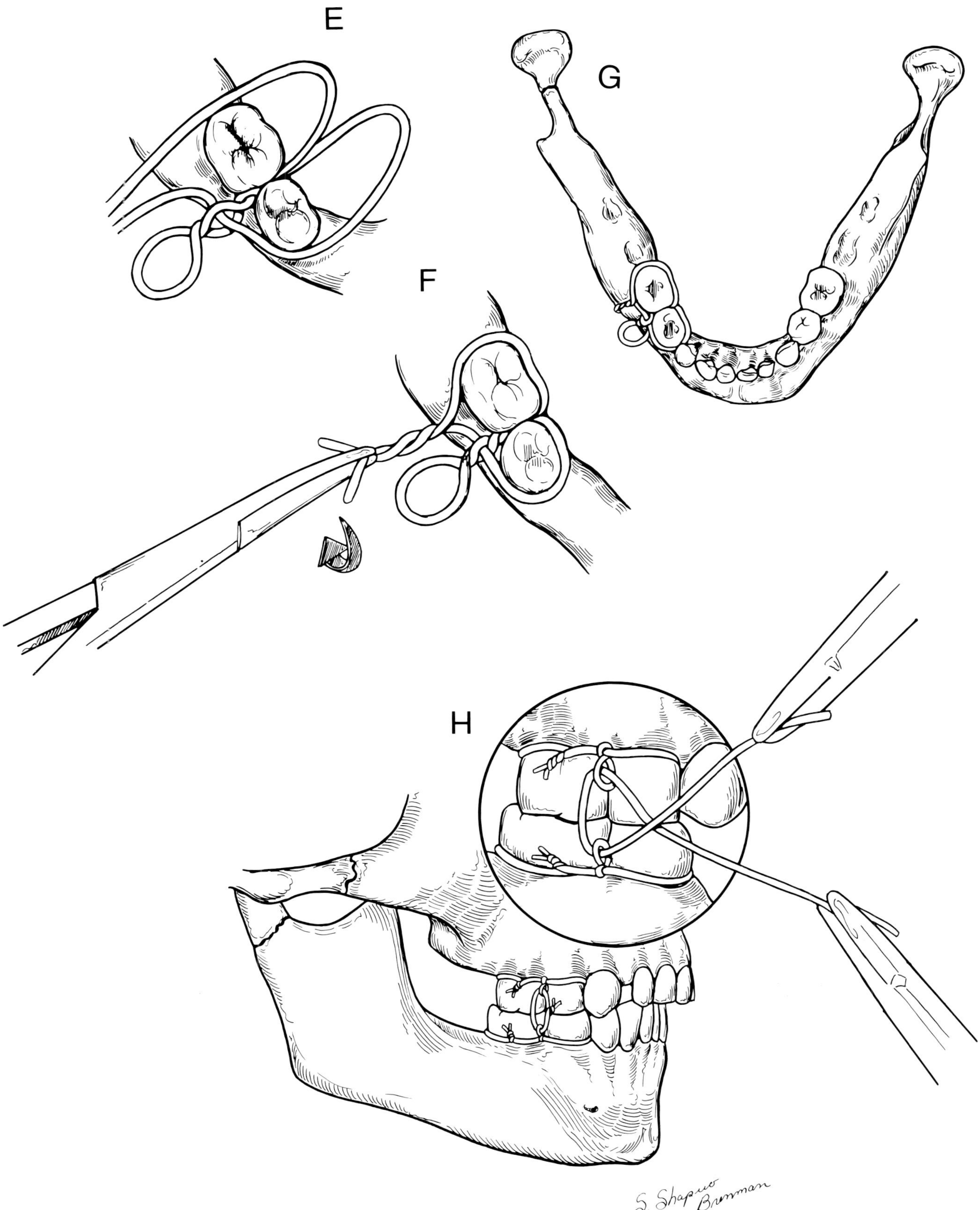


▶ **FIGURE 51-1**

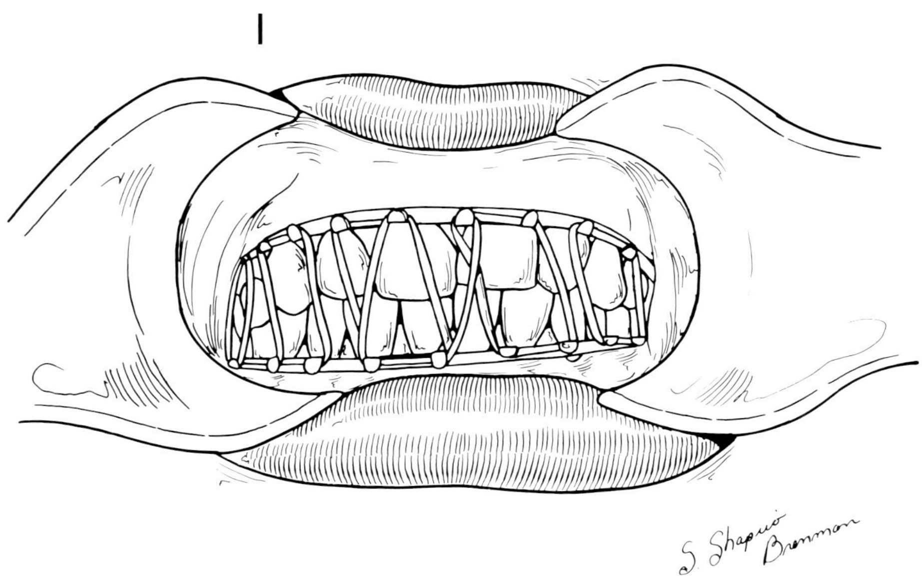


▶ **FIGURE 51-1**

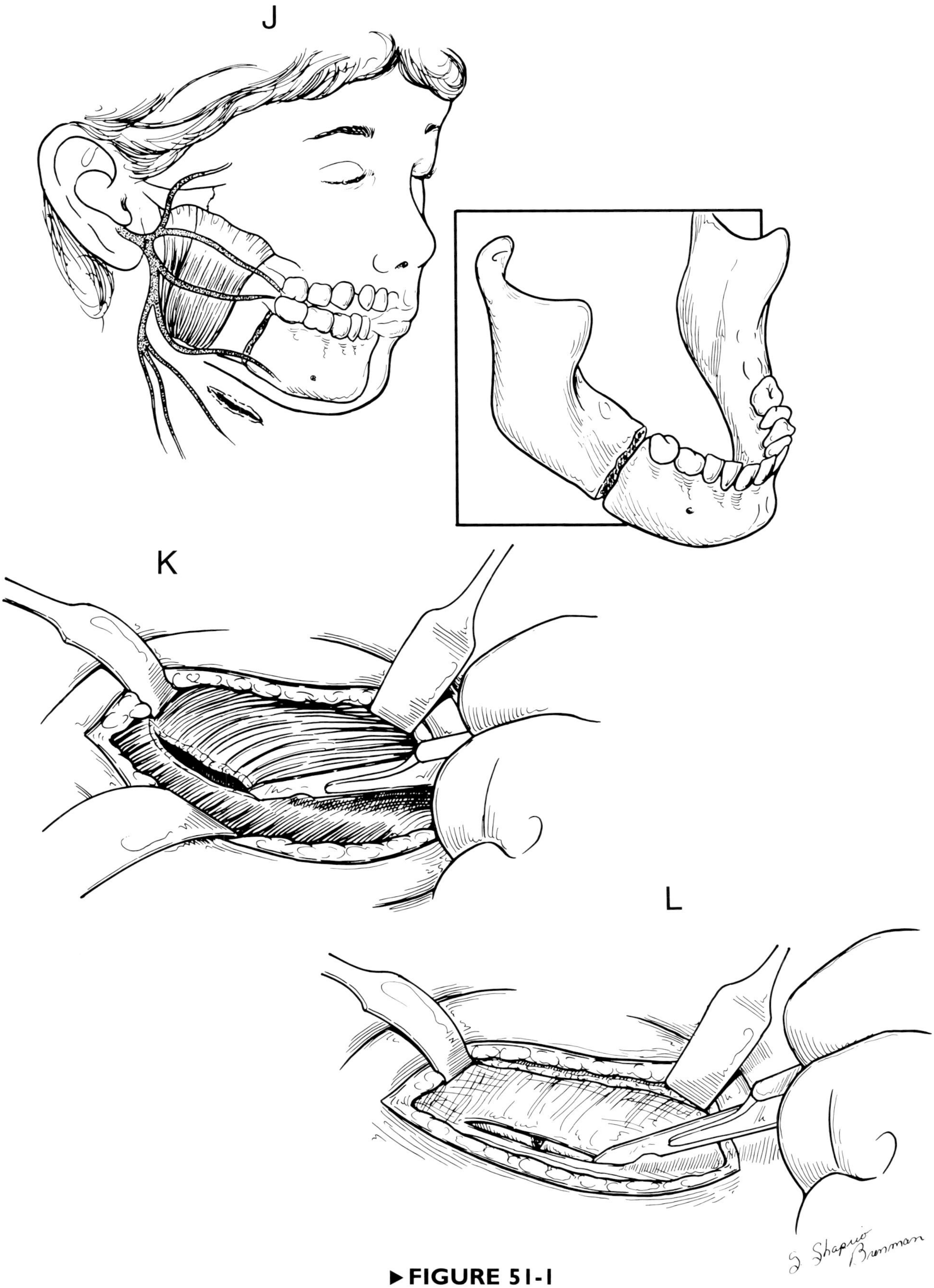


▶**FIGURE 51-1**

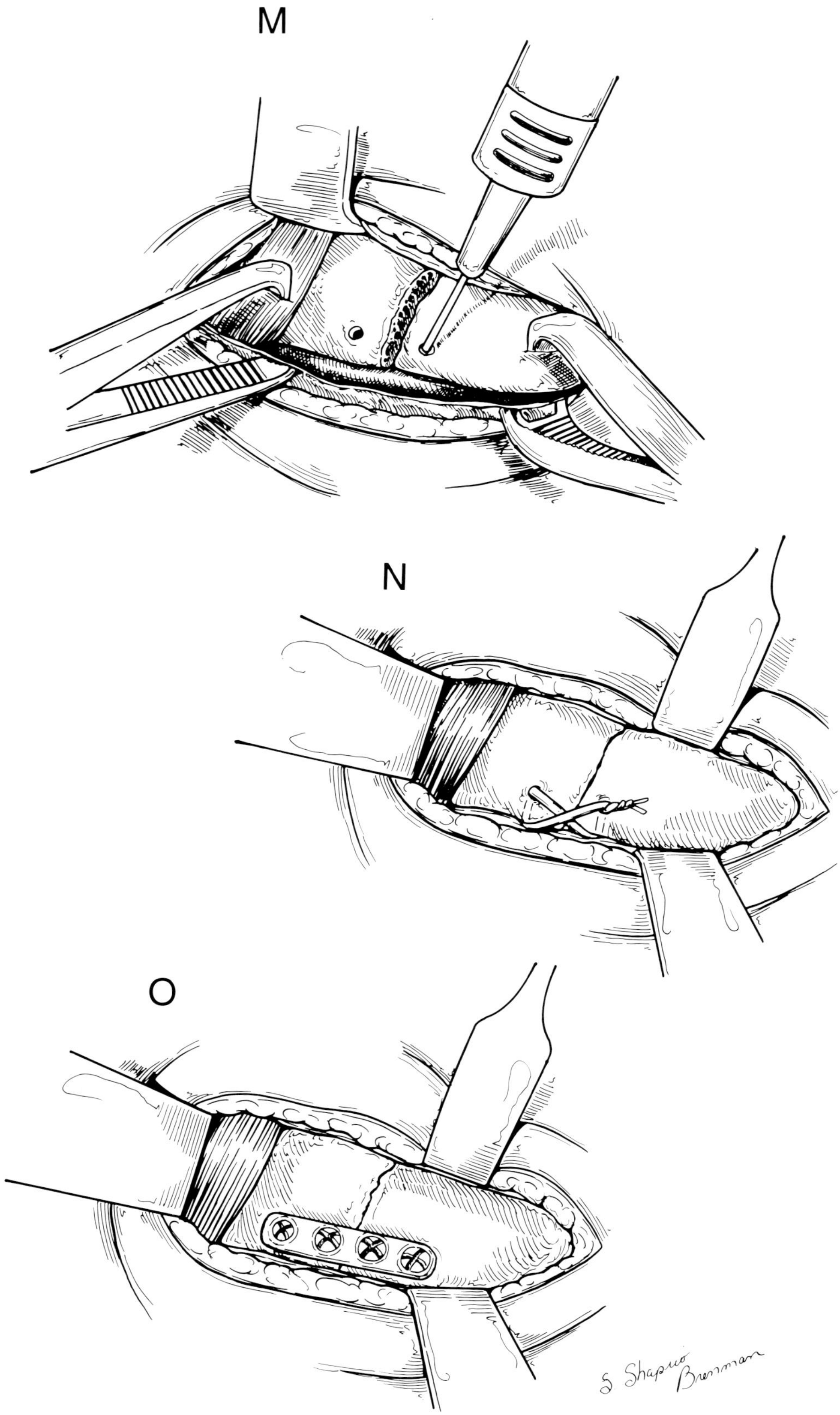


▶ **FIGURE 51-1**

# ▶ Index

*Numbers in italics indicate references to figures.*